Sport Nutrition

An Introduction to Energy Production and Performance

Asker Jeukendrup, MSc, PhD
University of Birmingham

Michael Gleeson, BSc, PhD
Loughborough University

Human Kinetics

Library of Congress Cataloging-in-Publication Data

Jeukendrup, Asker E., 1969-
  Sport nutrition : an introduction to energy production and performance / Asker Jeukendrup, Michael Gleeson.
    p. cm.
  Includes bibliographical references and index.
  ISBN 0-7360-3404-8 (soft cover)
  1. Athletes--Nutrition. I. Gleeson, Michael, 1956- II. Title.
  TX361.A8J48 2004
  613.2'024'796--dc22

                              2004005192

ISBN: 0-7360-3404-8

Acquisitions Editor: Michael S. Bahrke, PhD; **Developmental Editor:** D.K. Bihler; **Managing Editor:** Amanda S. Ewing; **Copyeditor:** Ozzievelt Owens; **Proofreader:** Red Inc.; **Indexer:** Writer's Anonymous; **Permission Manager:** Dalene Reeder; **Graphic Designer:** Nancy Rasmus; **Graphic Artist:** Denise Lowry; **Photo Manager:** Kareema McLendon; **Cover Designer:** Keith Blomberg; **Photographer (cover):** Mike Egerton/Empics; **Art Manager:** Kelly Hendren; **Illustrators:** Argosy and Denise Lowry; **Printer:** United Graphics

Printed in the United States of America   10   9   8   7   6   5   4   3   2

Human Kinetics
Web site: www.HumanKinetics.com

United States: Human Kinetics, P.O. Box 5076, Champaign, IL 61825-5076
800-747-4457
e-mail: humank@hkusa.com

Canada: Human Kinetics, 475 Devonshire Road Unit 100, Windsor, ON N8Y 2L5
800-465-7301 (in Canada only)
e-mail: orders@hkcanada.com

Europe: Human Kinetics, 107 Bradford Road, Stanningley, Leeds LS28 6AT, United Kingdom
+44 (0) 113 255 5665
e-mail: hk@hkeurope.com

Australia: Human Kinetics, 57A Price Avenue, Lower Mitcham, South Australia 5062
08 8277 1555
e-mail: liaw@hkaustralia.com

New Zealand: Human Kinetics, Division of Sports Distributors NZ Ltd., P.O. Box 300 226 Albany, North Shore City, Auckland
0064 9 448 1207
e-mail: blairc@hknewz.com

Contents

Contents

Chapter 13   Nutrition and Immune Function in Athletes   301

Functions of the Immune System and Its Cellular Components • General Mechanism of the Immune Response • Effects of Exercise on the Immune System • Nutritional Manipulations to Decrease Immunodepression in Athletes • Mechanisms of Nutritional Influences on Immune Function in Athletes • Conclusions and Recommendations • Key Points • Key Terms • Recommended Readings

Preface

The topic of sport nutrition has received considerable attention over the past few decades, and it is likely to get more attention, given that nutrition plays such an important—and sometimes crucial—role in an athlete's performance. Indeed, nutrition influences nearly every process in the body involved in energy production and recovery from exercise. To understand and apply the principles of sport nutrition, some basic understanding of nutrition is necessary, as well as some knowledge of the biochemical and physiological processes that occur in different cells and tissues and how these processes are integrated throughout the body.

We have written this book primarily for undergraduate students of sport science, exercise physiology, and other sport-related or exercise-related degree programs. Many degree courses in sport-related subjects now include some coverage of nutrition, and the aim of this book is to introduce students, as well as athletes and coaches, to the principles that underpin sport nutrition and its relation to sport performance. Because this background information is often lacking in current texts, understanding the reasoning behind particular nutritional guidelines can be difficult. Indeed, the whole market of sport nutrition products and manufacturers' claims can be very confusing. In contrast, with a few notable exceptions, very little confusion exists among scientists in most areas of sport nutrition, which perhaps emphasizes the importance of providing accurate and adequate information to students, athletes, and coaches. Thus, a book is needed that provides a scientific underpinning of sport nutrition guidelines and advice at a level appropriate for undergraduate study. In this book, we attempt to provide a scientific basis for sport nutrition that covers the principles, background, and rationale for current nutrition guidelines for athletes.

Readers of this book do not need a deep understanding of biochemistry, biology, chemistry, or physiology, but they should be familiar with some of the main concepts because the physical, chemical and biochemical properties of cells and tissues determine the physiological responses to exercise and the impact that nutrition has on these responses. Readers who are unfamiliar with or a bit rusty on fundamental concepts are advised to read appendix A before starting on the chapters of this book. Appendix A contains a brief explanation of the basic physical, chemical, and biological processes and structures. Any confusion over terms used in this book can be overcome by reference to the extensive glossary, which defines many of the terms and commonly used abbreviations in nutrition, physiology, and metabolism.

How This Book Is Organized

In each chapter, we have tried to explain the specific role of nutrition in enhancing exercise performance, as well as providing the reader with up-to-date findings from the most current research. Topics discussed in this book include the following:

- General Principles of Nutrition
- Fuel Sources for Muscle and Exercise Metabolism
- Energy Requirements of Different Sports
- The Digestion and Absorption of Food
- The Macronutrients: Carbohydrates, Fats, and Proteins
- Water Requirements and Fluid Balance
- The Micronutrients: Vitamins and Minerals
- Nutrition Supplements
- Weight Management and Eating Disorders in Athletes
- Nutrition and Immune Function in Athletes

First we explain some of the important principles of nutrition, including definitions and descriptions of the various terms used to describe such appropriate intakes as the recommended daily allowance (RDA). Second, we cover the biochemistry of exercise, with particular emphasis on the metabolic pathways that provide muscles with energy to perform physical work. This topic is followed by consideration of how the energy content of foods and the energy needs of athletes in different sports can be estimated. A full chapter, chapter 4, is devoted to explaining how food is digested and absorbed in the gastrointestinal tract and how exercise can influence these processes. The role of each of the major macronutrients—carbohydrate, fat, and protein—and the importance of adequate fluid intake in relation to exercise performance is discussed in the chapters that follow.

Nutrition supplements are sometimes considered synonymous with sport nutrition. However, as the name suggests, they should only supplement a normal diet, not replace it. This topic is surrounded by much confusion and many questions. The chapter on supplements gives some guidance on how to distinguish fact from fallacy and discusses the claims and scientific evidence that either supports or refutes the claims of a large number of supplements. The book also contains some more specialized chapters that delve into other nutrition-related issues that are important for athletes, including weight management, eating disorders, and the effects of nutrition and exercise on immune function.

The material presented follows a logical sequence. For example, to understand the importance of carbohydrate intake for endurance performance, we first describe what carbohydrates are, how they are stored in the body, how they are broken down to supply energy, and how they are obtained from the diet via the gastrointestinal tract. The micronutrients—vitamins and minerals—are combined into functional groupings (e.g., those that are important in forming tissues, transporting oxygen, as essential factors in energy metabolism and immune function, and as body fluid electrolytes) that provide a framework for understanding why they are needed for exercise performance and maintenance of health.

Special Chapter Elements

Each chapter begins with a list of objectives that explain what students should learn from the chapter. These objectives can be used for previewing the chapter and for checking after reading the chapter that these objectives have been met. Key terms are identified in bold font, defined in the text, and listed for review at the end of each chapter. These terms, as well as many other terms that may not be familiar to readers without a science background, are defined in the glossary. Chapters are organized to promote learning of concepts and ideas rather than simple memorization of facts and figures. The illustrations and tables used in each chapter help accomplish this goal, as do occasional sidebars, which provide more detailed or in-depth coverage of selected topics.

At the end of every chapter, a listing of the key points reemphasizes the important facts students should take away from that chapter. The appendixes provide some useful definitions of units and tables that students can use to convert from one system of measure to another (e.g., from kilojoules to kilocalories, from grams to ounces, and from liters into fluid ounces) and provide at-a-glance information on the RDAs or their equivalents in the USA, the UK, and Australia.

After reading this book, you should have a comprehensive understanding of the basics of nutrition as it relates to sport. You should also have an excellent grasp of how nutrition can influence exercise performance, training, and recovery from exercise. Thus, you should be able to give adequate sport nutrition advice to athletes or coaches, while understanding the mechanisms and reasoning underlying these recommendations. Of course, every sport has specific nutritional requirements, and, furthermore, these requirements may also be influenced by environmental factors and differences among individuals (e.g., gender, body mass). To offer a few examples, this book will help you understand why endurance athletes benefit from carbohydrate feedings during competition, whereas weightlifters do not. On the other hand, you will also be able to explain why creatine supplements benefit games players and athletes in strength sports, whereas in endurance sports, creatine supplements may have no effect on performance. In addition, you will be able to appreciate why, in prolonged exercise, fluid intake can influence performance, whereas in events lasting less than 30 minutes, fluid intake during exercise is unlikely to affect performance.

Notes for Instructors

Our approach in writing this book comes from years of experience in teaching sport nutrition at the university level. Thus, we have been conscious of the needs of course instructors. Above all, we wanted to create a book that will be a useful resource to students and instructors alike. Hence, the chapters of the book are constructed in the way we would deliver a lecture on the subject matter of each chapter. The diagrams, figures, and tables that we present in the book are similar to the ones we use in our own lectures and tutorials to illustrate important concepts, methods, and research findings.

The content of the book provides a broad coverage of nutrition as it relates to sport, including some unique aspects, such as the issue of nutrition, exercise, and immunity. We have attempted to provide an appropriate depth of content for students at the undergraduate level; thus, we describe the main findings of influential research studies without going into too much detail (except where absolutely necessary) about experimental protocols, and we critique some of the limitations of these studies. Although most of the text is based on appropriate scientific studies, not every statement is referenced by a bibliographic source, as too many citations tend to interrupt the flow of the text. We have used references selectively so that students can be directed to look at appropriate primary sources of information and find out more details about the experimental studies for themselves, without being overwhelmed by extensive reference lists.

The sequence of the chapters also follows the design of courses we have adopted to teach modules in sport nutrition that take place over one or two semesters.

These unique features of our book, we hope, will help instructors to deliver a better course and spend less time in preparing lectures and tutorials.

We hope that this book inspires instructors as well as students, coaches, and athletes to achieve their potential in many ways, be it academic or athletic. Most of all, we hope that you enjoy reading our book on this fascinating subject.

Acknowledgments

We are very grateful to many people who have contributed to this book. In particular, we acknowledge the expertise and assistance of Professor Anton Wagenmakers in the writing of the chapter on protein and amino acid metabolism. Similarly, we thank Dr. Stella Volpe for her comments that helped to shape the chapter on micronutrients.

We also thank Dr. Juul Achten and Dr. Roy Jentjens for proofreading parts of this book and for their help in the preparation phase of this book. Professor Hans Hoppeler (University of Berne) kindly provided an electron microscopic photograph for use in chapter 6. We acknowledge the discussions with many of our colleagues who have inspired us to write this book and with whom we had the pleasure to interact both socially and academically: Nicolette Bishop, Louise Burke, Andrew Coggan, Edward Coyle, Jacques Decombaz, Mark Febbraio, Martin Gibala, Jose Gonzales-Alonso, Bret Goodpaster, Paul Greenhaff, Mark Hargreaves, John Hawley, Jorn Helge, Peter Hespel, Matthijs Hesselink, Hans Hoppeler, John Ivy, David Jones, Bente Kiens, John Leiper, Luc van Loon, David Martin, Ronald Maughan, Timothy Noakes, Stuart Phillips, Wim Saris, Susan Shirreffs, Lawrence Spriet, Mark Tarnopolsky, Kevin Tipton, Kostas Tsintzas, Stella Volpe, Anton Wagenmakers, and Clyde Williams.

We also thank the dedicated team at Human Kinetics, in particular Mike Bahrke, D.K. Bihler, Amanda Ewing, and Dalene Reeder who have been very professional, patient, and helpful throughout the editorial process. Finally, we thank our wives, Antoinette and Laura, for their love and patience and for putting up with the many hours we spent writing this book.

Chapter 1

General Principles of Nutrition

© Dan Wendt

Objectives

After studying this chapter, you should be able to do the following:

- Describe the main functions of food
- Describe the main classes of nutrients
- Describe the different types of carbohydrates (monosaccharides, disaccharides, polysaccharides, and dietary fiber) and their relationship with health
- Describe the main composition of the average Western diet
- Describe the chemical properties of various lipids (fats), including the differences between saturated and unsaturated fatty acids and between *cis* and *trans* fatty acids, the functions of dietary lipids, and their effects on health
- Describe the chemical properties of amino acids and proteins and the functions of protein in the body
- Discuss the recommended daily intake of protein
- Discuss the role and importance of water in the body
- Describe the role of vitamins and minerals in the body
- Discuss the differences between essential and nonessential nutrients
- Discuss the differences in the various methods of assessing food intake and diet composition and their advantages and disadvantages

Nutrition is often defined as the total of the processes of ingestion, digestion, absorption, and metabolism of food and the subsequent assimilation of **nutrient** materials into the tissues. This chapter discusses some of the general principles of nutrition, and subsequent chapters discuss the specific nutritional needs of athletes and other physically active people. These needs are often higher than those for relatively sedentary individuals, and, in preparation for and during competition, different nutrition guidelines apply to athletes compared with the general public. However, in principle, the guidelines for healthy nutrition apply to both the general public and to athletes. In a few cases or situations, guidelines for athletes and for the general public will not match, though usually, during periods of training, guidelines given for the general public will also apply to athletes. However, to optimize athletic performance, the guidelines may be modified somewhat. For example, a high fiber intake is often recommended because it protects against cardiovascular disease and also possibly against some forms of cancer. However, dietary fiber consumed in the hours before or during prolonged endurance exercise may reduce gastric emptying and increase the risk of gastrointestinal problems and may be detrimental to athletic performance. Therefore, fiber should be consumed on training days, when performance is usually less critical, and avoided before and during exercise.

Function of Food

Food provides nutrients that have one or more physiological or biochemical functions in the body. Nutrients are usually divided into six different categories: **carbohydrates, fats, proteins, vitamins, minerals,** and **water.** Often the functions of nutrients are divided into three main categories:

- Promotion of growth and development. This function is mainly performed by proteins. Muscle, soft tissues, and organs consist largely of protein, and for any tissue growth or repair, protein is required. In addition, calcium and phosphorus are also important as building blocks of the skeleton.

- Provision of energy. This function is predominantly performed by carbohydrates and fats. Although protein can also function as a fuel, its contribution to energy expenditure is usually limited, and energy provision is not a primary function of protein.

- Regulation of metabolism. Nutrients used in this function are vitamins, minerals, and protein. Enzymes are proteins and play an important role as catalysts, allowing metabolic reactions to proceed at far higher rates than they would do spontaneously. An example is phosphorylase that breaks down carbohydrate stores in the liver and muscles. Another example of an important protein is hemoglobin, which is found in erythrocytes (red blood cells). Erythrocytes are essential for the transport of oxygen from the lungs to the tissues, and the hemoglobin molecule acts as an oxygen carrier. The hemoglobin molecule is a complex of protein (polypeptide chains) and non-protein groups (porphyrin rings) that hold iron (to which oxygen molecules can be bound). For the synthesis of this complex, other enzymes, minerals, and vitamins are required. Thus, the interaction between vitamins, minerals, and proteins in the regulation of metabolism can be quite complex.

The body requires substantial amounts of certain nutrients every day, whereas other nutrients may be ingested in only small amounts. Nutrients for which the daily intake is more than a few grams are usually referred to as **macronutrients** (see figure 1.1). Macronutrients are carbohydrates, fat, protein, and water. Nutrients that are needed in only small amounts (less than 1 g/day) are referred to as **micronutrients.** Most nutrients are micronutrients, and they consist of vitamins, minerals, and trace elements.

Macronutrients	**Micronutrients**
Carbohydrate	Vitamins
Fat	Minerals
Protein	Trace elements
Water	

Figure 1.1 Different categories of nutrients. Macronutrients are present in relatively large amounts in the human diet; micronutrients are present in very small amounts.

Dietary Carbohydrate

The name **carbohydrate** indicates molecules built of carbon (carbo), hydrogen, and oxygen (hydrate; water). The general formula of carbohydrate is (CH_2O). In other words, the molar ratio of carbon, hydrogen, and oxygen is 1:2:1 in all carbohydrates. A carbohydrate can be one or a combination of many of these CH_2O units, and this is often written as $(CH_2O)n$, where n is the number of CH_2O units. For example, in glucose, n = 6; thus, a molecule of glucose contains 6 carbon atoms, 12 hydrogen atoms, and 6 oxygen atoms $(C_6H_{12}O_6)$. The chemical structure of glucose is depicted in figure 1.2. Glucose is formed

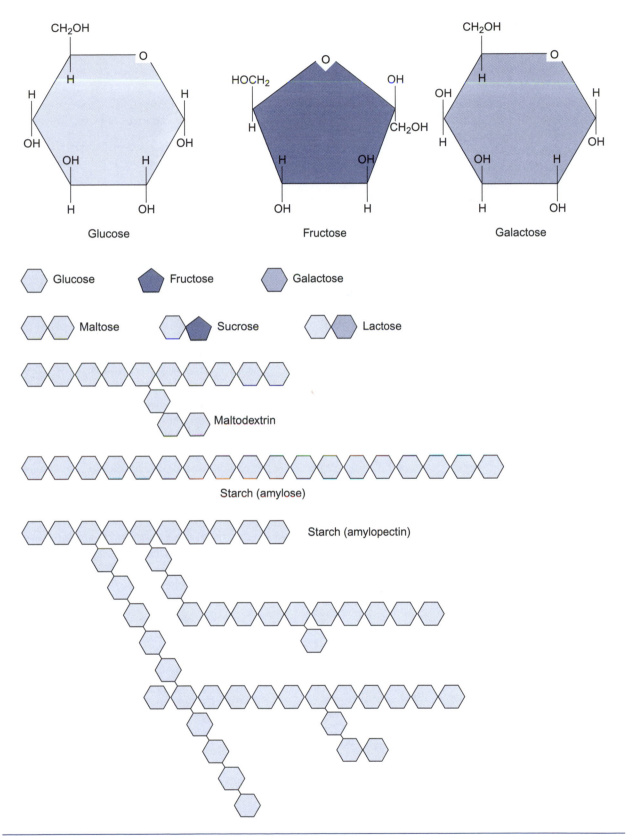

Figure 1.2 Carbohydrates and their structures. The three monosaccharides (glucose, fructose, and galactose) and three disaccharides (maltose, sucrose, and lactose) are common in human nutrition. Glucose polymers (maltodextrins) and starch are a series of coupled glucose molecules.

From A.E. Jeukendrup and R. Jentjens, 2000.

during photosynthesis, and we obtain almost all our carbohydrates from plants. Carbohydrates, however, can be found in all living cells.

Carbohydrate plays a crucial role during exercise. It also plays a major role in an athlete's overall diet as well as in the specific preparation for competition. Carbohydrate, in the form of glucose, fructose, sucrose, glucose polymers (maltodextrins), or starch (amylopectin), is one of the main ingredients of sports drinks. Carbohydrates are typically divided into monosaccharides, disaccharides, oligosaccharides, and polysaccharides.

- Monosaccharides. The monosaccharides represent the basic unit of a carbohydrate, and three monosaccharides, glucose, fructose, and galactose, are present in our diet. These three monosaccharides have a similar structure and an identical number of carbon, hydrogen, and oxygen atoms. However, slightly different carbon-hydrogen-oxygen linkages give these molecules different biochemical characteristics (see figure 1.2). Glucose is the only carbohydrate that can be oxidized in muscle. Fructose and galactose must be converted into glucose before they can be oxidized. The conversion of fructose and galactose into glucose occurs in the liver at relatively slow rates. Galactose is usually only present in small amounts in our diet but relatively large amounts are released after the digestion of the disaccharide milk sugar (lactose).

- Disaccharides. Disaccharides are a combination of two monosaccharides. Disaccharides and monosaccharides are collectively called sugars, simple sugars, or simple carbohydrates. The most important disaccharides are sucrose, lactose, and maltose. Sucrose is by far the most abundant dietary disaccharide and provides about 20% to 25% of the daily energy intake in the Western world. It is composed of a glucose and a fructose molecule. Foods that contain sucrose include beet and cane sugar, brown sugar, table sugar, maple syrup, and honey. Lactose, or milk sugar, is found in milk and consists of glucose and galactose. Maltose, or malt sugar, is present in beer, in cereals, and in germinating seeds and consists of two glucose molecules. Maltose is only present in small amounts in our diet.

- Oligosaccharides and polysaccharides. Oligosaccharides are three to nine monosaccharides combined and can be found in most vegetables. Polysaccharides contain 10 or more monosaccharides combined in one molecule. Polysaccharides can contain 10 to 20 monosaccharides (often referred to as glucose polymers or maltodextrins) or up to thousands of monosaccharides (starch, glycogen, or fiber). Starch, glycogen, and fiber are the predominant forms of polysaccharides. Essentially, these polysaccharides are the storage forms of carbohydrate.

- Starch. Starches, or complex carbohydrates, are present in seeds, rice, corn, and various grains that make bread, cereal, pasta, and pastries. Starch is the storage form of carbohydrates in plants. The two apparently differently forms of starch are amylopectin and amylose. Amylopectin is a highly branched molecule consisting of a large number of glucose molecules, whereas amylose is a long chain of glucose molecules (200-4000) twisted into a helical coil. Starches with a relatively large amount of amylopectin are rapidly digested and absorbed, whereas those with a high amylose content are digested more slowly. Most starches contain both amylase and amylopectin, and the relative contribution determines the properties of the food. For example, the quantity of amylose in rice kernels has a big impact on the properties of cooked rice kernels. That is, rice with little amylose will be sticky and soft. But rice with a large amount of amylose will be harder and not sticky. Approximately 50% of our total daily carbohydrate intake are starches.

- Glycogen. Glycogen is the storage form of carbohydrate in animals, including humans. It is stored in the liver (80 to 100 g) and in skeletal muscles (300 to 900 g), and its structure is comparable to amylopectin. (See chapters 2 and 5 for detailed discussions.)

- Fiber. Fiber consists of structural plant polysaccharides, such as cellulose, which cannot be digested by the human gastrointestinal tract. Other types of fiber include gums, hemicellulose, and pectin. The two types of dietary fiber are soluble and insoluble. Soluble fiber dissolves very well in water, whereas insoluble does not. Fiber intake has several effects on nutrient digestion and absorption. It reduces the rate of gastric emptying and can influence the absorption of various micronutrients (e.g., fiber can reduce the absorption of calcium and several trace minerals). It makes the food bulky, which increases satiety, and it can reduce energy intake by 400 to 800 kJ/day (100 to 200 kcal/day).

Increasing the dietary fiber intake is often recommended because it can decrease the risk of cardiovascular diseases. Furthermore, diets with a high fiber content seem to protect against colon cancer. The mechanisms are largely unknown, but the reduced transit time of food (the time food spends in the gut) as a result of fiber intake has been speculated to reduce the uptake of carcinogenic substances. A second explanation is that the fiber itself absorbs some of these carcinogenic substances. Also, a change in fiber intake may be the result of an alteration in nutritional habits that reduce the presence of carcinogenic substances (i.e., an increase in fiber intake is often accompanied by a decrease in fat intake).

Functions of Carbohydrate

Carbohydrates have a very important role in energy provision and exercise performance. They are the predominant fuel during high-intensity exercise (see chapter 3). Muscle glycogen and blood-borne glucose can provide more than 130 kJ/min (32 kcal/min) during very-high-intensity exercise. Carbohydrate is stored in relatively small amounts in muscle and liver and can become completely depleted after prolonged strenuous exercise. Ingestion of carbohydrate will rapidly replenish carbohydrate stores, and excess carbohydrate is converted into fat and stored in adipose tissue.

In normal conditions, blood glucose is the only fuel used by the cells of the central nervous system. After prolonged fasting (about 3 days), ketone bodies are produced by the liver, which can serve as an alternative fuel for the central nervous system (especially after prolonged starvation). The central nervous system functions optimally when the blood glucose concentration is maintained above 4 mmol/L. The normal blood glucose concentration is about 5.5 mmol/L. At concentrations below 3 mmol/L, symptoms of hypoglycemia may develop, including weakness, hunger, dizziness, and shivering. Prolonged and severe hypoglycemia can result in unconsciousness and irreversible brain damage. Therefore, a very tight control of the blood glucose concentration is crucial. Blood glucose also provides fuel for the red and white blood cells.

Carbohydrate Intake

The carbohydrate intake varies enormously in different parts of the world. For instance, in many parts of Africa, a typical diet consists of 80% carbohydrate, whereas in the Western world, carbohydrate intake is often 40% to 50%. In Caribbean countries, the carbohydrate intake averages 65%, which is closer to the recommended daily carbohydrate intake. A carbohydrate intake of 40% to 50% is equal to about 300 g of carbohydrate a day in a relatively sedentary person. An athlete in a strenuous training program may consume as much as 1,000 g of carbohydrate a day. Athletes are usually encouraged to consume more than 60% of their total energy intake as carbohydrate. However (as will be discussed in chapter 5), carbohydrate needs of athletes are not always best expressed as percentages. Absolute amounts may be more appropriate.

In the Western diet, about 50% of the carbohydrate intake is in the form of simple sugars, especially sucrose and high-fructose corn syrups. Over the past century, the yearly intake of simple sugars has increased dramatically to approximately 50 kg per person—25 times more than 100 years ago.

The intake of large amounts of simple sugars has been linked to increased risk of obesity and cardiovascular disease. However, there is considerable debate about this topic (Gibson 1996) and the results of studies are not conclusive either way. Generally, diets low in fiber and high in simple sugars are associated with an increased risk of non–insulin-dependent diabetes mellitus (NIDDM), or type 2 diabetes. This disease is characterized by a resistance of different tissues to insulin, resulting in various metabolic and related complications. For example, insulin-stimulated glucose uptake into tissues is disturbed, and fasting blood glucose concentrations are often very high. Fat mobilization is normally inhibited by insulin, and reduced insulin action will therefore result in increased fatty acid concentrations in the blood. This reduced insulin sensitivity (or increased insulin resistance) has far-reaching consequences and may result in many serious clinical complications. A high intake of fiber-rich foods seems to protect against this disease.

One of the adverse effects of certain carbohydrates (primarily glucose, fructose, and sucrose) is dental caries (bacterial tooth decay). Sucrose in particular increases the prevalence and progression of dental caries (Depaola et al. 1999). Sugars are most detrimental if they are consumed between meals and in a form that is retained in the mouth for a long time. For example, sweets consist often of sucrose and will have a relatively long contact time with teeth (Kandelman 1997). If sugar is consumed in beverages with low pH (such as soft drinks or sports drinks), the risk of dental caries and teeth erosion is further increased.

Concern has been raised about the dramatic increases in the intake of added sugar over the past 30 years; that is, all sugars used as ingredients in processed and prepared foods such as bread, cake, soft drinks, jam, and ice cream as well as sugars eaten separately. Naturally occurring sugars, such as in milk and fruit, are excluded. Fruit drinks and other soft drinks (i.e., cola) are the most important sources of added sugars. Soft drinks commonly contain sugar in amounts of 10 to 20 g/100 ml. Soft drink consumption among children in the United States 2 to 17 years of age increased from 198 g a day in 1989–1991 to 279 g a day in 1994–1995 (Morton and Guthrie 1998). Based on another survey, consumption of soft drinks increased 130% from 144 g to 332 g between 1977 and 1996 (Tippett and Cleveland 1999). One of the main problems with this increased intake of soft drinks is that it is inversely related to the intake of milk. This problem has already resulted in an increased proportion of the population not meeting the recommended intake for calcium.

Consumption of diets high in total carbohydrate does not seem to adversely affect insulin sensitivity compared with a high-fat diet. Animal studies suggest that simple sugars, particularly fructose, have adverse effects on insulin action, but such effects have not been shown conclusively in humans. Increased intake of dietary fiber appears to improve insulin action and may offer protection against type 2 diabetes.

In the United States and Canada, a fiber intake of 10 to 13 g/4,200 kJ (1,000 kcal) of dietary energy intake is usually recommended. For most people, this intake would equal 20 to 35 g of fiber a day. The typical fiber intake in Western countries, however, is about 14 to 15 g a day (American Dietetic Association 1997). Again, in African countries, the intake of fiber is much higher, at about 40 to 150 g a day.

A high consumption of fruit and vegetables has been suggested to reduce the risk of numerous forms of cancer. This reduction has been linked to the high fiber intake with fruit and vegetables. However, recent studies have not confirmed a link between fiber intake and cancer. Earlier studies may have been confounded by the fact that populations with a high fiber intake generally were also poorer and had different nutritional habits (e.g., less meat intake). Evidence indicates that the reduced incidence of cancer with a high consumption of fruit and vegetables is related to folic acid rather than fiber intake (Willett 2000).

Dietary Lipids

Lipids are compounds that are soluble in organic solvents such as acetone, ether, and chloroform. The term lipid is derived from the Greek word lipos (meaning fat) and is a general name for oils, fats, waxes, and related compounds. Oils are liquid at room temperature, whereas fats are solid. Lipid molecules contain the same structural elements as carbohydrates but with little oxygen relative to carbon and hydrogen. A typical structure of a fatty acid is $CH_3(CH_2)_{14}COOH$ (palmitic acid or palmitate). Fatty acids have a carboxylic acid (COOH) at one end of the molecule and a methyl group (CH_3) at the other end, separated by a hydrocarbon chain that can vary in length (see figure 1.3).

Although the solubility of the different lipids varies considerably, they generally dissolve poorly in water. The three classes of lipids most commonly recognized are simple lipids, compound lipids, and derived lipids (see table 1.1). Triacylglycerols, or triglycerides, are the most abundant dietary lipids consumed by humans. They are composed of a three-carbon glycerol backbone esterified with three fatty acids. However, they differ in their fatty acid composition.

In humans, the chain length of fatty acids typically varies from C14 to C24, although shorter or longer chains may occur (see table 1.2). Fatty acids with a chain length of C8 or C10 are medium-chain fatty acids (MCFAs), and those with a chain length of C6 or less are short-chain fatty acids (SCFAs). The most abundant fatty acids are the long-chain fatty acids (LCFAs), with a chain length of C12 or more. Of the long-chain fatty acids, palmitic acid (C16) and oleic acid (C18, one double bond) are the most abundant. Fatty acids with no double bonds in their hydrocarbon chains are saturated fatty acids (SFA), and those with one or more double bonds are unsaturated fatty acids (UFA). Fatty acids with one double bond are monounsaturated fatty acids (MUFA), and those with two or more double bonds are polyunsaturated fatty acids (PUFA). Also, the position of the double bond is usually indicated. For example, C18:3 (n-3) means that this 18-carbon fatty acid with three double bonds has the first double bond starting at the third carbon counting from the terminal methyl (CH_3) group (see figure 1.3). Another way of indicating the fatty acid and the position of the double bond is C20:4 ω3. The latter is called an omega-3 fatty acid.

In the literature, different nomenclature is used with regard to fatty acids. To avoid misunderstandings or misinterpretations, the nomenclature in this book will be explained. Distinction must be made between fatty acids that are incorporated into triacylglycerols or other particles and fatty acids that are not incorporated into triacylglycerols. The fatty acids that are not esterified to form a monoacylglycerol, diacylglycerol, or triacylglycerol are so-called nonesterified fatty acids (NEFAs), or free fatty acids (FFAs). The term *free fatty acid* might be somewhat ambiguous

Figure 1.3 Lipids in the human body include fatty acids, triacylglycerols, lipoproteins, and phospholipids. Fatty acids differ in their chain length (number of carbons) and the number and location of double bonds.

because, for example, in plasma, these fatty acids are bound to albumin and are not "free." Only a very small fraction of fatty acids (less than 0.01% of the plasma fatty acid pool) are not bound to any other compound (non–protein bound fatty acids).

In this book, the term fatty acid (not free fatty acid) is used to designate fatty acids that are not esterified to monoacylglycerols, diacylglycerols, or triacylglycerols, but might be bound to albumin or fatty acid–binding proteins (FABPs). These plasma triacylglycerols (and cholesterol esters) are usually incorporated into the core of a lipoprotein with phospholipids, free cholesterol, and apolipoproteins surrounding it. Various lipoproteins differ in their density, triacylglycerol content, and cholesterol content, but they also fulfill different functions. Examples of such lipoproteins are chylomicrons, very-low-density lipoproteins (VLDLs), low-density lipoproteins (LDLs), intermediate-density lipoproteins (IDLs), and high-density lipoproteins (HDLs) (see figure 1.4).

Table 1.1 Classes of Lipids

Lipid	Examples
Simple lipids	
Neutral fat	Triacylglycerols (triglycerides)
Waxes	Beeswax
Compound lipids	
Phospholipids	Lecithins, cephalins, lipositols
Glycolipids	Cerebrosides, gangliosides
Lipoproteins	Chylomicrons, very-low-density lipoproteins (VLDL), low-density lipoproteins (LDL), high-density lipoproteins (HDL)
Derived lipids	
Fatty acids	Palmitic acid, oleic acid, stearic acid, linoleic acid
Steroids	Cholesterol, ergosterol, cortisol, bile acids, vitamin D, estrogens, progesterone, androgens
Hydrocarbons	Terpenes

Table 1.2 Different Fatty Acids (FA) and Their Nomenclature

FA	Double bonds	Common name	Chemical formula
2:0	–	acetic	CH_3COO-
4:0	–	butyric	$CH_3(CH_2)_2COO-$
6:0	–	capronic	$CH_3(CH_2)_4COO-$
8:0	–	caprylic	$CH_3(CH_2)_6COO-$
10:0	–	caprynic	$CH_3(CH_2)_8COO-$
12:0	–	lauric	$CH_3(CH_2)_{10}COO-$
14:0	–	myristic	$CH_3(CH_2)_{12}COO-$
16:0	–	palmitic	$CH_3(CH_2)_{14}COO-$
16:1	n-6	palmitoleic	$CH_3(CH_2)_5CH=CH(CH_2)_7COO-$
18:0	–	stearic	$CH_3(CH_2)_{16}COO-$
18:1	n-9	oleic	$CH_3(CH_2)_7CH=CH(CH_2)_7COO-$
18:2	n-6	linoleic	$CH_3(CH_2)_4(CH=CHCH_2)_2(CH_2)_6COO-$
18:3	n-6	γ-linolenic	$CH_3(CH_2)_4(CH=CHCH_2)_3(CH_2)_3COO-$
18:3	n-3	α-linolenic	$CH_3(CH_2)(CH=CHCH_2)_3(CH_2)_6COO-$
20:0	–	arachidic	$CH_3(CH_2)_{18}COO-$
20:2	n-6	eicosadinoic	$CH_3(CH_2)_4(CH=CHCH_2)_2(CH_2)_8COO-$
20:3	n-6	eicosatrinoic	$CH_3(CH_2)_4(CH=CHCH_2)_3(CH_2)_5COO-$
20:4	n-6	arachidonic	$CH_3(CH_2)_4(CH=CHCH_2)_4(CH_2)_2COO-$
20:5	n-3	eicosapentaenoic (EPA)	$CH_3(CH_2)(CH=CHCH_2)_5(CH_2)_2COO-$
22:0	–	behenic	$CH_3(CH_2)_{20}COO-$
22:5	n-3	docosapentaenoic	$CH_3(CH_2)(CH=CHCH_2)_5(CH_2)_4COO-$
22:6	n-3	docosahexaenoic (DHA)	$CH_3(CH_2)(CH=CHCH_2)_6(CH_2)COO-$
24:0	–	lignoceratic	$CH_3(CH_2)_{22}COO-$

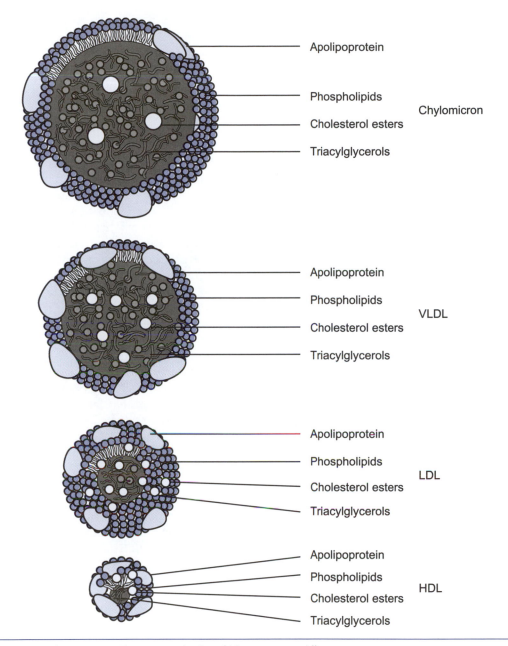

Apolipoprotein

Phospholipids

Cholesterol esters   Chylomicron

Triacylglycerols

Apolipoprotein

Phospholipids

VLDL

Cholesterol esters

Triacylglycerols

Apolipoprotein

Phospholipids

LDL

Cholesterol esters

Triacylglycerols

Apolipoprotein

Phospholipids

HDL

Cholesterol esters

Triacylglycerols

Figure 1.4   Various lipoproteins. The various shades of blue represent different components.

Functions of Lipids

Lipids are an important energy source, especially during prolonged exercise. Large amounts of fat can be stored in the body, mainly in subcutaneous adipose tissue, from which it is mobilized and transported to the organ that utilizes it. Skeletal muscle contains a directly accessible store of fat (intramuscular triacylglycerol). Lipids have many other important functions, including the following:

- They are a fuel to most cells and an important fuel for the contracting muscle.

- Fat protects vital organs such as the heart, liver, spleen, kidneys, brain, and spinal cord. These organs are covered by a layer of adipose tissue that protects the organ against trauma. About 2% to 4% of the total body fat is stored around vital organs.

- The intake of fat-soluble vitamins A, D, E, and K is dependent on the daily fat intake, and fats also provide the transport medium for these compounds in the body.

- Phospholipids and cholesterol are important constituents of cell membranes.

- Cholesterol is also an important precursor in the formation of bile and is itself an important component of bile.

- Cholesterol is a precursor for important hormones, in particular steroids such as testosterone.

- Linoleic acid plays an important role in the formation of eicosanoids, hormone-like substances formed in cells with a regulatory function. Eicosanoids play a role in the maintenance of blood pressure, platelet aggregation, intestinal motility, and immune function.

- Fat seems to suppress hunger feelings better than other macronutrients.

- Fat often makes food more tasty and attractive. It carries many aromatic substances and makes food more creamy and appetizing.

Lipids As Fuel

Oxidizable lipid fuels include fatty acids, intramuscular triacylglycerols (IMTG), and circulating plasma triacylglycerols (chylomicrons and VLDLs). VLDL, for instance, is the main transport form of triacylglycerols from the liver to adipose tissue and muscle while HDLs transport cholesterol from the peripheral tissues to the liver. Therefore, chylomicrons and VLDL may play a role in energy metabolism during exercise, but LDL, IDL, and HDL probably do not play a significant role in the energy provision for the muscle. Also fat-derived compounds such as ketone bodies (acetoacetate and β-hydroxybutyrate) can serve as a fuel, and glycerol can be converted into glucose in gluconeogenesis in the liver and subsequently oxidized.

Fat Intake in Western Countries

Fat intake represents 38% of total energy consumed in the average North American diet (Posner et al. 1993). Over 95% of the daily fat intake is in the form of triacylglycerols; the remainder are phospholipids, fatty acids, cholesterol, and plant sterols. The daily triacylglycerol intake in the North American diet is about 100 to 150 g/day. The average person in the United States consumes about 34% of fat from plant origin (vegetables) and 66% from animal sources. Saturated fatty acids typically represent 15% of the total energy intake.

Most cholesterol is found in eggs, red meat, organ meat (heart, liver, and kidney), shellfish, and dairy products such as whole milk, butter, cheese, and cream. Foods of plant origin contain no cholesterol. However, even if a cholesterol-free diet is consumed,

the body synthesizes 0.5 to 2.9 g of cholesterol a day.

Epidemiological research has shown that populations consuming diets high in saturated fats have relatively high levels of blood cholesterol and suffer a high prevalence of coronary heart disease (Hu et al. 1997; Kagan et al. 1974; Kromhout and de Lezenne Coulander 1984; Kromhout et al. 1995; Singh et al. 1998). Particularly, LDL cholesterol promotes the development of arteriosclerosis and predisposes one to cardiovascular disease. HDL cholesterol on the other hand seems to protect against cardiovascular disease. Reducing blood LDL cholesterol decreases the risk for coronary heart disease, thus providing evidence for a direct causal relationship. Various ways by which LDL cholesterol in the blood can be lowered seem effective in reducing the risk of cardiovascular disease, such as reducing the intake of saturated fat (Gordon 1995a, b), increasing physical activity, and consuming cholesterol-lowering drugs (Gould et al. 1998). For example, Gordon (1995a, b) analyzed the results of six studies in a meta-analysis (a large-scale statistical analysis based on data from studies available in the literature) and concluded that decreasing the intake of saturated fat reduces the incidence of coronary heart disease by 24% and decreases coronary mortality by 21%.

A large body of evidence indicates that *trans* fatty acid intake raises blood LDL cholesterol levels and lowers HDL cholesterol levels (Lichtenstein et al. 1999; Mensink and Katan 1990). *Trans* fatty acids have a slightly different configuration of their double bonds than *cis* fatty acids (see figure 1.5). A *trans* unsaturated fatty acid is formed when a hydrogen atom moves from its natural *cis* position to the opposite side of the double bond that separates two carbons (*trans* position). Most naturally occurring fatty acids contain *cis* double bonds, but *trans* fatty acids occur in processed foods (e.g., margarine). *Trans* fatty acids resemble saturated fatty acids more closely than do *cis* fatty acids.

Controversy exists over the health risks associated with regular consumption of butter compared with margarine. Although butter and margarine cannot be distinguished by their energy density or fat content, they can be distinguished by the composition of their fatty acids. Margarine is manufactured from plant-derived unsaturated fatty acids that are hydrogenated to convert the lipids into a hardened form (although not as hard as butter). About 20% of the fatty acids in margarine are *trans* fatty acids compared with 7% in butter. Margarine does not contain cholesterol, because it is manufactured from vegetable oil, whereas each gram of butter contains

Figure 1.5 *Trans* fatty acids have a slightly different chemical configuration than *cis* fatty acids and are recognized as a cardiovascular risk factor.

10 to 15 mg of cholesterol.

The issue of butter versus margarine is controversial because *trans* unsaturated fatty acids will increase blood LDL cholesterol concentrations while decreasing HDL cholesterol concentrations. The saturated fatty acids in butter will also raise LDL cholesterol but will not lower HDL cholesterol. High intake of *trans* fatty acids is known to increase the risk of cardiovascular disease. Reducing total fat intake will reduce the intake of saturated fat and *trans* fatty acids, which may also reduce the risk of several forms of cancer.

A high-fat intake has been linked with increased incidence of breast, colon, and prostate cancer and with increased body weight. Studies (Blundell et al. 1996; Bray and Popkin 1998; Golay and Bobbioni 1997) have suggested a correlation between high dietary fat intake and obesity. However, other studies, seem to raise questions about the effect of the percentage of energy from dietary fat on body weight (Rolls and Bell 1999; Rolls et al. 1999; Seidell 1997, 1998). Thus, the evidence that a high-fat intake contributes to obesity is not strong enough to make definitive recommendations for a very low-fat diet. Therefore, the most recent version of dietary guidelines for Americans states that fat intake should be moderate (rather than low).

In fact a very low-fat high-carbohydrate intake may have adverse health effects. Reducing dietary fat to below 20% of the energy intake results in elevated plasma triacylglycerols, increased LDL cholesterol, and decreased HDL cholesterol. As discussed, this lipoprotein pattern has been shown to predispose to coronary heart disease.

Fat intake is often related to the incidence of certain forms of cancer. Women with a high-fat and low-fiber intake are at increased risk for breast cancer. However, in Mediterranean countries, where people rely on olive oil (i.e., unsaturated fatty acids), the total fat intake is similar to that of people in the United States, yet the incidence of breast cancer is significantly lower. Epidemiological studies suggest that, as with cardiovascular diseases, the type of fat is very important to cancer risk. The associations between a high fat intake and cancer may be due to the intake of animal fat (saturated fat), not vegetable fat (unsaturated fat), raising the possibility that fat intake per se (and especially the percentage fat in the diet) is not the most important factor (Willett 2000). Omega-3-(n-3) fatty acids from fish seem to protect against cancer. For example, native Eskimos of Alaska and populations in Japan, who rely heavily on fish and thus have a relatively high intake of fish oil, have lower incidences of cancer.

Dietary Protein

Amino acids are the building blocks of all **proteins.** Most proteins are polypeptides combining up to 300 amino acids. Twenty different amino acids are commonly found in proteins. Each amino acid consists of a carbon atom bound to four chemical groups: a hydrogen atom; an amino group, which contains nitrogen; a carboxylic acid group; and a fourth group called a side chain, which varies in length and structure (see figure 1.6). Different side chains give different properties to the amino acid. The proteins actin,

Figure 1.6 Chemical structures and abbreviations of amino acids.

Nonessential amino acids	**Essential amino acids**
Alanine	Histidine
Arginine	Isoleucine
Asparagine	Leucine
Aspartate	Lysine
Cysteine	Methionine
Glutamate	Phenylalanine
Glutamine	Threonine
Glycine	Tryptophan
Proline	Valine
Serine	
Tyrosine	

Figure 1.7 Nonessential (dispensable) and essential (nondispensable) amino acids.

tropomyosin and troponin, and myosin make up the contractile apparatus in the muscle. (See chapter 2 for more detailed discussion.)

Of the 20 amino acids normally found in dietary protein, humans can synthesize 11. The other 9 amino acids cannot be manufactured in the human body. Those that can be synthesized are called nonessential amino acids. Those that cannot be synthesized and must be derived from the diet are called the essential amino acids. Figure 1.7 lists the different amino acids.

Amino acids have central roles in the metabolism of many organs and tissues. Amino acids are not only precursors for the synthesis of body proteins but also precursors and regulators of the synthesis of important metabolic mediators and compounds with a regulatory biological activity (e.g., neurotransmitters, hormones, DNA, and RNA).

Proteins provide structure to all cells in the human body. They are an integral part of the cell membrane, the cytoplasm, and the organelles. Muscle, skin, and hair are largely composed of protein. Bones and teeth are composed of minerals embedded in a protein framework. When a diet is deficient in protein, these structures break down, resulting in reduced muscle mass, loss of skin elasticity, and thinning hair. Many proteins are enzymes that increase the rate of metabolic reactions.

Unlike fat and carbohydrate, protein is not usually linked with diseases such as cancer, tooth caries, or arteriosclerosis. For this reason protein is often associated with health, and many companies use this association in their marketing strategies (e.g., protein shampoo). Indeed, in the developed world, where protein deficiency is uncommon, the dietary protein intake is less critical and not related to disease. However, in developing countries, protein deficiency is more common and can result in kwashiorkor (a pure protein deficiency, mainly in children, characterized by a bloated belly) or marasmus (a protein deficiency resulting from a total dietary energy deficiency, characterized by extreme muscle wasting).

Long-term consumption of high-protein diets have been hypothesized, but not proved, to result in impaired kidney function. The amino acids are speculated to break down, and the resulting (toxic) ammonia nitrogen is excreted mainly as urea via the kidneys.

Reference intakes are generally based on data from nitrogen balance studies (see chapter 7). Recommended dietary allowance (**RDA**) for protein varies worldwide between 0.8 to 1.2 g/kg b.w. Protein intake in the Western world is usually well in excess of the RDA and usually averages about 80 to 100 g/day. Because meat and fish are the most common sources of protein, vegetarians could be at risk for marginal protein intake. Vegetarians often compensate by eating more grains and legumes, which both are excellent protein sources. However they do not contain all the essential amino acids. Grains lack the essential amino acids lysine, and legumes lack methionine. An exception may be well-processed soybean protein, which is a very-high-quality protein comparable to protein from animal sources. Many cultures have a very high protein intake, and most Western countries have protein intakes between 10% and 15% of the total daily energy intake.

The data on which the RDA is based are typically obtained from studies in sedentary individuals. Are protein requirements for athletes involved in strenuous training programs increased? Interestingly, although many national committees recognize the possibility that strenuous daily activity may increase protein needs, most experts do not suggest an increased protein intake for active individuals. However, the diet of endurance-trained individuals often contains twice the RDA (see chapter 7), mainly because the increased energy intake also increases the protein intake.

As mentioned earlier, both the amount and the quality of protein are important. Proteins that contain all the essential amino acids are called complete, or high-quality, proteins. Proteins that are deficient in one or more amino acids are called incomplete proteins, and they are commonly referred to as low-quality proteins. Incomplete proteins are unable to support human life and growth. Animal proteins are generally of higher quality than plant proteins. However, the individual amino acids found in animal proteins and plant proteins are identical and of equal quality. The quality of the protein therefore depends purely on the kind of amino acids present in the protein. Animal protein is considered higher quality not only because all essential amino acids are present but also because the amino acids are present in larger quantities and in a more balanced proportion.

Because the metabolism of all amino acid is integrated, all 20 amino acids must be obtained by dietary intake. A short supply of any amino acid can interfere with normal protein synthesis. An appropriate selection of plant protein sources can provide an adequate supply of amino acids, but consumption of animal protein is more likely to ensure a balanced intake. By combining plant foods such as rice and beans, it is possible to obtain a balanced intake of amino acids. Essential amino acids that are deficient in one food can be obtained from another, so that in the overall diet, all amino acids are obtained. Proteins from sources that balance the amino acid intake are called complementary proteins.

Water

The adult body is about 60% water by weight. The percentage of water is highest in infants and generally decreases with age. Water content varies among different tissues of the body. Blood is about 90% water, muscle is about 75%, bone is about 25%, and adipose tissue is about 5%. The proportion of water in various body compartments also varies. About two-thirds of body water is found inside cells as intracellular fluid. The remaining one-third is found outside cells as extracellular fluid. Extracellular fluid includes water in the blood, lymph, and cerebrospinal fluid as well as in the fluid found between cells, which is called interstitial fluid. (See appendix A for detailed explanations.)

Water transports nutrients, provides protection, helps regulate body temperature, participates in biochemical reactions, and provides the medium in which these reactions take place. (Blood transports nutrients and oxygen to the different tissues and transports carbon dioxide and waste products away from the tissues.) Water in urine transports waste products such as urea, excess salt, and ketones out of the body.

Water's protective functions are lubrication, cleansing, and cushioning. Tears lubricate the eyes and wash away dirt. Synovial fluid lubricates the joints. Saliva lubricates the mouth, making chewing and swallowing food possible. Water inside the eyeballs and spinal cord acts as a cushion against shock. During pregnancy, water in the amniotic fluid provides a protective cushion for the fetus.

An important role of water during exercise is regulating body temperature (see chapter 8). When body temperature starts to rise above the normal temperature of around 37° C (98.6° F), the blood vessels in the skin dilate, causing blood to flow close to the surface of the body and release some of the heat. This release occurs with fevers and when the environmental temperature increases as well as with exercise. In a cold environment, blood vessels in the skin constrict, restricting blood flow near the surface and conserving body heat. The most obvious way that water helps regulate body temperature is through sweat. When body temperature increases, the sweat glands in the skin secrete sweat. As the sweat evaporates, heat is removed from the body surface.

Water also acts in the body as a solvent, a fluid in which solutes dissolve to form a solution. Water is an ideal solvent for some substances because it is polar, which means that the two sides, or poles, of the water molecule have different electrical charges. The oxygen side of a water molecule has a slightly negative charge, and the hydrogen side has a slightly positive charge. This polarity allows water to surround other charged molecules and disperse them. Table salt, which dissolves well in water, consists of a positively charged sodium ion bound to a negatively charged chloride ion. In water, the sodium and chloride ions dissociate because the positively charged sodium ion is attracted to the negative pole of the water molecule and the negatively charged chloride ion is attracted to the positive pole. Substances like sodium chloride, which dissociate in water to form positively and negatively charged ions, are known as electrolytes, so named because they can conduct an electrical current when dissolved in water.

As with all other nutrients, a regular and sufficient water intake is required to maintain health and good physical performance. The hydration status of the body is determined by the balance between water intake and water loss. Loss of water (through diarrhea or sweating) may result in dehydration; a failure to drink fluid for more than only a few days can result in death. With water losses of 3% of the total body weight, blood volume is decreased and exercise performance is negatively affected (see chapter 8). A 5% loss results in confusion and disorientation, and losses greater than 10% are life threatening. Dehydration is a frequently occurring problem in certain sports (see chapter 8 for a detailed discussion).

Water intake of an adult is typically 2.0 to 2.8 L/ day. Because water requirements are highly dependent on sweat rates, and sweat rates are dependent on energy expenditure, as a rule of thumb, fluid requirements are 1 ml for every 4 kJ of energy expended or 1 ml/kcal. Of the daily 2.0 to 2.8 L consumed, 1.0 to 1.5 L is usually in the form of fluids, and the rest is obtained from foods. Athletes training and competing in hot conditions may have fluid requirements greater than 15 L/day.

Vitamins, Minerals, and Trace Elements

Vitamins are organic compounds, and minerals and trace elements are inorganic compounds. Collectively known as micronutrients, these essential compounds have many biological functions. They serve as regulators and links in the processes of energy release from food. They are important cofactors in various chemical reactions and as such are important in maintaining homeostasis (relatively constant internal conditions). The general public often considers vitamin intake synonymous with good health (e.g., folic acid prevents birth defects, vitamin E protects the heart, and vitamin A prevents cancer), and some minerals also are reputed to have strong relations to health (e.g., calcium helps to prevent osteoporosis).

All of the 13 known vitamins have important functions in most metabolic processes in the body. Vitamins must be obtained from the diet, except vitamin D, which can be synthesized from sunlight, and vitamin K, which is synthesized by bacteria in the intestine. When a vitamin becomes unavailable in the diet, a deficiency may develop within 3 to 4 weeks. Vitamins are either water soluble or fat soluble (see figure 1.8). Water-soluble vitamins dissolve in water; fat-soluble vitamins dissolve in organic solvents and are usually ingested with fats. Minerals can be divided into macrominerals, requiring a daily intake of more than 100 mg or presence in the body in amounts greater than 0.01% of the body weight, and microminerals (trace elements), requiring a daily intake of less than 100 mg or presence in the body in amounts less than 0.01% of body weight. (See chapter 9 for a detailed discussion.)

Sodium, often ingested as sodium chloride (table salt), has various functions in the body, including some related to muscle contraction (see chapter 8). However, excess sodium intake is related to the development of high blood pressure (hypertension). Normal blood pressure (normotension) is about 120 mmHg (systolic) and 80 mmHg (diastolic). Blood pressure is largely regulated by the degree of constriction of blood vessels and by sodium and water retention in the kidney. When blood volume is increased or blood vessels are narrowed, blood pressure rises. If blood pressure is chronically above 140/90 (hypertension), risk of arteriosclerosis, heart attack, stroke, kidney disease, and early death increases.

Epidemiological studies have shown that a high sodium intake (more than 5.8 g/day) is associated with high blood pressure (Carvalho et al. 1989), and on the basis of these studies a low-sodium diet has been recommended. However, controversy surrounds this recommendation. Whether increased salt intake elevates blood pressure in people without existing hypertension is unclear. Salt reduction in normotensive individuals has little or no effect on blood pressure, and a high sodium intake does not affect blood pressure in all individuals (Graudal et al. 1998). About 50% of people may be "salt sensitive" and the other 50% are relatively unaffected by increased sodium intake. Because targeting only the individuals who are salt sensitive would be difficult, and because a moderate salt intake has no reported negative effects (Kumanyika and Cutler 1997), dietary guidelines recommend that people choose and prepare foods with less salt (USDA 2000). In recommendations, an upper limit for sodium intake is usually provided and this is typically 2,400 mg/day.

Water soluble	Fat soluble
Vitamin B$_1$ (thiamin)	Vitamin A
Vitamin B$_2$ (riboflavin)	Vitamin D
Vitamin B$_3$ (niacin)	Vitamin E (α-tocopherol)
Vitamin B$_6$ (pyridoxine)	Vitamin K
Vitamin B$_{12}$	
Biotin	
Pantothenic acid	
Folic acid	
Choline*	
Vitamin C (ascorbic acid)	

Figure 1.8 Fat-soluble and water-soluble vitamins. The asterisk (*) indicates that choline is not classed as an essential vitamin.

Alcohol

Alcohol, or ethanol, is a nutrient that provides 28 kJ of energy per gram (7 kcal/g) but is not essential in our diet. Alcohol is the most widely abused addictive drug and causes specific liver and other organ damage if consumed in excess. It is responsible for approximately 1 in 20 deaths in the United States (McGinnis and Foege 1993). However, alcohol may also have health benefits when ingested in moderation. Moderate alcohol consumption reduces stress and raises levels of HDL cholesterol, which has a protective effect against cardiovascular diseases. Protection may also be provided by phenols in red wine, antioxidant compounds that reduce lipoprotein oxidation and thereby prevent or reduce the formation of atherosclerotic plaques. However, a large intake of alcohol increases blood pressure, which outweighs the positive effects of alcohol consumption. Consumption of alcohol in any amount has been shown to increase the risk of oropharygeal, esophageal, and breast cancers.

Essential Nutrients

Although Hippocrates practiced a form of dietetic medicine in 400 B.C., this area has evolved exponentially over the past 200 to 250 years. Ancient peoples were already aware that certain food components could prevent disease or could be used to treat diseases. However, only during the past two centuries have some nutrients been recognized as essential for human life. In 1740, a British naval surgeon named James Lind discovered that the consumption of citrus fruits by sailors could prevent and cure scurvy. Other shipboard foods and medicine did not have this effect. Although at that time the effect was not related to vitamin C, the essentiality of certain nutrients for the maintenance of health was established.

Tragic studies with prisoners in Nazi death camps have revealed the importance of various vitamins and minerals. The prisoners received a diet deficient in a certain vitamin or mineral, and their health status was recorded. With diets deficient in certain nutrients, specific diseases developed and ultimately resulted in death. In early studies with rats, diets deficient in one or more nutrients retarded growth, and the animals experienced specific disease symptoms. However, when the animals were subsequently fed with the missing nutrient, they recovered completely and growth was promoted.

The nutrients that exhibited these health effects were classified as essential. According to more recent definitions (Harper 1999), a nutrient is defined as essential according to the following criteria:

- The substance is required in the diet for growth, health, and survival.
- Absence of the substance from the diet or inadequate intake results in characteristic signs of a deficiency disease and ultimately death.
- Growth failure and characteristic signs of deficiency are prevented only by the nutrient or a specific precursor of it and not by other substances.
- Below some critical level of intake of the nutrient, growth response and severity of signs of deficiency are proportional to the amount consumed.

- The substance is not synthesized in the body and is therefore required for some critical function throughout life.

A nutrient can be essential for the body but classified as nonessential because it can be synthesized within the body. To avoid confusion, nutritionists often prefer the terms *indispensable* (essential) and *dispensable* (nonessential). Here we will continue to use the terms *essential* and *nonessential*.

Some nutrients are classified as conditionally essential or conditionally indispensable. The term was introduced in 1984 because some nutrients that were normally not essential seemed to become essential under certain conditions. Conditionally essential nutrients must be supplied exogenously to specific populations that do not synthesize them in adequate amounts. The deficiency can be the result of a defect in the synthesis of a certain nutrient or (temporarily) an increased need for that nutrient. An example of the former condition is the genetic defect in the synthesis of carnitine. Without carnitine supplementation, individuals with this condition experience muscle-wasting disease (myopathy). However, when carnitine is supplemented, the condition is corrected. Muscle wasting may also occur in surgical patients in an intensive care unit. These patients usually have lower than normal plasma and muscle glutamine concentrations. This deficit is associated with a negative nitrogen balance, decreased protein synthesis, and increased protein breakdown, resulting in muscle wasting. The patients improve when glutamine is supplemented. Thus, glutamine is classified as conditionally essential.

Recommended Intake

Nowadays, the list of nutrients classified as indispensable is quite extensive (see figure 1.9). More than 40 nutrients meet the criteria. For many centuries people have tried to determine what the minimum and optimum intakes of various nutrients are. In 1941, the first Food and Nutrition Board was formed in the United States. In 1943, dietary standards for evaluating nutritional intakes of large populations and for planning of agricultural production were published. Since then, the guidelines have been revised several times (see appendix C). Previous recommendations did not maximize benefits from food components, especially with respect to chronic illnesses such as heart disease, osteoporosis (decreased bone density), and cancer.

The framework for a set of new recommendations is the dietary reference intake, or **DRI.** The DRI has been released in stages over the past few years. So far, DRIs have been set for all vitamins and miner-

Water	Minerals	Chloride
Amino Acids	Calcium	Vitamins
Histidine	Phosphorus	Ascorbic acid
Isoleucine	Magnesium	Vitamin A
Leucine	Iron	Vitamin D
Lysine	Trace Minerals	Vitamin E
Methionine	Zinc	Vitamin K
Phenylalanine	Copper	Thiamin
Threonine	Manganese	Riboflavin
Tryptophan	Iodine	Niacin
Valine	Selenium	Vitamin B_6 (pyridoxine)
Fatty Acids	Molybdenum	Pantothenic acid
Linoleic	Chromium	Folic acid
α-linoleic	Electrolytes	Biotin
(Linolenic acid)	Sodium	Vitamin B_{12} (cobalamin)
	Potassium	Ultratrace Elements

Figure 1.9 Essential (indispensable) nutrients.

als. Under the umbrella of DRIs, four standards have been developed: the estimated average requirement **(EAR)**, the recommended dietary allowance **(RDA)**, the adequate intake **(AI)**, and the tolerable upper intake level **(UL)**.

The EAR represents the amount of a nutrient that is deemed sufficient to meet the needs of the average individual in a certain age and gender group (see figure 1.10). If these people consume these levels of nutrients, they are unlikely to experience nutritional deficiencies.

The RDA has been prepared by the Food and Nutrition Board since 1941. The first edition was pub-

lished in 1943 to provide "standards to serve as a goal for good nutrition." The RDA is the level of intake of essential nutrients determined on the basis of scientific knowledge to be adequate to meet the known nutrient needs of practically all (97%) healthy persons (National Research Council 2001).

The RDA is a safe excess of nutrients that prevents nutritional deficiencies in the majority of the population. It is calculated as $RDA = EAR + 2\ STDEV_{EAR}$ (see figure 1.10). Meals in institutions will, generally speaking, be considered adequate if they achieve vitamin and mineral levels between the RDA and the EAR.

These recommendations vary depending on age, gender, and whether a woman is pregnant or lactating; they do not apply to other populations or to conditions that may have specific requirements. RDAs are currently available for energy intake, protein, 11 vitamins, and seven minerals (see appendix C). The RDA is based on the median heights and weights of a population, and thus groups of adults who weigh more or less than this median may have a slightly higher or lower requirement, respectively, than the RDA. Also, stress, disease, injuries, and total energy expenditure can influence the needs for certain nutrients.

When sufficient scientific evidence is not available to estimate an EAR, an AI will be set. Individuals should use the AI as a goal for intake where no RDAs exist. The AI is derived through experimental

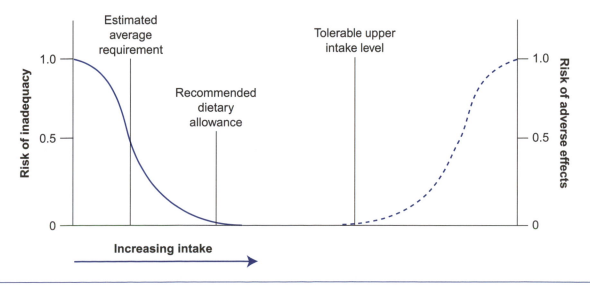

Figure 1.10 Determination of reference and threshold intakes from the mean observed requirements to meet the chosen criteria of 2 standard deviations around the mean and the cumulative distribution of requirements expressed as the probability that a given level of intake will meet an individual's requirements.

or observational data that show a mean intake that appears to sustain a desired indicator of health, such as calcium retention in bone for most members of a population. The AI has been set for two B vitamins, the vitamin-like choline, vitamin D, and some minerals such as calcium and fluoride (see appendix C).

UL is the maximum level of daily nutrient intake that is unlikely to pose health risks to the greatest number individuals in the group for whom it is designed (see figure 1.10). The UL is not intended to be a recommended level of intake; no benefit has been established for individuals to consume nutrients at levels above the RDA or AI. For most nutrients, the UL refers to total intakes from food, fortified food, and nutrient supplements. The need for setting the UL grew out of the increased practice of fortifying foods with nutrients and of the popularity of dietary supplements, resulting in high intakes of some nutrients.

DRIs are mainly intended for diet planning. Specifically, a diet should aim to meet any RDA set. If no RDA has been determined, AIs should be used as a guide for nutrient intake. The UL should not be exceeded. DRIs are based on averages of large populations and, thus, are not designed to detect nutrient deficiencies in individuals. Only a clinical and biochemical examination can determine whether an individual has a nutritional deficiency. Comparison of an individual's intake to the RDA, however, can help determine whether the person is at risk for a deficiency. If someone wants to determine whether the individual's nutrient intake meets the RDA, food intake should be measured over a period of 5 to 8 days. An individual whose diet does not contain the full RDA on one day is not necessarily at risk for deficiencies, because the inadequacy can be compensated for the next day. The RDA does not reflect the minimum requirements but a safe excess intake.

RDAs do not account for unusual requirements caused by disease or environmental stress. Also, the data used to determine the RDAs often did not include athletes, or the activity levels of the subjects were not reported. Therefore, the RDAs may not be an accurate means of evaluating the nutritional needs of individuals engaged in regular strenuous exercise.

The reference values used to determine RDAs are age-specific and gender-specific, and for food-labeling purposes an additional set of reference values had to be produced. Packages must be the same for men and women and for children and adults, so the RDA values had to be condensed into an acceptable recommendation for all groups.

Originally the labels contained the U.S. Recommended Daily Allowances (US RDA). The US RDA has been replaced by daily values (DV).

The US RDA, which was based on RDAs, was developed by the Food and Drug Administration (FDA) in 1973 for use in food labeling. The US RDA is a single number that does not vary with age and gender, except for children under 4 years of age and pregnant or lactating women, where the RDA is still the standard. The FDA usually picked the highest RDA level needed by age or gender group to determine the US RDA. This value was adopted not only for the sake of simplicity in food packaging but also to reflect the advances in scientific knowledge since 1968, with respect to essential nutrient requirements.

The DV has recently replaced the US RDA. The DV is based on two sets of references: (1) the RDI, which makes up most of the DVs and provides a set of dietary references for essential vitamins and minerals, and (2) the daily reference value (**DRV**), a standard for proteins and various dietary components that have no RDA or other established nutrient standard (e.g., cholesterol, total fat, carbohydrate, dietary fiber, sodium, and potassium) (see figure 1.11). On food labels all reference values are listed as DV although they can be either DRV or RDI. On current food labeling, the "% *Daily Value*" is the percentage of RDI or DRV available in a single serving.

Some countries have formulated recommendations with respect to the amount of each nutrient that should be consumed. Therefore, definitions of RDA differ slightly in different countries (see appendixes C, D, and E). The United Nations and the European Union have formulated their own reference intakes, as have many individual countries. In some countries, such as the United Kingdom (appendix D) and Germany, the RDA has been redefined as the reference nutrient intake (RNI) and in Australia as the recommended daily intake (**RDI**) (appendix E). Canada now uses the same system as the United

Food component	DRV 8 MJ (2,000 kcal)
Total fat	Less than 65 g (30% of energy intake)
Saturated fat	Less than 20 g (10% of energy intake)
Cholesterol	Less than 300 mg
Total carbohydrate	300 g (60% of energy intake)
Dietary fiber	25 g (11.5 g/1,000 kcal)
Sodium	Less than 2,400 mg
Potassium	3,500 mg
Protein	50 g (10% of energy intake)

Figure 1.11 Daily reference values (DRVs).

States, and that country's RNI is being replaced by the DRI.

United Kingdom

In the United Kingdom, the RNI, very similar to the original RDA, is the level of intake required to meet the known nutritional needs of more than 97.5% of healthy persons (see appendix D). The EAR in the United Kingdom is similar to the EAR in the United States, but unlike the United States, the United Kingdom also has a lower reference nutrient intake (LRNI) value. The LRNI represents an amount of a nutrient that is virtually certain to be inadequate. (Notably, the average intake of the trace element selenium in the UK falls well below the LRNI.)

Australia

The RDI is the level of intake of essential nutrients considered, by the National Health and Medical Research Council in Australia, on the basis of available scientific knowledge, to be adequate for the known nutritional needs of practically all healthy people (see appendix E). RDI values are derived from estimates of requirements for each age/gender category and incorporate generous factors to accommodate variations in absorption and metabolism. They therefore apply to group needs. RDIs exceed the actual nutrient requirements and are not synonymous with requirements. Note that the RDI in Australia is different from the RDI (Reference Daily Intakes) used in the United States.

The Food Guide Pyramid

Although the DRI may provide guidance on nutrient requirements, it is not a very practical way of informing people about appropriate food choices. For example, how does someone know if he or she is consuming about 0.8 g/kg b.w. of protein a day? Nutritionists addressed this question early in the twentieth century and developed several simple and comprehensive food guides, the most important guide of which is the food guide pyramid (see figure 1.12). The food guide pyramid has six categories of foods (see figure 1.13).

The foods in each category make a similar nutrient contribution. The food guide pyramid also

Figure 1.12 Food guide pyramid.

Food categories	**Essential nutrients**
Breads, cereals, rice, pasta	Thiamin, niacin, riboflavin, iron
Dairy products: milk, yogurt, cheese	Calcium, protein, riboflavin, vitamin A
Meat, poultry, fish, eggs, dry beans, nuts	Protein, thiamin, niacin, iron
Vegetables	Vitamin A, vitamin C
Fruit	Vitamin A, vitamin C
Fats, oils, sweets*	Vitamin A, vitamin D, vitamin E

Figure 1.13 Major nutrients in the six categories of the food guide pyramid and the most important nutrients they provide. The asterisk (*) indicates that a component mainly adds to energy intake and does not provide micronutrients.

recommends the number of servings from each category each day. The emphasis is on the base of the pyramid: bread, cereal, rice, and pasta (six to 11 servings), followed by vegetables and fruit (three to five servings and two to four servings a day, respectively). Two to three servings a day are recommended for the dairy product group and the meat and poultry group. Finally, fats, oils, and sweets should be used sparingly.

Food Labels

Food labels are another useful tool for diet planning or nutritional assessment (see figure 1.14). Food labels help consumers make choices by providing detailed information about the nutrient content of food and how that food fits into the overall diet. In the United States, food labeling is standardized as specified by the Nutrition Labeling and Education Act of 1990. All packaged foods, except those produced by small businesses and those in packages too small to fit the labeling information, must be labeled. Serving size and the format of the food labels are identical on all products to make comparing foods easier. In Canada, nutrition labeling is voluntary but standardized. In other parts of the world, the labels are not yet standardized. Food labeling laws regulate about 75% of all food consumed in the United States.

The information on food labels includes the name of the product; the name and contact details of the manufacturer, packager, or distributor; the net contents or weight of the package; and the date by which the product has to be sold. The label also contains information about the ingredients in the food, expressed per unit of weight of the whole product. For instance, whole milk contains 3.5 g of fat, 3.2 g of protein, 4.7 g of carbohydrate (all sugars), 120 mg of calcium, 0.4 µg of vitamin B_{12}, and 270 kJ (65 kcal) per 100 g of milk. In the United States, the ingredients are expressed per serving; in Europe, they are expressed per serving as well as per 100 g. In the United States, the ingredients are also expressed as a percentage of the daily recommended value.

Labels often contain information that might be of interest to the consumer such as "low fat," "reduced fat," "fat free," "light," and "lean." The use of these and other terms is also regulated, and definitions of these terms have been established (see table 1.3). When a consumer buys a product with "low fat" on the label, he or she can be sure that it meets the definition established by the FDA (less than 3 g of fat per serving).

Food labels also often contain health claims. For instance, calcium-rich products such as milk may claim to protect against osteoporosis. However, any and all claims are not allowed on food labels. Only the claims summarized in table 1.4 are legal (detailed information on health claims can be found on the FDA Web site). Health claims can only be used when a certain percentage of the DV is present in the food product, and the claims must be backed up by scientific evidence, usually derived from epidemiological studies.

Healthy Nutrition: Recommendations

As with deficiency of essential nutrients, excess intake of nutrients can also result in health problems and disease. Some of these effects may be acute, but excess intake of certain nutrients may also affect long-term health, and a reduced intake of these nutrients may lower the risk of several chronic diseases. Organizations such as the USDA have formulated dietary guidelines to improve or optimize health (USDA 2000). Although such guidelines are usually very clear, they may sometimes be difficult to incorporate into daily life.

These dietary guidelines reflect recommendations of health and nutrition experts, who agree that enough is known about the effect of diet on health to encourage certain eating practices. The guidelines are as follows:

Macaroni & Cheese

Nutrition Facts

Start here ➤ Serving Size 1 cup (228g)
Serving Per Container 2

Amount Per Serving

Calories 250   Calories from Fat 110

% Daily Value*

Total Fat 12g	**18%**
Saturated Fat 3g	**15%**
Cholesterol 30mg	**10%**
Sodium 470mg	**20%**
Total Carbohydrate 31g	**10%**
Dietary Fiber 0g	**0%**
Sugars 5g	
Protein 5g	

Vitamin A	4%
Vitamin C	2%
Calcium	20%
Iron	4%

Limit these nutrients

5% or less is low

20% or more is high

Get enough of these nutrients

*Percent Daily Values are based on a 2,000 calorie diet.
Your Daily Values may be higher or lower depending on your calorie needs:

	Calories	2,000	2,500
Total Fat	Less than	65g	80g
Sat Fat	Less than	20g	25g
Cholesterol	Less than	300mg	300mg
Sodium	Less than	2,400mg	2,400mg
Total Carbohydrate		300g	375g
Dietary Fiber		25g	30g

Footnote

Figure 1.14 How to read a food label.

- Eat a variety of foods to get the energy (calories), protein, vitamins, minerals, and fiber you need for good health.

- Maintain a healthy weight to reduce the risk of high blood pressure, heart disease, stroke, certain cancers, and diabetes.

- Choose a diet low in fat, saturated fat, and cholesterol to reduce your risk of heart disease and certain cancers. Because fat contains more than twice the calories of an equal amount of carbohydrate or protein, a low-fat diet low can help you maintain a healthy weight.

- Choose a diet with plenty of vegetables, fruits, and grain products that provide needed vitamins, minerals, fiber, and complex carbohydrates.

- Use sugars only in moderation. A sugar-rich diet has too many calories and too few nutrients and can contribute to tooth decay.

- Use salt and other forms of sodium only in moderation to reduce your risk of high blood pressure.

- Drink alcoholic beverages only in moderation. Alcoholic beverages supply calories but little

Table 1.3 Definitions of Nutrient Content Claims

Nutrient	Free (zero, no, without, trivial source of, negligible source of)	Low (little, few for calories, contains a small amount of, low source of)	Reduced/less (lower, fewer for calories)	Comments
Calories	*Calorie free*: Less than 5 cal per reference amount and per labeled serving	*Few calories*: 40 cal or less per reference amount (and per 50 g if reference amount is small); meals and main dishes: 120 cal or less per 100 g	*Fewer calories*: At least 25% fewer calories per reference amount than an appropriate reference food; reference food may not be "low calorie"	*"Light"* or *"lite"*: If 50% or more of the calories are from fat, fat must be reduced by at least 50% per reference amount; if less than 50% of calories are from fat, fat must be reduced at least 50% or calories reduced at least 1/3 per reference amount
Total fat	*Fat free*: Less than 0.5 g per reference amount and per labeled serving (or for meals and main dishes, less than 0.5 g per labeled serving)	*Low fat*: 3 g or less per reference amount (and per 50 g if reference amount is small); meals and main dishes: 3 g or less per 100 g and not more than 30% of calories from fat	*Reduced fat*: At least 25% less fat per reference amount than an appropriate reference food; reference food may not be "low fat"	*"_ % fat free"*: Allowed if meets the requirements for "low fat"; "100% fat free: food must be "fat free"
Sugars	*Sugar free*: Less than 0.5 g sugars per reference amount and per labeled serving (or for meals and main dishes, less than 0.5 g per labeled serving)	Not defined; no basis for recommended intake	*Reduced sugar*: At least 25% less sugars per reference amount than an appropriate reference food	*"No added sugars"* and *"without added sugars"*: Allowed if no sugar or sugar-containing ingredient is added during processing; state if food is not "low" or "reduced" calorie

Reference amount = reference amount customarily consumed. Small reference amount = reference amount of 30 g or less or 2 tablespoons or less (for dehydrated foods that are typically consumed when rehydrated with water or a diluent containing an insignificant amount of the pertinent nutrient).

Table 1.4 Health Claims Allowed on Food Labels

Health issue	Claim
Calcium and osteoporosis	Adequate calcium intake throughout life helps maintain bone health and reduce the risk of osteoporosis. A food must contain 20% or more of the DV for calcium.
Sodium and hypertension	Diets high in sodium may increase the risk of high blood pressure in some people, and, hence, a diet low in sodium may protect against hypertension.
Dietary fat and cancer	Diets high in fat increase the risk of some types of cancer, and, hence, low-fat diets may be protective
Saturated fat and cholesterol and risk of coronary heart disease	Diets high in saturated fat and cholesterol increase blood cholesterol and, thus, the risk of heart disease. A diet low in saturated fat may, therefore, reduce this risk.
Foods high in fiber and cancer	Diets low in fat and rich in fiber-containing grain products, fruits, and vegetables may reduce the risk of some types of cancer.
Foods high in fiber and risk of coronary heart disease	Diets low in saturated fat and cholesterol and rich in fruits, vegetables, and grain products that contain fiber, particularly soluble fiber, may reduce the risk of coronary heart disease.
Folic acid and birth defects	Adequate folic acid intake by the mother reduces the risk of birth defects of the brain or spinal cord in her baby.
Dietary sugar and dental carries	Sugar-free foods that are sweetened with sugar alcohols do not promote tooth decay and may reduce the risk of dental caries.

A food carrying a health claim must be a naturally good source (10% or more of the daily value) for one of six nutrients (vitamin A, vitamin C, protein, calcium, iron, or fiber) and must not contain more than 20% of the Daily Value for fat, saturated fat, cholesterol, or sodium.

or no nutrients. Alcohol consumption is the cause of many health problems and accidents and can lead to addiction.

Processed Food and Additives

The term "processed food" refers to food treated to extend storage life, or to improve taste, nutrition, color, or texture. "Processing" includes adding preservatives, colorings, or flavorings; fortifying, enriching, dehydrating, smoking, drying, or freezing; and a number of other treatments. Concern has been expressed that the nutritional quality of food has declined during recent years because the amount of processing has increased. Indeed, modern foods contain more refined sugar, extracted oils, or white flour, products from which nutrients are lost in the refinement process. In the bleaching of flour, for example, 22 known essential nutrients are lost. Artificially ripened fruit contains much smaller amounts of micronutrients than naturally ripened fruit.

Many products are completely artificial, such as synthetic fruit juices, soft drinks, and nondairy creamers. Refined or artificial products may contain little or no nutrients but have the same energy content as their natural counterparts. Thus, the nutrient density (the amount of essential nutrients per unit of energy) is very low. However, although some nutrients are lost during processing, modern techniques used by the majority of food manufacturers prevent major losses of nutrients. Frozen and canned vegetables, for example, contain similar amounts of essential nutrients to fresh vegetables. So although food processing can reduce nutrient density, the problem seems to be relatively small. In fact, most nutrients may be lost when the food is prepared at home. When vegetables are boiled or steamed, vitamins and minerals may end up in the water, or, with other cooking methods, heat-labile vitamins may be lost because of overcooking. The increased use of refined sugar, oils, unenriched white flour, salt, and questionable additives is a greater concern. Food labels can help us to make decisions about the quality of processed foods.

Food additives lengthen shelf lives; enhance color, texture, or taste; facilitate food preparation; or otherwise make food products more marketable. Certain additives, such as sugar, are derived from natural sources. Other additives, such as the artificial sweetener aspartame, are made synthetically. Although artificial sweeteners have been said to cause cancer, concrete evidence to support such claims has not been found. A selection of common artificial sweeteners is listed in table 1.5.

The color of food is an integral part of our culture. Even early civilizations such as the Romans recognized that people "eat with their eyes" as well as their palates. Saffron was often used to provide a rich yellow color to various foods. Butter has been colored

Table 1.5 Artificial Sweeteners and Their Characteristics

Sweetener	Sweetness × sucrose	Characteristics	Can be found in
Saccharin	300–500	• Not metabolized in the human body and is excreted in urine. • Fairly strong aftertaste.	Soft drinks, table top sweeteners, and a wide variety of foods (Sweet 'n Low)
Aspartame	180	• Derived from the two amino acids: phenylalanine and aspartate. • Contains 16 kJ (4 kcal) per g, but because such small amounts are needed it adds virtually no energy. • Aspartame is metabolized to its amino acids phenylalanine and aspartate. • The taste of aspartame can be quite pleasant, and it is therefore sometimes added to foods to improve taste.	Although aspartame is used in a wide variety of food products, the disadvantage of aspartame is that it cannot be used in foods that need to be heated. At high temperatures aspartame will denature. Aspartame also has limited stability in foods with a low pH such as soft drinks. Aspartame is sold under the brand name Nutrasweet.
Acesulfame potassium	200	• Not metabolized in the body and excreted in urine (noncaloric sweetener).	Sold under the brand name Sunnet
Sorbitol	0.5–0.7	• Is produced from sugar but contains only 10.4 kJ (2.6 kcal) per g compared with 16 kJ (4 kcal) for sucrose. • Excessive consumption of sorbitol (more than 50 g) can cause gastrointestinal problems.	Various food products
Sucralose	300–1000	• Discovered in 1976 and approved by the FDA in 1998. • A relatively new artificial sweetener synthesized from sucrose. • Sucralose is only absorbed in small quantities and the small amounts that are absorbed are excreted in urine.	Various food products
Xylitol	1	• Contains slightly less energy than sucrose (2.4 kcal per g).	Chewing gum, candy, and oral health products
Stevia	200	• Stevia sweetener is a natural sweetener that is made from an herbal plant extract (Stevia rebaudiana). • High stability at low pH and high temperature. • Can provide long shelf life; cooking and baking resistant.	Chewing gum, candy, ice cream, yogurt, and soft drinks

yellow as far back as the 1300s. Today, all food color additives are carefully regulated by the FDA to ensure that foods with such additives are accurately labeled and safe to eat. Food colorants are both natural and synthetic. Natural colorants include beta carotene, beet powder, carrot oil, carmine, fruit juice, paprika, riboflavin, saffron, and turmeric.

Fat Substitutes

Fat substitutes have one or more of the technical effects of fat in food but are not absorbed or metabolized as fat. The three types of fat substitutes include carbohydrate-based fat substitutes, which use plant polysaccharides in place of fat; proteins and microparticulated proteins, which block fat absorption; and fat-based fat substitutes, which also block fat absorption.

Examples of carbohydrate-based fat replacements are corn syrup solids, dextrin, maltodextrin, and modified food starch. These fat substitutes have very little or no taste and contain less energy than fat. Dietary fibers such cellulose gel, cellulose gum, guar gum, insulin, and pectin have some of the properties of fat but minimal absorption occurs. A protein-based fat substitute sold under the name Simplesse is approved for use in low-temperature foods such as ice cream. It contains 4 to 8 kJ (1 to 2 kcal) /g.

Probably the most studied fat substitute is Olestra (Olean). Olestra looks like fat, cooks like fat, and gives foods all the rich taste and "mouth feel" of ordinary fat. However, unlike ordinary fats and oils, Olestra is not digested or absorbed in the body and therefore contributes no fat or calories to the diet. Olestra is made from sucrose polyester, which is composed of sucrose with six to eight fatty acids bound to it. These fatty acids are from vegetable oils such as soybean or corn oil. Because the Olestra molecule is large in comparison to a fat molecule, it is not hydrolyzed by the body's digestive enzymes. It passes through the digestive system unchanged. Olestra is currently approved for snack foods such as chips and crackers. Because Olestra is not absorbed, the absorption of fat-soluble vitamins is reduced. Therefore, products containing Olestra are enriched with vitamins A, D, E, and K.

Although the fat substitutes already on the market are considered safe by the FDA, their long-term or cumulative health effects are unknown.

Assessing Nutrient and Energy Intake

Analyzing dietary intake can be useful for several reasons. The average intake in a group of athletes can be studied, and the data can be used in conjunction with biochemical or anthropometric data to inform them of the adequacy of their diet. Dietary intake data can also be used in conjunction with a medical report or to explain the incidence or prevalence of health problems. Such measurements can also be used for educational purposes, and the efficacy of nutritional advice or intervention programs can be investigated. Several methods have been developed to measure dietary intake (see table 1.6), and each method has advantages and disadvantages.

Three-Day Food Record

The three-day dietary survey, or diet record, is a relatively simple and reasonably accurate way to determine the total daily energy intake and the quality of food. The 3-day log should represent a normal eating pattern. Inclusion of 2 weekdays and 1 day during a weekend is recommended. Calculations of energy intake from records of daily food consumption are usually within 10% of the actual energy intake.

This method provides fairly reliable results for the intake of some nutrients such as carbohydrate and water, but longer periods may be required to get a more reliable classification of individual intake for nutrients such as cholesterol and fat and some of the micronutrients.

To obtain an accurate measure of food, common measuring tools may be used, including a ruler to measure the length, width, and height of food; standard measuring cups, teaspoons, tablespoons to determine volume, and a balance to determine weight to the nearest gram. A weighed food intake is a very accurate measurement, but individuals have to be very motivated to perform this activity. Poor compliance has been reported with weighed food records, and the use of household measuring devices is often the preferred method. However weighed food records may be the method of choice for use with highly motivated athletes.

All the foods consumed, including all beverages, should be recorded using the blank 3-day food logs on the pages of the **food diary** (see table 1.7). When completing a diet record, keep these sheets with you all the time and record the food intake while you are consuming the food. When the food log is completed, the energy intake and nutrient intakes can be calculated using either a software package or a food table. Use a software package or a food table of the country in which you live because many products are specific to different countries.

Most people are only vaguely aware of what they eat. Without instruction, food records will lack sufficient detail to be useful for most research purposes. Errors occur mainly because of memory failures. In general, the common foods are recorded accurately, but the uncommon foods are sometimes poorly registered. Most errors are made in reporting the frequency of consumption. Errors in estimating portion size are very common as well. If food is not weighed, the mass of various foods may be underestimated or overestimated considerably. Errors are sometimes as large as 50% for foods and 20% for particular nutrients (Burke and Deakin 2000; Shils et al. 1999). Training and instructing the persons who are registering their food intake can reduce errors, but the instructions should be repeated over and over again. On an individual level, the three-day food survey is generally accepted as one of the best methods to assess nutritional intake. However, this method also has disadvantages. Overweight people tend to underestimate their portion sizes, whereas underweight people tend to overestimate portions (Johansson et al. 1998). Individuals may not report their food intake accurately, which makes coding of the specific food

Table 1.6 Methods to Estimate Nutrient Intake

Method	Short description	Advantages	Disadvantages
Prospective methods			
3-day dietary survey	Recording all foods consumed for 3 days	• Fairly accurate • Inexpensive • Detailed information • Provides information about eating habits	• May not represent normal diet • Tends to underestimate energy intake
3-day weighed food record	Weighing and recording all foods consumed for 3 days	• Accurate • Inexpensive • Detailed information • Provides information about eating habits	• Demanding for respondent • Potential compliance problems • May not represent normal diet • Tends to underestimate energy intake
7-day dietary survey	Recording all foods consumed for 7 days	• Fairly accurate • Inexpensive • Detailed information • Provides information about eating habits	• Demanding for respondent • Compliance may be reduced after 4 days • May not represent normal diet • Tends to underestimate energy intake
7-day weighed food record	Weighing and recording all foods consumed for 7 days	• Accurate • Inexpensive • Detailed information • Provides information about eating habits	• Highly demanding for respondent • Compliance may be reduced after 4 days • May not represent normal diet • Tends to underestimate energy intake
Duplicate food collections	A duplicate of each meal/food is saved for chemical analysis	• Probably the most accurate method • Detailed information	• Expensive (analysis) • Time consuming • May affect food choice • Demanding for respondent • Likely to underestimate food intake
Retrospective methods			
24-hour recall	Questionnaire or interview to assess dietary intake in the previous 24 hours	• Good response rate • Relatively easy • Inexpensive • Can be used to rank nutrient intakes in groups of people	• May not represent usual food intake • Memory bias • Underestimates total energy intake • Does not provide quantitative data
Food frequency	Questionnaire or interview with questions about the frequency of intake of certain foods	• Good response rate • Relatively easy • Inexpensive • Can be used to rank nutrient intakes in groups of people in qualitative terms	• Memory bias • Underestimates total energy intake • Does not provide quantitative data • Overestimates at low energy intakes and underestimates at high energy intakes • The list of foods used may not represent the person's normal food intake
Diet history	A combination of the 24-hour recall and food frequency questionnaire	• Can be used to rank nutrient intakes in groups of people	• Requires trained interviewer • Takes longer to complete than 24-hour recall or food frequency questionnaire

Table 1.7 Sample of an Accurate Food Diary

Time	Place	Kind/brand	How prepared?	Amount
7:00 A.M. 9:00 A.M.	Home Office	Cornflakes/Kelloggs Whole milk Coffee Sugar	 Filter	1 small bowl 1 glass (200 ml) 1 cup 1 teaspoon

type difficult. For example, writing just "potatoes" is not very informative. Were the potatoes large or small? Were they boiled, baked, fried, or raw? Were the skins removed? Sometimes food records may be illegible, introducing more coding errors. Therefore, individuals must be carefully instructed to provide as much detail as possible.

Seven-Day Food Record

The seven-day dietary survey is identical to the three-day survey, except for the duration of the recording period. The extended recording time may allow for a more reliable classification of a person's normal diet and nutrient intake. The seven-day survey includes all weekdays and the 2 days of the weekend. The disadvantage of this method is that with such a long period of recording, persons may become tired of recording and forget to write down foods consumed, resulting in a less accurate nutritional assessment. Often, lack of compliance is reported after about 4 days. Besides the three-day and seven-day dietary surveys, other alternatives have been used, with 4, 5, or 6 days of recording and even up to 12 months of continuous recording.

Duplicate Food Collections

A very accurate method is the duplicate food collections method, which involves preparing two portions of food and saving a duplicate of everything that is eaten. These portions are then collected and put in a blender for chemical analysis of the nutrient content. This method has been used mainly for research purposes and is very expensive because of the costs of the chemical analyses, especially when a wide range of nutrients is investigated. The method also places a burden on the individual and is likely to affect food choices. This method may also result in underreporting of food intake.

24-Hour Recall

The most common technique of assessing food intake is the 24-hour recall. A trained interviewer asks participants on one or more occasions to describe the food, drinks, and dietary supplements they have consumed during the previous 24 hours. The data obtained may include information about time of food intake, preparation of food, and eating environment.

The advantages of the 24-hour recall technique are that it is easy to administer, it is time efficient, and it is inexpensive. On the other hand, disadvantages include underreporting, even when participants are interviewed by a skilled dietician; underestimating energy and nutrient intake, sometimes by as much as 20%; and tendencies by overweight individuals to underestimate their portions (underweight persons tend to overestimate portions) (Johansson et al. 1998). Also, this technique relies heavily on memory, which makes it unsuitable for certain groups, such as the elderly.

The data obtained from 24-hour recalls are more accurate when they are repeated several times at random. This approach also corrects somewhat for the day-to-day variation in food intake. The 24-hour recall method is a reasonably good way to estimate nutrient intake in a group of people, but it is less valuable for individual use. However, it can give a foundation for pursuing of a more detailed picture of someone's nutrient intake.

Food Frequency

A food frequency questionnaire (see table 1.8) is often used to get a general picture of someone's patterns of food intake. Individuals respond to a series of questions about the frequency of their food intake: How often do you eat red meat? How often do you eat fruit? How often do you drink milk? Questions about portion size, food preparation, and supplement use can be included, but it is not a standard procedure. A problem with this method is that the products mentioned in the questionnaire may not represent the respondent's actual food intake.

The food frequency questionnaire is a relatively easy and quick method, but it does not itemize a specific day's intake. The information obtained is

Table 1.8   Food Frequency Questionnaire

	Once a day	Twice or more a day	Once a week	Twice or more a week	Once a month	Twice or more a month
Milk Whole Reduced fat Nonfat		√	√			
Yogurt Whole Reduced fat Nonfat					√	
Cheese Hard Soft Reduced fat		√		√		
Ice cream Regular Reduced fat					√	

qualitative rather than quantitative. The food frequency questionnaire is regularly used in clinical or research settings. If investigators are only interested in one particular food item or food group, the food frequency questionnaire can be very useful.

Diet History

A diet history provides general information about dietary habits and patterns. This technique was originally described by Burke in 1947 and combines the 24-hour recall with a food frequency questionnaire. Combining these different methods usually gives a better view of a person's dietary habits by asking question of the following type: Do you always have breakfast? Do you skip lunch? Did you drink milk as an adolescent? Diet history can provide information about changes in dietary habits, including seasonal changes. A diet history takes about 20 minutes to complete. This method also requires quite a bit of skill from the interviewer, who must be a well-trained dietician.

Analyzing Nutrient Intake

Once the nutrient intake information is obtained, it can be compared with the recommendations. A simple but not very accurate comparison is with a guide such as the food guide pyramid. However, when a three-day to seven-day dietary survey is completed, the intake can be analyzed in more detail. To calculate the intake of specific nutrients, the food labels or one of many food composition databases can be used. In the United States the major source of information is the USDA Nutrient Database, which is available online (USDA 2003). Various software packages and some programs online use this database or other databases to calculate food intake. In all cases, the exact amount and kind of food must be entered in the computer program. If a food is not included in the database, an appropriate substitute should be chosen. Most such programs allow the user to add new products to the database, which can be done using information on the food label. The software will usually produce an average intake over 24 hours for all macronutrients and micronutrients. These values can than be compared with the recommended amounts.

Nutritional Requirements and Exercise

In the chapters that follow we will focus on exercise nutrition. In particular, we will examine the question of whether nutrition requirements change with exercise. In this introductory chapter, we have only discussed nutrition in the general population, assuming relatively low physical activity levels. In subsequent chapters, we will discuss the energy requirements of exercise and the specific needs for macronutrients and micronutrients.

Key Points

- The nutrients in food have three main functions: promotion of growth and development, provision of energy, and regulation of metabolism.

- Nutrients are usually divided into six different categories: carbohydrates, fats, proteins, vitamins, minerals, and water. Some of the functions of these nutrients are providing building blocks for cells (protein), repairing damaged cells (protein), providing energy (predominantly carbohydrate and fat), protecting organs (fat), and regulating metabolism (protein, vitamins, and minerals).

- Amino acids are the building blocks of all proteins. Most proteins are polypeptides combining up to 300 amino acids. Twenty different amino acids are commonly found in proteins.

- Proteins provide structure to all cells in the human body. They are an integral part of the cell membrane, the cytoplasm, and the organelles, but individual amino acids are also precursors and regulators of the synthesis of important metabolic mediators and compounds with a regulatory biological activity (e.g., neurotransmitters, hormones, DNA, and RNA).

- Recommended daily intakes for protein are generally based on data from nitrogen-balance studies and vary worldwide between 0.8 and 1.2 g/kg b.w.

- In adults, about 60% of body weight is water. The percentage is higher in infants and generally decreases with age. Water content varies among different tissues of the body: blood is about 90% water, muscle is about 75% water, bone is about 25% water, and adipose tissue is about 5% water.

- Loss of water (through diarrhea or sweating) may result in dehydration. With water losses of 3% of the total body weight, blood volume decreases and exercise performance is negatively affected. A 5% loss results in confusion and disorientation. Losses greater than 10% can be life threatening.

- Vitamins are organic compounds and minerals are inorganic compounds that are essential to the diet in small amounts.

- Essential nutrients cannot be synthesized in the body and are therefore required in the diet for growth, health, and survival. Absence from the diet or inadequate intake results in characteristic signs of a deficiency, disease, and ultimately death.

- Nonessential nutrients can be synthesized in the body from their precursors.

- Humans have an essential requirement for over 40 nutrients.

- Several methods are used to assess food intake and diet composition. These methods include diet history, 24-hour recalls, food frequency questionnaires, self-reported food records, and weighed food records. The methods differ substantially in their accuracy and practicality.

Key Terms

amino acids 11
carbohydrate 2
dietary reference intake (DRI) 16
DRV 18
fat 2
food diary 25

lipid 6
macronutrients 2
micronutrients 2
mineral 2
nutrient 2
nutrition 2

protein 11
recommended dietary allowance (RDA) 13
reference daily intake (RDI) 18
vitamin 2
water 2

Recommended Readings

Bender, D.A., and A.E. Bender. 1997. *Nutrition: A reference handbook.* Oxford University Press: Oxford.

Gibney, M.J., I. Macdonald, and H. Roche. 2003. *Nutrition and metabolism.* Blackwell Science: Oxford.

Gibney, M.J., H.H. Vorster, and F.J. Kok. 2002. *Introduction to human nutrition.* Blackwell Science: Oxford.

Mann, J., and A.S. Truswell. 2002. *Essentials of human nutrition.* Oxford University Press: Oxford.

Shils, M.E., J.A. Olson, M. Shike, and A.C. Ross. 1999. *Modern nutrition in health and disease.* Williams & Wilkins: Baltimore.

Chapter 2

Fuel Sources for Muscle and Exercise Metabolism

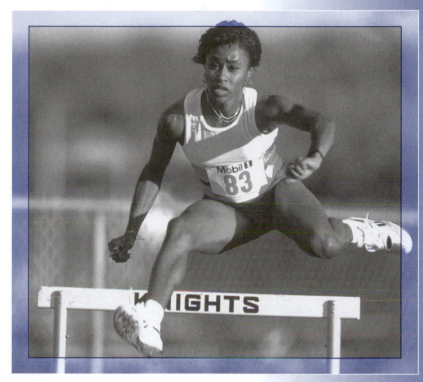

© Rob Tringali/SportsChrome USA

Objectives

After studying this chapter, you should be able to do the following:

- Describe the structure of skeletal muscle and explain the process of muscle contraction

- Describe the characteristics of the different muscle fiber types

- Describe the metabolic pathways that supply energy for muscle contraction

- Describe the nature and size of body fuel stores

- Describe the factors involved in the control of fuel mobilization and utilization

- Describe the metabolic responses and main causes of fatigue in moderate and high-intensity exercise

An in-depth understanding of sport nutrition requires some knowledge of biochemistry, which usually refers to the study of events such as reactions, energy transfer, and transport processes at the subcellular and molecular levels. If you think that you lack even a basic understanding of biochemistry and cell biology, refer to appendix A, in which some of the basic principles are explained. This chapter describes the sources of energy available for muscle force generation and explains how acute exercise modifies energy metabolism via intracellular effects and the action of **hormones** (for further details see the books by Maughan, Gleeson, and Greenhaff 1997 and Hargreaves 1995). The pre-exercise diet and feeding during exercise influence the hormonal and metabolic responses to exercise. Training also modifies the metabolic response to exercise, and training-induced adaptations encompass both biochemical responses (e.g., changes in enzyme activities in trained muscles) and physiological responses (e.g., changes in maximal cardiac output and maximal oxygen uptake, $\dot{V}O_2max$). These influences are also described in this chapter.

Subcellular Structure and Mechanism of Force Generation in Skeletal Muscle

Muscles are composed of long, cylindrical cells called fibers. These fibers contain the internal organelles and structures that allow muscle to contract and relax. Individual muscles are made up of many parallel fibers that may extend the entire length of the muscle. Inside the muscle fiber is the sarcoplasm (muscle cell cytoplasm), a red viscous fluid containing nuclei, **mitochondria**, myoglobin, and about 500 threadlike 1 mm to 3 mm thick **myofibrils** that are continuous from end to end in the muscle fiber. The red color is caused by myoglobin, an intracellular respiratory pigment. Surrounding the myofibrils is an elaborate baglike membranous structure called the sarcoplasmic reticulum. Its interconnecting membranous tubules lie in the narrow spaces between the myofibrils, surrounding and running parallel to them. Energy is stored in the sarcoplasm as fat (triacylglycerol droplets), **glycogen, phosphocreatine** (PCr), and **adenosine triphosphate** (ATP).

The myofibrils are composed of overlapping thin and thick filaments made of protein, and the arrangement of these filaments gives skeletal muscle its striated appearance when viewed through a microscope.

The thick filaments are composed of myosin molecules, each of which consists of a rodlike tail and a globular head. The latter contains **ATPase** activity sites and actin-binding sites. ATP is the energy currency of the cell. The breakdown of ATP to adenosine diphosphate (ADP) and inorganic phosphate (Pi) by the myosin ATPase provides the energy for muscle contraction. The thin filaments are composed of actin molecules and several regulatory proteins. Globular actin (G-actin) monomers are polymerized into long strands of fibrous actin (F-actin). Two F-actin strands twisted together in ropelike fashion form the backbone of each thin filament. Rod-shaped tropomyosin molecules spiral about the F-actin chains. The other main protein present in the thin filaments is troponin, which contains three subunits. One of these subunits, troponin-I, binds to actin; another subunit, troponin-T, binds to tropomyosin; and the third subunit, troponin-C, binds to calcium ions. A **sarcomere** is the smallest contractile unit, or segment, of a muscle fiber and is the region between two Z-lines (see figure 2.1).

Cross-Bridge Formation

When calcium and ATP are present in sufficient quantities, the filaments form actomyosin and shorten by sliding over each other. Sliding begins when the myosin heads form cross-bridges attached to active sites on the actin subunits of the thin filaments. Each cross-bridge attaches and detaches several times during a contraction, pulling the thin filaments toward the center of the sarcomere in a ratchet-like action. When a muscle fiber contracts, its sarcomeres shorten throughout the cell, and the whole muscle fiber shortens.

The attachment of the myosin cross-bridges requires the presence of calcium ions. In the relaxed muscle, calcium is sequestered in the sarcoplasmic reticulum. Without calcium, the myosin binding sites on actin are physically blocked by the tropomyosin rods, as illustrated in figure 2.1. Electrical excitation passing as an action potential along the muscle cell membrane (sarcolemma) and down the T tubules releases calcium from the sarcoplasmic reticulum into the sarcoplasm, subsequently causing activation and contraction of the filament array. The calcium ions bind to troponin, causing a change in its shape that physically moves tropomyosin away from the myosin binding sites on the underlying actin chain.

Excitation is initiated by the arrival of a nerve impulse at the muscle membrane via the motor end plate. Activated, or "cocked," myosin heads now bind to the actin, and the myosin head changes from

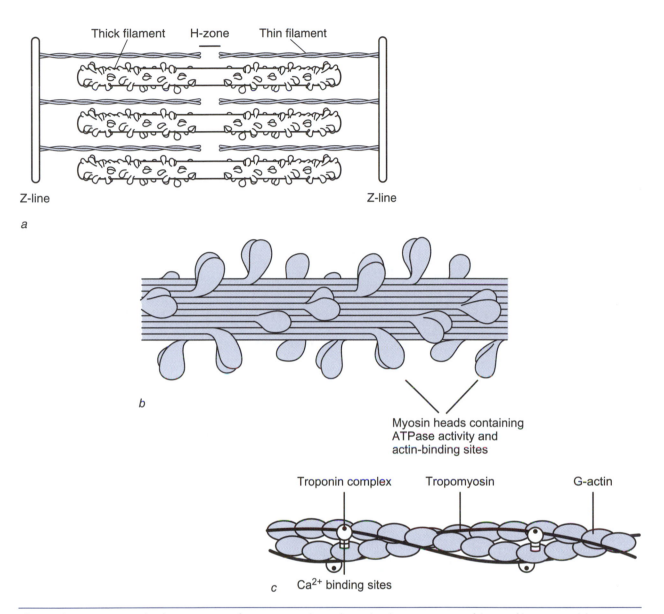

Thick filament   H-zone   Thin filament

Z-line   Z-line

a

b

Myosin heads containing
ATPase activity and
actin-binding sites

Troponin complex   Tropomyosin   G-actin

c   Ca²⁺ binding sites

Figure 2.1   *(a)* Longitudinal cross section of a sarcomere shows the molecular components of the myofilaments and the arrangement of the thick and thin filaments between 2 Z-lines in a myofibril. *(b)* The thick filaments are composed of myosin molecules. Each myosin molecule consists of a rodlike tail and a globular head. The latter contains ATPase activity sites and actin-binding sites. *(c)* The thin filaments are composed of actin molecules and the regulatory proteins tropomyosin and tropinin.

its activated configuration to its bent shape, which causes the head to pull on the thin filament, sliding it toward the center of the sarcomere. This action represents the power stroke of the cross-bridge cycle, and simultaneously ADP and inorganic phosphate (Pi) are released from the myosin head. As a new ATP molecule binds to the myosin head at the ATPase activity site, the myosin cross-bridge detaches from the actin. Hydrolysis of the ATP to ADP and Pi by the ATPase provides the energy required to return the myosin to its activated state, giving it the potential energy needed for the next cross-bridge cycle. ATP is

the only source of energy that can be used directly not only for muscle contraction but also for other energy requiring processes in the cell.

While the myosin is in the activated state, the ADP and Pi remain attached to the myosin head. The myosin head can attach to another actin unit farther along the thin filament, and the cross-bridge cycle is repeated. Sliding of the filaments continues as long as calcium is present in the sarcoplasm at a concentration in excess of 10 μmol/L. Removal and sequestration of the calcium by the ATP-dependent calcium pump (ATPase) of the sarcoplasmic reticulum restores the tropomyosin inhibition of cross-bridge formation and the muscle fiber relaxes.

Differences Between Fiber Types

The existence of different fiber types in skeletal muscle has long been recognized. On the basis of their contraction speed and metabolic characteristics, muscle fibers can be broadly classified as **type I fibers** or **type II fibers.** However, the physiological and biochemical bases for these differences and their functional significance have only recently been established. Much of the impetus for investigating these differences has come from the realization that success in athletic activities that require either the ability to generate a high power output or great endurance is dependent on the proportions of the fiber types in the muscles. The muscle fibers are, however, extremely plastic (i.e., adaptable), and although the distribution of fiber type is genetically determined and not easily altered, an appropriate training program will have a major effect on the metabolic potential of the muscle, regardless of the proportion of fiber types.

Human muscle fibers are commonly divided into types I, IIa, and IIX, which are analogous to animal muscle fibers that have been classified on the basis of direct observation as slow-twitch fibers, fast-twitch fatigue-resistant fibers, and fast-twitch fatigable fibers, respectively. The myosin of the different fiber types exists in different molecular forms (isoforms), and the myofibrillar ATPase activity of the different isoforms displays differential pH sensitivity that provides the basis for the differential chemical staining and identification of fiber types. The biochemical characteristics of the three fiber types are summarized in table 2.1.

Type I Fibers

Type I fibers are small-diameter red cells that contain relatively slow-acting myosin ATPases and hence contract slowly. The red color is caused by myoglobin, which is capable of binding oxygen and only releasing it at very low partial pressures. Type I fibers have numerous energy-producing mitochondria, mostly located close to the periphery of the fiber, near the blood capillaries that provide a rich supply of oxygen and nutrients. Type I fibers possess a high capacity for oxidative metabolism, are extremely fatigue resistant, and are specialized for repeated contractions over prolonged periods.

Type II Fibers

Type IIX fibers contain little myoglobin. They possess rapidly acting myosin ATPases, therefore their contraction (and relaxation) time is relatively fast. These fibers have fewer mitochondria and a poorer capillary supply, but they have greater glycogen and phosphocreatine stores compared with the type I fibers. High glycogenolytic and glycolytic enzyme activity gives

Table 2.1 Biochemical Characteristics of Human Muscle Fiber Types

Characteristic	Type I	Type IIa	Type IIX
Nomenclature	Slow, red Fatigue resistant Oxidative	Fast, red Fatigue resistant Oxidative/glycolytic	Fast, white Fatigable Glycolytic
Capillary density	1.0	0.8	0.6
Mitochondrial density	1.0	0.7	0.4
Myoglobin content	1.0	0.6	0.3
Phosphorylase activity	1.0	2.1	3.1
PFK activity	1.0	1.8	2.3
Citrate synthase activity	1.0	0.8	0.6
SDH activity	1.0	0.7	0.4
Glycogen content	1.0	1.3	1.5
Triacylglycerol content	1.0	0.4	0.2
Phosphocreatine content	1.0	1.2	1.2
Myosin ATPase activity	1.0	>2	>2

Values of metabolic characteristics of type II fibers are shown relative to those found in type I fibers. PFK = phosphofructokinase; SDH = succinate dehydrogenase.

type IIX fibers a high capacity for rapid (but relatively short-lived) ATP production in the absence of oxygen (**anaerobic** capacity). Lactic acid accumulates quickly in these fibers and they fatigue rapidly. Thus, these fibers are best suited for delivering rapid, powerful contractions for brief periods. The metabolic characteristics of type IIa fibers lie between the extreme properties of type I and type IIX fibers. Type IIa fibers contain fast-acting myosin ATPases like the type IIX fibers but have an oxidative capacity more like that of type I fibers.

The differences in activation threshold of the motor neurons supplying the different fiber types determine the order in which fibers are recruited during exercise, and in turn influence the metabolic response to exercise. During most forms of movement, an orderly hierarchy of motor unit recruitment occurs that roughly corresponds with a progression from type I to type IIa to type IIX. Light exercise utilizes mostly type I fibers, moderate exercise utilizes both type I and type IIa fibers, and more severe exercise utilizes all fiber types.

Muscle Fiber Composition

Muscles contain a mixture of the three different fiber types, although the proportions in which the types are found differ substantially among muscles and can also differ among individuals. For example, muscles involved in maintaining posture (e.g., soleus in the leg) have a high proportion (usually >70%) of type I fibers, which is in keeping with their function of maintaining prolonged but relatively weak contractions. Type II fibers, however, predominate in muscles that produce rapid movements, such as the muscles of the hand and the eye. Muscles such as the quadriceps group in the leg contain a variable mixture of fiber types. The vastus lateralis muscle in the quadriceps muscle group of successful marathon runners has a high percentage (about 80%) of type I fibers, whereas the same muscle in elite sprinters contains a higher percentage (about 60%) of the type II fibers. The fiber type composition of muscles is genetically determined and is not pliable to any significant degree by training. Hence, athletic capabilities are mostly in-born (assuming the genetic potential of the individual is realized through appropriate nutrition and training).

Sources of Energy for Muscle Force Generation

Energy is the potential for performing work or producing force. In muscle, energy from the hydrolysis of ATP by myosin ATPase activates specific sites on the contractile elements, as described previously, causing the muscle fiber to shorten. The hydrolysis of ATP yields approximately 31 kJ (7 kcal) of free energy per mole of ATP (a mole is equivalent to molecular weight in grams) degraded to ADP and Pi:

$$ATP + H_2O \rightarrow ADP + H^+ + Pi - 31 \text{ kJ per mole of ATP}$$

Active reuptake of calcium ions by the sarcoplasmic reticulum also requires ATP, as does the restoration of the muscle cell's membrane potential via the action of the Na^+/K^+-ATPase (commonly known as the sodium pump).

Three mechanisms are involved in the resynthesis of ATP for muscle force generation: (1) PCr hydrolysis, (2) **glycolysis,** which involves metabolism of glucose-6-phosphate, derived from muscle glycogen or blood-borne glucose, and produces ATP by substrate-level phosphorylation reactions, and (3) the products of carbohydrate, fat, protein, and alcohol metabolism enter the **tricarboxylic acid (TCA) cycle** in the mitochondria and are oxidized to carbon dioxide and water; this process is known as **oxidative phosphorylation** and yields energy for the synthesis of ATP.

These mechanisms regenerate ATP at sufficient rates to prevent a significant fall in the intramuscular ATP concentration. The resting concentration of ATP in skeletal muscle is about 4 mmol/kg to 5 mmol/kg wet weight (w.w.) of muscle, which can only provide enough energy to sustain a few seconds of intense exercise. PCr breakdown and glycolysis are anaerobic mechanisms that occur in the sarcoplasm. Each uses only one specific substrate for energy production PCr and glucose-6-phosphate, respectively. The **aerobic** processes in the mitochondria utilize a variety of different substrates, and the sarcoplasm contains a variety of enzymes that can convert carbohydrates, fats, and proteins into usable substrate, primarily a 2-carbon acetyl group linked to coenzyme A (acetyl-CoA), which can be completely oxidized in the mitochondria with the resultant production of ATP. A general summary of the main energy sources and pathways of energy metabolism is presented in figure 2.2.

Phosphocreatine in Anaerobic Metabolism

Some of the energy for ATP resynthesis is supplied rapidly and without the need for oxygen. Within the muscle fiber, the concentration of PCr is 3 to 4 times greater than that of ATP. When PCr is broken down to creatine and Pi by the action of the enzyme creatine kinase (CK), a large amount of free energy is

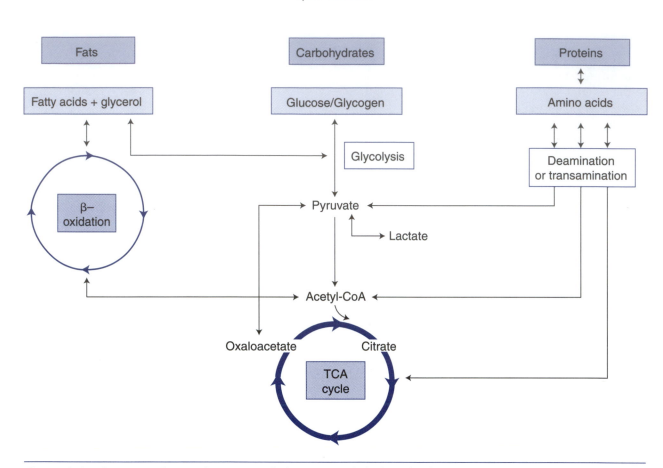

Figure 2.2 The main pathways of energy metabolism using carbohydrate, lipid, and protein as energy sources.

released (43 kJ [10.3 kcal] per mole of PCr). Because PCr has a higher free energy of hydrolysis than ATP, its phosphate is donated directly to the ADP molecule to re-form ATP. When the ATP content begins to fall during exercise, PCr is broken down, releasing energy for restoration of ATP. During very intense exercise, PCr can be almost completely depleted. However, the reactions of ATP and PCr hydrolysis are reversible, and when energy is readily available from other sources (oxidative phosphorylation), creatine and phosphate can be rejoined to form PCr:

$$ADP + PCr + H^+ \rightarrow ATP + Cr - 43 \text{ kJ per mole of PCr}$$

Note that the resynthesis of ATP via breakdown of PCr buffers some of the hydrogen ions formed as a result of ATP hydrolysis. This helps to prevent a rapid acidification of the muscle sarcoplasm, which could induce premature failure of the contractile mechanism.

The PCr in muscle is immediately available at the onset of exercise and can be used to resynthesize ATP quickly. This rapid energy transfer corresponds to the ability to produce a high-power output (see table 2.2). The major disadvantage of this process compared with other means of regenerating ATP is its limited capacity. The total amount of energy available is small (see table 2.3).

An additional pathway to regenerate ATP when ATP and PCr stores are depleted is through a kinase reaction that utilizes 2 molecules of ADP to generate 1 molecule of ATP (and 1 molecule of adenosine monophosphate [AMP]). This reaction is catalyzed by the enzyme myokinase:

$$ADP + ADP \rightarrow ATP + AMP - 31 \text{ kJ per mole of ADP}$$

This reaction only becomes important during high-intensity exercise. Even then, the amount of energy available in the form of ATP is extremely limited, and the real importance of the reaction may be the formation of AMP, which is a potent activator of a number of enzymes involved in energy metabolism.

The total adenylate pool can decline rapidly if the AMP concentration of the cell rises during muscle force generation. This decline occurs principally via deamination of AMP to inosine monophosphate (IMP), but it also occurs by the dephosphorylation of AMP to adenosine. The loss of AMP may initially appear counterproductive because of the

Table 2.2 Anaerobic Production of ATP

	Capacity (mmol ATP/kg w.w.)	Power (mmol ATP/kg w.w./s)
Phosphagen system	14–24	2.3
Glycolytic system	48–75	1.1
Combined	62–93	2.8

Values are expressed per kg wet weight (w.w.) of muscle and are based on estimates of ATP provision during high-intensity exercise of human vastus lateralis muscle.

Table 2.3 ATP Resynthesis From Anaerobic and Aerobic Metabolism

	Max rate of ATP resynthesis (mmol ATP/kg w.w./s)	Delay time*
Fat oxidation	0.25	>2 hours
Glucose (from blood) oxidation	0.35	~ 90 minutes
Glycogen oxidation	0.70	1–3 minutes
Glycolysis	1.10	5–10 seconds
PCr breakdown	2.25	Instantaneous

*Approximate delay time before maximal rates are attained after onset of exercise.

reduction in the total adenylate pool. However, the deamination of AMP to IMP only occurs under low ATP/ADP ratio conditions, and, by preventing excessive accumulation of ADP and AMP, it enables the adenylate kinase reactions to continue, resulting in an increase in the ATP/ADP ratio and continuing muscle force generation. Furthermore, the free energy of ATP hydrolysis possibly decreases when ADP and Pi accumulate, which could further impair muscle force generation. For these reasons, adenine nucleotide loss is important to muscle function during conditions of metabolic crisis, such as during maximal exercise or in the later stages of prolonged submaximal exercise when glycogen stores become depleted.

Glycolysis in Anaerobic Metabolism

Under normal conditions, muscle does not fatigue after only a few seconds of effort, so a source of energy other than ATP and PCr must be available. The source is glycolysis, which involves the breakdown of glucose (or glycogen) in a series of chemical reactions that yield pyruvate. This process does not require oxygen but does result in ATP being available to the muscle from reactions involving substrate-level phosphorylation. However, the pyruvate must be removed for the reactions to proceed. In low-intensity exercise, when adequate oxygen is available to the muscle, pyruvate is converted to carbon dioxide and water by oxidative metabolism in the mitochondria. In some situations when oxygen availability is limited (e.g., isometric exercise) or the rate of formation of pyruvate is very high (e.g., sprinting), the pyruvate can also be removed by conversion to lactate, a reaction that does not involve oxygen.

Muscle Uptake of Glucose From the Blood

A specific transporter protein, GLUT 4, carries glucose molecules across the cell membrane. Once the glucose molecule is inside the muscle cell, an irreversible phosphorylation (addition of a phosphate group), catalyzed by the enzyme hexokinase, occurs to prevent the loss of glucose from the cell. The glucose is converted to glucose-6-phosphate (G6P). The hexokinase reaction is an energy-consuming reaction, requiring the investment of one molecule of ATP for each molecule of glucose. This reaction also ensures a concentration gradient for glucose across the cell membrane, down which transport can occur. Hexokinase is inhibited by an accumulation of G6P, and during high-intensity exercise, the increasing concentration of G6P limits the contribution that the blood glucose can make to carbohydrate metabolism in the active muscles.

Muscle Glycogen Breakdown

If glycogen, rather than blood glucose, is the substrate for glycolysis, a single glucose molecule is split off by the enzyme glycogen phosphorylase, and the products are glucose-1-phosphate and a glycogen molecule that is one glucose residue shorter than the original. The substrates are glycogen and inorganic phosphate, so, unlike the hexokinase reaction, no breakdown of ATP occurs. Phosphorylase acts on the α-1,4 carbon bonds at the free ends of the glycogen molecule but cannot break the α-1,6 bonds forming the branch points. These bonds are hydrolyzed by the combined actions of a debranching enzyme and amylo-1,6-glucosidase, releasing free glucose, which is quickly phosphorylated to G6P by hexokinase. Free glucose accumulates within the muscle cell only in very-high-intensity exercise, where **glycogenolysis** is proceeding rapidly. Because relatively few α-1,6 bonds exist, no more than about 10% of the glucose residues appear as free glucose.

Glycolytic Pathway From Glucose-6-Phosphate to Pyruvate

The enzyme phosphoglucomutase rapidly converts the glucose-1-phosphate formed by the action of phosphorylase on glycogen to G6P, which then proceeds down the glycolytic pathway (see figure 2.3). After a further phosphorylation, the glucose molecule is cleaved to form 2 molecules of the 3-carbon sugar glyceraldehyde-3-phosphate. The second stage of glycolysis is the conversion of glyceraldehyde-3-phosphate into pyruvate, accompanied by the formation of ATP and reduction of nicotinamide adenine dinucleotide (NAD^+) to NADH.

The net effect of glycolysis is the conversion of 1 molecule of glucose to 3 molecules of pyruvate, with the formation of 2 molecules of ATP and the conversion of 2 molecules of NAD^+ to NADH. If glycogen rather than glucose is the starting substrate, 3 molecules of ATP are produced because no initial investment of ATP is made when the first phosphorylation step occurs. Although this net energy yield appears small, the relatively large carbohydrate store available and the rapid rate at which glycolysis proceeds makes energy supplied in this way crucial for the performance of intense exercise. The 800-meter runner, for example, obtains about 60% of the total energy requirement from anaerobic metabolism and may convert about 100 g of carbohydrate (mostly glycogen and equivalent to about 550 mmoles of glucose) to lactate in less than 2 minutes. The amount of ATP released in this way (3 ATP molecules per glucose molecule degraded, about 1,667 mmol of ATP in total)

far exceeds the ATP available from PCr hydrolysis. This high rate of anaerobic metabolism not only allows a faster "steady state" speed than is possible with aerobic metabolism alone but also allows a faster pace in the early stages, before the cardiovascular system has adjusted to the demands and the delivery and utilization of oxygen have increased in response to the exercise stimulus.

The reactions of glycolysis occur in the cytoplasm of the muscle cell, and some pyruvate will escape from active muscle tissues when the rate of glycolysis is high, but most is further metabolized. The fate of the pyruvate produced depends not only on factors such as exercise intensity but also on the metabolic capacity of the tissue. When glycolysis proceeds rapidly, the availability of NAD+, which is necessary as a cofactor in the glyceraldehyde 3-phosphate dehydrogenase reaction, becomes limiting.

Reduction of pyruvate to lactate will regenerate NAD^+ in muscle, and this reaction can proceed in the absence of oxygen. Lactate can accumulate within the muscle fibers, reaching much higher concentrations than those reached by any of the glycolytic intermediates. However, when lactate accumulates in high concentrations, the associated hydrogen ions cause intracellular pH to fall, inhibiting some enzymes such as phosphorylase and phosphofructokinase, and the contractile mechanism begins to fail. A low pH also stimulates free nerve endings in the muscle, causing the perception of pain. Although the negative effects of the acidosis resulting from lactate accumulation are often stressed, the energy made available by anaerobic glycolysis allows the performance of high-intensity exercise that would otherwise not be possible.

Carbohydrate Oxidation in Aerobic Metabolism

Pyruvate may also undergo oxidative metabolism to carbon dioxide (CO_2) and water. This process occurs within the **mitochondrion,** and pyruvate that is produced in the sarcoplasm is transported across the mitochondrial membrane by a specific carrier protein (monocarboxylic acid transporter). The 3-carbon pyruvate is converted by oxidative decarboxylation into a 2-carbon acetate group, which is linked by a thio-ester bond to coenzyme A (CoA) to form acetyl-CoA. This reaction, in which NAD^+ is converted to NADH, is catalyzed by the pyruvate dehydrogenase enzyme complex. Acetyl-CoA is also formed from the metabolism of fatty acids (FAs) within the mitochondria, in a metabolic process called **β-oxidation.** These processes are summarized in figure 2.4.

Figure 2.3 The glycolytic pathway. Glycolysis makes 2 molecules of ATP available for each molecule of glucose that passes through the pathway, or 3 molecules of ATP if muscle glycogen is the starting substrate.

Tricarboxylic Acid Cycle

Acetyl-CoA is oxidized to CO_2 in the TCA cycle (also known as the Krebs cycle and the citric acid cycle). The reactions involve combination of acetyl-CoA with oxaloacetate to form citrate, a 6-carbon tricarboxylic acid. A series of reactions lead to the sequential loss of hydrogen atoms and CO_2, resulting in the regeneration of oxaloacetate.

$$acetyl\text{-}CoA + ADP + Pi + 3NAD^+ + FAD + 3H_2O \rightarrow$$
$$2CO_2 + CoA + ATP + 3NADH + 3H^+ + FADH_2$$

Because acetyl-CoA is also a product of FA oxidation, the final steps of oxidative degradation are common to both fat and carbohydrate. The hydrogen atoms are carried by the reduced coenzymes NADH and flavin adenine dinucleotide ($FADH_2$). These coenzymes act as carriers and donate pairs of electrons

Figure 2.4 Formation of acetyl-CoA occurs from the catabolism of carbohydrates, fats, and protein. Acetyl-CoA is oxidized in the tricarboxylic acid (TCA) cycle, generating CO_2, reduced coenzymes, and ATP.

to the **electron transport chain,** allowing oxidative phosphorylation with the subsequent regeneration of ATP from ADP.

The reactions involved in the TCA cycle are shown in figure 2.5. The 2-carbon acetate units of acetyl-CoA are combined with the 4-carbon oxaloacetate to form 6-carbon citrate. The latter undergoes 2 successive decarboxylations (removal of CO_2) to yield 4-carbon succinate, which, in subsequent reactions, is converted to oxaloacetate, completing the TCA cycle. Molecular oxygen (O_2) does not participate directly in these reactions. The most important function of the TCA cycle is to generate hydrogen atoms for subsequent passage to the electron transport chain by means of NADH and $FADH_2$ (see figure 2.6).

Electron Transport Chain and Oxidative Phosphorylation

The aerobic process of electron transport and oxidative phosphorylation regenerates ATP from ADP, thus conserving some of the chemical energy contained within the original substrates in the form of high-energy phosphates. As long as the O_2 supply is adequate and substrate is available, NAD^+ and FAD are continuously regenerated and TCA metabolism proceeds. This process cannot occur without oxygen. For each molecule of NADH that enters the electron transport chain, 3 molecules of ATP are generated, and for each molecule of $FADH_2$, 2 molecules of ATP are formed. Thus, for each molecule of acetyl-CoA undergoing complete oxidation in the TCA cycle, a total of 12 ATP molecules are formed.

The transfer of electrons through the transport chain located on the inner mitochondrial membrane causes hydrogen ions, or protons (H^+), from the inner mitochondrial matrix to be pumped into the space between the inner and outer mitochondrial membranes. The high concentration of positively charged hydrogen ions in this outer chamber causes H^+ to flow back into the mitochondrial matrix through an ATP synthase protein complex embedded in the inner mitochondrial membrane. The flow of H^+ through this complex constitutes a proton-motive force that drives ATP synthesis. The overall reaction starting with glucose as the fuel can be summarized as follows:

$$Glucose + 6O_2 + 38ADP + 38Pi \rightarrow 6CO_2 + 6H_2O + 38ATP$$

The total ATP synthesis of 38 moles per mole of glucose oxidized is primarily from oxidation of reduced coenzymes in the terminal respiratory system as follows:

ATP synthesized	Source
2	Glycolysis
6	NADH by glycolysis
24	NADH
4	$FADH_2$
2	GTP

The reactions of oxidative phosphorylation occur within the mitochondria, whereas glycolysis takes place in the cytoplasm, and the inner mitochondrial membrane is impermeable to NADH and to NAD^+.

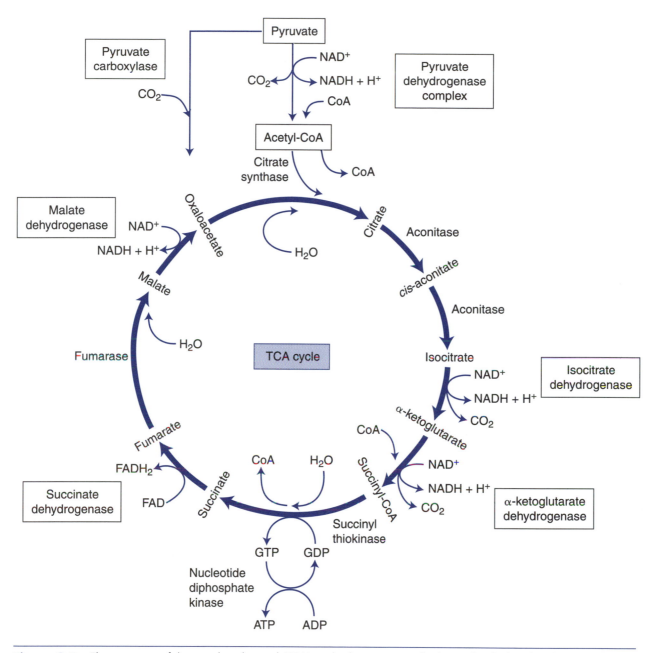

Figure 2.5 The reactions of the tricarboxylic acid (TCA) cycle showing sites of substrate-level phosphorylation and NAD$^+$ and FAD reduction.

Without regeneration of the NAD$^+$ in the cytoplasm, glycolysis will stop. Therefore a mechanism must exist for the effective oxidation of the NADH formed during glycolysis. This mechanism is provided by a number of substrate shuttles that transfer reducing equivalents into the mitochondrion.

Fat Oxidation in Aerobic Metabolism

Fat and carbohydrate are the major nutrients that provide energy for muscular contraction. Because acetyl-CoA is also a product of fat oxidation, the

sequence of reactions involving the TCA cycle and oxidative phosphorylation are common to both fat and carbohydrate.

Lipolysis

To generate the 2-carbon acetyl groups from fat, several metabolic steps must occur. The first step involves the breakdown of the storage form of fat, triacylglycerol, into its FA and glycerol components. This process is called **lipolysis,** and it begins with the hydrolytic removal of an FA molecule from the

Figure 2.6 The TCA cycle generates the reduced coenzymes NADH and $FADH_2$. Oxidation of these coenzymes in the electron transport chain releases energy that is used for the resynthesis of ATP. This process is called oxidative phosphorylation.

glycerol backbone at either position 1 or position 3. This step is catalyzed by a hormone-sensitive lipase (see figure 2.7). Insulin promotes triacylglycerol synthesis and inhibits lipolysis, whereas catecholamines (epinephrine and norepinephrine), glucagon, growth hormone, and cortisol stimulate lipolysis by activating the hormone-sensitive lipase. A specific lipase for the remaining diacylglycerol removes another FA and another specific lipase removes the last FA from the monoacylglycerol. Thus, from each molecule of triacylglycerol, 1 molecule of glycerol and 3 molecules of FA are produced. Glycerol may diffuse and FAs are transported out of the adipose cells and into the circulation. Both the rate of lipolysis and the rate of adipose tissue blood flow will influence the rate of entry of FA and glycerol into the circulation. During prolonged exercise at about 50% $\dot{V}O_2$max, adipose tissue blood flow increases. However, during intense exercise, sympathetic vasoconstriction causes a fall in adipose tissue blood flow, resulting in accumulation of FA within adipose tissue and effectively limiting the entry of FA (and glycerol) into the circulation. Another factor that limits fat mobilization during high-intensity exercise is the accumulation of lactate in the blood. Lactate promotes the re-esterification of FA back into triacylglycerol (see figure 2.7) and therefore limits the entry of FA into the bloodstream.

Glycerol in plasma can be taken up by the liver and phosphorylated to glycerol-3-phosphate, which can be used to form triacylglycerol as described earlier, or, alternatively, can be oxidized to dihydroxyacetone phosphate, which can enter the glycolytic pathway or be converted to glucose. FAs are very poorly soluble in water, and most of the FAs in plasma are transported loosely bound to albumin, the most abundant protein in plasma. The usual resting plasma concentration of FA is 0.2 to 0.4 mM. However, during (or shortly after) prolonged exercise, the plasma FA concentration may increase to about 2.0 mM.

FA Uptake into Muscle

Uptake of FA by muscle is directly related to the plasma FA concentration, and, hence, the mobilization of fat stores is an important step in ensuring an adequate nutrient supply for prolonged muscular

Figure 2.7 Lipolysis in adipose tissue mobilizes free fatty acids (FAs), which enter the circulation and thus become available for muscle to use as a fuel for exercise.

work. The normal plasma albumin concentration is about 45 g/L (approximately 0.7 mM). Each albumin molecule contains 3 high-affinity binding sites for FA (and 7 other low-affinity binding sites). When the 3 high-affinity binding sites are full (at an FA concentration of 2.0 mM or more) the concentration of FA not bound to albumin (i.e., FFAs) increases markedly, forming fatty-acid micelles, which are potentially damaging to tissues because of their detergent-like properties.

FA transport across the sarcolemmal membrane into the muscle fiber occurs via a carrier-mediated transport mechanism that becomes saturated at high-plasma unbound FA concentration (approximately equivalent to 1.5 mM total FA concentration). FA uptake into muscle will only occur if the intracellular FA concentration is less than that in true aqueous solution in the extracellular fluid (viz. < 10 μM). The low intracellular FA concentration is probably maintained by the presence of a FA-binding protein inside the cell, perhaps similar to the ones found in the cells of the small intestine and liver. Also, the rate of uptake of FA into muscle fibers will be proportional to the difference in their concentrations inside and outside the cell, until the plasma membrane transport mechanism becomes saturated. After the FAs enter the muscle cell, they are converted into a CoA derivative by the action of ATP-linked fatty acyl-CoA synthetase (also known as thiokinase), in preparation for β-**oxidation,** the major pathway for FA breakdown. Hence, the priming (activation) of each FA molecule requires the utilization of one molecule of ATP:

$$RCOOH + ATP + CoA\text{-}SH \rightarrow R\text{-}C(=O)\text{-}S\text{-}CoA + AMP + PPi$$

β-*Oxidation of Fatty Acids*

The process of β-oxidation occurs in the mitochondria and is the sequential removal of 2-carbon units from the FA chain in the form of acetyl-CoA, which can then enter the TCA cycle. Fatty acyl-CoA molecules in the muscle sarcoplasm are transported into the mitochondria via formation of an ester of the FA with carnitine, as illustrated in figure 2.8. The latter is synthesized in the liver and is normally abundant in tissues able to oxidize FAs. Concentrations of about 1.0 mM are found in muscle. The enzyme regulating the transport of FA via carnitine is carnitine acyl-transferase (CAT), two forms of which exist in muscle. One form (CAT-1) is located on the outer surface of the membrane (to generate acyl-carnitine), and the other form (CAT-2) is located on the inner surface of the inner mitochondrial membrane and regenerates the acyl-CoA and free carnitine (see figure 2.9). This transport process may be the main rate-limiting step in the utilization of FAs for energy production in muscle.

At high exercise intensities (above about 60% $\dot{V}O_2$max) the rate of fat oxidation cannot provide sufficient ATP for muscle contraction, and, increasingly, ATP is derived from carbohydrate oxidation and anaerobic glycolysis. Energy cannot be derived from fat via anaerobic pathways. Once released into the mitochondrial matrix, the fatty acyl-CoA is able to enter the β-oxidation pathway. Carnitine acyl-transferase is inhibited by malonyl-CoA, a precursor for FA synthesis. Hence, when the ATP supply is sufficient, surplus acetyl-CoA will be diverted away from the TCA cycle to malonyl-CoA, reducing catabolism of FAs and promoting their formation and subsequent triacylglycerol synthesis.

Figure 2.8 In the carnitine–fatty acyl-CoA transferase reaction, carnitine is linked to a FA.

Once inside the mitochondria, fatty acyl-CoA is oxidized via a series of reactions catalyzed by a multienzyme complex that releases a molecule of acetyl-CoA and a fatty acyl-CoA, which is now a 2-carbon unit shorter. This fatty acyl-CoA can now repeat the cycle, and the acetyl CoA formed can enter the TCA cycle. At each passage through the cycle, the FA chain loses a 2-carbon fragment as acetyl-CoA and 2 pairs of hydrogen atoms to specific acceptors. The 16-carbon palmitic acid thus undergoes a total of 7 such cycles, to yield in total 8 molecules of acetyl-CoA and 14 pairs of hydrogen atoms. The palmitic acid only needs to be primed or activated with CoA once because at the end of each cycle, the shortened FA appears as its CoA ester. The most common FAs oxidized contain 16 (e.g., palmitic acid) or 18 (e.g., oleic acid) carbons in the acyl chain. The 14 pairs of hydrogen atoms removed during β-oxidation of palmitic acid enter the mitochondrial respiratory chain, 7 pairs in the form of the reduced flavin coenzyme of fatty acyl-CoA dehydrogenase and 7 pairs in the form of NADH. The passage of electrons from $FADH_2$ to oxygen and from NADH to oxygen leads to the expected number of oxidative

phosphorylations of ADP (viz. 2 ATP molecules from each $FADH_2$ and 3 ATP molecules from each NADH). Hence, a total of 5 molecules of ATP are formed per molecule of acetyl-CoA cleaved:

$$\text{Palmitoyl-CoA} + 7\ \text{CoA} + 7\ O_2 + 35\ \text{ADP} + 35\ \text{Pi}$$
$$\rightarrow 8\ \text{acetyl-CoA} + 35\ \text{ATP} + 42\ H_2O$$

The 8 molecules of acetyl-CoA can enter the TCA cycle, and the following equation represents the result of their oxidation and the coupled phosphorylations:

$$8\ \text{acetyl-CoA} + 16\ O_2 + 96\ \text{ADP} + 96\ \text{Pi}$$
$$\rightarrow 8\ \text{CoA} + 96\ \text{ATP} + 104\ H_2O + 16\ CO_2$$

Combining the two previous equations gives the overall equation:

$$\text{Palmitoyl-CoA} + 23\ O_2 + 131\ \text{ADP} + 131\ \text{Pi}$$
$$\rightarrow \text{CoA} + 16\ CO_2 + 146\ H_2O + 131\ \text{ATP}$$

Because 1 molecule of ATP was required to initially activate the FA, the net yield for the complete oxidation of 1 molecule of palmitic acid is 130 molecules of ATP.

Figure 2.9 Carnitine aids the transport of long-chain FAs across the mitochondrial membrane. Inside the mitochondrion, carnitine is removed, and fatty acyl-CoA is re-formed, freeing carnitine to diffuse back across the mitochondrial membrane into the cytoplasm.

Fuel Stores in Skeletal Muscle

Carbohydrates are stored in the body as the glucose polymer glycogen. Skeletal muscle contains a significant store of glycogen in the sarcoplasm. The glycogen content of skeletal muscle at rest is approximately 13 g/kg w.w. to 18 g/kg w.w. (75 mmol glucosyl units/kg w.w. to 100 mmol glucosyl units/kg w.w.). For cycling and running, a total of about 300 g of glycogen is available in the leg muscles (see figure 2.10). About 100 g of glycogen are stored in the liver of an adult human in the postabsorptive state, which can be released into the circulation to maintain the blood glucose concentration at about 5 mmol/L (0.9 g/L). Fats are stored as triacylglycerol, mainly in white adipose tissue. Triacylglycerol molecules must be broken down by a lipase enzyme to release FA into the circulation for uptake by

working muscle. Skeletal muscle also contains some triacylglycerol that can be used as an energy source during exercise after lipolysis. Some of this intramuscular triacylglycerol may be contained in adipose cells dispersed among the muscle fibers in the tissue, but evidence from light and electron microscopy suggests the existence of triacylglycerol droplets located close to the mitochondria within the fibers themselves.

Early studies (Havel et al. 1967, Issekutz et al. 1964) of FA turnover during exercise using ^{14}C-labeled FAs showed that during prolonged exercise, plasma-derived FA could only account for about 50% of the total amount of fat oxidized, suggesting that intramuscular triacylglycerol could be providing a significant amount of the FA during prolonged exercise. Measurements of changes in intramuscular triacylglycerol content before and after exercise strongly support this view. Several studies have reported reductions of about 25% to 35% in triacylglycerol content after 1 hour to 2 hours of exercise at 55% to 70% $\dot{V}O_2$max. These changes have been observed in several studies despite the unreliable nature of triacylglycerol measurement in small biopsy samples of skeletal muscle (Turcotte et al. 1995).

Human skeletal muscle contains approximately 12 g/kg w.w. of triacylglycerol, and type I fibers contain more triacylglycerol than type II fibers. Between 12 MJ and 20 MJ of chemical potential energy is estimated to be available for oxidation after intramuscular lipolysis. The lipolysis is probably mediated by an intracellular lipase similar to the hormone-sensitive lipase of adipose tissue; evidence suggests that catecholamines regulate the mobilization of intramuscular triacylglycerol stores.

Fat stores in the body are far larger than carbohydrate stores, and fat is a more efficient form of energy storage, releasing 37 kJ/g (9 kcal/g) compared with 16 kJ/g (4 kcal/g) from carbohydrate. Each gram of

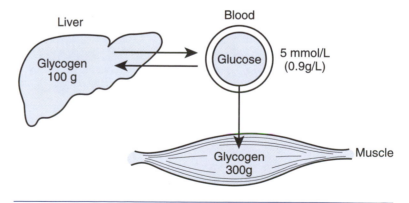

Figure 2.10 Carbohydrate availability for two-legged exercise (e.g., cycling and running) in liver, blood, and muscle.

carbohydrate stored also retains about 3 g of water, further decreasing the efficiency of carbohydrate as an energy source. However, the energy yield per liter of O_2 consumed during fat oxidation is about 8% to 10% less than for carbohydrate (about 19.5 kJ/L O_2 for fat compared with 20.9 kJ/L O_2 for carbohydrate). The energy cost of running a marathon is about 12,000 kJ (2,900 kcal); if this energy could be derived from the oxidation of fat alone, the total amount of fat required would be about 320 g, compared with 750 g of carbohydrate and an additional 2.3 kg of associated water. Aside from the weight that would have to be carried, this amount of carbohydrate exceeds the total amount normally stored in the liver, muscles, and blood combined. The total storage capacity for fat is extremely large, and for most practical purposes, the amount of energy stored in the form of fat far exceeds that required for any exercise task (see table 2.4).

The main problem associated with the utilization of fat as a fuel for exercise is the rate at which it can be taken up by muscle and oxidized to provide energy. Fat oxidation can only supply ATP at a rate sufficient to maintain exercise at an intensity of about 60% $\dot{V}O_2$max. To generate ATP to sustain higher exercise intensities, carbohydrate must be utilized. Both the oxidative pathway of carbohydrate utilization and the anaerobic pathway of glycolysis can supply ATP at a much faster rate than fat oxidation. During most forms of submaximal exercise, a mixture of fat and carbohydrate is oxidized to provide energy for muscular contraction. Obviously, the more fat that can be utilized will allow a greater sparing of the limited carbohydrate reserves, and exercise can be prolonged.

Protein is stored only as functionally important molecules (e.g., structural proteins, enzymes, ion channels, receptors, and contractile proteins), and the concentration of free amino acids in most extracellular and intracellular body fluids is quite low (e.g., total free amino acid concentration in muscle sarcoplasm is about 20 mmol/L). In most situations, carbohydrate

and fats supply most of the energy required to regenerate ATP to fuel muscular work. Protein catabolism contributes less than 5% of the energy provision for muscle contraction during physical activity. Protein catabolism can provide amino acids, some of which may eventually be oxidized (after removal of the amino group) in the TCA cycle. During starvation and when glycogen stores become depleted, protein catabolism may become an increasingly important source of energy for muscular work.

Regulation of Energy Metabolism

Experiments in which muscle biopsies were taken before and immediately after exercise indicate that the intramuscular ATP concentration remains fairly constant (Spriet 1995a). Thus, ATP is being continuously regenerated by other energy-liberating reactions at the same rate it is being used. This situation provides a sensitive mechanism for the control of energy metabolism within the cell. This control is exerted through changes in a number of intracellular factors, and further control is effected through the actions of the sympathetic nervous system and hormones that can also bring about changes in the activities of some enzymes involved in fuel mobilization and utilization (see figure 2.11).

Intramuscular factors		Hormones
ATP/ADP	Pi	Epinephrine (adrenaline)
AMP	Ca^{2+}	Insulin
Sympathetic nervous system		Glucagon
		Cortisol
Norepinephrine (noradrenaline)		Growth hormone

Figure 2.11 Factors that regulate the mobilization of fuels by altering the activities of enzymes.

Table 2.4 Energy Stores in the Average Man

	Mass (kg)	Energy (kJ)	Energy (kcal)	Exercise time (min)
Liver glycogen	0.10 (0.22 lb)	1,600	400	20
Muscle glycogen	0.40 (0.88 lb)	6,400	1,600	80
Blood glucose	0.01 (0.022 lb)	160	40	2
Fat	10.5 (23.0 lb)	390,000	93,000	4,900
Protein	8.5 (18.7 lb)	142,000	34,000	1,800

Assuming a body mass of 70 kg (154 lb), a fat content of 15% of body mass, and a protein content of about 12% of body mass. The value for blood glucose includes the glucose content of extracellular fluid. The exercise times are the approximate times these stores would last if they were the only source of energy available during exercise at marathon-running pace (equivalent to an energy expenditure of about 80 kJ/min [19 kcal/min]).

Intracellular Factors

Within the muscle fiber, several intracellular factors control the activity of key rate-limiting or flux-generating enzymes involved in energy metabolism, which allows a rapid (virtually instantaneous) alteration in the rate of ATP resynthesis to occur when such an alteration is needed, such as at the onset of exercise.

The decline in cellular concentration of ATP at the onset of muscle force generation and parallel increases in ADP and AMP concentrations (i.e., a decline in the energy charge) directly stimulate anaerobic and oxidative ATP resynthesis. The relatively low concentration of ATP (and ADP) inside the cell means that any increase in the rate of hydrolysis of ATP (e.g., at the onset of exercise) produces a rapid change in the ratio of ATP to ADP (and also increases the intracellular concentration of AMP). These changes, in turn, activate enzymes that immediately stimulate the breakdown of intramuscular fuel stores to provide energy for ATP resynthesis. In this way, energy metabolism increases rapidly after the start of exercise.

ATP, ADP, and AMP are activators or inhibitors of the enzymatic reactions involved in PCr, carbohydrate, and fat degradation and utilization (see figure 2.12). For example, CK, the enzyme responsible for the rapid rephosphorylation of ATP at the initiation of muscle force generation, is rapidly activated by an increase in cytoplasmic ADP concentration and is inhibited by an increase in cellular ATP concentration. Similarly, glycogen phosphorylase, the enzyme that catalyzes the conversion of glycogen to glucose-1-phosphate, is activated by increases in AMP and Pi (and calcium ion) concentration and is inhibited by an increase in ATP concentration.

The rate-limiting step in the glycolytic pathway is the conversion of fructose-6-phosphate to fructose-1,6-diphosphate, which is catalyzed by phosphofructokinase (PFK). The activity of this complex enzyme is affected by many intracellular factors, and it plays an important role in controlling flux through the pathway. The PFK reaction regulates the metabolism of both glucose and glycogen. The activity of PFK is stimulated by increased concentrations of ADP, AMP, Pi, ammonia, and fructose-6-phosphate and is inhibited by ATP, H^+, citrate, phosphoglycerate, and phosphoenolpyruvate. Thus, the rate of glycolysis is stimulated when ATP and glycogen breakdown are increased at the onset of exercise. Accumulation of citrate and, thus, inhibition of PFK may occur when the rate of the TCA cycle is high and provides a means whereby the limited stores of carbohydrate are spared when the availability of FAs is high. Inhibition of PFK also causes accumulation of G6P, which inhibits the activity of hexokinase and reduces the entry into the muscle of glucose, which is not needed.

Conversion of pyruvate to acetyl-CoA by the pyruvate dehydrogenase complex is the rate-limiting step in carbohydrate oxidation. It is stimulated by an increased intracellular concentration of calcium and decreased ratios of ATP/ADP, acetyl-CoA/free CoA, and $NADH/NAD^+$ and thus offers another site of regulation of the relative rates of fat and carbohydrate catabolism. If the rate of formation of acetyl-CoA from the β-oxidation of FAs is high, as after one hour to two hours of submaximal exercise, then this activity can reduce the amount of acetyl-CoA derived from pyruvate and cause accumulation of phosphoenolpyruvate and inhibition of PFK, thus slowing the rate of glycolysis and glycogenolysis. This process forms the basis of the "glucose-fatty acid cycle" proposed by Randle et al. (1963), which has for many years been accepted to be the key regulatory mechanism in the control of carbohydrate and fat utilization by skeletal muscle. However, recent work has challenged this hypothesis, and it seems likely that the regulation of the integration of fat and carbohydrate catabolism in exercising skeletal muscle must reside elsewhere; for example, at the level of glucose uptake into muscle, of glycogen breakdown by phosphorylase, or of the entry of FAs into the mitochondria (for further details see the books by Hargreaves 1995 and Maughan, Gleeson, and Greenhaff 1997).

A key regulatory point in the TCA cycle is the reaction catalyzed by citrate synthase. The activity of this enzyme is inhibited by ATP, NADH, succinyl-CoA and fatty acyl-CoA; the activity of the enzyme is also affected by citrate availability. Hence, when cellular energy levels are high, flux through the TCA cycle is relatively low but can be greatly increased when ATP and NADH utilization is increased, such as during exercise.

Hormones

Many hormones influence energy metabolism in the body (for a detailed review, see Galbo 1983). During exercise the interaction among insulin, glucagon, and the catecholamines (epinephrine and norepinephrine) is mostly responsible for fuel substrate availability and utilization; cortisol and growth hormone also have some significant effects.

Insulin

Insulin is secreted by the β cells of the islets of Langerhans in the pancreas. Its basic biological effects are to inhibit lipolysis and increase the uptake of glucose from the blood by the tissues, especially

Figure 2.12 Metabolic pathways important to energy provision during exercise. The main sites of regulation and the principal hormone and allosteric activators and inhibitors are shown. 1 and 2 = phosphorylase; 3 = hexokinase; 4 = phosphofructokinase; 5 = pyruvate dehydrogenase; 6 = hormone sensitive lipase; 7 = carnitine acyl transferase; 8 = fatty acyl-CoA dehydrogenase; 9 = citrate synthase; 10 = proteases.

skeletal muscle, liver, and adipose tissue. Cellular uptake of amino acids is also stimulated by insulin. These effects reduce the plasma glucose concentration, inhibit the release of glucose from the liver, promote the synthesis of glycogen (in liver and muscle), promote synthesis of fat and inhibit FA release (in adipose tissue), increase muscle amino acid uptake, and enhance protein synthesis. The primary stimulus for increased insulin secretion is a rise in the blood glucose concentration (e.g., after a meal). Plasma

Figure 2.13 Translocation of GLUT4 glucose transporters into the sarcolemmal membrane under the influence of insulin (important during rest) and calcium ions (important during exercise).

insulin concentration is usually depressed during exercise because the sympathetic nervous system and circulating catecholamines inhibit the release of insulin. However, the fall in the plasma insulin concentration during exercise does not reduce the uptake of glucose from the blood by active muscle, because the rise in intracellular Ca^{2+} concentration during muscle contractions also promotes the translocation of intracellular vesicles containing GLUT4 glucose transporters into the sarcolemma (see figure 2.13).

Glucagon

Glucagon is secreted by the α cells of the pancreatic islets and basically exerts effects that are opposite those of insulin. It raises the blood glucose level by increasing the rate of glycogen breakdown (glycogenolysis) in the liver. It also promotes the formation of glucose from noncarbohydrate precursors (**gluconeogenesis**) in the liver. The primary stimulus for increased secretion of glucagon is a decrease in the glucose concentration in the blood. During most types of exercise, the blood glucose concentration does not fall. However, during prolonged exercise, when liver glycogen stores become depleted, a drop in the blood glucose concentration (hypoglycemia) may occur.

The hormone-sensitive lipase in adipose tissue is activated by a cyclic AMP–dependent protein kinase. Binding of glucagon and epinephrine to plasma membrane receptors on adipocytes initiates the adenylate cyclase and the enzyme cascade that activates the lipase (see figure 2.14). Activation

of the hormone-sensitive lipase in adipose tissue and lipoprotein lipase occurs during exercise because of the actions of epinephrine and glucagon, which are released from the adrenal medulla and pancreatic islets, respectively. FAs thus released from triacylglycerols in the fat storage sites are delivered via the blood to muscle tissue and additional FA can be provided from the breakdown of intramuscular fat depots. These FAs provide a readily usable source of energy that is liberated through the process of β-oxidation and contributes significantly to the energy requirements of exercise.

During brief periods of light to moderate exercise, energy is derived equally from oxidation of carbohydrate and fat. If exercise is continued for an hour or more and carbohydrates become depleted, the quantity of fat used for energy gradually increases. In very prolonged exercise, fat (mainly as FA) may supply almost 80% of total energy. This condition probably arises because of a small fall in blood glucose concentration and a subsequent increase in glucagon (and decrease in insulin) release from the pancreas. Plasma concentrations of epinephrine and cortisol also increase as exercise progresses. These hormonal changes stimulate the mobilization and subsequent utilization of fat stores (see figure 2.7). The uptake of FA by working muscle rises during 1 to 4 hours of continuous moderate exercise. Lipolysis is stimulated by exercise, but this process only occurs gradually. Furthermore, it does not cease immediately after exercise has stopped.

The FA concentration in blood plasma reflects the balance between the FA release into the circulation (mainly from adipose tissue depots) and FA uptake by various tissues. Although the concentration of FAs in blood plasma is quite low (usually in the range of 0.2 mM to 2.0 mM), their plasma half-life is very short, less than 2 minutes in fact, indicating a rapid rate of uptake by tissues. At the onset of exercise, muscle capillaries open up, facilitating FA uptake, and this process is reversed shortly after the end of exercise. Consequently, plasma FA concentrations commonly fall in the early stages of exercise and then gradually increase. At the end of exercise, when muscle uptake abruptly falls but stimulation of lipolysis continues, plasma FA concentration rises sharply, reaching levels of up to 3 mM.

Figure 2.14 Mode of action of epinephrine (adrenaline).

Catecholamines

The catecholamines epinephrine (adrenaline) and norepinephrine (noradrenaline) are released from the adrenal medulla. Norepinephrine is also released from sympathetic nerve endings, and leakage from such synapses appears to be the main source of the norepinephrine in blood plasma. The catecholamines have many systemic effects, including stimulation of the heart rate and contractility and alteration of blood vessel diameters. These substances also influence substrate availability, with the effects of epinephrine being more important than those of norepinephrine. Epinephrine, like glucagon, promotes glycogenolysis in both liver and muscle. Epinephrine also promotes lipolysis in adipose tissue, increasing the availability of plasma FA, and inhibits insulin secretion. The primary stimulus for catecholamine secretion is the activation of the sympathetic nervous system by stressors such as exercise, hypotension, and hypoglycemia. Substantial increases in the plasma catecholamine concentration can occur within seconds of the onset of high-intensity exercise. However, the relative exercise intensity has to be above 50% $\dot{V}O_2$max to significantly elevate the plasma catecholamine concentration.

Growth Hormone and Cortisol

Growth hormone, secreted from the anterior pituitary gland, also stimulates mobilization of FA from adipose tissue, and increases in plasma growth hormone concentration are related to exercise intensity. During prolonged strenuous exercise, cortisol secretion from the adrenal cortex is increased. Cortisol, a steroid hormone, increases the effectiveness of catecholamines in some tissues (e.g., it promotes lipolysis in adipose tissue). However, its main effects are to promote protein degradation and amino acid release from muscle and to stimulate gluconeogenesis in the liver. The primary stimulus to cortisol secretion is stress-induced release of adrenocorticotrophic hormone (ACTH) from the anterior pituitary gland. Cortisol is derived from cholesterol, and its high fat solubility allows it to diffuse across cell membranes. Cortisol receptors in the cell cytoplasm translocate the hormone to the nucleus of the cell. Interaction of the hormone-receptor complex with specific sections of

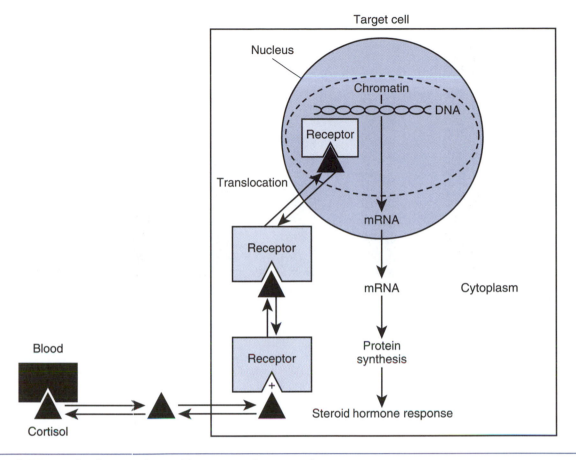

Figure 2.15 Mode of action of steroid hormones such as cortisol.

DNA switches on the transcription of specific genes and thus stimulates the synthesis of new proteins in the cell (see figure 2.15). This activity is common to all the steroid hormones (e.g., testosterone, estrogen, and aldosterone).

Metabolic Responses to Exercise

The most important factor influencing the metabolic response to exercise is exercise intensity. Physical fitness of the subject also modifies the metabolic response to exercise, and other factors—including exercise duration, substrate availability, nutritional status, diet, feeding during exercise, mode of exercise, prior exercise, drugs, environmental temperature, and altitude—are also important.

Causes of Fatigue in High-Intensity Exercise

ATP is the only fuel that can be used directly for skeletal muscle force generation, and the available ATP will fuel about 2 seconds of maximum-intensity exercise. Therefore, for muscle force generation to continue, ATP must be resynthesized very rapidly from ADP. During high-intensity exercise, the relatively low rate of ATP resynthesis from oxidative phosphorylation stimulates rapid anaerobic energy production from PCr and glycogen hydrolysis. PCr breakdown begins at the onset of contraction to buffer the rapid accumulation of ADP from ATP hydrolysis. However, the rate of PCr hydrolysis declines after only a few seconds of maximal force generation (see figure 2.16).

If high-intensity exercise is to continue beyond the first few seconds, a marked increase in the contribution from glycolysis to ATP resynthesis is necessary. Anaerobic glycolysis involves several more steps than PCr hydrolysis, although compared with oxidative phosphorylation, it is still very rapid. Anaerobic glycolysis starts at the onset of contraction, but unlike PCr hydrolysis, it does not reach a maximal rate until after 5 seconds of exercise, and it can be maintained at this level for several seconds during maximal muscle force generation (see figure 2.17). The mechanism(s) responsible for the eventual decline in glycolysis

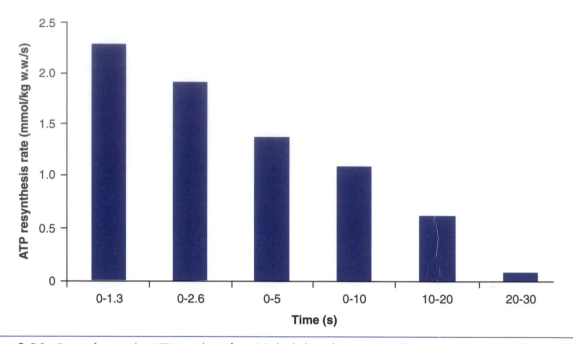

Figure 2.16 Rates of anaerobic ATP resynthesis from PCr hydrolysis during maximal isometric contraction in human skeletal muscle.

during maximal exercise have not been determined. Exercise at an intensity equivalent to 95% to 100% $\dot{V}O_2$max can be sustained for about 5 minutes before fatigue is experienced. Under these conditions, carbohydrate oxidation can make a significant contribution to ATP production, but its relative importance is often underestimated.

Fatigue is the inability to maintain a given or expected force or power output and is an inevitable feature of maximal exercise. Typically, the loss of power output or force production is likely to be in the region of 40% to 60% of the maximum observed during 30 seconds of all-out exercise. Many factors may contribute to fatigue. However, during maximal

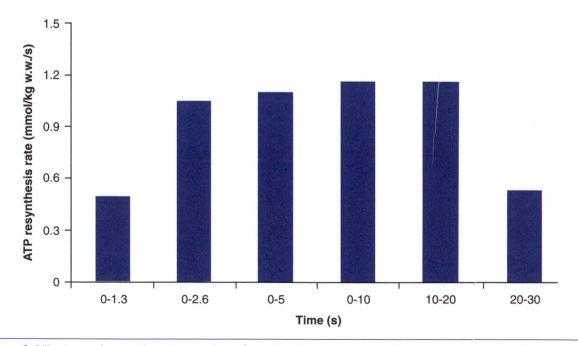

Figure 2.17 Rates of anaerobic ATP resynthesis from glycolysis during maximal isometric contraction in human skeletal muscle.

short-duration exercise, it will be caused primarily by a gradual decline in anaerobic ATP production or an increase in ADP accumulation caused by a depletion of PCr and a fall in the rate of glycolysis.

In high-intensity exercise lasting 1 minute to 5 minutes, lactic acid accumulation may contribute to the fatigue process. At physiological pH values, lactic acid almost completely dissociates into its constituent lactate and hydrogen ions, and studies using animal muscle preparations have demonstrated that direct inhibition of force production can be achieved by increasing hydrogen and lactate ion concentrations (Green 1995). A reduced muscle pH may cause some inhibition of PFK and phosphorylase, reducing the rate of ATP resynthesis from glycolysis. This development is unlikely to be important in exercising muscle, however, because the in vitro inhibition of PFK by a reduced pH is reversed in the presence of other activators such as AMP (Spriet 1991). Lactate and hydrogen ion accumulation also appear to result in muscle fatigue independent of one another, but the latter is the more commonly cited mechanism. However, although likely to be related to the fatigue process, it is unlikely that both lactate and hydrogen ion accumulation are wholly responsible for muscle fatigue. For example, studies involving human volunteers have demonstrated that muscle force generation after fatiguing exercise can recover rapidly, despite also having a very low muscle pH value. The general consensus appears to be that the maintenance of force production during high-intensity exercise is pH dependent, but the initial force generation is more related to PCr availability.

One of the consequences of rapid PCr hydrolysis during high-intensity exercise is the accumulation of Pi, which inhibits muscle contraction coupling directly. However, the simultaneous PCr depletion and Pi accumulation make in vivo separation of the effect of PCr depletion from the effect Pi accumulation difficult. This problem is further confounded by the parallel increases in hydrogen and lactate ions that occur during high-intensity exercise. All of these metabolites have been independently implicated with muscle fatigue.

Calcium release by the sarcoplasmic reticulum as a consequence of muscle depolarization is essential for the activation of muscle contraction coupling. During fatiguing contractions calcium transport slows and calcium transients become progressively smaller, which has been attributed to a reduction in calcium re-uptake by the sarcoplasmic reticulum or increased calcium binding. Strong evidence that a disruption of calcium handling is responsible for fatigue comes from studies showing that the stimulation of sarcoplasmic reticulum calcium release caused by the administration of caffeine to isolated muscle can improve muscle

force production, even in the presence of a low muscle pH (Green 1995). Alternatively, fatigue during high-intensity exercise may be associated with an excitation-coupling failure and possibly a reduced nervous drive caused by reflex inhibition at the spinal level. In the latter hypothesis, accumulation of interstitial potassium in muscle may play a major role.

When repeated bouts of maximal exercise are performed, the rates of muscle PCr hydrolysis and lactate accumulation decline. In the case of PCr, this response is thought to occur because of incomplete PCr resynthesis during recovery between successive exercise bouts. However, the mechanism(s) responsible for the fall in the rate of lactate accumulation is unclear.

Causes of Fatigue in Prolonged Exercise

The term *prolonged exercise* is usually used to describe exercise intensities that can be sustained for 30 minutes to 180 minutes. Because the rate of ATP demand is relatively low compared with high-intensity exercise, PCr, carbohydrate, and fat can all contribute to energy production. The different fuel sources available to resynthesize ATP are summarized in figure 2.18. The rates of PCr degradation and lactate production during the first minutes of prolonged exercise are closely related to the intensity of exercise performed, and energy production during this period would likely be compromised without this contribution from anaerobic metabolism. However, once a steady state has been reached, carbohydrate and fat oxidation become the principal means of resynthesizing ATP. Muscle glycogen is the principal fuel during the first 30 minutes of exercise at 60% to 80% $\dot{V}O_2$max. The rate of muscle glycogen utilization depends on the exercise intensity (see figure 2.19).

During the early stages of exercise, fat oxidation is limited by the delay in the mobilization of FAs from adipose tissue. At rest after an overnight fast, the plasma FA concentration is about 0.3 mmol/L to 0.4 mmol/L. This concentration is commonly observed to fall during the first hour of moderate-intensity exercise, followed by a progressive increase (see figure 2.20) as lipolysis is stimulated by the actions of catecholamines, glucagon, and cortisol. During very prolonged exercise, the plasma FA concentration can reach 1.5 mmol/L to 2.0 mmol/L, and muscle uptake of blood-borne FA is proportional to the plasma FA concentration.

The glycerol released from adipose tissue cannot be used directly by muscle, which lacks the enzyme glycerol kinase. However, glycerol (together with alanine and lactate) is taken up by the liver and used as a gluconeogenic precursor to help maintain liver

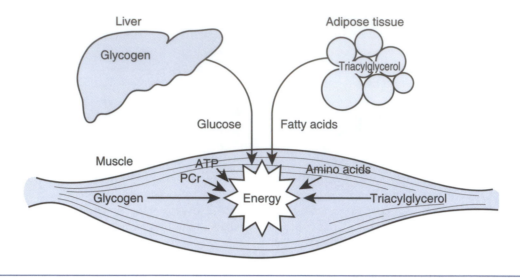

Figure 2.18 The main fuel sources available for exercise.

glucose output as liver glycogen levels decline. The utilization of blood glucose is greater at higher work rates and increases during prolonged submaximal exercise. At an exercise intensity of 60% $\dot{V}O_2$max, blood glucose uptake by muscle peaks after about 90 minutes (see figure 2.21). The decline in blood glucose uptake after 90 minutes is attributable to the increasing availability of plasma FA as fuel (which appears to directly inhibit muscle glucose uptake) and the depletion of liver glycogen stores.

At the marathon-running pace, muscle carbohydrate stores alone can fuel about 80 minutes of exercise before depletion (see table 2.4). However, the simultaneous utilization of body fat and hepatic carbohydrate stores enables ATP production to be maintained and exercise to continue. Figure 2.22 shows the contributions of fat oxidation, muscle glycogen, and blood glucose to energy expenditure during running at different speeds. At marathon-running pace, the muscle and hepatic carbohydrate stores will ultimately become depleted. At this point, ATP production becomes compromised because of the inability of fat oxidation to increase sufficiently to offset this deficit. The rate of ATP resynthesis from fat oxidation alone cannot meet the ATP requirement for exercise intensities higher than about 50% to 60% $\dot{V}O_2$max.

Figure 2.19 Effect of exercise intensity on rates of muscle glycogen utilization.

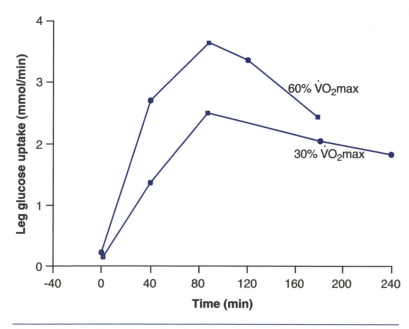

Figure 2.20 Changes in the concentrations of plasma glucose, plasma FAs, and muscle glycogen during continuous exercise at an intensity equivalent to 70% $\dot{V}O_2$max.

Figure 2.21 Rate of uptake of glucose from the blood by muscle during exercise at 30% $\dot{V}O_2$max and 60% $\dot{V}O_2$max. Peak uptake occurs after about 90 minutes of exercise.

The factor that limits the maximal rate of fat oxidation during exercise (i.e., why it cannot increase to compensate for carbohydrate depletion) is currently unknown, but it must precede acetyl-CoA formation because from this point, fat and carbohydrate share the same fate. The limitation may reside in the rate of uptake of FA into muscle from blood or the transport of FA into the mitochondria, rather than in the rate of β-oxidation of FA in the mitochondria.

The glucose-FA cycle partly regulates the integration of carbohydrate and fat oxidation during prolonged exercise. However, while this circumstance may be true of resting muscle, evidence (Dyke et al. 1993) suggests that the cycle does not operate in exercising muscle and that the site of regulation must reside elsewhere (e.g., at the level of phosphorylase or CAT-I). The integration of muscle carbohydrate and fat utilization during prolonged exercise is complex and unresolved.

During prolonged submaximal exercise, the main factors influencing the selection of fuel for muscular work are exercise intensity and duration. The effect of exercise duration on the contribution of different fuels during constant-load exercise at about 60% $\dot{V}O_2$max is illustrated in figure 2.23, and the effect of exercise intensity is summarized in figure 2.24.

In sedentary individuals, the glycogen store in muscle is fairly resistant to change. However, the combination of exercise and dietary manipulation can have dramatic effects on muscle glycogen storage. A clear positive relationship exists between muscle glycogen content and subsequent endurance performance. Furthermore, the ingestion of carbohydrate during prolonged exercise decreases muscle glycogen utilization and fat mobilization and oxidation, and it increases the rate of carbohydrate oxidation and endurance capacity. Therefore, the contribution of orally ingested carbohydrate to total ATP production under these conditions must be greater than that normally derived from fat oxidation. The precise biochemical mechanism by which muscle glycogen depletion causes fatigue is currently unresolved. However, the inability of muscle to maintain the rate of ATP synthesis in the glycogen-depleted state possibly results in ADP and Pi accumulation and consequently fatigue. Of course, a substantial fall in intramuscular ATP concentration is unlikely in this form of exercise, because very low ATP concentrations cause rigor and

Figure 2.22 Changes in the relative contributions of the major fuel sources to ATP resynthesis during running at different speeds. At the marathon-running speed for an elite endurance athlete, the rate of carbohydrate oxidation is about 3.5 g/min.

Figure 2.23 Changes in the relative contributions of the major fuel sources to ATP resynthesis during prolonged submaximal exercise at an intensity equivalent to about 60% V̇O₂max (approximately 10 times the resting metabolic rate).

irreversible damage to muscle fibers. Hence, some factor other than muscle glycogen depletion, but probably linked to low muscle glycogen concentrations, must act to constrain the activity of glycogen-depleted muscle before rigor can develop.

Starvation rapidly depletes the liver of carbohydrate. The rate of hepatic glucose release in resting, postabsorptive individuals is sufficient to match the carbohydrate demands of only the central nervous system. Approximately 70% of this release is derived from liver carbohydrate stores, and the remainder is derived from liver gluconeogenesis. During exercise,

the rate of hepatic glucose release is related to exercise intensity. Liver carbohydrate stores contribute 90% of this release, ultimately resulting in liver glycogen depletion.

Prolonged exercise, particularly after a period of fasting or a diet low in carbohydrate results in hypoglycemia, which may be a direct cause of fatigue. Alterations in liver rather than muscle glycogen concentrations could possibly be the more important determinant of the marked difference in exercise capacity induced by high-carbohydrate and low-carbohydrate diets. Hypoglycemia is detected

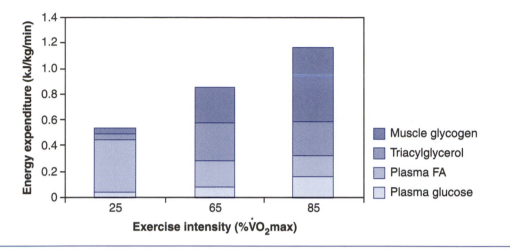

Figure 2.24 The contributions of different fuel sources to energy expenditure at three different exercise intensities.
From Romijn et al. 1995.

by the brain and causes symptoms of tiredness and dizziness. This central fatigue could then reduce the degree of skeletal muscle recruitment by the motor cortex, causing a fall in muscle force generation. Furthermore, afferent chemoreceptor information from both the hepatic portal system (monitoring hepatic portal blood glucose concentration) and the skeletal muscle (monitoring muscle glycogenolysis) possibly feeds back to the motor cortex. These signals increase as hypoglycemia develops, and the availability of muscle glycogen declines, inducing more central fatigue and causing the athletes to reduce their exercise intensity.

Thus, carbohydrate ingestion during exercise can also delay fatigue development by slowing the rate of liver glycogen depletion and helping to maintain the blood glucose concentration. Central fatigue is certainly a possibility during prolonged exercise, and undoubtedly the development of hypoglycemia contributes to this. Fatigue is a protective mechanism de-signed to prevent irreversible muscle damage, and—even more important—to prevent neural damage by hypoglycemia.

When exercise is performed with high initial muscle and liver glycogen levels, the hormonal response to exercise is attenuated

compared with when exercise is performed in a carbohydrate-depleted state (see figure 2.25). Similarly, carbohydrate feeding during exercise is associated with smaller rises in the plasma concentrations of

Figure 2.25 Influence of a high-carbohydrate or low-carbohydrate diet (for the preceding 3 days) on the hormonal response to prolonged exercise. Mean plasma hormone concentrations are shown for a group of 7 subjects running at 70% $\dot{V}O_2$max after 4 days on a low-carbohydrate or high-carbohydrate diet. At exhaustion (1), the subjects were encouraged to run for 10 minutes more (2) with glucose infusion.

Reprinted, by permission, from H. Galbo et al., 1979, "Exercise physiology: Humoral function," *Sport Science Review* 1: 65-93; adapted from Galbo et al., 1979, "The effect of different diets and of insulin on the hormonal response to prolonged exercise," *Acta Physiologica Scandanavica* 107: 19-32.

epinephrine, norepinephrine, glucagon, and cortisol. Because these hormones are involved in the stimulation of lipolysis, fat mobilization is delayed and the rate of fat oxidation is less when carbohydrate is consumed during exercise.

Metabolic Adaptation to Exercise Training

Muscle adaptations to aerobic endurance training include increases in capillary density and mitochondrial size and number. The activity of the TCA cycle and of other oxidative enzymes is increased, with a concomitant increase in the capacity to oxidize both fat and carbohydrate. Training adaptations in muscle affect substrate utilization. Endurance training also increases the relative cross-sectional area of type I fibers, increases intramuscular content of triacylglycerol, and increases the capacity to use fat as an energy source during submaximal exercise. Trained subjects also demonstrate an increased reliance on intramuscular triacylglycerol as an energy source. These effects and other physiological effects of training, including increased maximum cardiac output and $\dot{V}O_2$max, improved oxygen delivery to working muscle and attenuated hormonal responses to exercise (see figure 2.26), decrease the rate of muscle glycogen and blood glucose utilization, and decrease the rate of lactate accumulation during submaximal exercise. These adaptations contribute to the marked improvement in endurance capacity after training.

Alterations in substrate use with endurance training could be caused, at least in part, by less disturbance to ATP homeostasis during exercise. With an increased mitochondrial oxidative capacity after training, smaller decreases in ATP and PCr and smaller increases in ADP and Pi are needed to balance the rate of ATP synthesis with the rate of ATP utilization. In other words, with more mitochondria, the amount of oxygen as well as the ADP and Pi required per mitochondrion will be less after training than before training. The smaller increase in ADP concentration would result in formation of less AMP by the myokinase reaction, and also less IMP and ammonia would be formed by AMP deamination. Smaller increases in the concentrations of ADP, AMP, Pi, and ammonia could account for the slower rate of glycolysis and glycogenolysis in trained muscle compared with untrained muscle.

Training for strength, power, or speed has little if any effect on aerobic capacity. Heavy resistance training or sprinting brings about specific changes in the immediate (ATP and PCr) and short-term (glycolytic)

Figure 2.26 Influence of endurance training on the hormonal response to prolonged exercise.

Reprinted, by permission, from H. Galbo et al. 1979, "Exercise physiology: humoral function," *Sport Science Review* 1: 65-93; adapted from Kjaer et al., 1988, "Hormonal response to exercise in humans: Influence of hypoxia and physical training," *American Journal of Physiology* 254: R197-203.

energy delivery systems, increases in muscle buffering capacity, and improvements in strength or sprint performance. Several months of heavy resistance training causes hypertrophy of the muscle fibers, thus increasing total muscle mass and the possible maximum power output. Stretch, contraction, and damage to muscle fibers during exercise provide the stimuli for adaptation, which involves changes in the expression of different myosin isoforms.

Key Points

- Skeletal muscle cells are long, striated, multinucleated fibers. Myofibers are the contractile elements, composed of sarcomeres containing thin (actin) and thick (myosin) filaments arranged in a regular array. The heads of the myosin molecules form cross-bridges that bind reversibly to the actin filaments, causing the filaments to slide over each other toward the centers of the sarcomeres.

- The energy source for muscle contraction is ATP, which is continuously regenerated during exercise from phosphocreatine hydrolysis, anaerobic metabolism of glycogen or glucose, or aerobic metabolism of acetyl-CoA derived principally from breakdown of carbohydrate or fat. The carbon skeleton of amino acids can be used as a fuel for oxidative metabolism but is not a major fuel for energy production during exercise.

- Phosphocreatine is present in the sarcoplasm of muscle at about three times the concentration of ATP. Phosphocreatine hydrolysis is initiated at the immediate onset of contraction to buffer the rapid accumulation of ADP resulting from ATP hydrolysis. However, the rate of phosphocreatine hydrolysis begins to decline after only a few seconds of maximal force generation. The importance of phosphocreatine to muscle energy production and function lies in the extremely rapid rate at which it can resynthesize ATP.

- Carbohydrate provides energy by anaerobic metabolism, with lactate as the end product, or by complete oxidation to carbon dioxide and water. The net effect of glycolysis is conversion of 1 molecule of glucose to 2 molecules of pyruvate. This process makes 2 molecules of ATP available for each molecule of glucose that is broken down. If muscle glycogen is the starting substrate, 3 ATP molecules are generated for each glucose residue passing down the pathway.

- Glycolysis involves the reduction of NAD to NADH, depleting the intracellular pool of NAD. Reduction of pyruvate to lactate allows the NAD to be regenerated from NADH. The alternative pathway for NAD regeneration involves conversion of pyruvate to acetyl-CoA for subsequent oxidation in the TCA cycle.

- The TCA cycle and oxidative phosphorylation occur in the mitochondria. In the aerobic resynthesis of ATP, oxygen is the final electron acceptor in the electron transport chain, and it combines with hydrogen to form water.

- Carbohydrate stores are rapidly depleted during exercise (muscle glycogen) or during fasting (liver glycogen). Muscle glycogen stores are normally depleted after one hour to two hours of hard exercise. In very-high-intensity exercise, the muscle glycogen content falls rapidly but is not completely depleted at the point of fatigue.

- Carbohydrate is the major fuel for muscle activity in high-intensity exercise: when the muscle glycogen stores are depleted, only low-intensity exercise is possible. The time that a fixed exercise intensity can be sustained is related to the size of the pre-exercise glycogen store. The size of the store depends on the pattern of exercise and diet in the previous hours and days.

- A number of hormones are involved in the integration and control of carbohydrate metabolism, including (especially) insulin, which promotes carbohydrate storage, and glucagon, whose actions are generally antagonistic to those of insulin. Epinephrine and norepinephrine stimulate carbohydrate mobilization and metabolism at times of stress.

(continued)

(continued)

■ The principal storage form of fat in the body is triacylglycerol, most of which is located in white adipose tissue. Triacylglycerol stores are also found in liver and muscle and as lipoproteins in blood. Muscles cannot oxidize triacylglycerols directly. The triacylglycerol molecules must first be broken down into its FA and glycerol components by lipolysis. This process is activated during exercise by the actions of epinephrine, glucagon, and cortisol. The principal sources of fat fuels for exercise are blood-borne FA derived from adipose tissue and intramuscular triacylglycerol.

■ Several factors influence the type of substrate used to fuel muscular work, including substrate availability, diet, intensity and duration of exercise, training status, hormones, prior exercise, and environmental conditions. Fat oxidation makes an increasing contribution to ATP regeneration as exercise duration increases. In exercise lasting several hours, fat may supply almost 80% of the total energy required.

■ Endurance training increases the capacity of muscle to oxidize fat.

■ Fatigue is the inability to maintain a given or expected power output or force, and it is an inevitable feature of strenuous exercise. The onset of muscle fatigue has been associated with the disruption of energy supply, product inhibition, and factors preceding cross-bridge formation. It is likely a multifactoral process.

Key Terms

aerobic 35

anaerobic 35

adenosine triphosphate (ATP) 32

adenosine triphosphatase (ATPase) 32

β-oxidation 38

electron transport chain (ETC) 40

gluconeogenesis 49

glycogen 32

glycogenolysis 38

glycolysis 35

hormones 32

lipolysis 41

mitochondrion (plural mitochondria) 32

myofibril 32

oxidative phosphorylation 35

phosphocreatine, or creatine phosphate (PCr) 32

sarcomere 32

tricarboxylic acid (TCA) cycle 35

type I fibers 34

type II fibers 34

Recommended Readings

Åstrand, P.-O., K. Rodahl, H. Dahl, and S. Stromme. 2003. *Textbook of Work Physiology. Physiological Basis of Exercise.* Human Kinetics: Champaign, IL.

Bangsbo, J. 1997. Physiology of muscle fatigue during intense exercise. In *The Clinical Pharmacology of Sport and Exercise*, ed. T. Reilly and M. Orme, 123-133. Elsevier: Amsterdam.

Green, H.J. 1991. How important is endogenous muscle glycogen to fatigue in prolonged exercise? *Canadian Journal of Physiology and Pharmacology* 69: 290-297.

Greenhaff, P.L., and E. Hultman. 1999. The biochemical basis of exercise. In *Basic and Applied Sciences for Sports Medicine*, ed. R.J. Maughan, 69-89. Butterworth-Heinemann: Oxford.

Komi, P.V., and J. Karlsson. 1978. Skeletal muscle fibre types, enzyme activities and physical performance in young males and females. *Acta Physiologica Scandinavica* 103: 210-218.

Maughan, R.J., and M. Gleeson. 2004. *The Biochemical Basis of Sports Performance.* Oxford University Press: Oxford.

Sahlin, K., and S. Broberg. 1990. Adenine nucleotide depletion in human muscle during exercise: Causality and significance of AMP deamination. *International Journal of Sports Medicine* 11: S62-S67.

Saltin, B. 1985. Physiological adaptation to physical conditioning. *Acta Medica Scandinavica* (supplement) 711: 11-24.

Sjogaard, G. 1991. Role of exercise-induced potassium fluxes underlying muscle fatigue: A brief review. *Canadian Journal of Physiology and Pharmacology* 69: 238-245.

Chapter 3

Energy

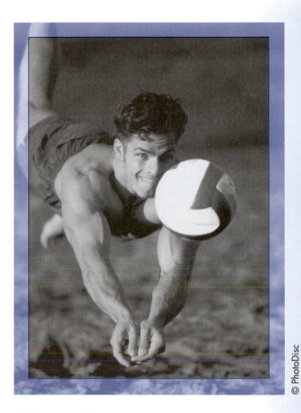

© PhotoDisc

Objectives

After studying this chapter, you should be able to do the following:

- Describe what energy is and how it is expressed and give an overview of the different types of energy

- Define the terms gross efficiency, net efficiency, delta efficiency, and economy

- Describe various ways to measure energy expenditure and explain the advantages and disadvantages of these methods

- Describe the various components of human energy expenditure and their respective contributions to energy expenditure in active and inactive persons

- Discuss the concept of energy balance and how it relates to body weight and physical performance

- Discuss the upper and lower limits of human energy expenditure and the practical problems associated with these energy expenditures

Cells need **energy** to function, muscle fibers need energy to contract, and ionic pumps in membranes need energy to transport ions across cell membranes. Although the human body has some energy reserves, most of its energy must be obtained through nutrition. During exercise, energy requirements increase and energy provision can become critical. Persons with a defect in energy metabolism have problems performing vigorous physical exercise. For instance, someone with McArdle's disease, who lacks the enzyme glycogen phosphorylase, cannot break down muscle glycogen and hence that person's energy provision and exercise capacity is severely impaired. In athletes, energy provision can be crucial, and energy depletion (carbohydrate depletion) is one of the most common causes of fatigue. Different types of exercise and different sports have different energy requirements. Therefore, athletes must adjust their food intake accordingly. This chapter describes the energy requirements and associated practical problems of some athletes.

What Is Energy?

Forms of energy range from light energy to chemical energy. Plants use light energy in the process of photosynthesis to produce carbohydrate, fat, or protein. The energy in food is stored in the chemical bonds of various molecules. Breaking these bonds releases this energy, and it becomes available for conversion into other forms of energy. For instance, when glucose is broken down during glycolysis, chemical energy is converted to another form of chemical energy (ATP) and ultimately transformed into mechanical energy (muscle contraction).

In physiology, energy represents the capacity to do work, which is often referred to as mechanical energy. Walking, running, throwing, and jumping require the production of mechanical energy. Work (energy) is the product of force times the vertical distance covered:

$$\text{work} = \text{force} \times \text{distance, or } W = F \times d$$

If work is expressed per unit of time, the term *power* (P) is used:

$$\text{power} = \text{work/time, or } P = W/t$$

Energy expenditure (EE) refers to energy expended (in kiloJoules [kJ] or kilocalories [kcal]) per unit of time to produce power. During conversion of one form of energy into another, no energy is lost. For example, in carbohydrate and fat combustion, chemical energy is converted into mechanical energy (muscle contraction) and heat energy.

The human body is not very efficient in its use of energy from the breakdown of carbohydrate and fat. During cycling exercise, for instance, only 20% of that energy is converted to power. The rest of the energy becomes heat. This heat can be partly used to maintain our body temperature at 37°C (98.6°F), but during exercise heat production may be excessive. To prevent the body temperature from rising too high, various heat-dissipating mechanisms must be activated (see chapter 8).

Energy is often expressed in calories (the English system) or Joules (the metric system). One calorie expresses the quantity of energy (heat) needed to raise the temperature of 1 g (1 ml) of water by 1°C (1.8° F) (from 14.5°C to 15.5°C [58.1°F to 59.9°F]). Thus, food containing 200 kcal (kilocalories) has enough energy potential to raise the temperature of 200 L of water by 1°C (1.8° F).

The SI (International Unit System) unit for energy is the Joule, named for the British scientist Sir Prescott Joule (1818–1889). One Joule of energy moves a mass of 1 g at a velocity of 1 m/s. A Joule is not a large amount of energy, and, therefore, kiloJoules are more often used. To convert calories to Joules or kilocalories to kiloJoules, the calorie value needs to be multiplied by 4.186.

1 calorie (cal) = 4.186 J

1 kcal = 4.186 kJ

1 kcal = 1,000 cal

1 kJ = 1,000 J

1 MJ = 1,000 kJ

When discussing energy expenditure or intake over 24 hours, megaJoules (MJ) are often used to avoid large numbers. Because Joules are not yet part of everyday language, both units are often mentioned on food labels. In this book kJ will be used, with the equivalent in kcal given in parentheses.

Energetic Efficiency

The effective work performed after muscle contraction, or **efficiency,** is expressed as the percentage of total work. As already mentioned, approximately 20% of all energy produced in the human body is used to accomplish work (movement). Therefore, humans are approximately 20% efficient. Most of the remaining 80% is used to maintain homeostasis and is wasted as heat. No system is 100% efficient. A gasoline engine is 20% to 30% efficient. A diesel engine is 30% to 40% efficient. An ordinary light bulb is about 20% efficient, and an energy saving bulb is about 80% efficient.

The precise definition of efficiency can vary. For example, gross efficiency (GE) is the ratio of the total work to energy expended:

$$GE\ (\%) = \frac{\text{work accomplished}}{\text{energy expended}} \times 100\%$$

However, as exercise intensity increases, the relative proportion of the energy expended as resting metabolism decreases, causing GE to increase with work rate. A solution for this problem is to subtract a baseline energy expenditure from the total energy expenditure. One way to calculate the baseline is to use net efficiency (NE), where the baseline is the energy expended at rest:

$$NE\ (\%) = \frac{\text{work accomplished}}{(\text{energy expended} - \text{resting energy expenditure})} \times 100\%$$

The second way to calculate the baseline is to use work efficiency (WE), where the baseline is the energy cost of unloaded (0 W) work (for example, unloaded cycling):

$$WE\ (\%) = \frac{\text{work accomplished}}{(\text{energy expended} - \text{energy expended in unloaded condition})} \times 100\%$$

Unfortunately, work efficiency is difficult or even impossible to determine reliably because of the unnatural nature of unloaded movements.

A fourth definition of efficiency is delta efficiency (DE), which expresses the change in energy expended per minute relative to the change in actual work accomplished per minute:

$$DE\ (\%) = \frac{\Delta \text{ work accomplished}}{\Delta \text{ energy expended}} \times 100\%$$

Delta efficiency may be the most accurate reflection of muscle efficiency, but it is more difficult to determine and is more variable. All four calculations of efficiency are commonly used in the literature and all have their limitations.

The term **economy** is typically expressed as the oxygen uptake required to exercise at a certain intensity. For runners, it is the oxygen uptake at a speed of 16 km/h. More efficient runners are usually better runners because they "waste" less energy. In other sports, such as cycling, such a strong relationship between efficiency and performance does not seem to exist.

Measuring the Energy Content of Food

Direct calorimetry is used to measure the energy content of food. The food is combusted (oxidized), and the resulting heat is used as a measure of the energy content. The measurement takes place in a bomb calorimeter (see figure 3.1).

Figure 3.1 Bomb calorimeter.

A weighed amount of food (about 1 g) is placed in a sealed steel chamber with a high oxygen pressure. The reaction is started through ignition by an electrical current. The food burns inside the chamber and produces heat, which is transferred through the metal walls of the chamber and heats the water that surrounds it. The rise in water temperature directly reflects the energy content of the food. If the water volume surrounding the chamber is 2 L and the temperature rises by 4.0° C (7.2° F), the energy content of that food is 2 × 4 = 8 kcal (or 8 × 4.186 = 33.5 kJ). If the weight of the food combusted was 1.2 g, the energy content of the food was 8/1.2 = 6.7 kcal/g (27.9 kJ/g). This measure is the gross energy value, or total energy content, of the food, and no distinction is made between carbohydrate, fat, and protein. Although the bomb calorimeter is probably the most accurate method of determining the energy content of food, it is expensive to run, and the results tend to overestimate actual calories absorbed because not all of the energy eaten can be digested or absorbed.

- Carbohydrates have varying energy content, depending on the type of carbohydrate and the arrangements of atoms within the carbohydrate. The combustion of glucose for instance gives 15.7 kJ/g (3.7 kcal/g), whereas the combustion of glycogen and starch is about 17.6 kJ/g (4.2 kcal/g). The latter figure is normally used as the energy value of carbohydrate (1 g carbohydrate = 17.6 kJ = 4.2 kcal).

- The energy content of fat is also dependent on the structure of the triacylglycerol or FA. A medium-chain FA, such as octanoate (8-carbon FA) may contain 36.0 kJ/g (8.6 kcal/g), whereas a long-chain FA may contain up to 40.2 kJ/g (9.6 kcal/g). The average energy content of fat in our diet is about 39.3 kJ/g (9.4 kcal/g).

- The energy content of protein depends on the type of protein and the nitrogen content. Nitrogen does not provide energy, and, therefore, proteins with a higher nitrogen density will contain less energy per gram. Nitrogen content in foods may vary from 15% (whole milk) to approximately 19% (nuts and seeds). On average, the proteins in our diet contain 23.7 kJ/g (5.65 kcal/g).

The gross energy value is not necessarily the amount of energy that would be available if the food was eaten, particularly in the case of protein. In the body, the nitrogen in amino acids is excreted by the kidneys as urea. The urea molecule consists of nitrogen, carbon, oxygen, and hydrogen, with the formula $CO(NH_2)_2$. Some of the hydrogen atoms present in the amino acid are excreted along with nitrogen and, thus, cannot provide energy. About 20% of the potential energy of the amino acid will be lost. If a bomb calorimeter shows that protein contains 23.7 kJ/g (5.65 kcal/g), in the human body, only 19.3 kJ/g (4.6 kcal/g) is available. This value is the net energy of food.

Food is sometimes not completely absorbed. Incomplete digestion and absorption will, of course, result in a decreased availability of energy. This fact was determined by Wilbur Olin Atwater (1844–1907), who was one of the pioneers in studying human energy balance. After measuring many different kinds of foods, Atwater came up with energy values for foods that accounted for differences in digestibility. Conveniently, these energy values were rounded to whole numbers. The energy contents of carbohydrate, fat, and protein were 4 kcal/g, 9 kcal/g, and 4 kcal/g, respectively (16 kJ/g, 36 kJ/g, and 16 kJ/g). These correction factors are often referred to as the **Atwater factors** or Atwater energy values.

The percentage of food energy that is actually absorbed is often expressed in a coefficient of digestibility. A coefficient of digestibility of 50 means that only half of the energy ingested was absorbed. Adding fiber to a meal generally reduces the coefficient of digestibility. Thus, when a food item is high in fiber, a smaller amount of the energy is available to the body than from a food item with identical energy content but low in fiber. Fiber causes the food to move faster through the gastrointestinal system, leaving less time for absorption processes. On average, 97% of carbohydrate is completely digested and absorbed. For fat, this value is 95%, and for protein, it is 92% (see table 3.1). On the other hand, the coefficient of digestibility of wheat bran protein is only 40%, and its protein calorie contribution is just 7.62 kJ/g (1.82 kcal/g), significantly less than the 16 kJ/g (4 kcal/g) estimated by Atwater. Furthermore, the coefficient of digestibility of wheat bran carbohydrate is 56%, and its calorie contribution is only 9.84 kJ/g (2.35 kcal/g), again, far below the 16 kJ/g (4 kcal/g) used by Atwater.

Atwater had begun to analyze the composition and the energy content of food. Nowadays a variety of extensive databases exist, usually compiled by governmental institutions. One of the largest and most comprehensible databases is the U.S. Nutrient Data Bank (USNDB), which is compiled by the U.S. Department of Agriculture's Consumer Nutrition Center. This database can be downloaded from the USDA Nutrient Laboratory database (http//www.nal.usda.gov/fnic/foodcomp/data/index). Software manufacturers base their programs on this database and comparable nutritional databases. Because each country has its own very specific products and brands, no one database covers all food items.

Measuring Energy Expenditure

The methods of measuring or estimating human energy expenditure range from direct but complex measurements of heat production (direct calorimetry), to relatively simple indirect metabolic measurements (indirect calorimetry), to very expensive tracer methods (doubly labeled water), to relatively cheap and convenient rough estimates (heart rate monitoring and accelerometry). Following are some of the available methods to measure human energy expenditure:

- Direct calorimetry
- Indirect calorimetry
- Closed circuit spirometry

Table 3.1 Energy Content of Nutrients and the Availability of Energy in the Body

	Energy of combustion per gram in kJ (kcal)	Energy available per gram in kJ (kcal)	Coefficient of digestibility
PROTEIN			
Animal food	**23.7 (5.65)**	**17.9 (4.27)**	**97**
Meats, fish, and poultry	23.7 (5.65)	17.9 (4.27)	97
Eggs	24.1 (5.75)	18.3 (4.37)	97
Dairy products	23.7 (5.65)	17.9 (4.27)	97
Plant food	**23.7 (5.65)**	**15.7 (3.74)**	**85**
Cereals	24.3 (5.80)	16.2 (3.87)	85
Legumes	23.9 (5.70)	14.5 (3.47)	78
Vegetables	20.9 (5.00)	13.0 (3.11)	83
Fruits	21.8 (5.20)	14.1 (3.36)	83
Average protein	*23.7 (5.65)*	*17.0 (4.05)*	*92*
FAT			
Animal food	**39.3 (9.40)**	**37.4 (8.93)**	**95**
Meat and eggs	39.8 (9.50)	37.8 (9.03)	95
Dairy products	38.7 (9.25)	36.8 (8.79)	95
Vegetable food	**38.9 (9.30)**	**35.0 (8.37)**	**90**
Average lipid	*39.3 (9.40)*	*37.4 (8.93)*	*95*
CARBOHYDRATE			
Animal food	**16.3 (3.90)**	**16.0 (3.82)**	**98**
Vegetable food	**17.4 (4.15)**	**16.9 (4.03)**	**97**
Cereals	17.6 (4.20)	17.2 (4.11)	98
Legumes	17.6 (4.20)	17.0 (4.07)	97
Vegetables	17.6 (4.20)	16.7 (3.99)	95
Fruits	16.7 (4.00)	15.1 (3.60)	90
Sugars	16.5 (3.95)	16.2 (3.87)	98
Average carbohydrate	*17.4 (4.15)*	*16.9 (4.03)*	*97*

The coefficient of digestibility reflects the percentage of energy in a nutrient that is actually available.

Adapted from A.L. Merrill and B.K. Watt, 1973, *Energy Value of Foods—Basis and Derivation*, (Washington, DC: US Department of Agriculture). Http://www.nal.usda.gov/fnic/foodcomp/Data/Classics/ah74.pdf.

- Open circuit spirometry
- Douglas bag technique
- Breath-by-breath technique
- Portable spirometry
- Doubly labeled water
- Labeled bicarbonate
- Heart rate monitoring
- Accelerometry
- Observations, records of physical activity, activity diaries, recall

Direct Calorimetry

Ultimately, all biochemical processes in the body result in heat production. This heat production can be measured in a similar manner as the heat production from combusting food. A human calorimeter is a small, well-insulated chamber with adequate ventilation (see figure 3.2). The top of the chamber consists of a series of coils through which a known amount of water flows. The water absorbs the heat radiated by the subject in the chamber, which reflects the metabolic rate of that person. The air is recirculated, and

Figure 3.2 Direct calorimetry chamber.

carbon dioxide and water are filtered out of the air before it reenters the chamber, together with added oxygen. This process prevents heat being lost from the chamber in the form of expired gases.

Although the direct calorimeter is based on a simple principle, the actual engineering and operation of the chamber are very complicated. Specially trained personnel are required to operate the device, and therefore it is not the most popular and most common way to measure energy expenditure. An important disadvantage of the direct calorimeter is that it is unsuitable for field studies and assessment of energy expenditure in most exercise and sport situations.

Direct Calorimeter Suit

To overcome some of the practical problems of the direct calorimeter chamber, a direct calorimeter suit was developed. This suit consists of a very long plastic tube through which a known amount of water flows. The tubing touches the skin and absorbs the body heat. Again, the rise in temperature of the water is directly related to the subject's heat production and thus to the metabolic rate. With this suit, measurements can be conducted outside the chamber, but

the suit may impair movements. The suit has been shown to be useful for walking exercise, but because it is heavy and not very flexible, it might impede more vigorous activities or faster movements. Nevertheless, the suit has been used successfully for these purposes as well.

Indirect Calorimetry

The energy for all biochemical reactions ultimately depends on the oxygen supply. The term *indirect* refers to the measurement of O_2 uptake and CO_2 production rather than to the measurement of heat transfer. This measurement requires a steady state CO_2 production and **respiratory exchange ratio** (RER = $\dot{V}CO_2/\dot{V}O_2$) and subjects with a normal acid-base balance. Studies with the bomb calorimeter have shown that the amount of oxygen required to combust carbohydrate, fat, and protein is directly related to the energy content. In fact, for every kJ, 50 ml of O_2 is required, or for every kcal, 207 ml of O_2 is required. In other words, the energy equivalent of 1 L of O_2 is 20.2 kJ (4.82 kcal). This energy equivalent of oxygen is relatively stable and fairly independent of the mixture of carbohydrate, fat, and protein oxidized. Indirect calorimetry is an indirect but accurate estimate of energy expenditure.

When $\dot{V}O_2$ is measured in L of O_2 at STPD (standard temperature [0° C, or 32° F], pressure [760 mm Hg], and dry) per minute, energy expenditure (EE) can be measured by

$$EE \text{ (kJ/min)} = 20.2 \times \dot{V}O_2$$

Energy expenditure can be estimated even more accurately if the RER is known because the energy equivalent for oxygen is 19.6 kJ/L at an RER of 0.7 (when 100% fat is being oxidized), rising to 20.9 kJ/L at a RER of 1.0 (when carbohydrate is the only fuel being oxidized). For these calculations, the relatively small contribution of protein oxidation is ignored.

Closed-Circuit and Open-Circuit Spirometry

Ways to measure O_2 uptake and CO_2 production included "closed-circuit" and "open-circuit" methods. The closed-circuit method is used to measure resting energy expenditure (see figure 3.3). The technique was developed in the late 1800s and is routinely used in clinical settings. The subject breathes through a mouthpiece into a spirometer that is prefilled with 100% oxygen. During each inspiration, some of the oxygen in the chamber of gas is consumed. Expired gas is passed back into the spirometer, and the CO_2 produced is trapped in a filter. The residual oxygen in the chamber is available for the next inspiration. As oxygen is consumed, the volume of oxygen in the spirometer decreases, and this change in volume is

measured. The oxygen taken up and energy expenditure can then be calculated. Closed-circuit spirometry is a good method in resting conditions, but it is not suitable during exercise, especially high-intensity exercise. When CO_2 production is very high, the trapping of CO_2 may become problematic. The subject breathes through a three-way valve from and into a spirometer, which is pre-filled with 100% oxygen. A recorder is connected so that the changes in volume are accurately measured.

With open-circuit spirometry (for research purposes the most common method of estimating energy expenditure), the subject inhales ambient air (0.03% CO_2 and 20.93% O_2 and 79.04% N_2). Energy expenditure is calculated from the difference in O_2 and CO_2 content between the inspired and expired gases and the ventilation rate. Such measurements can be made in a respiration chamber by so-called Douglas bags or online systems.

Respiration Chamber

For a measurement of a complete energy balance, a respiration chamber was developed. The respiration chamber (see figure 3.4) is comparable to the chamber used for direct calorimetry but without the coils to measure heat exchange and the insulation. Sufficient airflow into the respiration chamber prevents the chamber air from falling much below 20% oxygen, and the ventilation rate is carefully measured. Flow of air into the chamber is continuous. This flow is carefully monitored. In addition, the oxygen and carbon dioxide concentrations at the inlet and outlet of the chamber are recorded, from which oxygen uptake and carbon dioxide production can be calculated. Respiration chambers are usually designed like small hotel rooms, with a bed, chair, television, radio, and telephone, and measurements can be performed

Figure 3.3 Closed-circuit spirometry.

Figure 3.4 A respiration chamber.

over a period of several hours to several days. The chamber is ideal for measurements of **energy balance** because food intake can be accurately controlled, and all food is prepared by the investigators and handed to the subject through special hatches. Urine and feces can also be collected for further analysis, which is often done when a complete energy and nitrogen balance is required.

The advantage of this technique is that, besides accurate information about gas exchange (and thus energy expenditure), it allows accurate control over the energy intake, and potential energy losses in feces and urine can be analyzed. The main disadvantages of this technique are that it requires highly trained personnel and is very expensive. Also, the stay in the chamber interferes with every day life because not all activities can be performed inside the chamber. Furthermore, most chambers are not adapted to very high ventilation rates and are not suitable for vigorous exercise. However, modern respiration chambers with fast-response analyzers are capable of measuring energy expenditure during very-high-intensity exercise, and several studies have been performed of highly trained individuals performing vigorous exercise for prolonged periods of time.

Douglas Bag

A way to measure oxygen uptake and carbon dioxide production at the same time is by collecting the expired gases for a certain period of time and measuring the volume, the O_2 concentration, and the CO_2 concentration of this gas. The test subject inspires room air and expires through a mouthpiece connected to a high-flow, low-resistance valve into a large plastic bag. These Douglas bags are named after British scientist Claude Douglas (1882–1963), who was the first to use this method to measure gas exchange in humans (see figure 3.5).

After collection, the bags are closed until analysis. They are then emptied into a gas meter to measure the total volume. From the duration of collection (usually 1 minute) and the volume measurement, the ventilation rate can be calculated. A small sample of expired gas is collected from or in addition to the gas in this large Douglas bag for analysis of O_2 and CO_2 concentrations. From the difference between the inspired and expired O_2 and CO_2 concentration and the ventilation rate, the O_2 uptake and CO_2 production can be calculated. This relatively simple technique has been applied successfully for many years and is still used by exercise physiologists. Various versions of this technique are used, including methods where flow is measured directly from the expired or inspired air.

Breath-by-Breath Systems

Respiratory physiologists have taken the Douglas bag technique one step further, and computers and fast-response O_2 and CO_2 analyzers have made it

a   b

© Asker Jeukendrup

Figure 3.5 (a) Douglas bags and (b) dry gas meter (left) and oxygen/carbon dioxide analyzer (middle).

possible to develop an on-line breath-by-breath gas analysis system. This semiautomated or fully automated analyzer usually measures volume at the mouthpiece, and a small gas sample is collected every expiration for analysis of O_2 and CO_2 concentration (see figure 3.6). This technique enables respiratory physiologists to look at the time course of changes in various ventilatory variables. When averaged over periods of 20 seconds to several minutes, this technique gives similar values to those obtained with the Douglas bag technique. The big advantage of the breath-by-breath systems is that they can analyze every breath and are therefore able to register rapid changes and give instant feedback. Breath-by-breath systems are convenient, and most systems give a very accurate estimation of energy expenditure.

© Asker Jeukendrup

Figure 3.6 Automated breath-by-breath system.

However, the measurements are restricted to a laboratory situation because the equipment is bulky and sensitive and, therefore, difficult to move. Recently, manufacturers have tried to develop smaller and portable breath-by-breath systems for measurements in free-living conditions. These attempts have been fairly successful, and in the future smaller analyzers may replace some of the laboratory-based equipment.

Indirect Calorimetry and Substrate Utilization

Gas exchange measurements allow an estimation not only of the energy expenditure but also of the substrate mixture used. Krogh and Lindhard, in the beginning of the 20th century, used the inherent differences in chemical properties of carbohydrate, fat, and protein to obtain information about fuel utilization. The complete oxidation of carbohydrate, fat, and protein requires different amounts of O_2 and produces different amounts of CO_2. The oxidation of 1 g of glucose requires 0.746 L O_2 and produces 0.743 L of CO_2 and 3.868 kcal. The oxidation of 1 g of FA (palmitic acid) requires 2.009 L O_2 and produces 1.414 L CO_2 and 9.746 kcal. The substrate used, therefore, determines the total O_2 required and total CO_2 produced. The ratio of CO_2 production and O_2 consumption, or respiratory quotient (RQ), provides a convenient indication of the substrate that is being utilized during steady-state exercise.

$$RQ = VCO_2/VO_2$$

The complete oxidation of 1 molecule of glucose (1 mole = 180 g) will require 6 molecules of O_2 and will produce 6 molecules of CO_2. The number of oxygen molecules equals the number of CO_2 molecules, and the RQ for carbohydrate is therefore 1.

$$C_6H_{12}O_6 + 6\ O_2 \rightarrow 6\ CO_2 + 6\ H_2O$$
$$RQ = 6\ CO_2/6\ O_2 = 1$$

Lipids contain significantly fewer oxygen atoms compared with carbohydrate and, therefore, require more oxygen in the oxidation process. Lipids can have different chemical compositions, unlike carbohydrate, whose biochemical formula is always the same ($C_6H_{12}O_6$). The O_2 required and the CO_2 produced, therefore, depend somewhat on the type of lipid oxidized. Complete oxidation of 1 molecule of a typical (and most abundant) FA (palmitic acid; 1 mole = 256 g) in the human body oxidizes to CO_2 and H_2O using 23 molecules of O_2. It produces 16 molecules of CO_2 and 16 molecules of H_2O. The RQ of palmitic acid is, therefore, 16/23 = 0.696. This RQ value, however, may vary from 0.727 (octanoic acid C8:0) to 0.686 (lignoceric acid; C24:0), depending on the chain length of the FA oxidized:

$$C_{16}H_{32}O_2 + 23\ O_2 \rightarrow 16\ CO_2 + 16\ H_2O$$
$$RQ = 16\ CO_2/23\ O_2 = 0.696$$

In addition to carbon, oxygen, and hydrogen, proteins (amino acids) also contain nitrogen and sometimes sulfur, which cannot be oxidized. Proteins have to be deaminated (removal of nitrogen), and nitrogen (as urea) and sulfur will be excreted in urine and feces. The remaining carbon skeleton can be oxidized to CO_2 and H_2O in a similar manner to carbohydrate and fat. The O_2 required and the CO_2 produced depends somewhat on the type of protein. An example of the oxidation of a protein is:

$$(albumin) \; C_{72}H_{112}N_{18}O_{22}S + 77 O_2 \rightarrow 63 \; CO_2 +$$
$$38 \; H_2O + SO_3 + 9 \; CO(NH_2)_2 \; (urea)$$
$$RQ = 63 \; CO_2 / 77 O_2 = 0.818$$

If a mixture of carbohydrate and fat is oxidized, O_2 consumption will equal the sum of O_2 required to oxidize the carbohydrate plus that required for fat. Similarly, the CO_2 production will be the sum of CO_2 from carbohydrate and CO_2 production from fat. If, for instance, 100 g of carbohydrate and 50 g of fat is oxidized, the O_2 consumption is $(100 \times 0.746) + (50 \times 2.009) = 175$ L. The CO_2 production is $(100 \times 0.743) + (50 \times 1.414) = 145$ L. The RQ is $145/175 = 0.829$.

When experiments are performed using indirect calorimetry and measures of $\dot{V}O_2$ and $\dot{V}CO_2$ are obtained, the reverse calculation is used:

Rate of carbohydrate oxidation (g/min) $\times \; O_2$ (L/g) + rate of fat oxidation (g/min) $\times \; O_2$ (L/g) = $\dot{V}O_2$ (L/min)

Rate of carbohydrate oxidation (g/min) $\times \; CO_2$ (L/g) + rate of fat oxidation (g/min) $\times \; CO_2$ (L/g) = $\dot{V}CO_2$ (L/min)

These calculations give 2 equations and 2 unknown variables, which can be solved:

Carbohydrate oxidation (g/min) =
$4.585 \; \dot{V}CO_2 - 3.226 \; \dot{V}O_2$

Fat oxidation (g/min) = $1.695 \; \dot{V}O_2 - 1.701 \; \dot{V}CO_2$

These calculations assume that protein is not an important energy fuel. In some extreme conditions, protein may contribute up to 15% to the total energy expenditure (see chapter 6). In this case, correction for protein oxidation should be made. To make this correction, urine samples are collected, and protein oxidation is estimated from the nitrogen content. One gram of nitrogen in urine represents the oxidation of 6.25 of protein. This result is subtracted from the fat and carbohydrate oxidation rates:

Protein oxidation = $6.25 \times N$

Carbohydrate oxidation (g/min) =
$4.59 \; \dot{V}CO_2 - 3.25 \; \dot{V}O_2 - 3.68 \; N$

Fat oxidation (g/min) =
$1.69 \; \dot{V}O_2 - 1.69 \; \dot{V}CO_2 - 1.72 \; N$

Energy expenditure (kJ) =
$16.18 \; \dot{V}O_2 + 5.02 \; \dot{V}CO_2 - 5.99 \; N$

Energy expenditure (kcal) =
$3.87 \; \dot{V}O_2 + 1.20 \; \dot{V}CO_2 - 1.43 \; N$

Where N is the urinary nitrogen in grams.

As mentioned previously, because the energy equivalent for oxygen is slightly different, depending on what substrate is utilized, measuring both O_2 consumption and CO_2 production makes the estimation of energy expenditure more accurate. For instance, if $\dot{V}O_2$ is 600 L/day and $\dot{V}CO_2$ is 500 L/day and nitrogen excretion is 25 g/day, energy expenditure is 12.068 kJ (2,886 kcal). With the simple formula (i.e., ignoring protein oxidation) the result is 12.120 kJ (2,892 kcal), a difference of only 0.2%.

The application of RQ is based on the premise that exchange of O_2 and CO_2 at the mouth represents the processes that occur in the tissues that oxidize the fuels. This assumption is valid at rest and during light to fairly high-intensity exercise (up to about 85% $\dot{V}O_2$max). However, because RQ measured at the mouth does not always reflect the oxidation processes in cells, it is usually referred to as respiratory exchange ratio (RER, or R).

One common condition in which RER is different from RQ is hyperventilation. During hyperventilation excess amounts of CO_2 are expired. This CO_2 is not derived from metabolic processes but is simply an extra excretion of body CO_2 stores. (CO_2 is mainly stored in the form of bicarbonate in the extracellular body fluids.) Because very little change occurs in $\dot{V}O_2$ during hyperventilation, the RER increases, usually above 1.00, and clearly does not reflect metabolism in the cells anymore.

Another situation in which RER differs from RQ is during strenuous exercise at intensities above 80% $\dot{V}O_2$max. At these very high exercise intensities, high glycolytic rates in the muscle result in the production and accumulation of lactic acid. The hydrogen ions associated with this acid must be buffered. The body's bicarbonate buffer system neutralizes the acidity. Hydrogen ions bind with bicarbonate ions (HCO_3^-) to form H_2CO_3 and subsequently H_2O and CO_2:

$$H^+ + HCO_3^- \leftrightarrow H_2CO_3 \leftrightarrow H_2O + CO_2$$

This CO_2 is expired, and, as a result, the RER increases rapidly and can reach values between 1.00 and 1.30. This increase does not reflect the metabolism in the cell, and, therefore, calculation of energy expenditure or substrate utilization is only valid during steady-state exercise, when no accumulation of lactic acid occurs. Situations in which lipogenesis (i.e., the synthesis of fat from carbohydrate) and ketogenesis (the formation of ketone bodies) play a role are further examples of conditions in which RER may differ from RQ.

Doubly Labeled Water

The doubly labeled water technique is based on the administration of a bolus dose of 2 stable isotopes of water: ^2H_2O and $H_2^{18}O$. (For an explanation of stable isotopes, see appendix A.) These 2 isotopes are used as tracers and the slightly heavier atoms ^2H and ^{18}O can be measured in various body fluids (e.g., urine). ^2H is lost from the body in water alone, and ^{18}O is lost in water and as $C^{18}O_2$ in breath. The difference between the two tracer excretion rates, therefore, represents the CO_2 production rate (see figure 3.7). With the knowledge of the fuel mixture oxidized, energy expenditure can be calculated.

Figure 3.7 Doubly labeled water technique. Excretion of ^2H and ^{18}O occurs at different rates. The more rapid the drop in ^{18}O relative to the drop in ^2H, the higher the energy expenditure.

The main advantage of this technique is that it does not interfere with everyday life, and unbiased measurements of a free-living situation can be obtained. In addition, measurements can be conducted over prolonged periods of time, and, therefore, the values can be used to estimate the typical daily energy expenditure and, in turn, the energy needs of a free-living individual. The main disadvantages of the technique are the expense, the limited availability of the tracer, and the need for sophisticated equipment (mass spectrometer) to measure the isotopes. This method is only suitable for relatively long-term (days or weeks) estimation of energy expenditure.

Labeled Bicarbonate

Another method based on stable isotopes is the infusion of labeled bicarbonate (^{14}C or ^{13}C). When $H^{13}CO_3$ or $H^{14}CO_3$ (the latter is radioactive) is infused at a constant rate, it eventually reaches equilibrium with the body's CO_2 pool, after which, any change in the body's CO_2 production will result in a change in the percentage of labeled CO_2. The change in this so-called enrichment is, therefore, a direct indication of the total CO_2 production. This value can be used to calculate energy expenditure in a manner similar to the doubly labeled water technique. Samples are collected from expired gases, and tiny portions are needed for the analysis. Because $H^{13}CO_3$ has to be infused, this technique can only be applied for short periods of time (hours and, under some conditions, days). The bicarbonate labeling technique is relatively inexpensive but still requires sophisticated equipment and expertise.

Heart Rate Monitoring

To avoid some of the problems associated with the measurement of energy expenditure during free-living physical activity, various less complicated (and less accurate) methods have been developed. One of these methods is based on heart rate (HR), because of its linear relationship with oxygen uptake at submaximal exercise intensities. At very low and very high exercise intensities (supramaximal), this estimation is less reliable. To use HR for the estimation of energy expenditure, the individual relationship between HR and $\dot{V}O_2$ (and EE) must be determined. Measurements of oxygen uptake can then be used to calculate energy expenditure at several different HRs. The main limitation of the use of HR for measuring energy expenditure is the almost flat slope of the relationship at low levels of energy expenditure. At rest, slight movements can increase HR, while energy expenditure (i.e., oxygen consumption) remains almost the same. Emotions (e.g., anger or anxiety) may also cause HR to rise at rest with little or no change in oxygen uptake.

Although the HR method provides satisfactory estimates of average EE for a group, it is not necessarily accurate for individual subjects. For instance, Spurr et al. (1988) compared 24 hours of EE by calorimetry with EE by the HR method in 22 subjects. The maximum deviations of the values of EE between the two methods varied between +20% and –15% in individuals, but when the methods were compared statistically, no differences were found.

Also, the HR-$\dot{V}O_2$ relationship is influenced by several factors, including environmental conditions (temperature and humidity), altitude, body position, static (isometric) exercise, anxiety (at low-work rates), and so on. Nevertheless, in some conditions HR can provide a very convenient and relatively cheap estimate of energy expenditure.

Accelerometer

Another way of estimating activity level is through accelerometry. Accelerometers are small devices that can be attached to the body and register all accelerations the body makes. The number and the degree of the accelerations give an indication of activity level. Accelerometers can record accelerations along 1, 2, or 3 axes. A single-axis, or single-plane, accelerometer measures only acceleration in the vertical direction. Triaxial accelerometers measure accelerations along 3 axes and are likely to be more accurate. Generally, accelerometer readings (usually expressed as activity counts or in kJ [kcal]) correlate well with energy expenditure. However, for some movements, especially those in free-living conditions, the accelerometer tends to underestimate the true energy expenditure.

In the future, combined HR and accelerometer data may be used to estimate energy expenditure. Initial studies show promising results for simultaneous HR and motion measurements. Given the low weight and compactness of modern accelerometers, this instrument provides a very convenient and easy method of getting an estimation of activity level in a free-living situation. The disadvantage is of course that measurement provided is just a rough estimation (or indication) of the energy expenditure.

Activity Records

Activity records, physical activity diaries, or physical activity recall instruments are used to record activities during a 24-hour period, and from this information a rough estimation of the daily energy expenditure is obtained. Most of the existing questionnaires measure only some types of activities and may, therefore, not always be very accurate when used on an individual basis. Some individuals have a tendency to overestimate their physical activity, whereas others underestimate it. However, average physical activity scores reflecting a long-term period can be estimated satisfactorily using self-administered questionnaires.

Components of Energy Expenditure

Energy is needed for different processes in the body, including basal functions, digestion, absorption metabolism, and storage of food. In addition, active individuals expend energy during exercise. The three components, **resting metabolic rate,** diet-induced thermogenesis, and exercise-related energy expenditure will be discussed in this section.

Resting Metabolic Rate

The largest component (60% to 75%) of the daily energy expenditure (average daily metabolic rate, or ADMR) in a relatively inactive person is the resting metabolic rate (RMR), the energy required for the maintenance of normal body functions and homeostasis in resting conditions. Factors such as sympathetic nervous system activity, thyroid hormone activity, and sodium-potassium pump activity contribute to the RMR. Another measure is the basal metabolic rate (BMR). This test was developed for patients with thyroid disease and aimed at measuring the lowest oxygen uptake in resting thermoneutral conditions. Measurements were performed in the morning after a 12-hour to 18-hour fast. This measurement was inconvenient for many patients, and metabolism was affected because patients were disturbed in their sleep. Therefore, RMR has become the more popular measure, and the BMR is not often measured anymore. The RMR is primarily related to the fat-free mass (muscle mass) and is influenced by age, gender, body composition, and genetic factors. RMR seems to decrease with age (2% to 3% per decade), and males generally have a higher RMR than females (because of their larger body size). The following is a glossary of the most common abbreviations used in relation to energy expenditure:

ADMR—Average daily metabolic rate

BMR—Basal metabolic rate

RMR—Resting metabolic rate

REE—Resting energy expenditure (= RMR)

TEF—Thermic effect of food

DIT—Diet-induced thermogenesis

TEE—Thermic effect of exercise

EEA—Energy expenditure for physical activity

Diet-Induced Thermogenesis

The **diet-induced thermogenesis** (DIT), or thermic effect of food (TEF), is the increase in energy expenditure above RMR that occurs for several hours after ingestion of a meal. DIT is the result of digestion, absorption, metabolizing, and storage of food and normally represents about 10% of the total daily energy expenditure. The magnitude of the DIT depends on several factors, including the energy content of the food and the size and composition of the meal. DIT also depends on the metabolic fate of the ingested substrate. The cost of storing fat in adipose tissue is approximately 3% of the energy of the ingested meal, whereas if carbohydrate is stored as glycogen, about 7% of the energy is lost. The energy cost for the synthesis and breakdown of protein is approximately 24% of the available energy. Energy expenditure can be increased up to 8 hours. The sympathetic nervous system seems to play an important role in DIT. When the effects of the sympathetic nervous system are reduced by administering a β-adrenergic blocker (for instance, propanolol), DIT is also reduced. With increasing age, a small decline occurs in the DIT, possibly associated with a decrease in insulin sensitivity.

Thermic Effect of Exercise

The **thermic effect of exercise** (TEE), or energy expenditure for activity (EEA), is by far the most variable component of the daily energy expenditure. It includes all energy expended above the RER and DIT. The TEE often has a voluntary component (exercise) and an involuntary component (shivering, fidgeting, or postural control). In highly trained, very active individuals, the TEE can amount up to 32 MJ/day (8,000 kcal/day). In sedentary people, the TEE may be as low as 400 kJ/day (100 kcal/day). Figure 3.8 compares the various components of daily energy expenditure in a sedentary individual and an endurance athlete involved in heavy training. TEE can vary from an average of 30% of the daily energy expen-

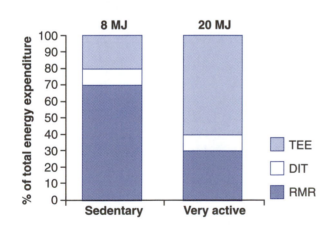

Figure 3.8 Energy expenditure and the relative contribution of its different components in a sedentary individual (energy expenditure 8 MJ/day or 2,000 kcal/day) and an athlete involved in heavy training (energy expenditure 20 MJ/day or 5,000 kcal/day). RMR = resting metabolic rate; DIT = diet-induced thermogenesis; TEE = energy expenditure during exercise.

diture up to 80% in extreme conditions during very heavy endurance training or competition. Exercise is, therefore, extremely important for the maintenance of the daily energy balance. It is not only the most variable component of 24-hour energy expenditure but also the component that can be controlled voluntarily.

Energy Balance

The energy balance is usually calculated over longer periods of time (days or weeks) and represents the difference between energy intake and energy expenditure. When the energy intake exceeds the energy expenditure, the energy balance is positive and will result in weight gain. When the energy intake is below the energy expenditure, the energy balance is negative and weight loss will result. Over the long term, energy balance is maintained in weight-stable individuals even though on a day-to-day basis this balance may be either positive and or negative. Individuals who want to lose weight should increase the energy expenditure relative to the energy intake.

In many activities in which body composition or body weight is believed to be important (gymnastics, dancing, body building, and weight category sports such as judo and boxing) participants often try to maintain a negative energy balance to lose weight. Thus, the energy intakes in these activities can be very low (see chapter 11). At the other extreme are endurance sports such as triathlon, cycling, cross-country skiing, and ultraendurance running that require extremely high energy expenditures and energy intakes. In these sports, maintaining energy balance on a day-to-day basis is crucial for performance. Both the upper and the lower limits of energy expenditure are discussed in the following sections.

Table 3.2 depicts the daily energy intake of a large number of Dutch elite female and male athletes in various sports. The data show that females generally have lower energy intakes than males. For females, energy intake ranged between 5.1 MJ (1,600 kcal) and 10.2 MJ (3,200 kcal). For males, energy intake ranged between 12.1 MJ (2,900 kcal) and 24.7 MJ (5,900 kcal). These differences in energy intake may be related to body size and weight, to body composition, and to the number of hours spent training on a daily basis. Athletes in team sports have a moderate energy intake, whereas some of the endurance athletes have very high energy intakes. In fact, only in endurance sports were energy intakes in excess of 12.6 MJ (3,000 kcal) for females and 16.7 MJ (4,000 kcal) for males.

Table 3.2 Energy Intake in Various Sports

Sports	Gender	Body mass in kg (lb)	kJ/kg	kcal/kg	MJ	kcal
Tour de France	m	70.8 (155.8)	347	83	24.6	5869
Tour de l'Avenir	m	73.7 (162.1)	316	75	23.3	5564
Triathlon	m	70.2 (154.4)	272	65	19.1	4561
Cycling, amateur	m	72.3 (159.1)	253	60	18.3	4370
Marathon speed skating	m	72.3 (159.1)	222	53	16.1	3834
Swimming	m	72.9 (160.4)	221	53	16.1	3849
Rowing	m	77.2 (169.8)	189	45	14.6	3486
Running	m	68.8 (151.4)	193	46	13.3	3172
Rowing	f	69.8 (153.6)	186	44	13.0	3101
Cycling, amateur	f	66.0 (145.2)	164	39	10.8	2586
Running	f	52.1 (114.6)	168	40	8.8	2091
Subtop swimming	f	43.6 (95.9)	200	48	8.7	2083
Bodybuilding	m	87.3 (192.1)	157	38	13.7	3274
Judo	m	82.5 (181.5)	157	38	13.0	3094
Weightlifting	m	76.4 (168.1)	167	40	12.8	3048
Judo	m	68.7 (151.1)	177	42	12.2	2905
Top gymnastics	f	46.9 (103.2)	158	38	7.4	1770
Subtop gymnastics	f	39.8 (87.6)	206	49	8.2	1959
Bodybuilding	f	56.0 (123.2)	110	26	6.2	1472
Water polo	m	85.5 (188.1)	194	46	16.6	3962
Soccer	m	74.5 (163.9)	192	46	14.3	3417
Hockey	m	75.0 (165.0)	181	43	13.6	3243
Volleyball	f	66.0 (145.2)	140	33	9.2	2207
Hockey	f	62.1 (136.6)	145	35	9.0	2151
Handball	f	63.2 (139.0)	142	34	9.0	2144

m = males; f = females.

International Journal of Sports Medicine: From Van Erp-Baart, W.H. Saris, R.A. Binkhorst, J.A. Vos, and J.W. Elvers, "Nationwide survey on nutritional habits in elite athletes," 1989, Vol. 10: 53-510. Reprinted by permission.

Energy Balance in Different Activities

Some physical activities require higher energy outputs than others, as shown in tables 3.3 and 3.4. Tennis, for example, has relatively low energy expenditure if played recreationally and could be classified as a light-to-moderate activity. Although during a game, the exercise can sometimes be very intense and energy expenditure during that short burst of intense exercise can be very high. However, because this high intensity is typically followed by a longer period of relatively low intensity (walking) or even standing, the average energy expenditure for this activity is relatively low. Tennis played at a high level will have shorter periods of rest, and the average intensity is much higher. On the other hand, in continuous sports such as cycling and running, in which there is usually little or no recovery during the activity, energy expenditures can be relatively high.

Lower Limits of Energy Expenditure

Female gymnasts, ballet dancers, and ice dancers often have energy intakes as low as 4 MJ (1,000 kcal) to 8 MJ (2,000 kcal). In some cases, this intake is only 1.2 to 1.4 times the RMR, which is lower than sedentary people who, on average, expend 1.4 to 1.6 times the RMR, despite the fact that these athletes

Table 3.3　Energy Costs of Different Activities

Activity	(kJ/min)	(kcal/min)	Examples
Resting	4	1	Sleeping, reclining while watching TV
Very light activities	12–20	3–5	Sitting and standing activities, driving, cooking, card playing, typing
Light activities	20–28	5–7	Walking (3 km/h to 5 km/h), baseball, bowling, horseback riding, golf
Moderate activities	28–36	7–9	Jogging, basketball, badminton, soccer, tennis, volleyball, walking (7 km/h to 8 km/h)
Strenuous activities	36–52	9–13	Running at 10 km/h to13 km/h, cross-country skiing (8 km/h to 10 km/h)
Very strenuous activities	>52	>13	Cycling at 35 km/h, running at >14 km/h, cross-country skiing >12 km/h

Table 3.4　Estimated Energy Cost of Activities in KiloJoules per Minute (Kilocalories per Minute)

	Body weight				
Activity	50 kg (110 lb)	60 kg (132 lb)	70 kg (154 lb)	80 kg (176 lb)	90 kg (198 lb)
Aerobics					
Beginners	22　(5.5)	26　(6.5)	30　(7.5)	34　(8.5)	39　(9.8)
Advanced	28　(7.0)	33　(8.3)	40 (10.0)	45 (11.3)	51 (12.8)
Badminton	20　(5.0)	24　(8.0)	28　(7.0)	33　(8.3)	37　(9.3)
Ballroom dancing	11　(2.8)	13　(3.3)	15　(3.8)	17　(4.3)	19　(4.8)
Basketball	29　(7.2)	35　(8.8)	40 (10.0)	46 (11.5)	52 (13.0)
Boxing					
Sparring in ring	46 (11.5)	56 (14.0)	65 (16.3)	74 (18.5)	84 (21.0)
	29　(7.2)	35　(8.8)	40 (10.0)	46 (11.5)	52 (13.0)
Canoeing					
Leisure	9　(2.3)	11　(2.8)	13　(3.3)	15　(3.8)	17　(4.3)
Racing	22　(5.5)	26　(6.5)	30　(7.5)	34　(8.5)	39　(9.8)
Circuit training	22　(5.5)	26　(6.5)	30　(7.5)	34　(8.5)	40 (10.0)
Cricket					
Batting	17　(4.3)	21　(5.3)	24　(6.0)	28　(7.0)	32　(8.0)
Bowling	19　(4.8)	22　(5.5)	26　(6.5)	30　(7.5)	34　(8.5)
Cycling					
9 km/h	13　(3.3)	16　(4.0)	18　(4.5)	21　(5.3)	24　(6.0)
15 km/h	21　(5.3)	24　(8.0)	28　(7.0)	33　(8.3)	38　(9.5)
racing	35　(8.8)	42 (10.5)	49 (12.3)	56 (14.0)	63　(5.8)
Football	28　(7.0)	33　(8.3)	39　(9.8)	44 (11.0)	50 (12.5)
Golf	18　(4.5)	21　(5.5)	25　(6.3)	28　(7.0)	32　(8.0)
Gymnastics	14　(3.5)	16　(4.0)	19　(4.8)	22　(5.5)	25　(6.3)
Hockey	18　(4.5)	20　(5.0)	24　(6.0)	29　(7.3)	33　(8.3)

(continued)

Table 3.4 (continued)

Activity	Body weight				
	50 kg (110 lb)	60 kg (132 lb)	70 kg (154 lb)	80 kg (176 lb)	90 kg (198 lb)
Judo	41 (10.3)	49 (12.3)	57 (14.3)	65 (16.3)	73 (18.3)
Running					
5.5 min/km	40 (10.0)	49 (12.3)	57 (14.3)	65 (16.3)	73 (18.3)
5 min/km	44 (11.0)	52 (13.0)	61 (15.3)	70 (17.5)	78 (19.5)
4.5 min/km	48 (12.0)	55 (13.8)	65 (16.3)	75 (18.8)	85 (21.3)
4 min/km	54 (13.5)	65 (16.3)	76 (19.0)	87 (21.8)	98 (24.5)
Skiing					
Cross-country	35 (8.8)	42 (10.5)	49 (12.3)	56 (14.0)	63 (15.8)
Down hill (easy)	18 (4.5)	21 (5.5)	25 (6.3)	29 (7.3)	33 (8.3)
Down hill (hard)	29 (7.3)	35 (8.8)	40 (10.0)	49 (12.3)	55 (13.8)
Squash	44 (11.0)	53 (13.3)	62 (15.5)	71 (17.8)	79 (19.8)
Swimming					
Freestyle	33 (8.3)	40 (10.0)	46 (11.5)	52 (13.0)	59 (14.8)
Backstroke	36 (9.0)	43 (10.8)	49 (12.3)	56 (14.0)	63 (15.8)
Breaststroke	34 (8.5)	41 (10.3)	47 (11.8)	54 (13.5)	61 (15.3)
Table tennis	14 (3.5)	17 (4.3)	19 (4.8)	23 (5.8)	26 (6.5)
Tennis					
Social	15 (3.8)	17 (4.3)	20 (5.0)	23 (5.8)	26 (6.5)
Competitive	37 (9.3)	44 (11.0)	50 (12.5)	58 (14.5)	65 (16.3)
Volleyball	10 (2.5)	12 (3.0)	15 (3.6)	17 (4.3)	19 (4.8)
Walking					
10 min/km	21 (5.3)	26 (6.5)	30 (7.5)	35 (8.8)	39 (9.8)
8 min/km	25 (6.3)	30 (7.5)	35 (8.8)	40 (10.0)	45 (11.3)
5 min/km	44 (11.0)	52 (13.0)	61 (15.3)	70 (17.5)	78 (19.5)

Note: All figures are approximate values only.

Adapted from F.I. Katch and W.O. McArdle, 1990, Recommended nutrient intakes, NHMRC: Australia. In *Nutrition, Weight Control, and Exercise* (Philadelphia, PA: Lea and Febiger).

and dancers may be involved in 3 hours to 4 hours of training a day. Although not all the time gymnasts and dancers spend in the gym or in the dance studio is high-intensity training, the metabolic rate is still expected to be higher, compared with the average sedentary individual. The food records of members of this group, who are striving for low body weight, may not be accurate and may represent an underestimation of the true energy intake. However, even when the reported intakes are corrected for this underestimation, the energy intakes are still very low. The lower limits of energy expenditure are determined by the sum of RMR, DIT, and a minimum of physical activity. The DIT is directly affected by the amount of food consumed. Reducing food intake will result in a decreased DIT, and it may also indirectly influence the RMR. One of the problems associated with reducing energy intake to very low levels is the possibility of marginal nutrition, particularly of essential nutrients such as fat-soluble vitamins, calcium, iron, and essential FAs. (See chapter 11.)

Upper Limits of Energy Expenditure

Energy-related problems in endurance sports are totally different from the problems discussed above. Well-trained endurance athletes can expend more than 4 MJ/h (1,000 kcal/h) for prolonged periods of time, resulting in very high daily energy expenditures. To maintain performance, energy stores must be replenished and energy balance must be restored, which means that these athletes must eat very large amounts in periods of heavy training or competition.

Scientists have studied whether an upper limit to human energy expenditure exists. The highest values reported are from sports such as cycling, triathlon, cross-country skiing, and ultraendurance running. The Tour de France is a 3-week, 20-stage cycling event in which the cyclists cover approximately 3,500 km, including various mountain stages. On some days, the cyclists spend up to 8 hours on their bicycles. Average energy expenditure in the Tour de France reached values of 24 MJ (6,000 kcal) when measured in weekly intervals. The highest recorded average energy intake during the entire 3 weeks of the Tour de France was 36 MJ/day (9,000 kcal/day) (see figure 3.9). Athletes involved in sports with such extreme energy expenditures on a daily basis face the problem of consuming large quantities if they want to maintain their body weight and performance. Figure 3.9 shows that generally such consumption is possible, but on days with very high energy expenditures, the cyclists tend to have a negative energy balance of about 4 MJ (1,000 kcal).

Thus, these cyclists do not face an easy task, because they have to consume an enormous amount of energy (mostly in the form of carbohydrate) to maintain energy balance. This requirement is often problematic for several reasons:

- Time for eating is limited, making consumption of large amounts of food during the 3-hour to 7-hour race difficult.
- Hunger feelings may be depressed for several hours after strenuous exercise.
- Especially during the last week of the Tour de France, gastrointestinal problems often make absorbing large quantities of food more difficult or even impossible.

Nevertheless, hardly any changes in body weight occur among participants during the Tour de France, indicating that these cyclists are indeed able to maintain energy balance. On the other hand, perhaps the cyclists who do not maintain their body weight drop out.

Although eating large amounts during the race is difficult, energy intake in the form of carbohydrate solutions has been shown to be crucial. During 2 days of high-intensity cycling, when 26 MJ (6,000 kcal) of energy expenditure were not supplemented with carbohydrate during the rides, cyclists were not able to maintain energy balance (5 to 10 MJ [1,200 to 2,400 kcal] negative energy balance). When the cyclists were given a 20% carbohydrate solution during exercise, from which they could drink as much as they liked, energy balance was maintained.

In some sports, even higher 24-hour energy expenditures may be reached. Using doubly labeled water, similar estimates of energy expenditure were made in Norwegian cross-country skiers during training. Energy expenditure amounted up to 36 MJ/day (8,600 kcal/day). A case report indicated that an ultraendurance runner expended 134 MJ (55,970 kcal) during a 1,000-km (600 mile) running race. The athlete ran for 5 days and 5 hours, during which he averaged an energy expenditure of 45 MJ/day (10,750 kcal/day). Interestingly, in both cases, the athletes' food intake was extremely high and almost matched the energy expenditure.

Figure 3.9 Energy balance during the Tour de France.

From A.M. Van Erp-Baart, W.H. Saris, R.A. Binkhorst, J.A. Vos, and J.W. Elvers, "Study on food intake and energy expenditure during the Tour de France," *International Journal of Sports Medicine* 1989, Vol. 10: S26-S31. Reprinted by permission.

Key Points

■ All biologic functions require energy, and although the human body has some energy reserves most of the energy must be obtained through nutrition.

■ Energy is the capacity to do work. The various forms of energy include light energy, chemical energy, heat, and electrical energy.

■ Energy is often expressed in calories (English system) or Joules (metric system) where 1 calorie equals 4.186 Joules.

■ Efficiency describes the effective work performed after muscle contraction and is usually expressed as the percentage of total work. Humans are approximately 20% efficient.

■ Gross efficiency (GE) is the ratio of the total work accomplished to the energy expended. Because resting metabolism is not accounted for, corrections have been made by subtracting baseline energy expenditure from the total energy expenditure. Net efficiency, work efficiency, and delta efficiency each take resting energy expenditure into account.

■ The energy content of 1 g of carbohydrate is 17.6 kJ (4.2 kcal). Fat contains between 36.0 kJ/g (8.6 kcal/g) and 40.2 kJ/g (9.6 kcal/g) (on average, about 39.3 kJ/g [9.4 kcal/g]), and protein contains about 23.7 kJ/g (5.65 kcal/g). The coefficient of digestibility represents the proportion of consumed food actually digested and absorbed by the body.

■ Coefficients of digestibility average about 97% for carbohydrates, 95% for lipids, and 92% for proteins. The net energy values of carbohydrate, fat, and protein are, therefore, 16 kJ (4 kcal), 36 kJ (9 kcal), and 16 kJ (4 kcal), respectively, and these are referred to as the Atwater energy values or Atwater factors.

■ Ways to measure (or estimate) human energy expenditure range from direct but complex measurements of heat production (direct calorimetry), to relatively simple indirect metabolic measurements (indirect calorimetry), to very expensive tracer methods (doubly labeled water), to relatively cheap and convenient rough estimations of energy expenditure (heart rate monitoring and accelerometry).

■ Human energy expenditure can be divided into different components: resting metabolic rate, thermic effect of food, and exercise-related energy expenditure. RMR is the largest component (60% to 75%) of the daily energy expenditure in relatively sedentary people, and the thermic effect of food represents about 10%, leaving 15% to 30% for exercise-related energy expenditure.

■ Respiratory exchange measurements can be used to calculate energy expenditure, as well as the contributions of carbohydrate and fat to energy expenditure.

■ The energy balance is usually calculated over longer periods of time (days or weeks) and represents the difference between energy intake and energy expenditure. When the energy intake exceeds the energy expenditure, a positive energy balance occurs, which will result in weight gain. When the energy intake is below the energy expenditure, a negative energy balance occurs, and weight loss will result.

■ Female gymnasts, ballet dancers, and ice dancers often have energy intakes between 4 MJ (1,000 kcal) and 8 MJ (2,000 kcal). In some cases this is only 1.2 to 1.4 times the resting metabolic rate. Such low energy intakes can result in nutritional deficiency.

■ Cycling, triathlon, and ultraendurance running are sports with energy expenditures as high as 36 MJ/day (8,600 kcal/day).

Key Terms

Atwater factor 64

diet-induced thermogenesis (DIT) 72

economy 63

efficiency 62

energy 62

energy balance 68

energy expenditure (EE) 62

respiratory exchange ratio 66

resting metabolic rate (RMR) 72

thermic effect of exercise (TEE) 73

Recommended Readings

Burke, L.M. 2001. Energy Needs of Athletes. *Canadian Journal of Applied Physiology* 26(suppl):S202-S219.

Roche, A.F., S.B. Heymsfield, and T.G. Lohman. 1996. *Human Body Composition*. Human Kinetics: Champaign, IL.

Chapter 4

Gastric Emptying, Digestion, and Absorption

© Sport the Library

Objectives

After studying this chapter, you should be able to do the following:

- Describe the functions of the gastrointestinal system and list its anatomical components and structures

- Describe the digestion processes of carbohydrate, fat, and protein

- Describe the absorption processes of carbohydrate, fat, and protein

- Describe the absorption process of water

- Describe the absorption processes of vitamins and minerals

- Describe the factors that regulate gastric emptying

- State the approximate transit times within each compartment of the gastrointestinal tract

- Describe the effects of exercise on gastric emptying and absorption

- Describe the gastrointestinal problems that may occur during exercise and know which factors may augment or reduce these problems

The primary function of the gastrointestinal (or alimentary) tract is to provide the body with nutrients, water, and electrolytes from ingested foodstuffs. When food moves through the gastrointestinal tract (see figure 4.1), it is broken down into very small units that can be absorbed in a process called **digestion. Absorption** (i.e., the transport of nutrients from the intestine into the blood or lymph system) takes place in various parts of the gastrointestinal tract for different nutrients. Here, we give an overview of the anatomy and physiology of the gastrointestinal tract, the various digestion and absorption processes that take place within it, and the changes that occur during exercise.

Organ	Function
Mouth	Mechanical digestion
Salivary glands	Secretion of fluid and digestive enzymes
Stomach	Secretion of HCl and protein-digesting enzymes (proteases)
Pancreas	Secretion of $NaHCO_3$ and digestive enzymes
Liver	Secretion of bile
Gallbladder	Temporary storage and concentration of bile
Small intestine	Digestion of food, absorption of water, nutrients, and electrolytes
Large intestine	Absorption of electrolytes

Figure 4.1 Major functions of different parts of the gastrointestinal tract.

Anatomy of the Gastrointestinal Tract

The gastrointestinal tract is a long tubular structure that reaches from the mouth to the anus and includes the esophagus, stomach, small intestine, large intestine, rectum and anus and several accessory digestive glands including the salivary glands, gall bladder, liver, and pancreas (see figure 4.2). In this 6 m to 8 m tube, digestion of food and absorption of nutrients takes place. The mouth and stomach, pancreas, and gall bladder have a predominantly digestive function, and most of the absorption occurs in the small and large intestine. After absorption, most nutrients are transported to the liver, and from there they enter the main circulation.

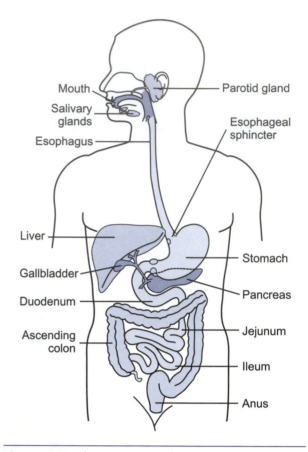

Figure 4.2 The gastrointestinal tract.

Mouth

Chewing (or masticating) of food is the first step of digestion. It is often referred to as mechanical digestion. The anterior teeth or incisors provide a very strong cutting action, and the posterior teeth (molars) are used for grinding. The forces applied to cut and grind the food can be as much as 25 kg on the incisors and 90 kg on the molars. Chewing of food serves three major purposes: (1) It mechanically makes the food particles smaller, which increases the rate of **gastric emptying.** (2) It increases the surface area of the food, which, in turn, increases the contact area for digestive enzymes that are released from the salivary glands and stomach (enzymatic digestion). Increasing the total surface area of the food increases the rate of digestion. (3) It mixes the food particles with saliva and digestive enzymes. The mouth has 3 pairs of salivary glands: the parotid glands, the sublingual glands, and the submandibular glands (see figure 4.3). Chewing is especially important for plant material (fruits and raw vegetables) because undigestible cellulose cell walls must be mechanically destroyed to release the nutrients.

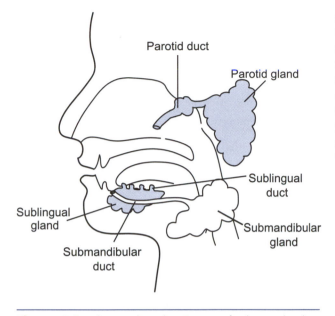

Figure 4.3 The mouth and its 3 pairs of salivary glands.

Esophagus

When the food is small and soft enough to swallow, it moves past the pharynx at the back of the mouth into the esophagus. The esophagus moves the food particles to the stomach. This transport process is caused by rhythmic contractions and relaxations of the esophagus. The esophagus contains an inner layer of smooth muscle consisting of circular bands and an outer layer of smooth muscle that runs longitudinally. Contraction of these muscles causes the peristalsis, a squeezing action involving progressive and recurring contractions, which mixes and moves the food to the stomach. This mechanism makes swallowing possible even when a person is hanging upside down or in space with zero gravity.

At the end of the esophagus, a valve of smooth muscle called the esophageal sphincter relaxes to allow food into the stomach. After some food particles have passed the esophageal sphincter, it contracts, preventing reflux of food or fluids from the stomach into the esophagus. People in whom this sphincter does not function properly may experience some acid leaking from the stomach, or heartburn. This gastrointestinal problem is common among runners and cyclists.

Stomach

The stomach, which is about 20 cm to 25 cm long, is divided in three parts (see figure 4.4): the corpus, or body, the antrum, and the fundus. The corpus

and the antrum have different physiological functions. Although the fundus is a different part of the stomach from an anatomical point of view, from a functional point of view it is considered part of the corpus. The end of the stomach is a circular valve called the pyloric sphincter (pylorus), which controls the emptying of food from the stomach into the small intestine. When this muscle relaxes, food leaves the stomach; when it contracts, food stays in the stomach. The functions of the stomach include

- storage of large quantities of food until it can be accommodated in the intestine,
- mixing of this food with gastric secretions to form a homogeneous, acidic, souplike liquid or a paste called **chyme,** and
- regulation of the emptying of the chyme into the duodenum (upper part of the small intestine) at a rate suitable for proper digestion and absorption.

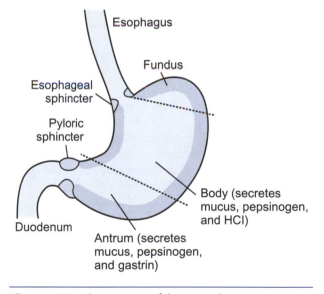

Figure 4.4 The anatomy of the stomach.

Normally, food that enters the stomach forms concentric circles in the corpus and fundus so that the latest food is closest to the esophagus and the oldest food nearest to the wall of the corpus. The stomach volume is normally around 1.5 L. However, this volume can change from almost nothing when the stomach is empty to about 6 L when the stomach is full. The muscular tone of the stomach wall decreases as soon as food enters the stomach, which allows the stomach wall to stretch outward to accommodate more food.

The wall of the corpus contains gastric glands that secrete digestive juices. These secretions come in contact with the food portions nearest to the stomach wall. The stomach can also contract and relax, which mixes the food into chyme. Chyme can be a fluid or a paste, depending on the relative amounts of food and secretions and the degree of digestion. The chyme is passed down to the small intestine by a strictly controlled process of gastric emptying. Very little absorption takes place in the stomach (with the exception of some water and alcohol).

Small Intestine

The small intestine is approximately 2 m to 3 m in length and 3 cm to 5 cm in diameter, and it can be divided into the duodenum (about 30 cm), the jejunum (next 1 m to 2 m), and the ileum (last 1 m). About 95% of all absorption takes place in the duodenum and jejunum. The intestinal mucosa of the duodenum and jejunum contains many folds called the folds of Kerkring (see figure 4.5). These folds increase the surface area of the intestine about three times that of a similarly sized flat internal lining. These folds are covered by millions of small fingerlike structures called villi, which project about 1 mm from the surface of the mucosa (see figure 4.6). The villi increase the total surface area of the small intestine another 10-fold. The intestinal cells that form the border of the villi are covered by a **brush border** consisting of about 600 microvilli approximately 1 μm long. These microvilli increase the total surface area a further 20-fold. The highly specialized construction of the small

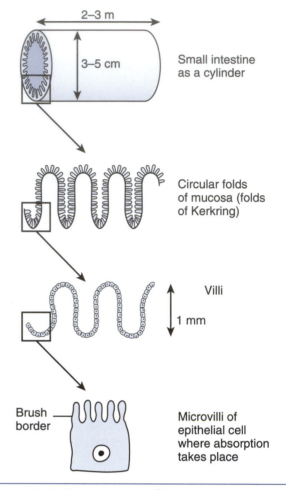

Figure 4.5 The organization of the small intestine increases the surface area about 600-fold over a simple tube with a flat internal surface.

Figure 4.6 Functional organization of the villus.

intestine, including the folds of Kerkring, the villi, and the microvilli, increases the absorption about 600-fold compared with a simple tube with a flat internal surface. The total surface area of the small intestine may be as large as 250 m².

ward before it advances. The function of these circular contractions is to mix the chyme with bile from the gall bladder, pancreatic juices, and intestinal juices. The juices get extra time to digest the food, and the contact time and area are increased.

Villi

Villi are finger-shaped and highly vascularized (see figure 4.6). The wall of a villus consists of a layer of epithelial cells, each with its own brush border. Water, water-soluble particles, and electrolytes require transport or diffusion across the luminal and contraluminal membrane of the epithelial cell into the blood vessels. These nutrients are then transported to the liver via the hepatic portal vein. Each villus also contains a lacteal, which is located in the central part of a villus. The lacteal transports particles that are not readily water soluble (e.g., long-chain FAs) via the lymphatic vessels. These vessels drain into large veins near the heart.

Gall Bladder

The gall bladder stores, concentrates, and releases bile. Bile, which is produced by liver cells, consists of water, electrolytes, bile salts, cholesterol, lecithin, and bilirubin. The gall bladder can store approximately 30 ml to 60 ml, but it secretes as much as 1,200 ml into the duodenum every day. The gall bladder stores up to 12 hours of bile secretion by concentrating the bile constituents. Bile facilitates the digestion and absorption of fat and is released through the hepatic duct, which joins the pancreatic duct just before entering the duodenum (see figure 4.7). Bile secretion is increased after a meal, especially when the meal contains a large amount of fat.

Motility and Transit Time

Food spends one day to three days in the gastrointestinal tract before it is eliminated. The time spent in a section of the gastrointestinal tract is the **transit time.** For instance, the transit time in the small intestine is approximately 3 hours to 10 hours, depending on the composition of the food and the **motility** (movement of food) of the gastrointestinal tract. The small intestine wall contains two layers of smooth muscle with longitudinal and circular muscle fibers that allows peristalsis and mixing contractions that push the chyme in the distal direction toward the large intestine (like squeezing toothpaste out of a tube). These contractions occur at a rate of 0.5 cm/s to 2.0 cm/s, with fastest movement in the proximal intestine and slowest movement in the distal intestine. The average speed of chyme along the small intestine is approximately 1 cm/s.

Peristalsis is increased after a meal and can be greatly increased after intense irritation of the intestinal mucosa, such as during infectious diarrhea. Mixing, or segmentation, contractions differ from peristalsis. The circular muscles contract, giving the small intestine the look of linked sausages. These intermittent contractions (8/min to 12/min) cause the chyme to move both forward and backward. The chyme moves back-

Pancreas

The pancreas is a large gland situated parallel to and just beneath the stomach (see figure 4.2 and 4.7). It secretes sodium bicarbonate to buffer the hydrochloric acid of the stomach and digestive enzymes to break down carbohydrate, protein, and fat. Pancreatic juice is mainly secreted in response to chyme in the upper portions of the small intestine. The regulatory mechanisms for sodium bicarbonate secretion and digestive enzyme secretion are different, and the secretion rate is highly dependent on the

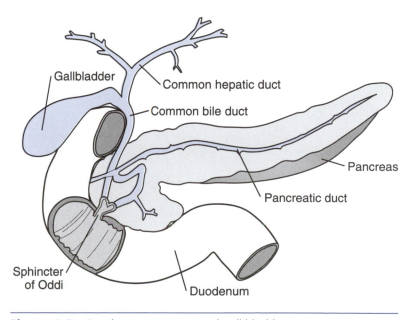

Figure 4.7 Duodenum, pancreas, and gall bladder.

type and amount of food ingested. The concentration of various enzymes in pancreatic juice to some extent is also dependent on the type of food ingested.

Ileocecal Valve

From the small intestine, the chyme moves into the large intestine through the ileocecal valve (see figure 4.8). This valve prevents backflow of undigestible fecal material into the small intestine. The valve can resist pressure equal to about 50 cm to 60 cm of water. The distal end of the small intestine, or ileum, has a thicker muscular coat that determines the emptying from the ileum. Contraction of the ileocecal sphincter is regulated by a variety of factors, including (1) distension of the cecum (a blind pouch, open only at one end, at the beginning of the large intestine), (2) irritating substances in the cecum, and (3) fluidity of the chyme. An inflamed appendix (a nonfunctional part of the intestine that is short, thin, and outpouching from the cecum) will restrict the emptying of the ileum. An increased fluidity of chyme, on the other hand, will increase emptying from the ileum.

Large Intestine

In the large intestine, the chyme is called feces. The large intestine consists of the colon, the rectum, and the anal canal. The colon is usually divided into the ascending colon, the transverse colon, the descending colon, and the sigmoid colon (see figure 4.8). The functions of the colon are (1) absorption of water and electrolytes from the chyme and (2) storage of feces until they can be expelled. Absorption takes place mainly in the first part of the colon, and storage mainly occurs in the distal parts. The peristaltic movements of the colon are slower than those of the small intestine. The colon also has circular and longitudinal smooth muscle layers and moves the feces towards the distal parts of the colon by rhythmic contractions. The fecal material is slowly rolled over and mixed so that the contact with the surface of the large intestine is increased and as much water as possible is absorbed. Normally only 80 ml to 150 ml of water are present in approximately 300 ml of the feces.

Regulation of the Gastrointestinal Tract

The gastrointestinal tract is innervated by both the sympathetic and parasympathetic components of the autonomic nervous system. Parasympathetic stimulation in general stimulates motility. The vagus nerve is the source of parasympathetic activity in the esophagus, stomach, pancreas, gall bladder, small intestine, and upper section of the large intestine. The lower portion of the large intestine receives parasympathetic innervation from spinal nerves in the sacral region (the lower end of the spine). Autonomic regulation, which is "extrinsic" to the gastrointestinal tract, is overruled by "intrinsic" modes of regulation. Sensory neurons in different parts of the gastrointestinal tract have their cell bodies in the gut wall but are not part of the autonomic system. In addition, hormonal regulation plays an important role. Endocrine glands secrete hormones into the circulation, whereas paracrine glands or cells secrete products that influence the secretion of another product secreted by a local gland or cell. For example, gastrin is a hormone secreted by the stomach that increases hydrochloric acid and pepsinogen secretion in the stomach. Another example is secretin, a hormone produced by the small intestine that increases water and bicarbonate secretion by the pancreas.

Substances within the tissues of the gastrointestinal tract and hormones released by organs in the gastrointestinal tract affect secretion and motility. An overview of the effects of gastrointestinal hormones and their functions is given in table 4.1.

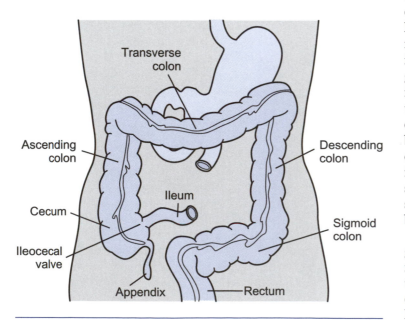

Figure 4.8 The ileocecal valve and large intestine.

Table 4.1 Effects of Gastrointestinal Hormones

Hormone	Secreted by	Effect
Gastrin	Stomach	Stimulates HCl production in the stomach; stimulates secretion of pepsinogen in the stomach
Secretin	Small intestine	Stimulates water and bicarbonate secretion in pancreatic juice
Cholecystokinin (CCK)	Small intestine	Stimulates secretion of enzymes in pancreatic juice; stimulates gallbladder contractions; inhibits gastric motility and secretion
Gastric inhibitory peptide (GIP)	Small intestine	Inhibits gastric motility and secretion
Glucagonlike peptide I (GLP-I)	Ileum and colon	Inhibits gastric motility and secretion
Guanylin	Ileum and colon	Causes removal of NaCl and water from feces

Digestion

Digestion starts the moment food is ingested and may take 4 hours to 6 hours to complete. Specific enzymes are responsible for the digestion of different macronutrients.

Carbohydrate Digestion

The digestion of carbohydrates starts in the mouth as saliva is added to the food. Saliva is secreted from the parotid glands, the sublingual glands, and the submandibular glands (see figure 4.3). The daily secretion of saliva normally ranges between 800 ml and 1,500 ml (see table 4.2). In the unstimulated state, saliva secretion rate is about 0.5 ml/min, but this rate can increase by up to 10-fold during the chewing of food. Saliva consists primarily of water (99.5%) derived from extracellular fluid. In addition, it contains -amylase (also referred to as ptyalin), an enzyme responsible for the breakdown of starch into smaller units; mucoid proteins; bicarbonate; electrolytes; lysozymes, enzymes that break down

Table 4.2 Daily Secretion of Intestinal Juices

Intestinal juices	Daily volume (ml)
Saliva	1,000
Gastric secretions	1,500
Pancreatic secretion	1,000
Bile	1,000
Small intestine	2,000
Large intestine	200
Total	6,700

proteins and attack bacteria; lingual lipase; and protein antibodies (immunoglobulin A [IgA]) that can help to destroy oral bacteria. Thus, besides a digestive function, saliva has a protective function against invading bacteria (see chapter 13). An overview of digestive enzymes is given in table 4.3.

The mucoid proteins give the saliva its viscous quality, which helps lubricate the food and make it easier to swallow. Chewing the food mixes the saliva with the food and increases the contact area so that amylase can start breaking down the glucose chain in starches. Prolonged chewing of a cracker will cause it to taste sweeter as some starch breaks down to disaccharide sugars such as maltose.

When the food is swallowed and arrives in the acid environment of the stomach, the amylase activity decreases. Carbohydrate digestion still takes place, but at a much slower rate. In the mouth and stomach, before the stomach content is completely mixed with gastric secretions, approximately 30% to 40% of the carbohydrate may be digested, predominantly to maltose, maltotrioses, and small oligosaccharides (see figure 4.9).

When the carbohydrates are emptied from the stomach into the duodenum and the acid is neutralized by sodium bicarbonate from the pancreas, digestion will proceed at a high rate again. In the duodenum, additional -amylase will be secreted in the pancreatic juice. This -amylase, like salivary amylase, hydrolyzes the starches into small glucose polymers (dextrins) and maltose (see figure 4.9). Almost complete hydrolysis of all starches to maltose has taken place when the chyme enters the ileum. The disaccharides and small polysaccharides are further digested by specific enzymes located in the brush borders of intestinal epithelial cells. As soon as disaccharides come in contact with the brush border, they are digested by the enzymes lactase, sucrase, and maltase (see figure 4.9). Lactase breaks lactose down

Table 4.3 Digestive Enzymes and Their Functions

Enzyme	Site of action	Source	Substrate	Product	Optimum pH
Carbohydrates					
Salivary amylase	Mouth	Salivary glands	Starch	Maltose	6.7
Pancreatic amylase	Duodenum	Pancreatic juice	Starch	Maltose, maltotriose, and oligosaccharides	6.7–7.0
Maltase	Small intestine	Brush border	Maltose	Glucose	5.0–7.0
Sucrase	Small intestine	Brush border	Sucrose	Glucose and fructose	5.0–7.0
Lactase	Small intestine	Brush border	Lactose	Glucose and galactose	5.8–6.2
Lipids					
Lingual lipase	Mouth	Lingual salivary glands	Starch	Maltose	3.5–6.0
Pancreatic lipase	Small intestine	Pancreatic juice	Triacylglycerols	Fatty acids and monoacylglycerols	8.0
Proteins					
Pepsin	Stomach	Gastric glands	Protein	Polypeptides	1.6–2.4
Trypsin	Small intestine	Pancreatic juice	Polypeptides	Amino acids, dipeptides, and tripeptides	8.0
Chymotrypsin	Small intestine	Pancreatic juice	Polypeptides	Amino acids, dipeptides, and tripeptides	8.0
Carboxypeptidase	Small intestine	Pancreatic juice	Polypeptides	Amino acids, dipeptides, and tripeptides	8.0
Elastase	Small intestine	Pancreatic juice	Polypeptides	Amino acids, dipeptides, and tripeptides	8.5

into glucose and galactose, sucrase breaks sucrose down into glucose and fructose, and maltase breaks maltose down into 2 glucose molecules.

Problems with the digestive process can result when a deficiency of one or more of these enzymes exists. Lactose intolerance is caused by an absence or deficiency of the intestinal enzyme lactase. When lactose, the main carbohydrate component of milk, is not digested, diarrhea and fluid loss result. In addition, bacteria in the large intestine will metabolize the lactose to produce large quantities of gas, which causes bloating and pain.

Fiber, a form of dietary carbohydrate, contains cellulose, which is a structural component of plant cells and is resistant to human digestive enzymes. Cellulose can be excreted in the feces. However, some of it is fermented by the bacteria present in the large intestine. Much like yeast ferments the sugars in grape juice to produce wine, the bacteria in the large intestine ferment cellulose to produce hydrogen and carbon dioxide gases, volatile FAs, and, in many instances, methane gas (which has an unpleasant odor). Changes in the diet or in the type of microorganisms can influence the amount of gas produced.

Peristaltic movements push undigested carbohydrates, including fibrous substances, to the colon, where more digestion occurs. Undigestible carbohydrates (predominantly cellulose) move to the rectum for expulsion though the anus.

Lipid Digestion

Digestion of lipids begins in the mouth because saliva contains small amounts of lingual lipase, the enzyme that splits triacylglycerols (triglycerides) into FAs and glycerol. In the stomach, this acid-stable lipase continues to hydrolyze the triacylglycerols (see figure 4.10). Hydrolysis, however, is slow because triacylglycerols are not soluble in water and, therefore, do not mix very well with the water fraction in which lipase is found. The lingual and gastric lipases act together but mainly on the short-chain (C4 to C6) and medium-chain triacylglycerols (C8 to C10), whereas the major-

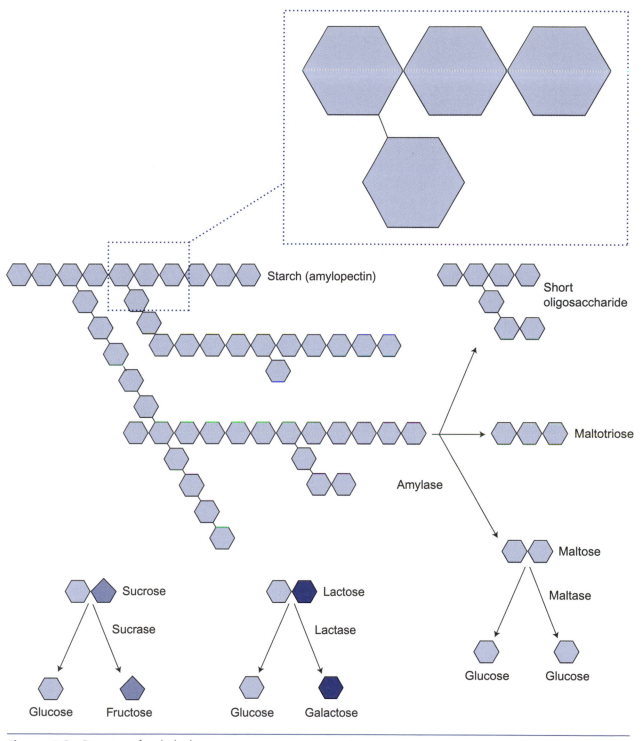

Figure 4.9 Digestion of carbohydrates.

ity of the fat (long-chain triacylglycerols; C12 to C24) is digested in the small intestine. Lingual lipase is responsible for 10% to 30% of the triacylglycerol digestion. When the chyme enters the duodenum, bile is added and it acts on the triacylglycerols, which, by this time, are organized into large lipid globules.

Pancreatic lipase is secreted into the duodenum and will further hydrolyze the triacylglycerols.

Once initial hydrolysis has started and the triglycerides are converted into FAs, monoglycerides and diglycerides organize themselves into small emulsion droplets. The fat-soluble part of the FA faces inward,

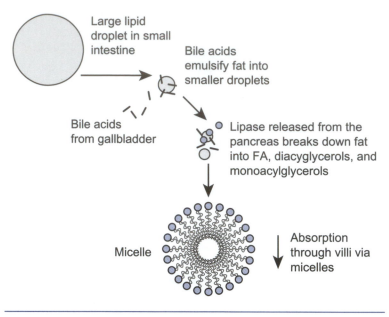

Figure 4.10 Digestion of fat.

structures with a disklike shape, on which phospholipids and FAs form a bilayer and the bile salts occupy the edge positions, rendering the edge of the disk hydrophilic (i.e., more attractive to water). The bile salts emulsify the lipids into small droplets, which increases the total surface area and, thus, makes hydrolysis (breakdown) of triacylglycerols by pancreatic lipase easier.

Protein Digestion

Protein digestion breaks down the ingested proteins into simple amino acids, dipeptides, and tripeptides for absorption across the intestinal mucosa (see figure 4.11). This process (protein hydrolysis) takes place within the stomach and small intestine and is dependent on specific protein-digesting enzymes (proteases) and the acidity of the stomach. Specific cells produce and secrete hydrochloric acid (HCl), a strong acid, into the stomach. These parietal cells secrete an isotonic 160 mM HCl solution with a

and the water-soluble part forms the core of these droplets. When bile salts (bile acids), stored in the gallbladder, are secreted into the duodenum, micelles are formed (see figure 4.10). Micelles are well-defined

Figure 4.11 Digestion of protein.

pH of about 0.8, illustrating its extreme acidity. The pH within the stomach and of the gastric contents is typically around 2.0.

HCl, and thereby the acidic ingested food, has various functions; among other things it

- activates the protease enzyme pepsin,
- kills many pathogenic organisms,
- increases the absorption of iron and calcium,
- inactivates hormones of plant and animal origin, and
- denatures (breaks down) food proteins, making them more vulnerable to enzyme action.

Proteases (see table 4.3) are often stored in the form of an inactive precursor, but as soon as it is released into the stomach or small intestine it becomes active. This mechanism prevents the digesting of the cells in which the proteases are produced and stored.

Pepsin (an important group of proteases), secreted as its precursor pepsinogen from the cells of the stomach wall, is initially inactive. As soon as pepsinogen comes in contact with the HCl of the stomach, it is automatically converted into the active pepsin that breaks down protein. Pepsin degrades the collagenous connective tissue fibers of meat. After dismantling these fibers, other proteases can effectively digest the remaining animal protein. Stomach enzymes and acids attack the long, complex protein strands and will hydrolyze approximately 10% to 20% of the ingested proteins. The low pH causes denaturation of the protein, meaning that the 3-dimensional structure of protein is uncoiled and breaks into smaller polypeptide and peptide units. When the chyme passes into the small intestine, pepsin becomes inactivated by the relatively high pH in the duodenum.

Other proteases (alkaline enzymes), including trypsin, are released and become active to digest the remaining proteins and polypeptides. The pancreatic juice is rich in precursors of endopeptidases, carboxypeptidases, enteropeptidases, trypsinogen, and trypsin (see figure 4.10). These proteases digest the polypeptides into tripeptides, dipeptides, and single amino acids. Amino acids, dipeptides, and tripeptides can be transported across the enterocyte.

Absorption

Absorption of nutrients across the intestinal walls occurs either by active transport or by simple diffusion. Active transport requires energy and usually takes place against a concentration gradient or an electrical potential. Active transport often requires specialized carrier proteins. Diffusion is the movement of substances across a membrane along, rather than against, an electrochemical gradient. Simple diffusion does not require transport proteins or energy in the form of ATP, but many nutrients are transported by facilitated diffusion, which does require a protein transporter or channel.

Absorption of Carbohydrates

The major monosaccharides that result from digestion of polysaccharides and disaccharides are glucose, fructose, and galactose. These monosaccharides are absorbed by carrier-mediated transport processes. The transporters that mediate the uptake of monosaccharides in the epithelial cell (see figure 4.12) are (1) a sodium monosaccharide cotransporter (most commonly sodium glucose transporter [SGLT]) and (2) a sodium-independent facilitated-diffusion transporter with specificity for fructose (GLUT 5). For each molecule of glucose, 2 sodium ions will be transported into the epithelial cell. The sodium is then actively transported back

Figure 4.12 Absorption of carbohydrate.

into the gut lumen through a Na+-K+-ATPase pump. Galactose also uses SGLT.

A separate monosaccharide transporter on the contraluminal side of the epithelial cell accepts all three monosaccharides (GLUT 2). The monosaccharides then enter the circulation in the hepatic portal vein, which will transport them to the liver.

Absorption of Fatty Acids

The monoacylglycerols and FAs incorporated into micelles are transported to the villi and move into the spaces between the microvilli. Here FAs diffuse across the membrane of the epithelium and enter the epithelial cell. The micelles then move away from the villi, incorporate new FAs and transport them to the villi. Micelles formed within the intestinal lumen, therefore, perform a very important ferrying function. In the presence of bile salts (and, thus, micelles), fat absorption is almost complete (97%), whereas in the absence of bile, only about 50% of the FAs are absorbed.

The absorption of FAs through the epithelial membranes is by diffusion (because they are highly soluble in the lipid membranes) (see figure 4.13). In the epithelial cell, FAs are re-esterified to triacylglycerols in the endoplasmatic reticulum. Once formed, triacylglycerols combine with cholesterol and phospholipids to form chylomicrons (see also figure 1.4). In this chylomicron, the fatty sides of the phospholipids face toward the center, and the polar parts form the surface. Chylomicrons make possible the transport of fat in the aqueous environment of the lymph and blood plasma. These large molecules move toward the central lacteal of the villi and are slowly transported through the lymphatic system, reaching the circulation in the subclavian veins.

Short-chain and medium-chain FAs are more water soluble than long-chain FAs and, therefore, follow a slightly different route of absorption. They enter the epithelial cell and, without being re-esterified to triacylglycerols, they directly diffuse through the contraluminal membrane into the portal blood, where they are bound to the plasma protein albumin and passed to the liver via the hepatic portal vein. The bile salts are reabsorbed again in the intestinal mucosa of the distal ileum. They enter the portal blood and pass to the liver. In the liver, they are resecreted into the bile. In this way, 94% of the bile salts are reutilized. The recirculation of bile salts is called the enterohepatic circulation.

Absorption of Amino Acids

Amino acids, dipeptides, and tripeptides are absorbed by active transport (coupled to the transport of sodium) in the small intestine and delivered to the liver via the hepatic portal vein. Dipeptides and tripeptides that have been transported across the epithelial membrane are broken down inside the cell into their amino acid constituents by specific dipeptidases and tripeptidases (see figure 4.11).

Most amino acids are transported across the epithelium against a concentration gradient, and, therefore, carrier-mediated transport is needed (see figure 4.14). At least 7 different brush border–specific transport proteins have been identified. The luminal membrane usually contains sodium-dependent transport systems, whereas the contraluminal membrane transport does not require sodium. The capacity of

Figure 4.13 Absorption of fat.

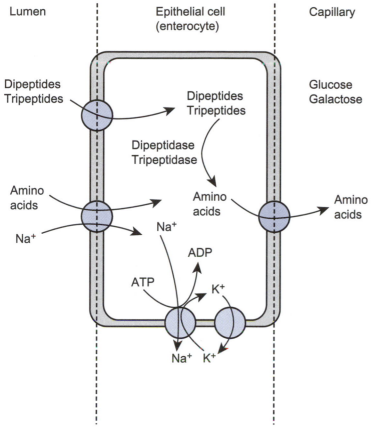

Lumen   Epithelial cell   Capillary
(enterocyte)

Figure 4.14 Absorption of amino acids.

the small intestine to absorb amino acids and small peptides is very large and effective. Less than 1% of the ingested protein is usually found in feces. Once amino acids have passed the epithelium, they are transported to the liver where they can be converted to glucose, fat, or protein, or they can be released into the bloodstream as free amino acids.

Absorption of Water

Most water absorption (99%) takes place in the small intestine, mainly in the duodenum (72%), entirely by simple diffusion. This absorption obeys the laws of osmosis (see figure 4.15). A membrane that is impermeable to solutes but permeable to water separates 2 compartments with the same amount of fluid but different numbers of solute particles. Water diffuses across this membrane in both directions, but relatively more water will flow towards the compartment with the lower water concentration (higher solute concentration). This net movement of water results eventually in a similar solute concentration on both sides of the membrane. The amount of water in compartment with the lower water concentration, however, has increased.

The term *osmole* describes the number of solute particles, and the solute particle density is expressed as mOsm/kg (osmolality) or mOsm/L (**osmolarity**). The osmolarity of most body fluids is around 290 mOsm/L (see table 4.4). Therefore, when the osmolarity of the chyme is low (< 280 mOsm/L), water moves toward the epithelial cell and the blood plasma in which the osmolarity is higher. If the

	Net water movement
	Water diffusion
	Impermeable solute

	A			B	
Solute	5 mOsm	15 mOsm	Solute	5 mOsm	15 mOsm
Volume	1 Liter	1 Liter	Volume	0.5 Liter	1.5 Liter
Osmolarity	5 mOsm/L	15 mOsm/L	Osmolarity	10 mOsm/L	10 mOsm/L

Figure 4.15 The process of osmosis.

osmolarity of the chyme is high (> 300 mOsm/L, as, for example, in a concentrated glucose solution), water moves into the gut lumen. With the absorption of solutes (e.g., glucose and sodium), the osmotic gradient changes and pulls water into the epithelium (a process known as solvent drag).

The secretions into the intestine can amount up to 7 L/day in a sedentary adult (see table 4.2). These 7 L of water are produced by the combined secretions of the salivary glands, stomach wall, gall bladder, pancreas, and intestine. Daily water intake may average 2 L, and the total daily water absorption may, therefore, be as high as 9 L. During exercise, especially in hot conditions when fluid losses and intakes are high, daily water absorption can easily exceed 10 L. With diarrhea, absorption of water is minimal, and the losses of fluid from the body can be high and, in some cases, life-threatening.

Table 4.4 Osmolarity of Body Fluids and Commercially Available Drinks

Solution	Osmolarity (mOsm/L)
Water	10–20
Sweat	170–220
Gastric fluids	280–303
Blood serum	300
Lucozade Sport	280
Isostar	296
Gatorade	349
Powerade (U.K.)	285
Powerade (U.S.)	381
Allsport	516
Pepsi-Cola	568
Coca-Cola	650
Fruit juice	450–690

Absorption of Vitamins

Most of the vitamin absorption takes place in the jejunum and ileum and is usually a passive process (diffusion). Fat-soluble vitamins (A, D, E, and K) are absorbed along with FAs. They are also incorporated into chylomicrons and transported through the lymph system into the systemic circulation to liver and other tissues. Most of the absorption of fat-soluble vitamins takes place in the small intestine.

Water-soluble vitamins are also mostly absorbed in the small intestine, via diffusion. The water-soluble vitamins are not retained to any great extent by different tissues, and when large amounts are ingested, they are mostly excreted in urine. Most vitamin C is absorbed in the distal portion of the small intestine. Excess intake of vitamin C (above approximately 1,200 mg/day) decreases the efficiency of renal reabsorption of vitamin C, and much of the excess intake appears in the urine. B vitamins are often ingested as part of coenzymes in food; digestion liberates the vitamins. For example, pantothenic acid is usually present in food as part of coenzyme A. Digestion releases the vitamin from its coenzyme, and absorption takes place. Thiamin and vitamin B_6 are mainly absorbed in the jejunum. Biotin and riboflavin are mainly absorbed in the proximal part of the small intestine. Niacin is partly absorbed in the stomach but mostly in the small intestine. Vitamin B_{12} is mainly absorbed in the ileum. Its absorption is more complex, involving binding to a specific protein (called intrinsic factor, which is secreted by the parietal cells of the gastric mucosa). Absorption of folic acid is dependent on the presence of the intestinal enzyme conjugase, which facilitates the absorption of folic acid in the small intestine. An overview of various vitamins and their absorption is given in table 4.5.

Absorption of Minerals

Minerals are not very well absorbed in the human intestine. The intake in food is, therefore, usually far in excess of the actual requirements. Mineral absorption often depends on its chemical form. The best-known example of this requirement is probably the difference in absorption between nonheme and heme iron. (Heme iron is found in meat; nonheme iron is obtained from plants). About 15% of all ingested heme iron is absorbed in the small intestine, whereas only 2% to 10% of nonheme iron is absorbed. Absorption of other minerals is also relatively poor. Only a maximum of 35% of ingested calcium is absorbed, 20% to 30% of ingested magnesium, 14% to 41% of ingested zinc, and less than 2% of ingested chromium. Besides the poor absorption, excretion rates via urine are also very high. About 65% of absorbed phosphorus is excreted via urine, and 50% of absorbed calcium is excreted. When the daily mineral intake is insufficient, an increased intake may result in increased retention. For example, many women in Western countries have an insufficient intake of iron and calcium, and increasing the intake generally increases the storage of these minerals.

Table 4.5 Absorption of Vitamins

Vitamin	Absorption mechanism
Vitamin C	Almost all absorption (90%) takes place in the distal portion of the small intestine.
Thiamine	Absorption occurs predominantly in the jejunum.
Riboflavin	Absorption occurs in the proximal part of the small intestine.
Niacin	Some absorption in the stomach, but most occurs in the small intestine.
Pantothenic acid	This vitamin exists as part of coenzyme A, but absorption occurs readily throughout the small intestine when the vitamin is released from CoA.
Biotin	Absorption occurs in upper one-third to one-half of the small intestine.
Folic acid	Absorption occurs in small intestine with the help of a specialized intestinal enzyme system called conjugase.
Vitamin B_6	Absorption occurs in the jejunum.
Vitamin B_{12}	Absorption occurs mainly in the ileum and requires an intrinsic factor secreted from parietal cells of the stomach.

Sodium is actively transported out of the epithelial cell into the portal circulation, a process requiring ATPase carrier enzymes and energy (in the form of ATP). The transport of sodium out of the epithelial cell creates a low sodium concentration in the cell, which increases diffusion of sodium from the gut lumen into the epithelial cell. About 30 g of sodium is secreted in intestinal secretions every day. Daily sodium ingestion is about 5 g to 8 g. Thus, about 25 g to 35 g of sodium must be reabsorbed each day, representing a large percentage of the body sodium stores. This requirement explains why extreme diarrhea results in large sodium losses, which can be dangerous and even life threatening.

Function of Bacteria in the Colon

The adult human gut contains about one kg of various bacteria (colon bacilli). These bacteria break down small amounts of cellulose. More importantly, however, is the production of vitamin K, vitamin B_{12}, thiamine, riboflavin, and other substances. Vitamin K is especially important because the daily vitamin K intake in foodstuffs is normally insufficient.

Regulation of Gastric Emptying

After the ingestion, food usually takes 1 hour to 4 hours to leave the stomach, depending on the content of the meal. Gastric motility and secretion are, to some extent, automatic. Contraction of the stomach increases the intragastric pressure to push chyme through the pyloric sphincter. Such contractions are initiated by pacemaker cells in the stomach wall. Gastric emptying is further controlled by a variety of signals directly from the stomach or the duodenum (see figure 4.16). The signals are either nervous signals or hormonal signals.

The stomach signals include (1) nervous signals caused by stretching and extension of the stomach wall and (2) the release of the hormone gastrin by the antral mucosa. Gastrin is released in response to both internal (thought of food and extension of the stomach) and external (sight and smell of food) stimuli. These signals from the stomach are always positive-feedback signals. The increased amount of food relaxes the pyloric sphincter and increases gastric emptying. Signals from the duodenum usually provide negative feedback (i.e., inhibit gastric emptying). The duodenum contains receptors that can detect acidity, distension of the duodenum, osmolarity, and possibly carbohydrate, fat, and protein. When these receptors are stimulated, the enterogastric reflex is initiated, which increases the contraction of the pylorus. This mechanism prevents dumping of an excessive amount of chyme into the small intestine. Too rapid delivery of the chyme into the intestine could mean insufficient time for digestion and absorption to take place, and some nutrients would be lost in the feces. Factors that have been suggested to affect gastric emptying include

- smell and sight of food,
- thought of food,
- volume of a drink,
- energy density of a drink,
- temperature of a drink,
- osmolarity of a drink,

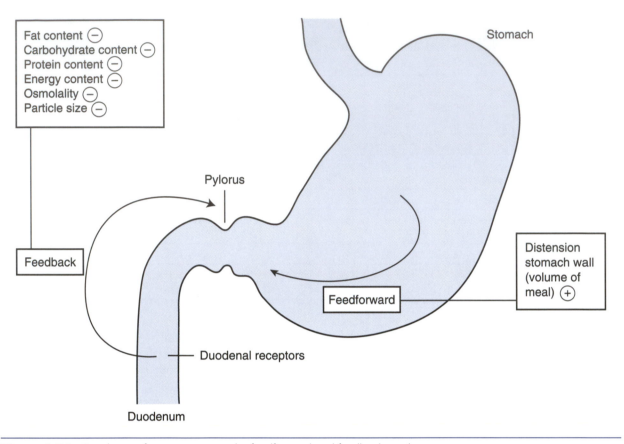

Figure 4.16 Regulation of gastric emptying by feedforward and feedback mechanisms.

- body temperature/dehydration,
- type of exercise,
- exercise intensity,
- gender, and
- psychological stress and anxiety.

These factors operate in the following ways:

- Volume of the food ingested. The stomach walls can extend to accommodate larger volumes, and as a result, the volume of the stomach increases without a change in pressure. When maximal distension is reached, the pressure will increase. The rate of gastric emptying of a fluid is highly dependent on the volume of the fluid in the stomach (Hunt and Donald 1954). Therefore, the rate of gastric emptying from a fluid bolus is exponential (see figure 4.17). The gastric-emptying phase is initially rapid, and when the volume is reduced, the rate of gastric emptying is reduced accordingly. The rate of gastric emptying is regulated through positive-feedback signals to the pyloric sphincter.
- Exercise intensity. The rate of gastric empty-ing is not affected by exercise intensity, up to

intensities of 80% $\dot{V}O_2$max. Above this inten-sity a reduction may occur in fluid and nutrient delivery to the small intestine (Sole and Noakes 1989; Costill and Saltin 1974). However, from a practical point of view, this reduction may not be very important, because exercise intensities of greater than 80% $\dot{V}O_2$max generally cannot be sustained long enough to cause a limitation in fluid or carbohydrate delivery. Eating and drinking at these high intensities is problem-atic anyway because of the exercise-induced hyperventilation. Gastric emptying of liquids is slowed during brief intermittent high-inten-sity exercise compared with rest or steady-state moderate exercise (Leiper et al. 2001a). Gastric emptying measured after a 5-a-side indoor soccer match was reduced even though the average intensity of the activity was only 54% to 63% $\dot{V}O_2$max (Leiper et al. 2001b). The relatively short bouts of very-high-intensity exercise were clearly enough to reduce gastric emptying.

- Osmolarity. Osmolarity has always been con-sidered an important factor controlling the rate of gastric emptying. Increased beverage osmolarity not only increases gastric secretions but also increases intestinal secretions. Osmolarity is therefore an important factor to consider when selecting a beverage for ingestion during exercise. Higher osmolarity may reduce gastric emptying and decrease water absorption. However, osmolarity and the concentration of simple carbohydrates are related. A high-energy or high-carbohydrate content is usually related to a high osmolarity, and the effects of concentration and osmolarity are, therefore, difficult to distinguish. Studies, however, suggest that, although osmolarity reduces the rate of gastric emptying, this factor is not important in beverages with osmolarities in the range of 200 mOsm/L to 400 mOsm/L (Brouns et al. 1995). This range is typical for most sports drinks (see table 4.4). Osmolarity possibly becomes more important in beverages with very high osmolarities (>500 mOsm/L).

- Energy density. The energy density has a very strong effect on the rate of gastric emptying. Whether this effect is an effect of energy density per se or of specific nutrients is not totally clear. Several nutrients exert a strong inhibitory effect on gastric emptying. For example, fat is a very strong inhibitor of gastric emptying. Increasing the carbohydrate or protein content of a beverage, however, will also slow gastric emptying. Carbohydrate-electrolyte solutions with 2% carbohydrate do already show a tendency to empty slower than water (Vist and Maughan 1994), but solutions of 8% or more will inhibit gastric emptying significantly. The energy content of the solution is a more important factor than the osmolarity (Vist and Maughan 1995).

- Meal or beverage temperature. The effect of meal or beverage temperature is probably physiologically not important. Lambert et al. 1999 showed that after ingestion of a ^2H_2O-containing beverage, deuterium (^2H) accumulation in plasma was similar in drinks at varying temperatures. Gastric emptying was not different, despite the differences in beverage temperature. This study reflects the findings in the literature that, generally, no effects of meal temperature have been found on the rate of gastric emptying. Some studies, however, have found a reduction in the rate of gastric emptying with very cold or very hot drinks, and gastric emptying may be influenced by the beverage temperature when the intragastric temperature is much higher or lower than the body temperature.

- Psychological stress. Stress affects gastrointestinal motility and the rate of gastric emptying.

This reduction in the rate of gastric emptying is usually related to changes in circulating hormone concentrations as a result of stress. Some of these hormones (e.g., epinephrine) reduce the blood flow to the gastrointestinal tract.

- Other factors. In addition to the factors mentioned earlier, other factors may also affect gastric emptying. Studies in hot conditions have shown that dehydration and hyperthermia can cause a slowing of gastric emptying (Rehrer et al. 1990; Neufer et al. 1989). Because subjects in these studies became dehydrated and hyperthermic at the same time, determining what the mechanisms were and whether dehydration, hyperthermia, or a combination of the two was responsible for the reduced gastric-emptying rate is not possible.

Figure 4.17 An example of a gastric-emptying curve.

Women have slower gastric-emptying rates than men (Notivol et al. 1984), although gastric-emptying rates seemed to be increased somewhat during ovulation. Women are reported to be more prone to gastrointestinal complaints after prolonged endurance exercise. This finding could be related to a slower rate of gastric emptying.

Considerable differences exist in the rate of gastric emptying between individuals. Some individuals may empty 70% to 80% of a solution in 15 minutes, whereas others empty only 20% to 30% of that same solution in 15 minutes. The reasons for these individual differences are not known, but diet has been suggested as an important factor. The gastrointestinal tract possibly adapts to the intake of certain nutrients, and, for instance, a high habitual fat intake may result in a high gastric-emptying rate of fat. Whatever the mechanisms, they highlight the importance of individual fluid intake recommendations.

Gastrointestinal Problems

Endurance athletes have a high prevalence of gastrointestinal complaints (see Brouns et al. 1987 and Brouns 1991). These complaints include abdominal pains, abnormal defecation, nausea, heartburn, and vomiting (see figure 4.18). Exercise must influence the functioning of the gastrointestinal tract. Therefore, factors that increase the risk of these symptoms must be understood. Various studies investigated the incidence of gastrointestinal symptoms during competition, usually running events or triathlons.

Prevalence of Gastrointestinal Problems

A study by Keeffe et al. (1984) surveyed 1,700 participants after a marathon race. Lower gastrointestinal symptoms, such as diarrhea, abdominal cramps, urge to defecate, flatulence, and gastrointestinal bleeding were found to be more common than upper gastrointestinal symptoms, such as nausea, vomiting, heartburn, bloating, and side ache (stitch). The most common symptom experienced was the urge to defecate (36% to 39% of the participants), both during and immediately after running. Bowel movements (35%) and diarrhea (19%) were reported quite frequently immediately after running. During the race, some runners (16% to 18%) had to stop to defecate, and some runners (8% to 10%) had to stop because of diarrhea. Bloody bowel movements were reported by 1% to 2% of the participants. Similar results were obtained by Jeukendrup, Vet-Joop, et al. (2000), who found that 93% of the participants of a long-distance triathlon reported at least one symptom of gastrointestinal discomfort; 29% of these symptoms were rated as serious (complaints that will affect exercise performance).

Lower gastrointestinal symptoms are more often observed in women than in men, and some symptoms are more frequently reported by younger compared with older participants. Problems seem to occur more frequently during running than during activities such as cycling or swimming, possibly because of the vertical (i.e., up and down) movements of the gut during running.

Prevention of Gastrointestinal Problems

At present, the cause of gastrointestinal symptoms is not entirely clear. Although some risk factors have been identified, which mechanism is responsible for which complaints and why some individuals seem to be more prone to such problems is not obvious. A study by Rehrer, van Kemenade, et al. (1992), demonstrated a link between nutritional practices and gastrointestinal complaints during a half–Ironman distance triathlon. Gastrointestinal problems were more likely to occur with the ingestion of fiber, fat, protein, and concentrated carbohydrate solutions during the triathlon. Beverages with high osmolarities (>500 mOsm/L) seemed especially to be responsible for some of the reported complaints. The intake of dairy products may also be linked to the occurrence of gastrointestinal distress. Mild lactose intolerance is fairly common and could result in increased bowel activity and mild diarrhea (Noakes 1986). To minimize gastrointestinal distress, all these risk factors must be taken into account, and milk products, fiber, high fat, and high protein must be avoided 24 hours before competition and during exercise.

Upper gastrointestinal symptoms	Lower gastrointestinal symptoms	Related symptoms
Vomiting	Diarrhea	Urge to urinate
Heartburn	Bleeding	Urge to defecate
Bloating		Side ache ("stitch")
		Nausea
		Dizziness

Figure 4.18 Frequently reported gastrointestinal and related problems.

Key Points

■ The primary function of the gastrointestinal (or alimentary) tract, a 6 m to 8 m long tubular structure that reaches from the mouth to the anus, is to provide the body with nutrients.

■ Chewing food makes the food particles smaller and increases the surface area of the food, thereby increasing the contact area for digestive enzymes. Chewing also mixes the food particles with saliva and digestive enzymes.

■ In the stomach, food is mixed with gastric secretions (hydrochloric acid and digestive enzymes).

■ Gastric emptying is influenced by volume of food, energy density, osmolarity, dehydration, psychological stress and anxiety, and to a lesser degree, possibly by exercise intensity, meal temperature, and gender.

■ Pancreatic juices and bile are added to the chyme in the duodenum to digest the carbohydrates, fat, and protein. Specialized enzymes split these macronutrients into the smallest subunits for absorption. Bile is added to emulsify lipid droplets and facilitate digestion and absorption.

■ About 90% to 95% of all absorption takes place in the duodenum and jejunum (first parts of the small intestine).

■ The large intestine is a storage place for undigested food residues, and the final water and electrolyte absorption occurs here.

■ Gastrointestinal problems are a common phenomenon, mainly among endurance athletes, and the incidence is increased by ingestion of concentrated carbohydrate drinks during the race, a high-fiber or high-fat intake before the race, and dehydration.

Key Terms

absorption 82
brush border 84

chyme 83
digestion 82

gastric emptying 82
motility 85

osmolarity 93
transit time 85

Recommended Readings

Brouns, F., and E. Beckers. 1993. Is the gut an athletic organ? Digestion, absorption and exercise. *Sports Medicine* 15: 242-257.

Guyton, A.C., and J.E. Hall. 2000. *Textbook of Medical Physiology*, 10th edition. W.B. Saunders: Philadelphia.

Chapter 5

Carbohydrate

© PhotoDisc

Objectives

After studying this chapter, you should be able to do the following:

- Describe the main biochemical pathways involved in carbohydrate metabolism

- Describe the changes that occur in carbohydrate metabolism at different intensities of exercise

- Describe how blood glucose concentrations are maintained and regulated

- Describe the metabolic and performance effects of carbohydrate ingestion 3 hours to 4 hours before exercise

- Describe the metabolic and performance effects of carbohydrate ingestion 1 hour before exercise

- Describe the metabolic and performance effects of carbohydrate ingestion during exercise

- Describe the mechanisms involved in glycogen synthesis

- Give generally accepted guidelines for carbohydrate intake before and during exercise

- Give generally accepted guidelines for carbohydrate intake to improve recovery in the short term and long term

- Describe the dietary requirements for carbohydrate in a variety of sports

Whereas 100 years ago beef was believed to be the most important component of an athlete's diet, nowadays pasta seems to be most important. Athletes are often advised to eat a high-carbohydrate diet, consume carbohydrate before exercise, ensure adequate carbohydrate intake during exercise, and replenish carbohydrate stores as soon as possible after exercise.

Since the beginning of the 20th century, carbohydrate intake has been known to be related to exercise performance. The availability of carbohydrate as a substrate for skeletal muscle contraction and the central nervous system (i.e., the brain) is important for endurance exercise performance. However, not only the performance of prolonged exercise but also the performance in intermittent-intensity and high-intensity exercise may be influenced by carbohydrate availability. Because carbohydrate is the most important fuel for the central nervous system, various cognitive tasks and motor skills that play a crucial role in skill sports may also be affected by carbohydrate availability.

Carbohydrate is, therefore, a very important component of the athlete's diet, and various strategies have been developed over the past 30 years to optimize carbohydrate availability and, hence, performance. Generally, these goals can be achieved by (1) carbohydrate feedings before exercise to replenish muscle and liver glycogen stores and (2) carbohydrate feeding during exercise to maintain blood glucose levels and, hence, high rates of glucose oxidation derived from the plasma. In this chapter, the effects of carbohydrate on exercise metabolism and performance are explained. The results of some classic experimental studies will be discussed, along with the practical implications arising from this work. This chapter is subdivided into four distinct sections:

- Carbohydrate in the days before competition (or training);
- Carbohydrate in the hours before competition;
- Carbohydrate during competition or training; and
- Carbohydrate after training or competition.

First, however, we start with a short historical tour, beginning with the first studies that linked carbohydrate with exercise performance.

History

Krogh and Lindhardt (1920) were probably the first investigators to recognize the importance of carbohydrate as a fuel during exercise. In their study, subjects consumed a high-fat diet for three days (bacon, butter, cream, eggs, and cabbage), followed by three days on a high-carbohydrate diet (potatoes, flour, bread, cake, marmalade, and sugar). The subjects performed a 2-hour exercise test and reported various symptoms of fatigue when they consumed the high-fat diet. However, when they consumed the high-carbohydrate diet, the exercise was reported as "easy." The investigators also demonstrated that after several days of a low-carbohydrate, high-fat diet, the average respiratory exchange ratio (RER) during 2 hours of cycling was reduced to 0.80 as compared with 0.85 to 0.90 when a mixed diet was consumed. Conversely, when subjects ate a high-carbohydrate, low-fat diet, RER was increased to 0.95.

Important observations were also made by Levine, Gordon, and Derick (1924). They measured blood glucose in some of the participants of the 1923 Boston Marathon and observed that in most runners, glucose concentrations markedly declined after the race. These investigators suggested that low blood glucose levels were a cause of fatigue. To test that hypothesis, they encouraged several participants of the same marathon one year later to consume carbohydrates during the race. This practice, in combination with a high-carbohydrate diet before the race, prevented hypoglycemia (low blood glucose) and significantly improved running performance (i.e., time to complete the race).

The importance of carbohydrate for improving exercise capacity was further demonstrated by Dill, Edwards, and Talbott (1932). These investigators let their dogs, Joe and Sally, run without feeding them carbohydrates. The dogs became hypoglycemic and fatigued after 4 hours to 6 hours. When the test was repeated with the only difference that the dogs were fed carbohydrates during exercise, the dogs ran for 17 hours to 23 hours.

Christensen (1932) showed that with increasing exercise intensity, the proportion of carbohydrate utilized increased. This work was expanded in the late 1960s, with the reintroduction of the muscle biopsy technique by a group of Scandinavian scientists (Bergstrom and Hultman 1966, 1967). These studies indicated the critical role of muscle glycogen. The improved performance after a high-carbohydrate diet was linked with the higher muscle glycogen concentrations observed after such a diet. A high-carbohydrate diet (approximately 70% of dietary energy from carbohydrate) elevated muscle glycogen stores and seemed to enhance endurance capacity compared with a normal-carbohydrate (~50%) and a low-carbohydrate (~10%) diet. These observations have led to the recommendations to carbohydrate-load (i.e., eat high-carbohydrate diets) before competition (Costill and Miller 1980; Sherman and Costill 1984).

In the 1980s, the effects of carbohydrate feeding during exercise on exercise performance and metabolism were further investigated (Coyle and Coggan 1984; Coyle et al. 1983; Coyle et al. 1986). Costill et al. (1973) were the first to study the contribution of ingested carbohydrate to total energy expenditure, and in the following years, studies were conducted using isotopic tracers (i.e., ^{14}C-glucose or ^{13}C-glucose) to investigate differences in oxidation rates and metabolism of different types of carbohydrate, different amounts of carbohydrate, different feeding schedules, and various other factors that influence the efficacy of carbohydrate ingestion. Although Costill et al. (1973) concluded that ingested carbohydrates were not oxidized to any major extent, later studies have convincingly shown that ingested carbohydrates are a very important energy source during prolonged exercise.

Role of Carbohydrate

As discussed in chapter 1, carbohydrate plays many roles in the human body, but one of its main functions is to provide energy for the contracting muscle. Glycogen is the storage form of carbohydrate and is found mainly in muscle and liver.

Muscle Glycogen

Muscle glycogen is a readily available energy source for the working muscle. The glycogen content of skeletal muscle at rest is approximately 12 g/kg to 16 g/kg w.w. (65 mmol glucosyl units/kg w.w. to 90 mmol glucosyl units/kg w.w. [see the sidebar]), equating to a total of about 300 g to 400 g of carbohydrate (see chapter 2). The rate at which muscle glycogen is oxidized is highly dependent on the exercise intensity. At low to moderate exercise intensities, most of the energy can be obtained from oxidative phosphorylation of acetyl-CoA derived from both carbohydrate and fat. As the exercise intensity increases to high levels, the energy requirements cannot be met by only the oxidation of carbohydrate and fat. Muscle glycogen becomes the most important substrate, as anaerobic energy delivery (ATP resynthesis from glycolysis) is mostly derived from the breakdown of muscle glycogen. In figure 5.1, the effects of exercise intensity on muscle glycogen breakdown are shown. At very high exercise intensities, muscle glycogen is broken down very rapidly and becomes nearly depleted in a relatively short period of time when this type of exercise is performed intermittently.

Figure 5.1　The effects of exercise intensity (shown as percentage V̇O₂max) on muscle glycogen breakdown.

Adapted, by permission, from P.D. Gollnick, K. Piehl, and B. Saltin, 1974, "Selective glycogen depletion pattern in human muscle fibers after exercise of varying intensity and at varying pedaling rates," *Journal of Physiology* 214(1): 45-57.

MUSCLE GLYCOGEN

In the literature, muscle glycogen is expressed in various ways, making possible comparison of results of different studies. The units used most frequently are mmol glycosyl (glucose) units per kilogram dry mass or per kilogram wet mass. To express the results per kg dry mass, the muscle biopsy sample must be freeze-dried. All the water is removed by placing the frozen biopsy sample in a freeze dryer. Muscle contains approximately 75% to 80% water, and to convert values from wet mass to dry mass the concentration is usually multiplied by 4.5.

Liver Glycogen

The main role of glycogen in the liver is to maintain a constant blood glucose level. Glucose is the main, and in normal circumstances the only, fuel used by the brain. The liver is often referred to as the glucoregulator or glucostat—the organ responsible for the regulation of the blood glucose concentration. An average liver weighs approximately 1.5 kg, and approximately 80 g to 110 g of glycogen is stored in the liver of an adult human in the postabsorptive state. The glycogen is broken down in the liver to glucose and then released into the circulatory system. The kidneys also store some glycogen and release glucose into the blood, but, from a quantitative point of view, the kidneys are far less important than the liver. In this book, the terms liver glucose output or **hepatic glucose output** includes the release of glucose from the liver and kidneys. This release is also often called endogenous glucose production. Glycogen that is broken down in the muscle is not released as glucose into the circulation, because muscle lacks the enzyme glucose-6-phosphatase (the enzyme that removes a phosphate group from glucose-6-phosphate). Once glucose has been phosphorylated in the muscle cell by the enzyme hexokinase (the enzyme that attaches a phosphate group to glucose), it cannot be dephosphorylated (see chapter 2).

The liver has a much higher concentration of glycogen (per kg tissue) than does muscle. Only because of the much larger mass of muscle does muscle contain more glycogen than the liver (in absolute terms, 300 g to 600 g versus 80 g to 110 g). After an overnight fast, the liver glycogen content can be reduced to very low levels (<20 g) because tissues such as the brain use glucose at a rate of about 0.1 g/min in resting conditions. During exercise, the rate of glucose utilization by tissues other than muscle does not change very much (~ 0.1 g/min).

Circulation (of blood) can be regarded as a sink (see figure 5.2) from which various tissues, and especially exercising muscle, can tap glucose. However, a very precise mechanism regulates the blood glucose concentration in this sink at 4.0 to 4.5 mmol/L. (This is equivalent to a plasma glucose concentration of 5 to 6 mmol/L because the concentration of free glucose inside the red blood cells is somewhat less than that in the plasma; see the sidebar.) When the blood glucose concentration drops, the liver releases glucose. If the demands for glucose are less, the liver produces less glucose or even takes up glucose from the bloodstream to synthesize glycogen. After a meal, for instance, when a large amount of glucose enters the liver through the hepatic portal vein, the liver uses this glucose to synthesize glycogen. Despite the changes in glucose flux, both after feeding and during exercise (or fasting), normoglycemia is usually nicely maintained.

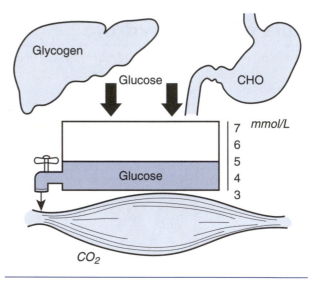

Figure 5.2 The bloodstream can be regarded as a sink in which the blood glucose concentration is accurately controlled. During exercise, muscle glucose uptake will increase dramatically, and to prevent the blood glucose concentration from dropping, the liver must produce glucose at an equally high rate.

DIFFERENCES BETWEEN WHOLE BLOOD, PLASMA, AND SERUM

Blood refers to the red liquid in our arteries and veins. It is composed of cells (red blood cells or erythrocytes, white blood cells or leukocytes, and cell fragments called platelets or thrombocytes) that are suspended in a fluid called plasma. The plasma contains proteins, lipoproteins, electrolytes, and small organic molecules such as glucose, fatty acids, glycerol, lactate, and amino acids, but by weight it is about 93% water. After taking a blood sample from a person, plasma can be separated from the cellular components by centrifugation, provided that an anticoagulant (a substance that pre-

(continued)

(continued)

vents the activation of clot formation) is added to the blood sample soon after it is collected. Typical anticoagulants that can be used include heparin, oxalate, citrate, and ethylene-diamine-tetraacetate (EDTA). If an anticoagulant is not added, the blood will clot within a matter of minutes. Centrifuging the clotted blood will separate the cellular elements and the insoluble clotting protein fibrin from the fluid; this fluid is called serum.

Hence, the difference between plasma and serum is that plasma has an anticoagulant in it and still contains soluble fibrinogen, whereas serum does not. Substances such as glucose can be measured in whole blood (after lysing all the blood cells), plasma, or serum. However, the glucose concentrations measured in each of these fluids will be a little different because the concentration of free glucose inside the red blood cells is somewhat less than that in the plasma. This means that whole blood will have a lower glucose concentration than plasma or serum. The concentration of most substances in plasma is pretty much the same as in serum, providing that the blood is not left too long to clot before centrifugation takes place. If left at room temperature, blood cell metabolism will use up glucose at a rate of about 0.5 mmol/L/h. In this situation, the serum glucose concentration will be less than that in plasma if the latter was obtained by centrifugation immediately after blood sampling.

Early studies in Scandinavia showed with liver biopsies that liver glycogen is decreased by about 50% after 1 hour of exercise at 75% $\dot{V}O_2$max. Later studies have used stable isotopes to indirectly measure the oxidation of liver glucose. These studies clearly show that liver glycogen is a significant substrate during exercise, and its importance (in absolute terms) increases when exercise intensity increases (Jeukendrup et al. 1999; Romijn 1993).

The liver can also produce glucose through gluconeogenesis. Substrates such as lactate, glycerol, pyruvate, alanine, glutamine, and some other amino acids can be used for the synthesis of glucose. These substrates are usually formed in other organs of the body and transported to the liver. For example, most of the lactate is formed in skeletal muscle, and most of the glycerol is from adipose tissue.

In resting conditions, the glucose output by the liver is approximately 150 mg/min (0.8 mmol/min). About 60% of this output (90 mg/min) is derived from the breakdown of liver glycogen, and about 40% (60 mg/min) is newly formed glucose (gluconeogenesis) (Hultman and Nilsson 1971; Nilsson and Hultman 1973). During exercise, the liver glucose output increases dramatically. During high-intensity exercise (>75% $\dot{V}O_2$max), liver glucose output increases to about 1 g/min, and the majority of this glucose is derived from the breakdown of liver glycogen (>90%). The rate of gluconeogenesis is only marginally increased during exercise compared with resting conditions. Gluconeogenesis is increased in the presence of high plasma concentrations of cortisol, epinephrine (adrenaline), and glucagon, whereas insulin has the opposite effect. The longer the exercise, the greater the relative contribution of gluconeogenesis to liver glucose production and output. During periods of starvation gluconeogenesis is increased, whereas after carbohydrate feeding gluconeogenesis is suppressed.

Regulation of Glucose Concentration

Blood glucose concentrations are normally maintained within a very narrow range (a normal resting blood glucose concentration is usually between 4.0 mmol/L and 4.5 mmol/L; plasma glucose concentrations are between 5 mmol/L and 6 mmol/L). Hormones play a key role in this regulation. In resting conditions, insulin is the most important glucoregulatory hormone. It increases the uptake of glucose into various tissues. After a meal, plasma insulin concentrations increase, and, as a result, glucose uptake by muscle, liver, and other tissues increases. Insulin promotes not only the uptake but also the storage of the glucose. Glycogen synthase activity is increased, and glycogen phosphorylase (the enzyme responsible for the breakdown of glycogen) is inhibited. Glucagon is the most important counteractive hormone. Secretion of glucagon causes the breakdown of liver glycogen and release of glucose into the circulation. Several other hormones may have a role in the regulation of blood glucose concentrations, including growth hormone, cortisol, somatostatin, and catecholamines.

During exercise, catecholamine release reduces the secretion of insulin by the pancreas, and plasma insulin concentrations can decrease to very low levels. Muscle glucose uptake is enhanced by contraction-stimulated glucose transport. As mentioned previously, however, despite dramatically increased glucose uptake by the muscle during exercise, blood glucose levels are well maintained in most conditions.

However, a situation in which a mismatch between glucose uptake and glucose production by the liver occurs is during high-intensity exercise. At an intensity of approximately 80% $\dot{V}O_2$max or more, the liver produces glucose at a higher rate than it is taken up by the muscle. This increased hepatic glucose release is most likely caused by neural feedforward mechanisms and results in slightly elevated blood glucose concentration compared with rest. Another situation in which a mismatch occurs is during the later stages of prolonged exercise. As liver glycogen becomes depleted, the rate of glucose production may become insufficient to compensate for the glucose uptake by the muscle and other tissues. As a result, hypoglycemia develops, with blood glucose levels sometimes dropping below 3 mmol/L.

Hypoglycemia

If blood glucose concentrations drop below a critical level (often 3 mmol/L), the rate of glucose uptake by the brain is insufficient to meet its metabolic requirements, and symptoms of hypoglycemia results. Hypoglycemia is characterized by a variety of symptoms, including dizziness, nausea, cold sweat, reduced mental alertness and ability to concentrate, loss of motor skill, increased heart rate, excessive hunger, and disorientation. Hypoglycemia is a common problem in exercise and sport and can be treated simply by carbohydrate consumption. Hypoglycemia has received considerable attention

because pre-exercise carbohydrate feeding seemed to induce a **rebound hypoglycemia.**

Carbohydrate Before Exercise

Carbohydrate can play an important role in the preparation for competition. Carbohydrate intake in the days before competition will mainly replenish muscle glycogen stores, whereas carbohydrate intake in the hours before competition will optimize liver glycogen stores. Because carbohydrate intake in the days before competition has distinctly different effects than carbohydrate immediately before competition, these will be discussed separately.

Carbohydrate in the Days Leading Up to Competition

Carbohydrate consumption in the days leading up to competition allows muscle glycogen stores to be fully replenished. Scandinavian researchers discovered that muscle glycogen could be supercompensated by changes in diet and exercise (Bergstrom and Hultman 1967). In a series of studies, they developed a so-called **supercompensation** protocol, which resulted in very high muscle glycogen concentrations. This diet and exercise regimen started with a glycogen depleting exercise bout (see figure 5.3a). The exercise was then followed by three days of a high-protein,

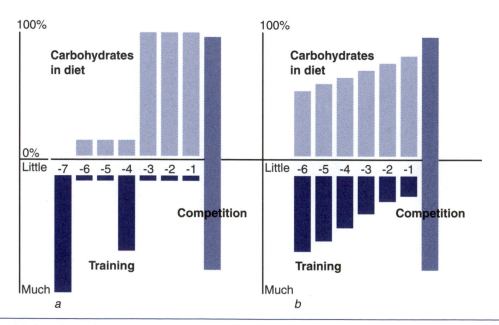

Figure 5.3 (a) The "classical supercompensation protocols" consisting of a glycogen-depleting exercise bout followed by 3 days of a high-protein, high-fat diet and another exhausting exercise bout on day 4, followed by a 3-day high-carbohydrate diet. (b) A more moderate protocol was later suggested to be almost as effective.

high-fat diet. Another exhausting exercise bout was performed on day 4, after which the subjects were placed on a high-carbohydrate diet for three days. Another group of subjects followed the same exercise protocol, but their diets were in reverse order.

Interestingly, this study revealed that the subjects who received the high-protein, high-fat, low-carbohydrate diet first followed by the high-carbohydrate diet had higher rates of muscle glycogen resynthesis. The authors, therefore, concluded that a period of carbohydrate deprivation further stimulated glycogen resynthesis when carbohydrates were given after exercise.

The regimen that was proposed is generally referred to as the "classical supercompensation protocol" (see figure 5.3a). It has been used successfully by several top athletes, including the legendary British runner Ron Hill. In fact, nowadays many marathon runners use this method to optimize their performance. Although the supercompensation protocol has been very effective in increasing muscle glycogen to very high concentrations, it also has several important (potential) disadvantages of which athletes should be aware:

- Hypoglycemia during the low-carbohydrate period
- Practical problems (difficulty in preparing such extreme diets)
- Gastrointestinal problems (especially on the low-carbohydrate diet)
- Poor recovery when no carbohydrate is ingested
- Athletes do not feel comfortable during a week without training
- Increased risk of injury
- Mood disturbances (lethargy and irritability) during low-carbohydrate period

The main problem may be the incidence of gastrointestinal problems when using this regimen. Diarrhea has often been reported on the days when the high-protein, high-fat diet is consumed. During the first three days, athletes may also experience hypoglycemia, and they may not recover very well from the exhausting exercise bout when no carbohydrate is ingested. Also, the fact that athletes cannot train in the week before an event is not ideal, because the worst punishment for most athletes seems to be asking them to avoid training. These factors may also have an impact on the mental preparation for an event.

Because of the numerous disadvantages of the classical supercompensation protocol, studies have focused on a more moderate protocol that would

achieve similar results. Sherman et al. (1981) studied three types of muscle glycogen supercompensation regimens in runners. The subjects slowly reduced their training over a 6-day period from 90 minutes running at 75% $\dot{V}O_2$max to complete rest on the last day. During each taper, they ingested one of the following three diets:

- A mixed diet with 50% carbohydrate
- A low-carbohydrate diet (25% carbohydrate) for the first 3 days, followed by 3 days of a high-carbohydrate diet (70%) (classical supercompensation protocol)
- A mixed diet for the first 3 days (50% carbohydrate) followed by 3 days of a high-carbohydrate diet (70%) (moderate supercompensation protocol)

The classical protocol resulted in very high muscle glycogen stores (211 mmol/kg w.w.), thus, confirming the results of earlier studies. However, the moderate approach produced very similar muscle glycogen levels (204 mmol/kg w.w.) and therefore, a normal training taper in conjunction with a moderate-carbohydrate to high-carbohydrate diet proved just as effective as the classical supercompensation protocol. A slightly modified and commonly applied strategy of the moderate supercompensation protocol is depicted in figure 5.3b. The moderate supercompensation protocol does not have the disadvantages of the classical protocol and is the preferred regimen.

Carbohydrate loading, or increased carbohydrate stores, increases time to exhaustion (endurance capacity) on average by about 20% and reduces the time taken to complete a set task (time trial; endurance performance) by 2% to 3% (Hawley et al. 1997). However, the available studies seem to suggest that the duration of exercise has to be at least 90 minutes before performance benefits can be demonstrated. Carbohydrate loading seems to have no effect on sprint performance and high-intensity exercise up to about 30 minutes compared with normal diets (~50% carbohydrate). This finding is not unexpected, because, at these high intensities, glycogen depletion is probably not the performance-limiting factor. However, several days on a very low (<10%) carbohydrate diet after a prolonged cycle ride to exhaustion has been shown to impair endurance capacity at 100% $\dot{V}O_2$max (Maughan, Greenhaff, et al. 1997).

Carbohydrate loading has also been reported to improve performance in team sports involving high-intensity intermittent exercise and skills, such as soccer and hockey (Balsom et al. 1999), although this result has not always been confirmed. A study was performed in elite Swedish soccer players who played 2 matches separated by 3 days (Saltin 1973). One group consumed a high-carbohydrate diet, and the other group consumed a normal diet between the matches. Before the second match, muscle glycogen concentrations were 50% lower in the group that consumed the control diet. At halftime (after 45 minutes), muscle glycogen was virtually depleted in this group, whereas the high-carbohydrate group still had some glycogen left (see table 5.1). This glycogen status was related to the distance covered during the match, which was significantly lower with the control diet and low muscle glycogen concentrations. The players also spent less time sprinting and thus were believed to have impaired running performance.

Supercompensation Strategies in Sport

Although muscle glycogen is important in most endurance sports, supercompensation strategies are not always applicable. For instance in cycling, stage races consist of several days of consecutive competition. Although a supercompensation regimen can theoretically be followed before the first stage, the nature of the sport does not allow the athletes to prepare for a week. Similar problems occur in sports where consecutive competitions follow each other within 1 day to 5 days. This supercompensation protocol, however, seems very suitable for marathon running and triathlon.

Muscle glycogen supercompensation is not of great importance to individuals involved in high-intensity exercise. Muscle glycogen availability per se is not usually responsible for fatigue during high-intensity exercise, provided that the pre-exercise glycogen store is not depleted to below 25 mmol/kg w.w. (4 g/kg w.w.). Even so, athletes involved in high-intensity training do need to consume sufficient carbohydrate in their diet. It has been shown that diets very low in carbohydrate content can compromise exercise performance at intensities around 95% to 100% of the maximum oxygen uptake (Maughan, Greenhaff, et al. 1997). Glycogen availability probably does not limit performance during repeated bouts of high intensity exercise because rates of glycogenolysis and lactate production decline under these conditions.

It must also be noted that every gram of carbohydrate is stored with approximately 3 g of water, which means that storage of 500g (8,000 kJ or 2,000 kcal) of carbohydrate is accompanied by an increase in body mass of approximately 2 kg. In some sports or disciplines (especially weight-bearing activities) this increase in body mass may not be desirable.

Carbohydrate Intake 3 Hours to 5 Hours Before Exercise

Athletes should have the last fairly large meal 3 hours to 5 hours before competition. Often this meal is a breakfast, which can be very important after an overnight fast when the liver is almost depleted of glycogen. The advantages of a meal in the hours before exercise are related to the increased carbohydrate availability in muscle and liver. In the 3 hours to 5 hours before exercise, some carbohydrate is incorporated into muscle glycogen. Carbohydrate intake in the last hour before competition will not affect muscle glycogen but still has an effect on liver glycogen and increases the delivery of carbohydrate to the muscle during exercise.

Ingestion of a carbohydrate-rich meal (containing 140 to approximately 330 g carbohydrate) 3 hours to 5 hours before exercise increases muscle glycogen levels (Coyle et al. 1985) and improves exercise performance (Neufer et al. 1987). Such a meal could include carbohydrate sources such as bread and jam or honey, cereals, porridge, bananas, canned fruit,

Table 5.1 Diet and Performance in Soccer

Glycogen concentration (g/kg ww muscle)			
	Before	**Halftime**	**End**	
High-carbohydrate diet	15	4	1	
Normal diet	7	1	0	
Distance covered				
	1st half (m)	**2nd half (m)**	**Walk (%)**	**Sprint (%)**
High-carbohydrate diet	6,100	5,900	27	24
Normal diet	5,600	4,100	50	15

Reprinted, by permission, from B. Saltin, 1973, "Metabolic fundamentals in exercise," *Medicine and Science in Sports and Exercise* 5: 137-146.

and fruit juice. Following is an example of a daily diet containing 150 g of carbohydrate representing at least 80% of the energy intake:

- Meal 1: 1 large bowl of porridge with skim milk, 1 banana, 1 glass (250 ml) of sweetened orange juice
- Meal 2: 4 slices of bread with jam or honey, 1 can of a soft drink
- Meal 3: 3 cups of rice made into a light stir fry with small amounts of lean ham or chicken, peas, corn, mushrooms, and onion, and 1 glass (250 ml) of fruit juice

The enhanced performance observed in research studies is likely related to small increases in pre-exercise muscle glycogen. However, replenishing the liver glycogen levels may be even more important. Liver glycogen concentrations are substantially reduced after an overnight fast. Ingestion of carbohydrate increases these reserves and contributes, together with any ongoing absorption of the ingested carbohydrate, to the maintenance of blood glucose concentrations during the subsequent exercise bout. Plasma glucose and insulin concentrations return to basal levels within 30 minutes to 60 minutes after ingestion. However, ingestion of carbohydrate in the hours before exercise has three important effects:

- Transient fall in plasma glucose with the onset of exercise
- Increased carbohydrate oxidation and accelerated glycogen breakdown
- Blunting of FA mobilization and fat oxidation

The effects on FA mobilization can persist for a long time after carbohydrate ingestion. Montain et al. (1991) showed a blunting of FA mobilization 6 hours after ingestion of a carbohydrate meal.

These metabolic changes, however, do not appear to be detrimental to exercise performance, with an increased carbohydrate availability compensating for the greater carbohydrate utilization. No differences in exercise performance were observed after ingestion of meals that produced marked differences in plasma glucose and insulin levels (Wee et al. 1999; Jentjens and Jeukendrup 2003a; Jentjens, Cale, et al. 2003; Moseley et al. 2001). From a practical perspective, if access to carbohydrate during exercise is limited or nonexistent, ingestion of 200 g to 300 g of carbohydrate 3 hours to 4 hours before exercise may be an effective strategy for enhancing carbohydrate availability during the subsequent exercise period.

Carbohydrate Intake 30 Minutes to 60 Minutes Before Exercise

The ingestion of carbohydrate in the hour before exercise results in a large rise in plasma glucose and insulin. With the onset of exercise, however, a rapid fall in blood glucose occurs. This fall is caused by a combination of several metabolic events. First, hyperinsulinemia stimulates glucose uptake, and in addition, contractile activity further stimulates muscle glucose uptake. The exercise-induced increase in the normal liver glucose output is inhibited by carbohydrate ingestion (Marmy-Conus et al. 1996), despite ongoing absorption of the ingested carbohydrate. An enhanced uptake and oxidation of blood glucose by skeletal muscle may account for the increased carbohydrate oxidation after pre-exercise carbohydrate ingestion. In addition, in some studies, an increase in muscle glycogen degradation has been observed.

The increase in plasma FA with exercise is attenuated after pre-exercise carbohydrate ingestion as a consequence of insulin-mediated inhibition of lipolysis (Horowitz et al. 1997). Even small increases in plasma insulin (e.g., after fructose ingestion) can result in a marked reduction of lipolysis. Fat oxidation is reduced not only because of the lower plasma FA availability (Horowitz et al. 1997) but also because of inhibition of fat oxidation in skeletal muscle. Artificially increased plasma FA availability did not completely return fat oxidation to levels seen during exercise in the fasted state (Horowitz et al. 1997). Some evidence indicates that the hyperinsulinemia and hyperglycemia reduce the uptake of FA into the mitochondria (Coyle et al. 1997).

Because the metabolic effects of pre-exercise carbohydrate ingestion are a consequence of hyperglycemia and hyperinsulinemia, interest has developed in strategies that minimize the changes in plasma glucose and insulin before exercise. These strategies include the ingestion of fructose or carbohydrate types other than glucose that have a lower **glycemic index** (see the side bar for an explanation of glycemic index), varying the carbohydrate load or the ingestion schedule, the addition of fat, and the inclusion of warm-up exercise in the pre-exercise period. In general, although these various interventions do modify the metabolic response to exercise, blunting the pre-exercise glycemic and insulinemic responses appears to offer no advantage for exercise performance.

GLYCEMIC INDEX

The glycemic index (GI) refers to the increase in blood glucose and insulin in response to a standard amount of food and is determined by measuring the area under the glucose curve. The GI measurements are usually based on the ingestion of 50 g of carbohydrate and measurements of blood glucose over a 2-hour period. The greater the glucose response and the greater the area under the curve, the greater the GI of a food. A greater GI indicates a rapid absorption and delivery of the carbohydrate into the circulation. The GI is calculated using the following formula:

$$GI = \text{area under the glucose curve of test food}/$$
$$\text{area under the glucose curve of reference food} \times 100$$

The reference food is usually glucose or white bread and has a glycemic index of 100. Foods are generally divided into low-GI foods, moderate-GI foods, and high-GI foods. Low-GI foods have a GI of 55 or less, moderate-GI foods have a GI between 56 and 70, and high-GI foods have a GI of 71 or higher. Apples or lentils, for example, will result in a slow and small rise of the blood glucose concentration, whereas white bread or potatoes will result in a rapid rise in the blood glucose concentration. The apples and the lentils, therefore, are classified as low-GI foods and bread and potatoes are classified as high-GI foods. A list of high-GI, moderate-GI, and low-GI foods is given in table 5.2.

Table 5.2 Glycemic Index (GI) and Glycemic Load (GL)

Food	GI	Serving size (g)	Available carbohydrate (g)	GL (per serving)
High GI (>70)				
Boiled potato	101	150	17	17
Glucose	99	10	10	10
Baked potato	85	150	30	26
Lucozade, original	95	250 (ml)	42	40
Pancakes, buckwheat	102	77	22	22
Pretzels	83	30	20	16
Scones	92	25	9	7
Gatorade	78	250 (ml)	15	12
Isostar	70	250 (ml)	18	13
Bagel	72	70	35	25
Baguette, white, plain	95	70	37	27
Cheerios cereals	74	30	20	15
Corn flakes	81	30	26	21
Shredded wheat	75	30	20	15
K-time strawberry crunch bar	77	30	25	19
Puffed rice cakes	78	25	21	17
Watermelon	72	120	6	4
Popcorn	72	20	11	8
Stir fried vegetables	73	360	75	55

(continued)

Food	GI	Serving size (g)	Available carbohydrate (g)	GL (per serving)
Moderate GI (56–70)				
Doughnut	67	47	23	17
Croissant	67	57	26	17
Blueberry muffin	60	57	29	17
Coca-Cola	58	250 (ml)	26	16
French baguette with butter and strawberry jam	62	70	41	26
Porridge	58	250 (ml)	22	13
Rice, white, boiled	64	150	36	23
Long-grain rice, boiled	56	150	41	23
Digestives (cookies)	59	25	16	10
Oreo cookies	64	40	32	20
Ice cream, regular	61	50	13	8
Fruit cocktail, canned	55	120	16	9
Mars bar	65	60	40	26
Snickers bar	55	60	35	19
Power bar, chocolate	56	65	42	24
Ironman PR bar	39	65	26	10
Low GI (<55)				
Honey	55	25	18	10
Potato crisps/chips	54	50	21	11
Sweet corn	54	80	17	9
Pizza Super supreme (Pizza Hut)	36	100	24	9
Wheat bread	53	30	20	11
Carrots	47	80	6	3
Orange juice	50	250 (ml)	26	13
Apple juice	40	250 (ml)	29	12
Rye bread	41	30	12	5
All Bran cereal	42	30	23	9
Baked beans	48	150	15	7
Kidney beans	28	150	25	7
Lentils	30	150	17	5
Smoothie, raspberry	33	250 (ml)	41	14
M&Ms (peanut)	33	30	17	6
Muesli	49	30	20	10
Prince Fourre chocolate cookies	52	45	30	16
Ice cream, low-fat, vanilla	50	50	6	3
Spaghetti, boiled	38	180	48	18
Chocolate milk, plain	43	50	28	12
Skim milk	32	250 (ml)	13	4
Milk, full-fat	27	250 (ml)	12	3

(continued)

(continued)

Table 5.2 *(continued)*

Food	GI	Serving size (g)	Available carbohydrate (g)	GL (per serving)
Low GI (<55)				
Yogurt	36	200	9	3
Low-fat yogurt	24	200	14	3
Apple	38	120	15	6
Banana	52	120	24	12
Orange	42	120	11	5
Grapes	46	120	18	8
Peach	42	120	11	5
Peanuts	14	50	6	1
Fructose	19	10	10	2

Reprinted, by permission, from K. Foster-Powell and J.C. Brand-Miller, "International table of glycemic index and glycemic load values: 2002," *American Journal of Clinical Nutrition.* July 76(1): 5-56.

The use of the GI as a tool is quite controversial, mainly because the GI for any given food might vary considerably between individuals. The tables usually provide an average figure that is not necessarily useful in controlling an individual's blood glucose concentration. The GI of foods is also sometimes confusing. In general, foods with large amounts of refined sugar (simple carbohydrates) have a high GI and sugars with a high fiber content and complex carbohydrates have a lower GI. However, some complex carbohydrates (starches) can have a high GI. On the other hand, adding relatively small amounts of fat to a high-GI carbohydrate can lower the GI of the food substantially. Therefore, the GI must be interpreted and used with caution. It can probably be a useful tool if its limitations and pitfalls are well understood.

The **glycemic load** (GL) is a relatively new way to assess the impact of carbohydrate consumption that takes the GI into account but gives a fuller picture than does GI alone. A GI value indicates only how rapidly a particular carbohydrate appears as glucose in the circulation but does not take into account the amount of the food that is normally consumed. For example, the carbohydrate in watermelon has a high GI, but there is not a lot of it, so watermelon's GL is relatively low. A GL of 20 or more is high, a GL of 11 to 19 is medium, and a GL of 10 or less is low. Foods that have a low GL almost always have a low GI. Foods with an intermediate or high GL range from a very low to a very high GI. The GL is calculated by multiplying the GI by the amount of carbohydrate (g) in one serving, and dividing by 100.

For example, a carrot weighing 60 g contains only 4 g of carbohydrate. To get 50 g, you would have to eat about 750 g of carrots. GL takes the GI value and multiplies it by the actual amount of carbohydrates in a serving. A GL is low if it is between 1 and 10, medium if it is between 11 and 19, and high if it is 20 or higher.

The glycemic responses during exercise after carbohydrate ingestion are determined by a number of factors related to the delivery of carbohydrate into the circulation, as well as the uptake from the circulation. Some of the factors that determine the glycemic response during exercise are

- the combined stimulatory effects of insulin and contractile activity on muscle glucose uptake;

- the balance of inhibitory and stimulatory effects of insulin and catecholamines on liver glucose output; and

- the magnitude of ongoing intestinal absorption of glucose from the ingested carbohydrate.

The metabolic alterations associated with ingestion of carbohydrate in the 30 minutes to 60 minutes before exercise have the potential to influence exercise performance. The increase in muscle glycogenolysis observed previously possibly results in an earlier onset of fatigue during exercise as suggested in a study by Foster, Costill, and Fink (1979). In contrast, the vast majority of such studies have shown either unchanged or enhanced endurance exercise performance after ingestion of carbohydrate in the hour before exercise.

Thus, the well-documented metabolic effects of pre-exercise carbohydrate ingestion and the possibility of negative consequences in susceptible individuals notwithstanding, little evidence appears to support the practice of avoiding carbohydrate ingestion in the hour before exercise, provided sufficient carbohydrate is ingested. Individual practice must be determined on the basis of individual experience with various pre-exercise carbohydrate ingestion protocols.

Finally, when carbohydrate is ingested during prolonged exercise, the potential negative effects of the pre-exercise carbohydrate feedings is reduced. When a high-GI food is ingested before exercise, it has little or no effect on metabolism and performance if carbohydrate is ingested during exercise (Burke et al. 1998).

Carbohydrate During Exercise

There is convincing evidence from numerous studies that carbohydrate feeding during exercise of about 45 minutes or longer (Jeukendrup et al. 1997; Coyle et al. 1986) can improve endurance capacity and performance. Studies have also addressed questions of which carbohydrates are most effective, what is the most effective feeding schedule, and what is the optimal amount of carbohydrate to consume. Other studies have looked at factors that could possibly influence the oxidation of ingested carbohydrate, such as muscle glycogen levels, diet, and exercise intensity. Mechanisms by which carbohydrate feeding during exercise may improve endurance performance include the following.

- Maintaining blood glucose and high levels of carbohydrate oxidation. Coyle et al. 1986 demonstrated that carbohydrate feeding during exercise at 70% $\dot{V}O_2$max prevents the drop in blood glucose that was observed when water (placebo) was ingested. In the placebo trials, the glucose concentration started to drop after 1 hour of exercise and reached extremely low concentrations (2.5 mmol/L) at exhaustion after 3 hours. With carbohydrate feeding, glucose concentrations were maintained above 3 mmol/L,

and subjects continued to exercise for 4 hours at the same intensity. Total-carbohydrate oxidation rates followed a similar pattern. A drop in carbohydrate oxidation occurred after about 1.5 hours of exercise with placebo, and high rates of carbohydrate oxidation were maintained with carbohydrate feeding. Interestingly, when subjects ingested only water and exercised to exhaustion, they were able to continue again when glucose was ingested or infused intravenously. These studies showed the importance of plasma glucose as a substrate during exercise.

- Glycogen sparing. Carbohydrate feedings during exercise "spare" liver glycogen (Bosch, Dennis, and Noakes 1994; Jeukendrup et al. 1999), and Tsintzas and Williams (1998) discussed a potential muscle glycogen sparing effect. Generally, muscle glycogen sparing is not found during cycling (Coyle et al. 1986; Jeukendrup et al. 1999), but it may be important during running (Tsintzas et al. 1995).

- Promoting glycogen synthesis during exercise. After intermittent exercise, muscle glycogen concentrations were higher when carbohydrate was ingested than when water was ingested (Yaspelkis et al. 1993). This finding could indicate a reduced muscle glycogen breakdown. However, the ingested carbohydrate was possibly used to synthesize muscle glycogen during the low-intensity exercise periods (Kuipers et al. 1986; Keizer et al. 1987).

- Affecting motor skills. Few studies have attempted to study the effect of carbohydrate drinks on motor skills. One such study investigated 13 trained tennis players and observed that when players ingested carbohydrate during a 2-hour training session (Vergauwen, Brouns, and Hespel 1998), stroke quality was improved during the final stages of prolonged play. This effect was most noticeable when the situations required fast running speed, rapid movement, and explosiveness.

- Affecting the central nervous system. Carbohydrate may also have central nervous system effects. Although direct evidence for such an effect is lacking, the brain can sense changes in the composition of the mouth and stomach contents. Evidence, for instance, suggests that taste influences mood and may also influence perception of effort. An interesting observation provides support for a central nervous system effect. When a hypoglycemic person bites a candy bar, that person's symptoms are almost immediately reduced, and the person feels better again long before the carbohydrate has reached the systemic circulation and the brain. The central nervous system effect may also explain why some studies report positive effects of carbohydrate during exercise on performance lasting approximately 1 hour (Jeukendrup et al. 1997). During exercise of such short duration, only a small amount of the carbohydrate becomes available as a substrate. Most of the ingested carbohydrate is still in the stomach or intestine. Whether the central nervous system effects of glucose feeding are mediated by sensory detection of glucose or perception of sweetness is not known, although studies with placebo solutions with identical taste to glucose solutions suggest that sweetness is not the key factor.

Feeding Strategies and Exogenous Carbohydrate Oxidation

A greater contribution of exogenous (external) fuel sources (carbohydrate) spares endogenous (internal) sources, and the notion that a greater contribution from exogenous sources increases endurance capacity is enticing. The contribution of exogenous substrates can be measured using stable (or radioactive) isotopic tracers. The principle of this technique is quite simple: The ingested substrate (e.g., glucose) is labeled and the label can be measured in expired gas after the substrate has been oxidized. The more the ingested substrate has been oxidized, the more of the label

(tracer) will be recovered in the expired gas. Knowing the amount of tracer ingested, the amount of tracer in the expired gas, and the total CO_2 production enables us to calculate exogenous substrate oxidation rates.

The typical pattern of exogenous glucose oxidation rates is shown in figure 5.4. The labeled CO_2 starts to appear 5 minutes after ingestion of the labeled carbohydrate. During the first 75 minutes to 90 minutes of exercise, **exogenous carbohydrate oxidation** continues to rise as more and more carbohydrate is emptied from the stomach and absorbed in the intestine. After 75 minutes to 90 minutes a leveling-off occurs, and the exogenous carbohydrate oxidation rate reaches its maximum value and does not increase further. Several factors have been suggested to influence exogenous carbohydrate oxidation including feeding schedule, type and amount of carbohydrate ingested, and the exercise intensity.

Feeding Schedule

The timing of carbohydrate feedings seems to have relatively little effect on exogenous carbohydrate oxidation rates. Studies in which a large bolus (100 g) of a carbohydrate in solution was given produced similar exogenous carbohydrate oxidation rates to studies in which 100 g carbohydrate was ingested at regular intervals.

Amount of Carbohydrate

From a practical point of view, the amount of carbohydrate that needs to be ingested to attain optimal

Figure 5.4 Exogenous carbohydrate oxidation during exercise. The curve shows the typical pattern of the oxidation of carbohydrate ingested at regular intervals.

Reprinted, by permission, from A.E. Jeukendrup and R. Jentjens, 2000, "Oxidation of carbohydrate feedings during prolonged exercise: Current thoughts, guidelines, and directions for future research," *Sports Medicine* 29(6): 407-424.

performance is important. The optimal amount is likely to be the amount that results in maximal exogenous oxidation rates without causing gastrointestinal problems. Rehrer, Wagenmakers, et al. (1992) studied the oxidation of different amounts of carbohydrate ingested during 80 minutes of cycling exercise at 70% $\dot{V}O_2$max. Subjects received either a 4.5% glucose solution (a total of 58 g glucose during 80 minutes of exercise) or a 17% glucose solution (220 g during 80 minutes of exercise). Total exogenous carbohydrate oxidation was measured and found to be slightly higher with the larger carbohydrate dose (42 g versus 32 g in 80 minutes). So, even though the amount of carbohydrate ingested was increased almost fourfold, the oxidation rate was barely affected. Jeukendrup et al. (1999) investigated the oxidation rates of carbohydrate intakes up to 3.00 g/min and found oxidation rates of up to 0.94 g/min at the end of 120 minutes of cycling exercise.

The results from a large number of studies were used to construct figure 5.5 (Jeukendrup and Jentjens 2000). The peak exogenous carbohydrate oxidation rates are plotted against the rate of ingestion. The maximal rate at which a single ingested carbohydrate can be oxidized is about 1.0 g/min. The horizontal line depicts the absolute maximum just below 1.1 g/min. The dotted line represents the line of identity where the rate of carbohydrate ingestion equals the rate of exogenous carbohydrate oxidation. This graph suggests that oxidation of orally ingested carbohydrate may already be optimal at ingestion rates around 1.2 g/min. Thus, athletes should ensure a carbohydrate intake of about 70 g/h for optimal

carbohydrate delivery. Adopting an ingestion rate of 70 g/h optimizes exogenous carbohydrate oxidation. Ingesting more than this amount of a single carbohydrate does not result in higher carbohydrate oxidation rates and is more likely to cause gastrointestinal discomfort. This amount of carbohydrate can be found in the following sources:

- 1 L sports drink (Gatorade, Powerade, Isostar, Lucozade Sport)
- 600 ml cola drink
- 1.5 Power bar
- 1.5 Gatorade energy bar
- Three medium bananas
- 120 g to 150 g wine gums

Type of Carbohydrate

Studies have compared the oxidation rates of various types of carbohydrate to the oxidation of ingested glucose during exercise (Jeukendrup and Jentjens 2000). Glucose is oxidized at relatively high rates (up to about 1 g/min). The other two monosaccharides, fructose and galactose, are oxidized at much lower rates because they have to be converted into glucose in the liver before they can be metabolized. They are, therefore, a relatively slow energy source.

The oxidation rates of maltose, sucrose, and glucose polymers (maltodextrins) are comparable to those of glucose. Starches with a relatively large amount of amylopectin are rapidly digested and absorbed, whereas those with a high amylose content

Figure 5.5 Maximal exogenous carbohydrate oxidation versus the rate of ingestion.

Reprinted, by permission, from A.E. Jeukendrup and R. Jentjens, 2000, "Oxidation of carbohydrate feedings during prolonged exercise: Current thoughts, guidelines, and directions for future research," *Sports Medicine* 29(6): 407-424.

have a relatively slow rate of hydrolysis. Ingested amylopectin is oxidized at very high rates (similar to glucose), whereas amylose is oxidized at very low rates. Carbohydrates are divided into two categories according to the rate at which they are oxidized: a higher rate group (~1 g/min) and a lower rate (~0.6 g/min). These two categories of carbohydrates are listed in figure 5.6.

Oxidized at rates of up to ~1 g/min	Oxidized at rates of up to ~0.6 g/min
Glucose	Fructose
Maltose	Galactose
Sucrose	Amylose
Maltodextrins	
Amylopectin	

Figure 5.6 Oxidation rates of ingested carbohydrate during exercise.

Reprinted, by permission, from K. Foster-Powell and J.C. Brand-Miller, "International table of glycemic index and glycemic load values: 2002," *American Journal of Clinical Nutrition* July 76(1): 5-56.

Shi et al. (1995) suggest that the inclusion of 2 or 3 different carbohydrates (glucose, fructose, and sucrose) in a drink may increase water and carbohydrate absorption despite the increased osmolality. This effect is attributed to the separate transport mechanisms across the intestinal wall for glucose, fructose, and sucrose. The monosaccharides glucose and galactose are transported across the luminal membrane by a glucose transporter called SGLT1 (see chapter 3) and fructose is transported by GLUT5. Interestingly, fructose absorption from a certain amount of the disaccharide sucrose is more

rapid than the absorption of the same amount of fructose. If a combination of glucose and fructose is ingested, more carbohydrate will be absorbed and made available for oxidation. Ingestion of relatively large amounts of glucose and fructose can result in exogenous carbohydrate oxidation rates well over 1 g/min (Jentjens et al. 2004) (see figure 5.7).

Exercise Intensity

With increasing exercise intensity, the active muscle mass becomes more dependent on carbohydrate as a source of energy. Both an increased muscle glycogenolysis and an increased plasma glucose oxidation contribute to the increased energy demands (Romijn et al. 1993). Therefore exogenous carbohydrate oxidation increases with increasing exercise intensities. Indeed, Pirnay et al. (1982) reported lower exogenous carbohydrate oxidation rates at low exercise intensities compared with moderate intensities, but exogenous carbohydrate oxidation tended to level off between 51% and 64% $\dot{V}O_2$max. However, when the exercise intensity was increased from 60% to 75% $\dot{V}O_2$max, exogenous carbohydrate oxidation rates leveled off or even decreased (Pirnay et al. 1995).

Lower exogenous carbohydrate oxidation rates possibly are only observed at very low exercise intensities when the reliance on carbohydrate as an energy source is minimal. In this situation, part of the ingested carbohydrate may be directed toward nonoxidative glucose disposal (storage in the liver or muscle) rather than toward oxidation. Studies with carbohydrate ingestion during intermittent exercise have suggested that during low-intensity exercise, glycogen can be resynthesized (Kuipers et al. 1989).

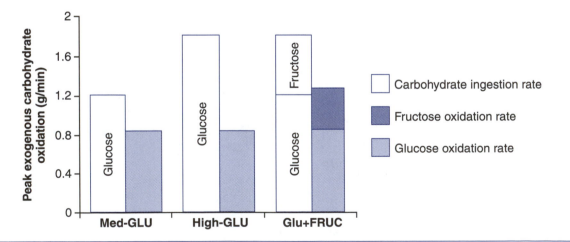

Figure 5.7 The oxidation rate of glucose plus fructose in a combined drink is higher than the oxidation rate of similar amounts of either glucose or fructose alone.

Reprinted, by permission, from A.E. Jeukendrup and R. Jentjens, 2000, "Oxidation of carbohydrate feedings during prolonged exercise: Current thoughts, guidelines, and directions for future research," *Sports Med* 29(6): 407-424.

Thus, at exercise intensities below 50% $\dot{V}O_2$max, exogenous carbohydrate oxidation increases with increasing total carbohydrate oxidation rates. Usually above approximately 60% $\dot{V}O_2$max, oxidation rates will not further increase.

Limitations to Exogenous Carbohydrate Oxidation

As discussed earlier, exogenous carbohydrate oxidation seems to be limited to rates of 1.0 g/min to 1.1 g/min (see figure 5.5). This finding is supported by most of the studies using either radioactive or stable isotopes to quantify exogenous carbohydrate oxidation during exercise. One limiting factor could be the rate of gastric emptying (see figure 5.8). However, some studies indicate that gastric emptying is unlikely to affect exogenous carbohydrate oxidation rates (Rehrer, Wagenmakers et al. 1992; Saris et al. 1993). Because in these studies only 32% to 48% of the carbohydrate delivered to the intestine was oxidized, gastric emptying was determined not to be limiting exogenous carbohydrate oxidation.

Another potential limiting factor is the rate of absorption of carbohydrate into the systemic circulation from the small intestine. Studies using a triple-lumen technique have measured glucose absorption and estimated whole-body intestinal absorption rates of a 6% glucose-electrolyte solution (Duchman et al. 1997). The estimated maximal absorption rate of the intestine ranged from 1.2 g/min to 1.7 g/min. Studies, using stable isotopes have observed a reduction in the glucose output by the liver when carbohydrate is ingested. When very large amounts of glucose are ingested, hepatic glucose output can be blocked completely (Jeukendrup et al. 1999). At low to moderate ingestion rates, no net storage of glucose occurs in the liver. Instead, all ingested glucose appears in the bloodstream. The glucose output from the liver can vary from nothing to approximately 1 g/min, when no carbohydrate is ingested, the intensity of exercise is high enough (>60% $\dot{V}O_2$max), and the duration long enough (>1 hour).

Glucose appearing in the bloodstream was taken up at rates similar to its rate of appearance (Ra), and 90% to 95% of this glucose was oxidized during exercise. When a larger dose of carbohydrate was ingested (3 g/min), the rate of appearance of glucose from the intestine was one-third of the rate of carbohydrate ingestion (0.96 g/min to 1.04 g/min). Thus, only part of the ingested carbohydrate entered the systemic circulation. However, a large proportion of the glucose appearing in the blood was taken up by tissues (presumably mainly by the muscle) and 90% to 95% was oxidized. Therefore, entrance into the systemic circulation is a limiting factor for exogenous glucose oxidation, rather than intramuscular factors. Hawley et al. (1994) bypassed both intestinal absorption and hepatic glucose uptake by infusing glucose into the circulation of subjects exercising at 70% $\dot{V}O_2$max. When large amounts of glucose were infused and subjects were hyperglycemic (10 mmol/L),

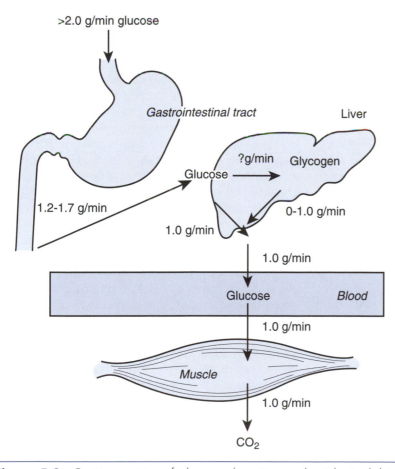

>2.0 g/min glucose

Gastrointestinal tract   Liver

?g/min   Glycogen

Glucose

1.2-1.7 g/min   0-1.0 g/min

1.0 g/min

1.0 g/min

Glucose   *Blood*

1.0 g/min

Muscle

1.0 g/min

CO_2

Figure 5.8 Gastric emptying of glucose, absorption, and uptake in skeletal muscle. Glucose travels from the gut after ingestion to the muscle. The suggested maximal flux at each of the stages is indicated.

Reprinted, by permission, from L.P.G. Jentjens and A.E. Jeukendrup, 2003, "Glycogen resynthesis after exercise," *Sports Medicine* 33(2): 117-144.

blood glucose oxidation rate increased substantially above 1 g/min.

Exogenous carbohydrate oxidation is limited by the rate of digestion, absorption, and subsequent transport of glucose into the systemic circulation. During high-intensity exercise (e.g., >80% $\dot{V}O_2$max), a reduced blood flow to the gut may result in a decreased absorption of glucose and water (Brouns and Beckers 1993) and hence a low rate of absorption relative to the rate of ingestion. Taken together, this information suggests that intestinal absorption is a contributing factor in limiting the oxidation of ingested carbohydrate at rates higher than 1.1 g/min, but it may not be the sole factor. The liver may also play an additional important role. Hepatic glucose output is highly regulated, and the glucose output derived from the intestine and from hepatic glycogenolysis and gluconeogenesis possibly does not exceed 1.1 g/min, even though the maximal rate of glucose absorption is slightly in excess of this rate. If supply from the intestine is too large (>1.0 g/min), glycogen synthesis may be stimulated in the liver.

Metabolic Effects of Carbohydrate Intake During Exercise

The metabolic effects of carbohydrate intake during exercise depend on various factors, including the amount ingested, the timing of the intake, and the intensity and duration of exercise. Generally, carbohydrate ingestion early in exercise has large effects on the insulin response, fat mobilization, and substrate utilization, whereas ingestion late in exercise has relatively little effect. If carbohydrate is ingested at the onset of exercise, plasma insulin concentrations rise in the first minutes of exercise and lipolysis is suppressed. FA availability is lowered and this condition may partly explain the lower fat oxidation rates observed in this situation. However, carbohydrate intake during exercise also inhibits fat oxidation by hindering the transport of FA into the mitochondria.

When carbohydrate is ingested later in exercise, the already raised catecholamine levels blunt the insulin response, and, hence, fat oxidation is less affected. Similarly, when a small amount of carbohydrate is ingested during exercise, the effect on the plasma insulin concentration is also small, whereas larger intakes result in an increased insulin response. Exercise intensity may be an important factor as well. Studies suggest that the suppressive effect of carbohydrate feeding on fat metabolism is greater at low exercise intensities than at high exercise intensities.

Carbohydrate After Exercise

The main purpose of carbohydrate intake after physical activity is to replenish depleted stores of liver and muscle glycogen. The replenishment of muscle glycogen is directly related to recovery of endurance capacity, and glycogen loading, or **carboloading,** in between training sessions has become common practice among endurance athletes.

Regulation of Glucose Uptake and Glycogen Synthesis

Glucose uptake in the muscle is through facilitated diffusion via the glucose transporter GLUT-4, which is largely responsible for transporting glucose across the sarcolemma. GLUT-4 is normally stored in intracellular vesicles but can translocate to the cell membrane, merge with the cell membrane, and allow increased transport of glucose into the cell (see figure 5.9). Both muscle contraction (through Ca^{2+} ions) and insulin secretion will stimulate the translocation of GLUT-4 and, hence, glucose transport into the cell.

After its transport across the sarcolemma, glucose is phosphorylated to glucose-6-phosphate (G6P) by the enzyme hexokinase (see figure 5.9). After phosphorylation, glucose is trapped in the muscle because the sarcolemma is impermeable to phosphorylated glucose and no transporters for G6P exists. G6P is next converted to glucose-1-phosphate (G1P) by the enzyme phosphoglucomutase, and G1P is combined with uridine triphosphate to form uridine diphosphate (UDP)–glucose and pyrophosphate (PPi) in a reaction catalyzed by 1-phosphate uridyltransferase. UDP is a carrier of glucose units and takes the glucose molecule to the terminal glucose residue of a preexisting glycogen molecule. UDP-glucose can be considered an activated glucose molecule. The UDP-glucose then forms an α-1,4 glycosidic bond, a reaction catalyzed by glycogen synthase, resulting in one long straight chain of glucose molecules. However, branch points (α-1,6 glycosidic bond) are introduced into the glycogen structure by a branching enzyme. When the length of a chain is about 12 glucose residues long, the branching enzyme detaches a chain about 7 residues long and reattaches it to a neighboring chain by an α-1,6 glycosidic bond. Branching results in the formation of a very large but compact glycogen molecule.

The rate of glycogen synthesis depends on several factors, including the activity of enzymes (especially glycogen synthase) and the transport of glucose into the cell, which, in turn, are influenced by muscle glycogen concentration and insulin. As

Figure 5.9 Mechanisms of glucose transport into the muscle and the synthesis of glycogen.

Reprinted, by permission, from L.P.G. Jentjens and A.E. Jeukendrup, 2003, "Glycogen resynthesis after exercise," *Sports Medicine* 33(2): 117-144.

a result of the changing activity of these enzymes and the effectiveness of these transport mechanisms, two phases can be distinguished in the process of glycogen synthesis after exercise. These phases are the initial, insulin-independent, or rapid, phase and the insulin-dependent, or slow, phase.

Rapid Phase of Glycogen Synthesis After Exercise

The rate-limiting enzyme for glycogen resynthesis after exercise, glycogen synthase, exists in an inactive D-form and an active I-form. More glycogen synthase is present in the active I-form when muscle glycogen concentrations are low (Kochan et al. 1979). As glycogen stores are replenished, more glycogen synthase

is transformed back into the D-form. Exercise activates glycogen synthase (immediately after exercise, as much as 80% of all glycogen synthase may be in the active I-form), but glycogen can only be formed if the substrate (UDP-glucose) is available. Another important factor in glycogen resynthesis, therefore, is the availability of glucose, which is mainly dependent on the glucose transport across the sarcolemma. During exercise and in the first hour after exercise, an abundance of GLUT-4 is available at the cell membrane, and glucose uptake into the muscle is facilitated. This exercise-induced effect on glucose transport, however, will last only a few hours in the absence of insulin. The increase in the permeability of the sarcolemma for glucose after exercise seems to be directly related to the amount of glycogen in the muscle. When muscle glycogen concentrations are very low, the enhanced glucose uptake may last longer. With high muscle glycogen concentrations, the effect is rapidly reversed.

Slow Phase of Glycogen Synthesis After Exercise

When the effect of the exercise-induced increase in glucose transport wears off, glycogen resynthesis occurs at a much slower rate. The rate at which glycogen synthesis occurs during the slow phase is highly dependent on the circulating insulin concentration, which will increase GLUT-4 translocation to the cell membrane and increase glucose transport into the muscle cell.

In addition, muscle contraction increases insulin sensitivity and this effect may last for several hours. This increased insulin sensitivity after exercise is thought to be an important component of the slow phase of glycogen synthesis. The glycogen synthase activity decreases during this phase as muscle glycogen is restored.

Once inside the muscle cell glucose is directed toward muscle glycogen rather than oxidation. This effect is mediated by an increased glycogen synthase activity. An increase in the amount of GLUT-4 present in the cell may also contribute to higher glycogen synthesis rates (Ren et al. 1994). After exercise, a rapid increase in GLUT-4 expression may occur, resulting in an increased synthesis of this protein, which, in turn, results in a proportional increase in insulin-stimulated glucose uptake and glycogen synthesis.

Postexercise Feeding and Rapid Recovery

A high rate of glycogen synthesis in the hours after exercise depends on the availability of substrate. In the absence of carbohydrate ingestion, glycogen resynthesis rates are very low, despite increased insulin sensitivity, increased glycogen synthase activity, and increased permeability of the sarcolemma to glucose (Ivy, Lee, et al. 1988). Often, the time to recover between successive athletic competitions or training sessions is very short. In such cases, rapid glycogen synthesis is even more important. Although muscle glycogen concentrations are unlikely to be completely restored to pre-exercise levels, all methods of carbohydrate supplementation that maximize glycogen restoration may benefit performance. Four factors have been recognized as potentially important in promoting restoration of muscle glycogen stores: (1) timing of carbohydrate intake, (2) rate of carbohydrate ingestion,

(3) the type of carbohydrate ingested, and (4) ingestion of protein and carbohydrate after exercise.

Timing of Carbohydrate Intake

The timing of carbohydrate intake can have an important effect on the rate of muscle glycogen synthesis after exercise (Ivy, Katz, et al. 1988). When carbohydrate intake is delayed until 2 hours after exercise, muscle glycogen concentration after 4 hours is 45% lower compared with ingestion of the same amount of carbohydrate immediately after exercise. Average glycogen resynthesis rates in the 2 hours after ingestion are 3 mmol/kg w.w./h to 4 mmol/kg w.w./h when carbohydrate is ingested after 2 hours and 5 mmol/kg w.w./h to 6 mmol/kg w.w./h when it is ingested immediately after exercise (see figure 5.10). When carbohydrate intake is delayed until after the rapid phase, less glucose is taken up and stored as glycogen, primarily because of decreasing insulin sensitivity after the first few hours after exercise. A substantial intake of carbohydrate immediately after exercise seems to prevent this developing insulin resistance quite effectively.

Figure 5.10 Effect of timing on muscle glycogen resynthesis.

Adapted, by permission, from J.L. Ivy, A.L. Katz, C.L. Cutler, W.M. Sherman, E.F. Cole, 1998, "Muscle glycogen synthesis after exercise: Effect of time of carbohydrate ingestion," *Journal of Applied Physiology* 64: 1480-1485.

Rate of Carbohydrate Ingestion

When no carbohydrate is ingested after exercise, the rate of muscle glycogen synthesis is extremely low (1 mmol/kg w.w./h to 2 mmol/kg w.w./h) (Ivy et al. 1988b). The ingestion of carbohydrate, especially in the first hours after exercise, results in enhanced muscle glycogen restoration, and glycogen is generally synthesized at a rate between 4.5 mmol/kg w.w./h and 11 mmol/kg w.w./h. In figure 5.11, the results of a large number of studies performed in different laboratories have been compiled. The rate of muscle glycogen synthesis plotted against the ingestion rate shows that with an increase in intake, an increase in synthesis also occurs in the first 3 hours to 5 hours after exercise. This graph shows a trend toward a higher glycogen synthesis rate when more carbohydrate is ingested, up to intakes of about 1.4 g/min, which is higher than previously suggested (Blom et al. 1987). At a given rate of carbohydrate intake, large variability exists in the rate of glycogen synthesis, probably indicating that other factors such as timing, type of carbohydrate ingested, and training are also important.

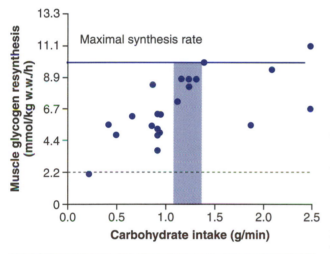

Figure 5.11 Muscle glycogen resynthesis after exercise as a function of the carbohydrate intake.

Adapted, by permission, from J.L. Ivy et al., 1988, "Muscle glycogen synthesis after exercise: Effect of time of carbohydrate ingestion," *Journal of Applied Physiology* 64: 1480-1485.

Type of Carbohydrate Ingested

Ingestion of different types of carbohydrate has different effects on glycogen synthesis. Blom et al. (1987) demonstrated that fructose ingestion resulted in slower rates of muscle glycogen synthesis after exercise compared with glucose or sucrose ingestion. Fructose must be converted to glucose in the liver before it can be used for glycogen synthesis in the muscle. Because this process takes time, glycogen synthesis occurs at a lower rate compared with a directly available carbohydrate source such as glucose. Other studies confirmed that glycogen synthesis from fructose occurs at only 50% of the rate of glycogen synthesis from glucose. In the study by Blom et al. (1987), sucrose intake resulted in similar

muscle glycogen levels 4 hours after exercise as glucose intake.

Glycogen synthesis is dependent on the GI of the meal consumed after exercise. After 6 hours of recovery, muscle glycogen is more restored with a high-GI meal compared with a low-GI meal. Thus, the absorption rate and the availability of glucose seem to be very important factors for glycogen synthesis. Low-GI foods result in lower glycogen resynthesis in the first hours after exercise.

Protein and Carbohydrate Ingestion After Exercise

Certain amino acids have a potent effect on the secretion of insulin. The effects of adding amino acids and proteins to a carbohydrate solution have been investigated to optimize glycogen synthesis. Zawadzki et al. (1992) compared glycogen resynthesis rates after ingestion of carbohydrate, protein, or carbohydrate plus protein. As expected, very little glycogen was stored when protein alone was ingested. Glycogen storage was increased when carbohydrate was ingested. However, most interestingly, glycogen storage was further increased when carbohydrate was ingested together with protein.

The increased glycogen synthesis also coincided with higher insulin levels. Van Loon et al. (2000) used a protein hydrolysate and amino acid mixture (0.8 g/kg/h carbohydrate plus 0.4 g/kg/h of protein/amino acid) that had previously been shown to result in a marked insulin response in combination with carbohydrate. When subjects ingested carbohydrate plus this protein/amino acid mixture, they observed higher glycogen resynthesis rates than when only carbohydrate was ingested. In this study, subjects also ingested an isoenergetic carbohydrate solution. Despite a larger insulin response with the added protein, glycogen resynthesis was highest with the isoenergetic amount of carbohydrate (see figure 5.12). These results suggest that insulin is an important factor, but the main limiting factor is the availability of carbohydrate. When a protein/amino acid mixture (0.4 g/kg/h) was added to a very large amount of carbohydrate (1.2 g/kg/h carbohydrate), insulin concentrations increased, but the increase did not further increase glycogen resynthesis (Jentjens et al. 2001). These studies are summarized in figure 5.12. The maximal capacity to store muscle glycogen is likely reached and, therefore, no additional effect of elevated insulin concentration is found. Thus, to achieve rapid muscle glycogen replenishment ingesting an adequate amount of carbohydrate is more important than adding protein or amino acid mixtures to a recovery meal or drink.

Figure 5.12 The rate of muscle glycogen synthesis after ingestion of different carbohydrate and carbohydrate-protein beverages. The synthesis rate for a drink containing 0.8 g/kg/h of carbohydrate is set at 100%, and all other synthesis rates are expressed relative to this baseline.

Solid Versus Liquid

Few studies have investigated the effect of solid versus liquid carbohydrate foods on glycogen synthesis in the early hours after exercise. Keizer et al. (1987) demonstrated that glycogen synthesis rates were similar after consumption of either a liquid or solid carbohydrate meal. However, the solid meal in this study contained slightly more carbohydrate compared with the liquid meal, and differences in fat and protein content between the two meals were substantial. Other investigators also found no difference in the rate of muscle glycogen storage between liquid and solid carbohydrate feedings. Therefore, no difference in glycogen synthesis with solid or liquid feedings is believed to exist. In the studies mentioned previously the investigators used a high-GI carbohydrate, probably resulting in a rapid delivery of glucose. Low-GI solid meals are likely to result in lower rates of glycogen synthesis compared with carbohydrate solutions. For further reading about glycogen synthesis after exercise, see reviews by Jentjens and Jeukendrup (2003b), Ivy (1998), and Ivy and Kuo (1998).

Muscle Glycogen, Diet, and Repeated Days of Training

Often, athletes compete or train on consecutive days, in which case, rapid replenishment of muscle glycogen appears crucial. Costill et al (1971) reported that in subjects running 16.1 km on 3 consecutive days,

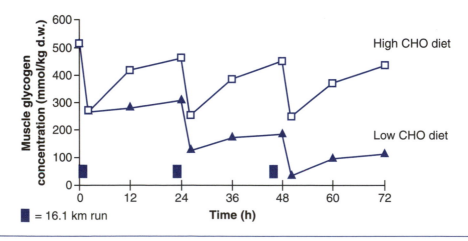

Figure 5.13 Muscle glycogen concentration after repeated bouts of running.

Reprinted, by permission, from D.L. Costill, R. Bowers, G. Branam, K. Sparks, 1971, "Muscle glycogen utilization during prolonged exercise on successive days," *Journal of Applied Physiology* 31: 834-838.

a diet containing only moderate amounts of carbohydrate (40% to 50%) may not be enough to fully restore muscle glycogen (see figure 5.13). A marked decrease in muscle glycogen occurred immediately after the run, and although some glycogen was synthesized before the run the next day, the starting muscle glycogen concentrations were lower. After 3 days of running, the muscle glycogen concentration had dropped considerably.

Sherman et al. (1993) fed subjects a diet containing either 5 g/kg b.w./day or 10 g/kg b.w./day during seven days of training. The diet containing 5 g carbohydrate/kg b.w./day resulted in a decline in muscle glycogen concentration in the first five days, which was then maintained for the remainder of the study. With the high-carbohydrate diet (10 g/kg b.w./day), muscle glycogen concentrations were maintained despite daily training.

In another study, well-trained cyclists exercised 2 hours a day at 65% $\dot{V}O_2$max (Coyle et al. 2001). They ingested a diet containing 581 g, 718 g, or 901 g of carbohydrate. These high-carbohydrate intakes made maintaining very high muscle glycogen concentrations possible (120 mmol/kg w.w., 155 mmol/kg w.w., and 185 mmol/kg w.w., respectively). The muscle glycogen concentrations were even higher than the values reported after the classical supercompensation diet. The amount of carbohydrate ingested between two exercise bouts on consecutive days is, therefore, very important in determining the total amount of muscle glycogen stored. A higher carbohydrate intake can also reduce some symptoms of overreaching (an early stage of overtraining) such as changes in mood state and feelings of fatigue, although it cannot completely prevent them. Achten, Halson, et al. (2003) observed such an effect in runners who increased their training volume and intensity and controlled their carbohydrate intake at either 5.4 g/kg b.w./day or 8.5 g/kg b.w./day.

Muscle Glycogen Restoration

Unless large amounts of carbohydrate are ingested, muscle glycogen does not normalize on a day-to-day basis (Costill et al. 1971). How much carbohydrate must we eat to replenish our glycogen stores within 24 hours? Costill et al. (1981) suggested that increasing carbohydrate intake from 150 g to 650 g results in a proportional increases in muscle glycogen. However, intakes higher than 600 g/24 h do not result in a further increase in glycogen resynthesis. More recent studies seem to suggest that with daily exercise, an almost linear increase in glycogen storage occurs in relation to carbohydrate intake (Coyle et al. 2001). These findings and others have led sports nutrition

experts to recommend increasing carbohydrate intake to 10 g/kg b.w./day to 13 g/kg b.w./day when exercising for 3 hours or more on a daily basis.

Carbohydrate Type and Long-Term Recovery

To stimulate glycogen resynthesis after exercise, the amount of carbohydrate ingested may be the most important factor, but the type of carbohydrate may also play a role. One study investigated the effects of the GI on muscle glycogen resynthesis. Subjects performed a bout of exercise that depleted their glycogen stores on two occasions and received a diet of high-GI carbohydrate on one occasion and a diet of low-GI carbohydrate on the other (Burke, Collier, and Hargreaves 1993). The total carbohydrate intake over 24 hours was 10 g/kg b.w. The increase in muscle glycogen was more than 50% greater when the high-GI carbohydrates were consumed. Therefore, high-GI foods are important for complete muscle glycogen resynthesis within 24 hours. The higher insulin responses of the high-GI meals are likely responsible for the increased glycogen synthesis.

Glycogen Loading and Long-Term Recovery

Often guidelines are expressed in percentages, which has confused the advice given to athletes. For example, a 50% carbohydrate diet may contain a very large amount of carbohydrate for a triathlete or cyclist who expends 6,000 kcal/day but contain only a small amount of carbohydrate for a distance runner who has an intake of 2,000 kcal/day. A more sensible expression of carbohydrate intake is grams/kilogram bodyweight/day.

As a general guideline, 5 g/kg b.w./day to 7 g/kg b.w./day during moderate-intensity training and 7 g/kg b.w./day to 10 g/kg b.w./day during increased training are recommended. Endurance athletes involved in extreme training programs should increase carbohydrate intake to 10 g/kg b.w./day to 13 g/kg b.w./day when exercising daily. This intake enables them to restore muscle glycogen even though they may become depleted in a training session. Recommendations for long-term recovery include

- ingesting 5-7 g/kg b.w./day during moderate intensity training;
- ingesting at least 7 g/kg b.w./day to 10 g /kg b.w./day of carbohydrate during prolonged hard training;

- ingesting 10 g/kg b.w./day to13 g /kg b.w./day of carbohydrate when performing very prolonged very hard exercise;
- choosing high-GI carbohydrates; and
- consuming sports drink to provides a convenient source of carbohydrate in the first hour after exercise when appetite is suppressed.

For optimal glycogen resynthesis, a large proportion of the carbohydrate intake should consist of high-GI foods (see table 5.2). Carbohydrate solutions have the advantage of providing fluid that will help restore fluid balance (see chapter 8).

A significant amount of ingested carbohydrate may be directed to the liver. Unfortunately, liver glycogen is very difficult to measure, and although some studies using liver biopsies were performed in the 1960s, very limited information is available about liver glycogen synthesis after exercise and its potential effect on performance. A noninvasive technique that has been used to address this problem is nuclear magnetic resonance (NMR) imaging. Using ^{13}C-NMR, Casey et al. (2000) measured liver glycogen concentrations after exercise and during 4 hours of recovery. They observed that liver glycogen resynthesis was evident after glucose and sucrose ingestion but not with water. Relatively small amounts of carbohydrate were ingested (1 g/kg b.w.), and these amounts were sufficient to initiate postexercise liver glycogen resynthesis.

What Athletes Really Do

What do athletes actually do in real life about carbohydrate intake? The many reports of dietary intake among athletes in a variety of sports are beyond the scope of this book. The interested reader is referred to an excellent publication (Burke 2001) in which this topic is discussed in great detail. The publication concluded that most male athletes achieve a dietary intake of 5 g/kg b.w./day to 7 g/kg b.w./day for regular training needs and 7 g/kg b.w./day to 10 g/kg b.w./day during periods of increased training or competition. Female athletes, in particular endurance runners, are less likely to achieve their specific carbohydrate intake targets because they sometimes try to reduce the energy intake to achieve or maintain low levels of body fat, without paying enough attention to carbohydrate intake.

Key Points

- Muscle glycogen is a readily available energy source for the working muscle. The glycogen content of skeletal muscle at rest is approximately 54 g/kg d.m. to 72 g/kg d.m. (65 mmol glucosyl units/kg w.w. to 90 mmol glucosyl units/kg w.w.), equating to a total of about 300 g to 600 g of carbohydrate.

- The main role of glycogen in the liver is to maintain a constant blood glucose level. An average liver weighs approximately 1.5 kg, and approximately 80 g to 110 g of glycogen is stored in the liver of an adult human in the postabsorptive state.

- In resting conditions, the glucose output of the liver is approximately 150 mg/min, of which 60% is derived from the breakdown of liver glycogen and about 40% is derived from gluconeogenesis. During exercise, the liver glucose output increases dramatically, up to about 1 g/min, and the majority of this glucose (>90%) is derived from the breakdown of liver glycogen.

- The classical supercompensation protocol results in very high muscle glycogen stores. However, a moderate approach results in similar muscle glycogen levels without the disadvantages of the classical protocol and is therefore the preferred regimen.

- The brain is highly dependent on glucose as a fuel. As blood glucose concentrations drop, hypoglycemia may develop, resulting in dizziness, nausea, cold sweat, reduced mental alertness and ability to concentrate, loss of motor skill, increased heart rate, excessive hunger, and disorientation.

- The primary role of carbohydrate in the days leading up to competition is to fully replenish muscle glycogen stores.

(continued)

(continued)

- Carbohydrate loading, or increased carbohydrate stores, increases time to exhaustion (endurance capacity) on average by about 20% and reduces time taken to complete a set task (time trial; endurance performance) by 2% to 3%.

- In the 3 hours to 5 hours before exercise, some carbohydrate may be incorporated into muscle glycogen, but the majority will be stored as liver glycogen.

- Carbohydrate intake in the hours before exercise results in a transient fall in plasma glucose with the onset of exercise, increases carbohydrate oxidation and accelerated glycogen breakdown, and results in a blunting of fatty acid mobilization and fat oxidation.

- Carbohydrate feeding during exercise of about 45 minutes or longer is believed to improve endurance capacity and performance. The mechanisms may be by maintaining of blood glucose levels and high carbohydrate oxidation rates, glycogen sparing, or central nervous system effects.

- Oxidation of ingested carbohydrate during exercise is dependent on the type of carbohydrate, the amount ingested, and the exercise intensity, but the maximum oxidation rate seems to be about 1 g/min.

- Ingestion of 70 g of carbohydrate per hour (1.2 g/min) is recommended during prolonged exercise.

- Multiple transportable carbohydrates (e.g. glucose and fructose) in a beverage can increase oxidation rates during exercise.

- Two phases can be distinguished in the process of glycogen synthesis after exercise, which have often been referred to as the initial, insulin-independent, or rapid phase, and the insulin-dependent, or slow, phase.

- Restoration of muscle glycogen stores after exercise may depend on the timing of carbohydrate intake, the rate of carbohydrate ingestion, the type of carbohydrate consumed, and the addition of other macronutrients (e.g., protein).

- As a general guideline, the recommended carbohydrate ingestion during periods of moderate-training intensity is 5 g/kg b.w./day to 7 g/kg b.w./day and 7 g/kg b.w./day to 10 g/kg b.w./day when training is increased. For endurance athletes who are involved in extreme training programs, increasing carbohydrate intake to 10 g/kg b.w./day to 13 g/kg b.w./day when exercising daily is generally recommended.

Key Terms

carboloading 118	glycemic load 112	rebound hypoglycemia 106
exogenous carbohydrate oxidation 114	hepatic glucose output 104	supercompensation 106
glycemic index 109		

Recommended Readings

Hargreaves, M., J.A. Hawley, and A.E. Jeukendrup. 2004. Pre-exercise carbohydrate and fat ingestion: Effects on metabolism and performance. *Journal of Sports Sciences* 22: 31-38.

Hawley, J.A., E.J. Schabort, T.D. Noakes, and S.C. Dennis. 1997. Carbohydrate loading and exercise performance: An update. *Sports Medicine* 24: 73-81.

Ivy, J. 1998. Glycogen resynthesis after exercise: Effect of carbohydrate intake. *International Journal of Sports Medicine* 19: S142-S145.

Ivy, J.L., and C.-H. Kuo. 1998. Regulation of GLUT4 protein and glycogen synthase during muscle glycogen synthesis after exercise. *Acta Physiologica Scandinavica* 162: 295-304.

Jentjens, L.P.G., and A.E. Jeukendrup. 2003. Glycogen resynthesis after exercise. *Sports Medicine* 33(2): 117-144.

Jeukendrup, A.E., and R. Jentjens. 2000. Oxidation of carbohydrate feedings during prolonged exercise: Current thoughts, guidelines and directions for future research. *Sports Medicine* 29 (6): 407-424.

Maughan, R.J., and M. Gleeson. 2004. *The Biochemical Basis of Sports Performance*. Oxford University Press: Oxford.

Chapter 6

Fat

© Digital Vision Online

Objectives

After studying this chapter, you should be able to do the following:

- Describe the main biochemical pathways in fat metabolism

- Describe the changes that occur in fat metabolism at different intensities of exercise

- Discuss the factors that limit fat oxidation

- Describe the interactions between carbohydrate and fat metabolism at rest and in response to exercise

- Describe the metabolic and performance effects of fat intake 3 hours to 4 hours before exercise

- Describe the metabolic and performance effects of short-term high-fat diets

- Describe the metabolic and performance effects of long-term high-fat diets

Dietary fat is often considered the "bad guy," and excess intakes are often believed to be detrimental to performance and to cause weight gain and deterioration of health. Dietary fat, however, is also very important for athletic performance and health. Fat is an extremely important fuel for endurance exercise, along with carbohydrate, and some fat intake is required for optimal health. Dietary fat provides the essential fatty acids (EFA) that cannot be synthesized in the body.

The body's fat stores are very large in comparison with carbohydrate stores. In some forms of exercise (e.g., prolonged cycling or running), carbohydrate depletion is possibly a cause of fatigue and depletion can occur within 1 hour to 2 hours of strenuous exercise (see chapter 5). The total amount of energy stored as glycogen in the muscles and liver has been estimated to be 8,000 kJ (2,000 kcal). Fat stores can contain more than 50 times the amount of energy in carbohydrate stores. A person with a body mass of 80 kg and 15% body fat has 12 kg of fat (see table 6.1). Most of this fat is stored in subcutaneous adipose tissue, but some fat can also be found in muscle as **intramuscular triacylglycerol** (IMTG). In theory, the fat stores could provide sufficient energy for a runner to run at least 1,300 km.

Ideally, athletes would like to tap into their fat stores as much as possible and save the carbohydrate for later in a competition. Researchers, coaches, and athletes have therefore tried to devise nutritional strategies to enhance fat metabolism, spare carbohydrate stores, and, hence, improve endurance performance. Understanding the effects of various nutritional strategies requires an understanding of fat metabolism and the factors that regulate fat oxidation during exercise. This chapter, therefore, describes fat metabolism in detail and discusses different ways in which researchers and athletes have tried to enhance fat metabolism by nutritional manipulation. Finally, the effects of both low-fat and high-fat diets on metabolism, exercise performance, and health are discussed.

Fat Metabolism During Exercise

FAs that are oxidized in the mitochondria of skeletal muscle during exercise are derived from various sources. The main two sources are adipose tissue and muscle triacylglycerols. A third fuel, plasma triacylglycerol may also be utilized, but the importance of this fuel is subject to debate. Figure 6.1 gives an overview of the fat substrates and their journey to the muscle. Triacylglycerols in adipose tissue are split into FAs and glycerol. The glycerol is released into the circulation, along with some of the FAs. A small percentage of FAs is not released into the circulation but is used to form new triacylglycerols within the adipose tissue, a process called **re-esterification.** The other FAs are transported to the other tissues and taken up by skeletal muscle during exercise. Glycerol is transported to the liver, where it serves as a gluconeogenic substrate to form new glucose.

Besides the FAs in plasma, two other sources of FAs for oxidation in skeletal muscle are available. Circulating triacylglycerols (for example in **VLDL**) can temporarily bind to lipoprotein lipase (LPL), which splits off FAs that can then be taken up by the muscle. A source of fat exists inside the muscle in the form of intramuscular triacylglycerol. These triacylglycerols are split by a **hormone-sensitive lipase** (HSL), and FAs are transported into the mitochondria for oxidation in the same way FAs from plasma and plasma triacylglycerol are utilized.

Table 6.1 Availability of Substrates in the Human Body

Substrate	Weight (kg)	Energy kJ (kcal)	
Carbohydrates			
Plasma glucose	0.01	160	(40)
Liver glycogen	0.1	1,600	(400)
Muscle glycogen	0.4	6,400	(1,600)
Total (approximately)	0.51	8,000	(2,000)
Fat			
Plasma fatty acid	0.0004	16	(4)
Plasma triacylglycerols	0.004	160	(40)
Adipose tissue	12.0	430,000	(108,000)
Intramuscular triacylglycerols	0.3	11,000	(2,700)
Total (approximately)	12.3	442,000	(111,000)

Values given are estimates for a "normal" man of 80 kg (176 lb) and 15% body fat and not those of an athlete, who might be leaner and have more stored glycogen. The amount of protein in the body is not mentioned, but it would be about 10 kg (22 lb [40,000 kcal or 167,440 kJ]), mainly located in the muscles.

International Journal of Sports Medicine: From A.E. Jeukendrup et al., "Fat metabolism during exercise. Part I. Fatty acid mobilization and muscle metabolism," 1998, 19(4): 231-244. Adapted by permission.

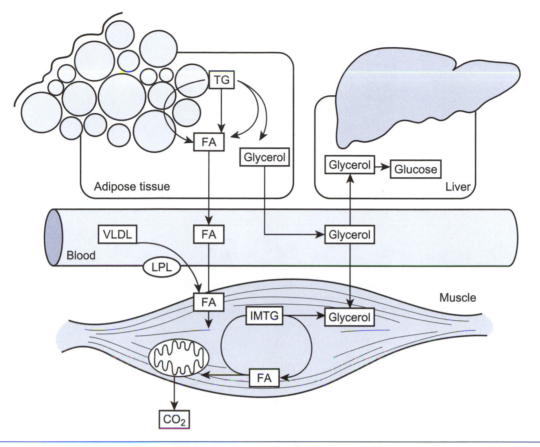

Figure 6.1 Overview of fat metabolism and the main organs involved. TG = triacylglycerol; FA = fatty acid; IMTG = intramuscular triacylglycerol; LPL = lipoprotein lipase; VLDL = very-low-density lipoprotein.

What Limits Fat Oxidation

Despite the fact that humans have large fat stores, in many situations utilizing these large amounts of fat as a fuel seems impossible. Why can fat not be oxidized at higher rates in some conditions? Because the FAs cannot be mobilized, or do other factors play a role? To find the factor that causes this limitation, we examine all the steps that are important in the process of fat oxidation: from the mobilization of FAs to the transport and the oxidation of FAs in the mitochondria itself. The steps that could potentially limit fat oxidation are

- **lipolysis,** the breakdown of triacylglycerols to FAs and glycerol;
- removal of FAs from the fat cell;
- transport of fat by the bloodstream;
- transport of FAs into the muscle cell;
- transport of FAs into the mitochondria; and
- oxidation of FAs in the β-oxidation pathway and TCA cycle.

Lipolysis in Adipocytes

Most FAs are stored in the form of triacylglycerols in subcutaneous adipose tissue. Before these FAs are oxidized, they must be mobilized and transported to the site of oxidation. The adipocyte contains hormone sensitive lipase (HSL), which splits triacylglycerols into FAs and glycerol and, as its name implies, is regulated by hormones (see figure 6.2). Conversion of the inactive form of HSL into the active form mainly depends on the sympathetic nervous system and circulating epinephrine. Insulin is probably the most important counterregulatory hormone. The glycerol released by this reaction diffuses freely into the blood. The adipocyte cannot reuse it, because the enzyme glycerokinase, which is required to phosphorylate the glycerol before re-esterification with FAs, is only present in very low concentrations. Therefore, almost all the glycerol produced by lipolysis is released into the plasma, and the measurement of glycerol in the blood is often used as a measure of lipolysis. FAs released by lipolysis are either re-esterified within the adipocyte or transported into the bloodstream for use in other tissues (see figure 6.3).

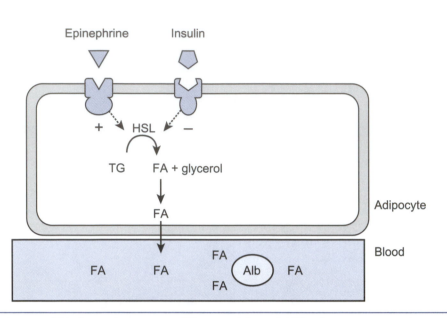

Figure 6.2 Mobilization of FAs from adipose tissue. TG = triacylglycerol; HSL = hormone-sensitive lipase; Alb = albumin.

Figure 6.3 Lipolysis of triacylglycerol and re-esterification of FAs.

Adapted, by permission, from A.E. Jeukendrup et al., 1998, "Fat metabolism during exercise. Part I. Fatty acid mobilization and muscle metabolism," *International Journal of Sports Medicine* 19(4): 231-244.

At rest, approximately 70% of all FAs released during lipolysis are re-esterified (Wolfe et al. 1990). During exercise, re-esterification is suppressed, which results in an increased availability of FAs in the adipocyte. The availability of FAs is even more increased because lipolysis is stimulated via β-adrenoreceptors during exercise. Catecholamines released from the adrenal gland stimulate lipolysis during exercise. Lipolysis is usually in excess of the demand for FAs both at rest and during exercise. Re-esterification is, therefore, believed to play a very important role in regulating the FA mobilization. Re-esterification is

dependent on the rate at which FAs are removed from the adipocyte by the blood and the rate of glycerol-3-phosphate production. Because glycerol cannot be recycled to any major extent in human adipocytes (or myocytes), the backbone for a triacylglycerol molecule is derived from glycerol-3-phosphate, an intermediate of the glycolytic pathway.

FAs are not soluble in the aqueous environment of the adipocyte cytoplasm. They are, therefore, bound to so-called FA-binding proteins (FABP) that transport the FAs to the cell membrane. At least during low-intensity to moderate-intensity exercise, the increase in lipolysis and the reduction in esterification of FAs result in a substantially increased level of FAs in the blood (Romijn et al. 1993; Wolfe et al. 1990).

Removal of FAs and Transport in the Blood

The removal of FAs from the adipocyte into the bloodstream depends on several factors, the most important being blood flow to the adipose tissue, the albumin concentration in the blood, and the number of free binding sites for FAs on the albumin molecule. Albumin is a plasma carrier protein that transports FAs. When it arrives at the target tissue (for example muscle) it binds to specific albumin-binding proteins (ABP). Binding to this protein then aids the release of FAs from albumin and their uptake.

A typical plasma albumin concentration is around 0.7 mmol/L (45 g/L) and albumin has at least three high-affinity binding sites for FAs, which provide a large capacity to bind FAs. Therefore, most FAs in the blood are bound to albumin (>99.9%) and only a small fraction (<0.1%), dissolved in the plasma water, circulate freely. Under most conditions, only a fraction of the total number of binding sites of albumin are occupied. However, during very prolonged exercise, the FA concentration in the blood can rise up to about 2 mmol/L. At this concentration the maximum capacity of albumin to bind FAs may be reached. When the FA concentration further rises, the percentage of unbound FAs increases, which is believed to be toxic for cells because of detergent-like properties of unbound FAs. These very high FA levels, however, are unusual, and the body seems to have protective mechanisms to prevent rises above 2 mmol/L. One of these mechanisms could be increased incorporation of FAs into plasma triacylglycerol. During every pass through the liver, a fraction of the FAs is extracted from the circulation and incorporated into VLDL particles.

Plasma Lipoproteins

Triacylglycerols bound to lipoproteins (VLDLs and chylomicrons) are another potential source of FAs (Havel et al. 1967). The enzyme lipoprotein lipase (LPL) in the vascular wall hydrolyzes some of the triacylglycerols in circulating lipoproteins passing through the capillary bed. As a result, FAs are released that the muscle can take up and use for oxidation. However, the FA uptake from plasma lipoprotein triacylglycerols occurs slowly and accounts for fewer than 3% of the energy expenditure during prolonged exercise (Havel et al. 1967; Issekutz et al. 1964). Therefore, it is generally believed that plasma triacylglycerols contribute only minimally to energy production during exercise. Some interesting observations need further investigation. For instance, LPL activity is significantly increased after training and after a high-fat diet; in both situations, fat oxidation is markedly increased. In addition, acute exercise also stimulates LPL activity.

Transport of FAs into the Muscle Cell

For a long time, the transport of FAs into the muscle cell was believed to be a passive process. This belief was based on early observations that FA uptake increased linearly with FA concentration. However, recently, specific carrier proteins have been identified (see figure 6.4). In the sarcolemma, at least two proteins are involved in the transport of FAs across the membrane, a specific plasma membrane FA-binding protein (FABPpm) and an FA transporter (FAT/CD36) protein. These proteins are likely to be responsible for the transport of most FAs across the sarcolemma. Animal studies indicate that the transporters become saturated at plasma FA concentrations around 1.5 mmol/L. FAT/CD36 can translocate from intracellular vesicles to the cell membrane in a similar manner as the GLUT-4 protein, indicating that FA transport can also be regulated acutely (Bonen et al. 2000). Muscle contraction increases plasma membrane FAT/CD36 and decreases the concentration of FAT/CD36 in the sarcoplasma. Along with a higher density of FAT/CD36 at the cell membrane, an increased FA transport into the cell was observed. What triggers the translocation of the FAT/CD36 to the cell membrane is currently not known. However, similar factors that result in GLUT-4 translocation might also be responsible for the translocation of FAT/CD36.

In the sarcoplasm (cytoplasm of muscle cells), the FAs are bound to another specific cytoplasmic FA-binding protein (FABPc). FABPc is thought to be responsible for the transport of FAs from the sarcolemma to the mitochondria. At present, little is known about the roles of these FA-binding proteins and transporters, and whether they are a limiting factor for fat oxidation is unknown.

Intramuscular Triacylglycerols

Another source of FAs are the IMTG stores in the muscle itself. Type I muscle fibers have higher contents of IMTG than type II muscle fibers. IMTG stores, usually located adjacent to the mitochondria as lipid

Figure 6.4 Presentation of the transport of glucose and FAs from the blood into the mitochondria. CoASH = free coenzyme A; CPT I = carnitine palmitoyl transferase I; CPT II = carnitine palmitoyl transferase II; FABP = fatty acid binding protein; IMTG = intramuscular triacylglycerol.

Reprinted, by permission, from A.E. Jeukendrup, 2002, "Regulation of skeletal muscle fat metabolism," *New York Academy of Sciences* 967: 1-19.

droplets (see figure 6.5), have been recognized as an important energy source during exercise. Studies in which muscle samples were investigated under a microscope revealed that the size of these lipid droplets decreases during exercise. Also, indirect measures of IMTG breakdown provide evidence for its use during exercise (Martin et al. 1993). The location of the droplets seems to be important as well. In trained muscle, the lipid droplets are believed to be located next to the mitochondria, whereas in untrained muscle, the lipid droplets do not seem to be linked with mitochondria at all.

Like adipose tissue, muscle contains a HSL that is activated by β-adrenergic stimulation and inhib-ited by insulin. FAs liberated from IMTGs may be released into the blood, re-esterified, or oxidized within the muscle. Because, at least in trained muscle, the lipid droplets are located close to the mitochondria, most of the FAs released after lipolysis are assumed to be oxidized. The FAs released are bound to FABPc until they are transported into the mitochondria.

Transport of FAs into the Mitochondria

FAs in the cytoplasm may be activated by the enzyme acyl-CoA synthethase or thiokinase to form an acyl-CoA complex (often referred to as an activated FA)

Figure 6.5 An electromyograph of skeletal muscle showing intramuscular triacylglycerols. A large lipid droplit (li) is located adjacent to the mitochondria (mi). Compare the enormous stores of lipid with the small stores of glycogen (gl) in this muscle.

International Journal of Sports Medicine: From A.E. Jeukendrup et al., "Fat metabolism during exercise PartI. Fatty acid mobilization and muscle metabolism," 1998, 19(4): 231-244. Adapted by permission.

(see figure 6.6). This acyl-CoA complex is used for the synthesis of IMTGs, or it is bound to carnitine under the influence of the enzyme **carnitine palmitoyl transferase** I (CPT I; which is also known as carnitine acyl transferase I or CAT I), which is located at the outside of the outer mitochondrial membrane.

The bonding between carnitine and the activated FA is the first step in the transport of the FA into the mitochondria. As carnitine binds to the FA, free CoA is released. The fatty acyl-carnitine complex is transported with a translocase and reconverted into fatty acyl-CoA at the matrix side of the inner mitochondrial membrane by the enzyme carnitine palmitoyl transferase II (CPT II). The carnitine that is released diffuses back across the mitochondrial membrane into the cytoplasm and thus becomes available again for the transport of other FAs. Fatty acyl-carnitine crosses the inner membrane in a 1:1 exchange with a molecule of free carnitine. Although short-chain FAs (SCFAs) and **medium-chain FAs** (MCFAs) are believed to freely diffuse into the mitochondrial matrix, carrier proteins with a specific maximum affinity for short-chain or medium-chain acyl-CoA transport at least some of these FAs.

β-Oxidation

Once in the mitochondrial matrix, the fatty acyl-CoA is subjected to β-oxidation, a series of reactions that splits a 2-carbon acetyl-CoA molecule of the multiple carbon FA chain (see figure 6.7). The β-oxidation pathway uses oxygen and generates some ATP through substrate-level phosphorylation. The acetyl-CoA is then oxidized in the tricarboxylic acid (TCA) cycle. The complete oxidation of FAs in the mitochondria depends on several factors, including the activity of enzymes of the β-oxidation pathway, the concentration of TCA-cycle intermediates and activity of enzymes in the TCA cycle (these factors determine the total TCA-cycle activity), and the presence of oxygen.

Figure 6.6 Transport of FAs into the mitochondria.

Figure 6.7 The β-oxidation process.

Fat As a Fuel During Exercise

Carbohydrate and fat are always oxidized as a mixture, and whether carbohydrate or fat is the predominant fuel depends on a variety of factors, including the intensity and duration of exercise, the level of aerobic fitness, diet, and carbohydrate intake before or during exercise. The changes in fat metabolism that occur in the transition from rest to exercise as well as the various factors that influence fat mobilization and oxidation will be discussed in the following sections.

Fat Utilization at Rest and During Exercise

After an overnight fast, most of the energy requirement is covered by the oxidation of FAs derived from adipose tissue. The rate of lipolysis in adipose tissue mostly depends on the circulating concentrations of hormones (epinephrine stimulates lipolysis and insulin inhibits lipolysis). It seems that most of the FAs liberated after lipolysis are re-esterified within the adipocyte. Some FAs enter the bloodstream, but only about half of them are oxidized. Resting plasma FA concentrations are typically between 0.2 mmol/L and 0.4 mmol/L.

When exercise is initiated, the rate of lipolysis and the rate of FA release from adipose tissue are increased. During moderate-intensity exercise, lipolysis increases approximately threefold, mainly because of an increased β-adrenergic stimulation (by catecholamines). In addition, during moderate-intensity exercise, the blood flow to adipose tissue is doubled and the rate of re-esterification is halved. Blood flow in skeletal muscle is increased dramatically, and, therefore, the delivery of FAs to the muscle is increased.

During the first 15 minutes of exercise, plasma FA concentrations usually decrease because the rate of FA uptake by the muscle exceeds the rate of FA appearance from lipolysis. Thereafter, the rate of appearance is in excess of the utilization by muscle, and plasma FA concentrations increase. The rise in FA depends on the exercise intensity. During moderate-intensity exercise, FA concentrations may reach 1 mmol/L within 60 minutes of exercise, but at higher exercise intensities, the rise in plasma FAs is very small or may even be absent.

Fat Oxidation and Exercise Duration

Fat oxidation increases as the exercise duration increases. Edwards et al. (1934) reported fat oxidation rates of over 1.0 g/min after 6 hours of running. Christensen and Hansen (1939) observed that the contribution of fat could even increase to levels as high as 90% of energy expenditure when a fatty meal was consumed, leading to fat oxidation rates of 1.5 g/min. The mechanism of this increased fat oxidation as exercise duration increases is not entirely clear but seems to be linked to the decrease in muscle glycogen stores.

Fat Oxidation and Exercise Intensity

Fat oxidation is usually the predominant fuel at low exercise intensities, whereas during high exercise intensities, carbohydrates are the major fuel. In absolute terms, fat oxidation increases as the exercise intensity increases from low to moderate intensities, even though the percentage contribution of fat may actually decrease (see figure 6.8). For the transition from light-intensity to moderate-intensity exercise, the increased fat oxidation is a direct result of the increased energy expenditure. At higher intensities of exercise (>75% $\dot{V}O_2$max) fat oxidation is inhibited and both the relative and absolute rates of fat oxidation decrease to negligible values. Achten et al. (2002, 2003) studied this relationship over a wide range of exercise intensities in a group of trained subjects and found that, on average, the maximal rates of fat oxidation were observed at 62-63% $\dot{V}O_2$max.

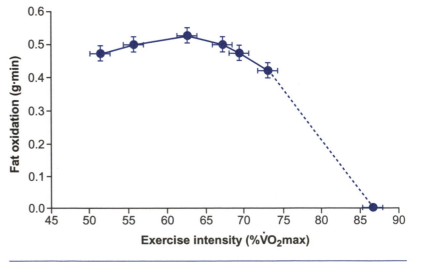

Figure 6.8 Fat oxidation as a function of exercise intensity.

International Journal of Sports Medicine: From J. Achten and A.G. Jeukendrup. Maximal fat oxidation during exercise in trained men. 2003; 24(8): 603-608. Reprinted by permission.

During exercise at 25% $\dot{V}O_2$max, most of the fat oxidized is derived from plasma FAs, and only small amounts comes from IMTGs. (Romijn et al. 1993) (see figure 6.9). However, during moderate exercise intensity (65% $\dot{V}O_2$max), the contribution of plasma FAs declines, whereas the contribution of IMTGs increases and provides about half of the FAs used for total fat oxidation (Romijn et al. 1993). Training also decreases the contribution of plasma FAs, despite a dramatic increase in total fat oxidation. This decrease in plasma FA oxidation is accounted for by a marked increase in the contribution of muscle triacylglycerols to energy expenditure.

When the exercise intensity is further increased, fat oxidation decreases, even though the rate of lipolysis is still high. The blood flow to the adipose tissue may be decreased (because of sympathetic vasoconstriction), which may result in a decreased removal of FAs from adipose tissue. During high-intensity exercise, lactate accumulation may also increase the

rate of re-esterification of FAs. As a result, plasma FA concentrations are usually low during intense exercise. However, this decreased availability of FAs can only partially explain the reduced fat oxidation observed in these conditions. When Romijn et al. (1995) restored FA concentrations to levels observed at moderate exercise intensities by infusing triacylglycerols (Intralipid) and heparin, fat oxidation was only slightly increased but still lower than at moderate intensities (see the sidebar and figure 6.10). Therefore, an additional mechanism in the muscle must be responsible for the decreased fat oxidation observed during high-intensity exercise.

Sidossis et al. (1997) and Coyle et al. (1997) suggested that the decreased fat oxidation is related to the transport of FAs into the mitochondria. They observed that during high-intensity exercise, the oxidation of **long-chain FAs** is impaired, whereas the oxidation of medium chain FAs is unaffected. Because the medium-chain FAs are less dependent on

Figure 6.9 Substrate utilization at different exercise intensities.

Reprinted, by permission, from J.A. Romijn et al., 1993, "Regulation of endogenous fat and carbohydrate metabolism in relation to exercise intensity and duration," *Journal of Applied Physiology* 265: E380-E391.

TRIACYLGLYCEROL AND HEPARIN INFUSION

In order to increase plasma FA concentrations for experimental purposes, researchers have used the infusion of triacylglycerol and heparin. Because FAs are not soluble in water (plasma), they cannot be infused directly. Therefore a lipid emulsion is used (often Intralipid) in combination with a heparin injection. Heparin releases lipoprotein lipase (LPL) from the capillaries. Once LPL becomes freely available in the circulation, it starts to break down the plasma triacylglycerol, and FA concentrations rise rapidly.

(continued)

(continued)

Figure 6.10 FA concentrations are usually low at high exercise intensities (>85% V̇O₂max), which could explain the relatively low oxidation rates of fat compared with moderate exercise intensities (gray bars). When lipid and heparin are infused, high plasma FA concentrations are achieved but do not restore fat oxidation to the levels observed at moderate exercise intensities (65% V̇O₂max).

Reprinted, by permission, from J.A. Romijn et al., 1995, "Relationship between fatty acid delivery and fatty acid oxidation during strenuous exercise," *Journal of Applied Physiology* 79(6): 1939-1945.

transport mechanisms into the mitochondria, these data provide evidence that carnitine-dependent FA transport is a limiting factor.

Fat Oxidation and Aerobic Capacity

Endurance training affects both substrate utilization and exercise capacity. Studies involving both animals and humans have established a marked adaptive increase in oxidative potential in response to increased regular physical activity (Holloszy and Booth 1976; Holloszy and Coyle 1984). A consequence and probably contributing factor to the enhanced exercise capacity after endurance training is the metabolic shift to a greater use of fat and a concomitant sparing of glycogen. The contribution of fat to total energy expenditure increases after training at both the relative and the absolute exercise intensities. The adaptations that contribute to a stimulation of fat oxidation in trained subjects include:

- increased mitochondrial density and an increase in the number of oxidative enzymes in trained muscle, which increases the capacity to oxidize fat;
- increased capillary density, which enhances FA delivery to the muscle;

- increased FABP concentrations, which may facilitate uptake of FAs across the sarcolemma; and
- increased CPT concentration, which facilitates the transport of FAs into the mitochondria.

One factor that does not seem to be influenced by training is lipolysis in adipose tissue (Klein et al. 1994) (see figure 6.11). After training, the rate of lipolysis at the same absolute exercise intensity does not seem to be affected. At the same relative exercise intensity, the rate of lipolysis is increased after training (Klein et al. 1996). An increased lipolysis of IMTG likely contributes to this increased whole-body lipolysis.

Fat Oxidation and Diet

Diet also has marked effects on fat oxidation. Generally a high-carbohydrate, low-fat diet reduces fat oxidation, whereas a high-fat, low-carbohydrate diet increases fat oxidation. Some scientists have argued that the results seen in most of these studies are the effects of the last meal, which is known to influence substrate utilization. However, Burke et al. (1999) showed that a high-fat, low-carbohydrate diet had a similar effect on substrate utilization, even after a day on a high-carbohydrate diet. The results indicate that some chronic effects of diet cannot be directly

Figure 6.11 Whole-body lipolysis in trained and untrained subjects.

Reprinted, by permission, from S. Klein, E.F. Coyle, and R.R. Wolfe, 1994, "Fat metabolism during low-intensity exercise in endurance trained and untrained men," *Journal of Applied Physiology* 267: E934-E940.

explained by substrate availability. In the study by Burke et al. (1999), for example, subjects consumed a high-fat diet or a high-carbohydrate diet for 5 days followed by 1 day on a high-carbohydrate diet. The one-day high-carbohydrate intake replenished glycogen stores in both conditions, and muscle glycogen concentrations were identical. Yet large differences existed in substrate utilization between the two diets. The respiratory exchange ratio (RER) changed from 0.90 to 0.82 after 5 days on a high-fat diet. After consuming a high-carbohydrate diet for one day, RER was still lower compared with baseline values (0.87). Because these changes were not caused by alterations in substrate availability, they are likely to be related to metabolic adaptations in the muscle.

Chronic diets can have marked effects on metabolism. These effects seem only partly related to the effects of diets on substrate availability. Adaptations at the muscular level, which result in changes in substrate utilization in response to a diet, may occur already after five days.

Response to Carbohydrate Feeding

The fastest way to alter fat metabolism during exercise is probably by carbohydrate feeding. Carbohydrate increases the plasma insulin concentration, which reduces lipolysis and causes a marked reduction in FA availability. In a study by Horowitz et al. (1997), carbohydrate was ingested 1 hour before exercise. Both lipolysis and fat oxidation were reduced. Plasma

FA concentrations decreased to very low levels during exercise. However, when Intralipid was infused and heparin was injected to increase the plasma FA concentrations, fat oxidation was only partially restored. These findings indicate that a reduced availability of FAs is indeed a factor that limits fat oxidation. However, because increasing the plasma FA concentrations does not completely restore fat oxidation, other factors must play a role as well. These factors must be located inside the muscle itself.

When a large amount of glucose is ingested 1 hour before exercise, plasma insulin levels are very high at the start of exercise, whereas plasma FA and glycerol concentrations are very low (Coyle et al. 1997). This results in a 30% reduction in fat oxidation compared with no carbohydrate intake. In a study by Coyle et al. (1997), trace amounts of labeled medium-chain or long-chain FAs were infused, and the oxidation rates of these FAs were determined. The oxidation of long-chain FAs appeared to be reduced, whereas the oxidation of medium-chain FAs appeared to be unaffected (see figure 6.12). Because medium-chain FAs are not as dependent on transport mechanisms into the mitochondria, but the long-chain FAs are highly dependent on this mechanism, these results provide evidence that this transport is an important regulatory step. Although the exact mechanisms are still unclear, carbohydrate feeding before exercise reduces fat oxidation by reducing lipolysis and plasma FA availability and exerts an inhibitory effect on carnitine-dependent FA transport into the mitochondria.

Regulation of Carbohydrate and Fat Metabolism

In all situations, carbohydrate and fat together constitute most, if not all, of the energy provision. The percentage contribution of these two fuels, however, varies depending on the factors discussed previously. The rate of carbohydrate utilization during prolonged strenuous exercise is closely related to the energy needs of the working muscle. In contrast, fat utilization during exercise is not tightly regulated. No mechanisms closely match the metabolism of FAs to energy expenditure. Fat oxidation is therefore mainly influenced by fat availability and the rate of carbohydrate utilization.

Some evidence suggests that increases in plasma FA concentration can cause a decrease in the rate of muscle glycogen breakdown. This action could theoretically be beneficial, because muscle glycogen depletion is one of the prime causes of fatigue. Researchers have artificially elevated plasma FA concentrations by raising plasma triacylglycerol

| ¹³C-LCFA Fasted 86% | ¹³C-LCFA Glucose 70% | ¹³C-MCFA Fasted 99% | ¹³C-MCFA Glucose 98% |

Figure 6.12 Oxidation of medium-chain FAs (MCFAs) and long-chain FAs (LCFAs) in the mitochondria during fasted and fed conditions (glucose). Glucose intake reduced the oxidation of LCFAs but not MCFAs. Because LCFAs use a transport protein to enter the mitochondria, and MCFAs are less dependent on this protein, glucose availability possibly regulates the entry of FA into the mitochondria.

Reprinted, by permission, from E.F. Coyle et al., 1997, "Fatty acid oxidation is directly regulated by carbohydrate metabolism during exercise," *American Journal of Physiology* 273: E268-E275.

concentrations by means of a fat meal or intravenous infusion of triacylglycerol (Intralipid), followed by a heparin injection. Using this method, it has been repeatedly shown that an increase in FA concentration can reduce carbohydrate dependence.

In a study by Costill et al. (1977), Intralipid was infused and heparin was injected during exercise at 70% $\dot{V}O_2$max. After 60 minutes, a muscle biopsy was taken and muscle glycogen was measured before and after the exercise bout. Muscle glycogen breakdown was reduced with the elevated plasma FA concentrations (see figure 6.13). Similar results were obtained when a fat feeding was given in combination with heparin infusion (Vukovich et al. 1993). Although elevating FA levels seems to reduce muscle glycogen breakdown during exercise, the mechanisms are still incompletely understood.

The classical glucose-FA cycle was originally thought to explain this interaction between carbohydrate and fat metabolism (see figure 6.14). This theory states that with an increase in plasma FA concentration, uptake of FAs increases and these FAs undergo β-oxidation in the mitochondria, in which they are broken down to acetyl-CoA. An increasing concentration of acetyl-CoA (or increased acetyl-CoA/CoA ratio) inhibits the pyruvate dehydrogenase complex that breaks down pyruvate to acetyl-CoA. Also, increased formation of acetyl-CoA from FA oxidation

Figure 6.13 Glycogen "sparing" with increased FA availability. This increased availability of FAs was achieved by infusing a triacylglycerol emulsion with heparin.

Data from D.L. Costill et al., 1977.

in the mitochondria increases muscle citrate levels, and after diffusing into the sarcoplasm, citrate could inhibit phosphofructokinase, the rate-limiting enzyme in glycolysis. The effect of increased acetyl-CoA and citrate levels is therefore a reduction in the rate of glycolysis. This reduced glycolysis, in turn, may cause accumulation of glucose-6-phosphate (G6P) in the muscle sarcoplasm, which inhibits hexokinase activity and thus reduces muscle glucose uptake.

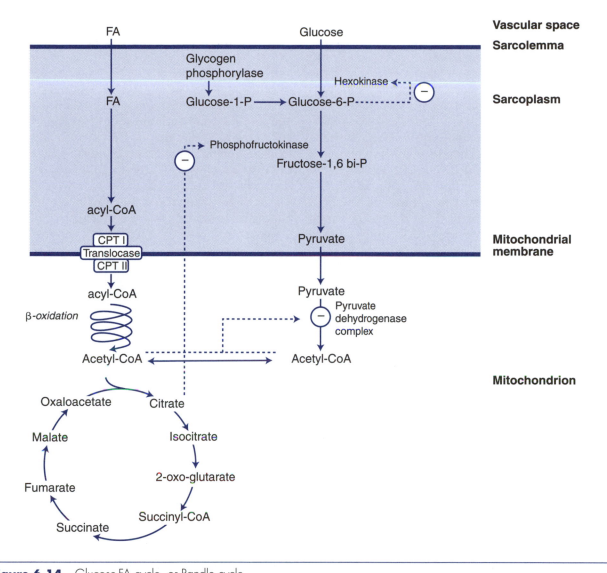

Figure 6.14 Glucose-FA cycle, or Randle cycle.

Reprinted, by permission, from A.E. Jeukendrup, 2002, "Regulation of fat metabolism in skeletal muscle," New York Academy of Sciences 967: 217-235.

With increased fat availability the disturbance in the cellular homeostasis is less. Increasing FA availability decreases intramuscular inorganic phosphate (Pi) and adenosine monophosphate (AMP) accumulation during exercise, possibly because of a greater accumulation of mitochondrial reduced nicotinamide adenine dinucleotide (NADH) (Dyck et al. 1996; Dyck et al. 1993). Pi and AMP are energy sensing signals; high concentrations indicate low energy status, whereas low concentrations reflect ample energy availability. Because Pi and AMP are known to stimulate the enzyme glycogen phosphorylase, the reduction in Pi and AMP levels may be at least partially responsible for the reduced muscle glycogen breakdown.

An alternative explanation for reduced muscle glycogen breakdown after elevation of plasma FA concentrations is given in some studies. When studied in more detail, the plasma FA concentrations appear significantly elevated (by infusion of TG and injection of heparin) compared with the control condition. The FA concentrations in the control condition, however, were below 0.2 mmol/L. Conceivably, these FA levels are too low to provide the muscle with sufficient fat substrate. As a result, muscle glycogen breakdown may have been increased in the control condition. Therefore, the observed "sparing" of glycogen with the high FA concentrations could have been caused by an increased breakdown of glycogen in the control condition. Blocking lipolysis and reducing FA availability by giving nicotinic acid or a derivative increases muscle glycogen breakdown during exercise.

A more recent theory about the regulation of carbohydrate and fat metabolism proposes that fat does not regulate carbohydrate metabolism, but rather carbohydrate regulates fat metabolism. An increase in the rate of glycolysis decreases fat oxidation. Figure 6.15 shows some of the factors that regulate carbohydrate and fat metabolism.

Regulation of fat metabolism involves the transport of FAs into the mitochondria, which is controlled mainly by the activity of CPT I. CPT I is regulated by several factors, including the malonyl-CoA (a precursor of FA synthesis) concentration. The high rate of glycogenolysis during high-intensity exercise increases the amount of acetyl-CoA in the muscle cell, and some of this acetyl-CoA is converted to malonyl-CoA by the enzyme acetyl CoA carboxylase (ACC). Malonyl-CoA inhibits CPT I and could thus reduce the transport of FAs into the mitochondria. Although evidence suggests that malonyl-CoA may be an important regulator at rest, studies in exercising humans indicate no important role of malonyl-CoA (Odland et al. 1998; Odland et al. 1996). Reductions in intramuscular pH that may occur during high-intensity exercise may also inhibit CPT I and, hence, FA transport into the mitochondria (Starritt et al. 2000).

Another explanation is that a reduced free carnitine concentration plays a role. When glycogenolysis is accelerated, acetyl-CoA accumulates during intense

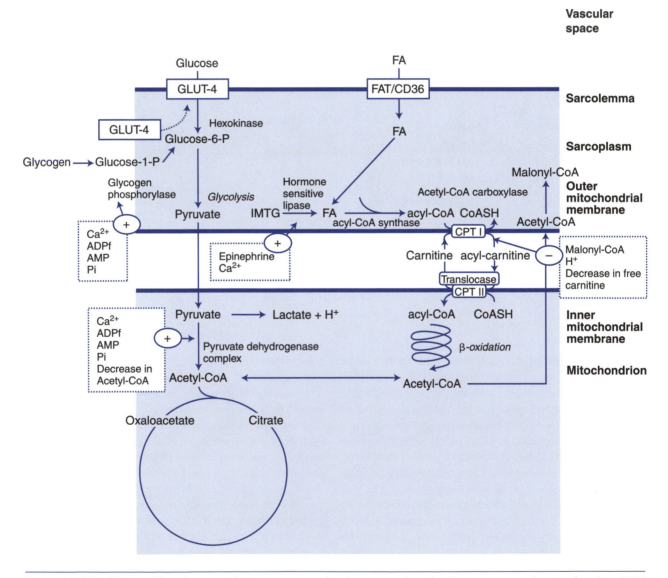

Figure 6.15 Glucose FA cycle reversed. An increase in glycolysis can reduce the FA transport into the mitochondria. CPT I = carnitine palmitoyl transferase I; CPT II = carnitine palmitoyl transferase II; ADPf = free ADP.

Reprinted, by permission, from A.E. Jeukendrup, 2002, "Regulation of metabolism in skeletal muscle," New York Academy of Sciences 967: 217-235.

exercise and some of this acetyl-CoA is bound to carnitine. As a result, the free carnitine concentration drops, and less carnitine is available to transport FAs into the mitochondria (Greenhaff and Timmons 1998). Finally, it has been proposed that pyruvate-derived acetyl-CoA competes with the FA-derived acetyl-CoA for entrance into the TCA cycle.

The rate of carbohydrate utilization during prolonged strenuous exercise is closely related to the energy needs of the working muscle. In contrast, fat utilization during exercise is not tightly regulated. No mechanisms closely match the metabolism of FAs to energy expenditure. Fat oxidation is, therefore, mainly influenced by fat availability and the rate of carbohydrate utilization. The importance of each of these factors may depend on the situation. For example, carbohydrate utilization may be a more important factor during exercise, whereas the availability of FAs may be more important at rest.

Fat Supplementation and Exercise

The effects of eating fat before or during exercise have been studied as a method to increase FA availability and increase fat oxidation in order to reduce muscle glycogen breakdown. Initial studies looked at fatty meals consisting mainly of long-chain triacylglyerols (LCTs); later studies have also looked at alternative lipid fuels such as medium-chain triacylglycerols (MCTs).

Ingestion of Long-Chain Triacylglycerols

Nutritional fats include triacylglycerols (containing mostly C16 and C18 FAs), phospholipids, and cholesterol, of which only triacylglycerols can contribute to any extent to energy provision during exercise. In contrast to carbohydrates, nutritional fats only reach the circulation slowly because they are potent inhibitors of gastric emptying. Furthermore, the digestion in the gut and absorption of fat are also rather slow processes compared with the digestion and absorption of carbohydrates.

Bile salts, produced by the liver, and lipase, secreted by the pancreas, are needed for lipolysis of the long-chain triacylglycerols (LCTs) into glycerol and 3 LCFAs or monoacylglycerol and 2 FAs. The FAs diffuse into the intestinal mucosa cells and are re-esterified in the cytoplasm to form LCTs. These LCTs are encapsulated by a coat of proteins—forming chylomicrons—to make them water soluble. These chylomicrons are then released in the lymphatic

system, which ultimately drains in the systemic circulation. Exogenous LCTs enter the systemic circulation much more slowly than carbohydrates, which are absorbed as glucose (or to minor extents, as fructose or galactose) and directly enter the main circulation through the portal vein. Long-chain dietary FAs typically enter the blood 3 to 4 hours after ingestion.

The fact that these LCFAs enter the circulation in chylomicrons is also important, and the rate of breakdown of chylomicron-bound triacylglycerols by muscle is generally believed to be relatively low. The primary role of these triacylglycerols in chylomicrons may be the replenishment of IMTG stores after exercise (Oscai et al. 1990). The intake of fat during exercise should, therefore, be avoided. Many so-called "sports bars" or "energy bars," however, contain relatively large amounts of fat. Food labels of these products should be checked when choosing an energy bar.

Ingestion of Medium-Chain Triacylglycerols

Medium-chain triacylglycerols (MCTs) contain FAs with a chain length of C8 or C10. MCTs are normally present in our diet in very small quantities and they have few natural sources. Intake via these sources is small and, therefore, MCTs are often consumed as a supplement. MCTs are sold as a supplement to replace normal fat because MCTs are not stored in the body and, therefore, could help athletes lose body fat. MCT supplements are fairly popular among body builders and have been used as an alternative fuel source during exercise. (See chapter 10.)

Ingestion of Fish Oil

Fish oil is a natural source of long-chain omega-3 FAs. It contains both docosahexaenoic (DHA) and eicosapentaenoic acid (EPA). Fish oil is said to improve membrane characteristics and improve membrane function when more of these omega-3 FAs are incorporated into the lipid bilayer of the membrane. (See chapter 10.)

Effect of Diet on Fat Metabolism and Performance

Another strategy that has been used to increase fat oxidation and reduce reliance on carbohydrate stores has involved longer-term manipulations of the diet lasting days or weeks. These methods included fasting and high-fat, low-carbohydrate diets.

Fasting

Fasting has been proposed as a way to increase fat utilization, spare muscle glycogen, and improve exercise performance. In rats, short-term fasting increases plasma epinephrine and norepinephrine concentrations, stimulates lipolysis, and increases the concentration of circulating plasma FAs. These effects, in turn, increase fat oxidation and "spare" muscle glycogen, leading to a similar (Koubi et al. 1991), or even increased, running time to exhaustion in rats (Dohm et al. 1983). In humans, fasting also results in an increased concentration of circulating catecholamines, increased lipolysis, increased concentration of plasma FAs (Dohm et al. 1986), and a decreased glucose turnover (Knapik et al. 1988). Muscle glycogen concentrations, however, are unaffected by fasting for 24 hours when no strenuous exercise is performed (Knapik et al. 1988; Loy et al. 1986). Although fasting has been reported to have no effect on endurance capacity at low exercise intensities (45% $\dot{V}O_2$max), decreases in performance have been observed for exercise intensities between 50% and 100% $\dot{V}O_2$max. The observed decreased performance was not reversible by carbohydrate ingestion during exercise (Riley et al. 1988).

Some investigators argued that the effects observed in most of these studies were seen because, in the control situation, the last meal was provided 3 hours before the exercise to exhaustion. The effects, therefore, are of the feeding before exercise improving endurance capacity rather than of decreased performance after fasting. However, the studies that compared a prolonged fast (>24 hours) to a 12-hour fast also reported decreased performance (Knapik et al. 1988; Maughan and Gleeson 1988; Zinker et al. 1990) and, thus, the conclusion that fasting decreases endurance capacity seems justified. The mechanism remains unclear, although certainly liver glycogen stores are substantially depleted after a 24-hour fast. Thus, euglycemia may not be as well maintained during exercise. Some degree of metabolic acidosis may also be observed after prolonged fasting. When hepatic glycogen stores are exhausted (e.g., after 12 hours to 24 hours of total fasting), the liver produces ketone bodies (acetoacetate, β-hydroxybutyrate, and acetone) to provide an energy substrate for peripheral tissues. These keto-acids lower blood pH, although the acidosis is usually only mild.

Effects of a Short-Term High-Fat Diet

Christensen and Hansen (1939) showed that short-term exposure to a high-fat diet resulted in impaired fatigue resistance. After muscle biopsy techniques were redeveloped, a high-fat, low-carbohydrate diet was shown to result in decreased muscle glycogen levels, and this was the main factor causing lack of fatigue resistance during prolonged exercise (Bergstrom and Hultman 1967; Hultman 1967). Plasma FA concentrations are increased at rest and increase more rapidly when a low-carbohydrate diet is consumed (Conlee et al. 1990; Martin et al. 1978; Maughan et al. 1978). These changes in plasma FA concentrations are attributed to changes in the rate of lipolysis. Not only plasma FAs but also plasma glycerol concentrations are increased after a low-carbohydrate diet.

Jansson and Kaijser (1982) reported that the uptake of FAs by the muscle during 25 minutes of cycling at 65% $\dot{V}O_2$max was 82% higher in subjects receiving a low-carbohydrate diet (5%) for 5 days, compared with subjects receiving a high-carbohydrate diet (75%) for 5 days. Plasma FAs contributed 24% and 14%, respectively, to energy expenditure. Increased FA concentrations in the blood after a period of carbohydrate restriction leads to an increased ketogenesis with elevated plasma levels of β-hydroxybutyrate and acetoacetate. After a few days of high-fat feeding, the ketone body production increases 5-fold (Fery and Balasse 1983) and the arterial concentration of ketone bodies may increase 10-fold to 20-fold (Fery and Balasse 1983). During the first phase of light to moderate exercise, ketone body concentrations usually decline, and after 30 minutes to 90 minutes, they increase again (Fery and Balasse 1983; Knapik et al. 1988; Zinker et al. 1990). However, the observed plasma concentrations under those conditions are still higher after a high-fat diet compared with those associated with low-fat diets. Carbohydrate-restricted diets may also lead to an increased breakdown of muscle triacylglycerols.

Effects of a Long-Term High-Fat Diet

A 3-day to 4-day alteration in the dietary composition has been suggested to be an insufficient time to induce an adaptive response to the changed diet. A high-fat diet over a prolonged period, however, may result in a decreased utilization of carbohydrates and an increased contribution of fat to energy metabolism. In rats, adaptation to a high-fat diet leads to considerable improvements in endurance capacity (Miller et al. 1984; Simi et al. 1991) (see figure 6.16). These adaptations can be attributed to the increased number of oxidative enzymes and a decreased degradation of liver glycogen during exercise (Simi et al. 1991). The results suggest that after adaptation to a high-fat diet, the capacity to oxidize FAs instead of carbohydrates is increased because of an adaptation of the oxidative enzymes in the muscle cell. These

Figure 6.16 Running performance with high-fat diets in rats.

Reprinted, by permission, from W.C. Miller, R. Bryce, and R.K. Conlee, 1984, "Adaptation to a high-fat diet that increase exercise endurance in male rats" *Journal of Applied Physiology* 56(1): 78-83.

adaptations are much like the adaptations seen after endurance training.

One of the first studies that investigated the effects of prolonged high-fat diets on humans was conducted by Phinney et al. (1980). They investigated exercise performance in obese subjects who followed a high-fat diet (90% of energy intake from fat) for 6 weeks. Before and after the diet, subjects exercised at 75% $\dot{V}O_2$max until exhaustion. Subjects were able to exercise as long on the high-fat diet as they did on their normal diet, but after the high-fat diet, fat became the main substrate. Results of this study, however, may have been influenced by the fact that these subjects were not in energy balance and lost 11 kg of body weight. So, although no differences were seen in the absolute $\dot{V}O_2$max before and after the dietary period, considerable differences were apparent in the relative exercise intensity.

The observed improvement in performance may have been an artifact rather than a positive effect of the adaptation period. Therefore, Phinney and colleagues (Phinney, Bistrian, Evans, et al. 1983; Phinney, Bistrian, Wolfe, and Blackburn 1983) conducted a follow-up study in which trained subjects were studied before and after a four-week high-fat diet (<20 g/day of carbohydrates). The diet reduced the pre-exercise muscle glycogen concentration by 50%, but no difference in the average time to exhaustion at 62% to 64% $\dot{V}O_2$max before and after the diet was found. However, the results are difficult to interpret because of the large variability of the subjects' performance times (times to exhaustion). One subject exercised 57% longer, whereas other subjects showed no improvement or even had decreased times to exhaustion. Also, the exercise intensity was rela-

tively low and subjects' reliance on carbohydrates during exercise at 62% to 64% $\dot{V}O_2$max was low. In such a situation, reduced carbohydrate stores may not be limiting. Possibly at higher exercise intensities, performance would have been impaired. Nevertheless, the fact that performance was not reduced in all subjects, even though muscle glycogen levels measured before exercise were decreased by almost 50% and fat oxidation during exercise was markedly increased, is remarkable. These observations have been attributed to enzymatic adaptations (including a 44% increase in carnitine palmitoyl transferase activity and a 46% decrease in hexokinase activity) (Phinney, Bistrian, Evans, et al. 1983). In subsequent studies, a maintained or improved performance was seen at relatively low exercise intensities (60% to 65% $\dot{V}O_2$max), which are far below the intensities observed during competition. How these results translate into practical applications in training and competition for most athletes is unclear.

Eating large amounts of fat has been associated with the development of obesity and cardiovascular disease. Whether this association is also true for athletes is not known. Few studies have described the effects of high-fat diets on cardiovascular risk factors in athletes who train regularly. Pendergast et al. (1996) reported no changes in plasma LDL, HDL, or total cholesterol levels in male and female runners with diets in the range of 17% to 40% fat. Although the risk of obesity and cardiovascular disease increases with the consumption of high-fat diets in sedentary people, regular exercise or endurance training seems to attenuate these risks (Sarna and Kaprio 1994). Exposure to high-fat diets has also been associated with insulin resistance, which has recently been linked to an effect of the IMTG pools on glucose uptake (Pan et al. 1997). However, this observation was made in obese subjects, and whether these results can be extrapolated to athletes is not clear, especially because athletes seem to have larger IMTG stores and increased insulin sensitivity. Because little information is available about the negative effects of high-fat diets on athletes, and since the effects of these diets on performance are unclear, we suggest caution when recommending high-fat diets to athletes.

Although chronic high-fat diets induce persistent enzymatic adaptations in skeletal muscle that favor fat oxidation, the effects on performance may not be visible because muscle glycogen levels are suboptimal. A period of adaptation to a high-fat diet, followed by acute carbohydrate feeding, might theoretically induce the enzymatic adaptations in the muscle while also allowing optimizing of pre-exercise glycogen stores. If the high glycogen levels are accompanied by a slightly lower rate of glycogenolysis, an improvement in exercise capacity is expected. Indeed, in rats after 3 weeks to 8 weeks of adaptation to a high-fat diet (0% to 25% carbohydrate) followed by 3 days of carbohydrate feeding (70% carbohydrate), muscle and liver glycogen were restored to very high levels.

In humans, Helge et al. (1998) studied trained subjects who, after 7 weeks of adaptation to a high-fat diet (62% fat, 21% carbohydrate), changed to a high-carbohydrate diet (65% carbohydrate, 20% fat) for 1 week (see figure 6.17). A control group followed a high-carbohydrate diet for 8 weeks. Although exercise time to exhaustion increased from week 7 to week 8 in the group that received a high-fat diet followed by the high-carbohydrate diet, performance was less compared with the group that received the high-

carbohydrate diet for 8 weeks. Because switching to a high-carbohydrate diet after 7 weeks of a high-fat diet did not reverse the negative effects, these authors concluded that the negative effects of 7 weeks of a high-fat diet on performance are not simply caused by a lack of carbohydrate as a fuel, but rather by suboptimal adaptations to the training (i.e., improvements in endurance capacity were smaller compared with the high-carbohydrate diet).

In another study by Burke et al. (1999), trained cyclists received a high-fat diet for a relatively short period (5 days), followed by a day of carbohydrate loading on day 6. On day 7, substrate oxidation during exercise was measured, followed by a performance ride. No significant performance improvement was observed. The potential benefits of an adaptation period to a high-fat diet followed by a period of carbohydrate loading are not clear. A fat-adaptation period beyond four weeks may decrease exercise performance, which cannot be reversed by a week on a high-carbohydrate diet.

Although the hypothesis that chronic high-fat diets may increase the capacity to oxidize fat and improve exercise performance during competition is attractive, little evidence indicates that it is true. The available studies that indicate a positive effect on performance were conducted at exercise intensities lower than the normal intensities during competition. Therefore, more well-controlled studies are needed to clarify the importance of the effect of dietary carbohydrate and fat content on athletic performance and, at this time, because little information is available about the negative effects of high-fat diets for athletes, caution should be exercised when recommending a high-fat diet to athletes.

Figure 6.17 High-fat diets and performance improvements during training in humans.

Data from J.W. Helge et al., 1998 and J.W. Helge et al., 1996.

Supplements That Increase Fat Oxidation

Several nutritional supplements on the market are claimed to increase fat oxidation, increase fat loss and lean body mass, and help weight loss. Supplements that have been associated with fat oxidation are caffeine, carnitine, pyruvate, and dihydroxyacetone (see figure 6.18).

Caffeine is thought to stimulate lipolysis and the mobilization of FAs. Carnitine is believed to help transport FAs into the mitochondria. Pyruvate and dihydroxyacetone are often sold as supplements to

Caffeine   Pyruvate

Carnitine   Vanadium (vanadyl-sulphate)

Chromium   Yohimbine

Dihydroxyacetone

Figure 6.18 Supplements that are claimed to increase fat oxidation.

increase fat oxidation. Similarly, the trace elements chromium and vanadium are claimed to promote fat oxidation and help weight loss. (See chapter 10 for further details.)

Key Points

- In contrast to carbohydrate stores, fat stores are large in humans and are regarded as practically unlimited. The stores of fat are mainly located in adipose tissue but significant amounts also exist as IMTGs.

- The steps that could potentially limit fat oxidation are lipolysis, removal of FAs from the fat cell, transport of fat by the bloodstream, transport of FAs into the muscle cell, transport of FAs into the mitochondria, or oxidation of FAs in the β-oxidation pathway and TCA cycle.

- The majority of FAs are stored in the form of triacylglycerols in subcutaneous adipose tissue, and FAs are released along with glycerol after the breakdown of triacylglycerols (lipolysis) by the enzyme hormone-sensitive lipase.

- Most FAs in the blood are bound to albumin (>99.9%).

- Transporter proteins (FAT/CD36) have been identified that are likely to be responsible for most of the transport of FAs across the sarcolemma. Once in the muscle cell, FAs are bound to FA-binding proteins.

- In the muscle, FAs are stored as IMTG, which can provide an important fuel during exercise.

- The enzyme CPT I plays a crucial role in the transport of FAs into the mitochondria.

- Carbohydrate and fat are always oxidized as a mixture, and the relative contribution of these two substrates depends on the exercise intensity and duration, the level of aerobic fitness, diet, and the carbohydrate intake before and during exercise.

- In absolute terms, fat oxidation increases as the exercise intensity increases from low to moderate intensities, even though the percentage contribution of fat may actually decrease. At higher intensities of exercise (>75% $\dot{V}O_2max$) fat oxidation is inhibited and both the relative and absolute rates of fat oxidation decrease to negligible values. In trained individuals, the maximal rates of fat oxidation were observed at 63% $\dot{V}O_2max$.

- Diet also has marked effects on fat oxidation. Generally a high-carbohydrate, low-fat diet reduces fat oxidation, whereas a high-fat, low-carbohydrate diet increases fat oxidation.

- Carbohydrate feeding before exercise reduces fat oxidation by reducing lipolysis and plasma FA availability and by an inhibition of the carnitine-dependent FA transport into the mitochondria.

(continued)

(continued)

■ The rate of carbohydrate utilization during prolonged strenuous exercise is closely related to the energy needs of the working muscle. In contrast, fat utilization during exercise is not tightly regulated. No mechanisms exist that closely match the metabolism of FAs to energy expenditure. Fat oxidation is, therefore, mainly influences by fat availability and the rate of carbohydrate utilization.

■ Long-chain triacylglycerol ingestion during exercise is not desirable, because they slow gastric emptying, they only slowly appear in the systemic circulation, and they enter the systemic circulation in chylomicrons, which are believed to be an insignificant fuel source during exercise.

■ Medium-chain triacylglycerols (MCTs) are rapidly emptied from the stomach, absorbed, and oxidized, but the ingestion of larger amounts of MCTs resulted in gastrointestinal distress. When ingested in smaller amounts MCTs do not appear to have the positive effects on performance that are often claimed.

■ Fasting increases the availability of lipid substrates, resulting in increased oxidation of FAs at rest and during exercise. However, because the liver glycogen stores are not maintained, fatigue resistance and exercise performance are impaired.

■ High-fat diets for 3 days to 5 days increase the availability of lipid substrates, but reduce the storage of glycogen. As a result, fat oxidation increases during exercise, but fatigue resistance and exercise performance are compromised.

■ Although the hypothesis that chronic high-fat diets may increase the capacity to oxidize fat and improve exercise performance during competition is attractive, little evidence indicates that the hypothesis is true.

Key Terms

carnitine palmitoyl transferase (CPT) 133

hormone-sensitive lipase 128

intramuscular triacylglycerol (IMTG) 128

lipolysis 129

long-chain FA (LCFA) 135

medium-chain FA (MCFA) 133

re-esterification 128

very low-density lipoprotein 128

Recommended Readings

Hawley, J.A., F. Brouns, and A. Jeukendrup. 1998. Strategies to enhance fat utilization during exercise. *Sports Medicine* 26:241-257.

Jeukendrup, A.E. 1999. Dietary fat and physical performance. *Current Opinion in Clinical Nutrition Metabolic Care* 2:521-526.

Jeukendrup, A.E. 2002. Regulation of skeletal muscle fat metabolism. *Annals of the New York Academy of Science* 967:217-35.

Jeukendrup, A.E. 2003. Modulation of carbohydrate and fat utilization by diet, exercise and environment. *Biochemical Society Transactions* 31: 270-1273.

Jeukendrup, A.E., W.H.M. Saris, and A.J.M. Wagenmakers. 1998. Fat metabolism during exercise: A review. Part I:

Fatty acid mobilization and muscle metabolism. *International Journal of Sports Medicine* 19:231-244.

Jeukendrup, A.E., W.H.M. Saris, and A.J.M. Wagenmakers. 1998. Fat metabolism during exercise: A review. Part II: Regulation of metabolism and the effects of training. *International Journal of Sports Medicine* 19:293-302.

Jeukendrup, A.E., W.H.M. Saris, and A.J.M. Wagenmakers. 1998. Fat metabolism during exercise: A review. Part III: Effects of nutritional interventions. *International Journal of Sports Medicine* 19:371-379.

Van der Vusse, G.J., and R.S. Reneman. 1996. Lipid metabolism in muscle. In *Handbook of Physiology*, Section 12. ed. L.B. Rowell and J.T. Shephard. Oxford University Press: New York.

Chapter 7

Protein and Amino Acids

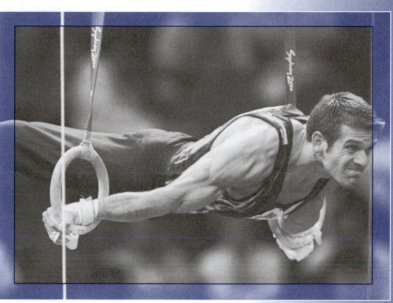

© Rob Tringali/SportsChrome USA

Objectives

After studying this chapter, you should be able to do the following:

- Give a general description of amino acids and protein metabolism and describe the potential fate of amino acids

- Understand the functions of protein and identify the most abundant amino acids

- Describe the effects of training on body proteins

- List techniques available to study protein metabolism and to discuss the advantages and disadvantages of these techniques

- Discuss the contribution of protein to energy expenditure at rest and during exercise

- Discuss the effect of feeding on protein synthesis and breakdown

- Describe the recommendations generally given for strength and endurance athletes

- Discuss the need for protein supplementation in athletes

- Describe the potential health hazards of excess intake of protein

- Discuss the effects of ingesting single amino acids

Debate has always raged over how much dietary protein is required for optimal athletic performance, partly because muscle contains a large proportion of the protein in a human body (about 40%). Muscle also accounts for 25% to 35% of all protein turnover in the body. Both the structural proteins that make up the myofibrils and the proteins that act as enzymes within a muscle cell change as an adaptation to exercise training. Indeed, muscle mass, muscle protein content, and muscle protein composition change in response to training.

Interest in protein consumption is very high among amateur and professional athletes. Therefore, the fact that meat, which contains high-quality protein, is a very popular protein source for athletes (especially strength athletes) is not surprising. This preference for meat probably dates back to ancient Greece where athletes in preparation for Olympic games consumed large quantities of meat.

A strong belief, especially among strength athletes, is that a large protein intake or certain protein or amino acid supplements increases muscle mass and strength. Despite the long history of protein use in sport, debate continues even over questions such as whether protein requirements are increased in athletes. Protein and amino acid metabolism is very complex, and many organs and tissues are involved. Thus, no uniform opinion exists as to what should be measured as an endpoint. For example, the effectiveness of protein intake or supplements could be assessed by measuring performance, muscle mass, or strength, or it could be measured by **nitrogen balance** over several days or by short-term methods involving the incorporation of labeled amino acids into muscle proteins.

The use of different techniques to estimate protein turnover may give different results. Therefore, the principles of the techniques and their limitations must be understood. This chapter discusses the various techniques available to investigate protein metabolism. Then, a brief overview of protein and amino acid metabolism is given. Subsequently, protein metabolism during exercise and dietary protein needs for endurance and strength-training athletes are examined. Finally, the effects of individually supplementing the diet with various amino acids is discussed.

Amino Acids

The most abundant proteins in muscle are the contractile proteins actin and myosin. Together they account for approximately 80% to 90% of all muscle protein. Muscle contains all the naturally occurring amino acids, and, thus, meat is a very valuable food.

The most abundant amino acids are the **branched-chain amino acids** (BCAAs) leucine, valine, and isoleucine, which together account for 20% of the total amino acids found in muscle protein.

Amino Acid Transport

The concentrations of amino acids in muscle and in the blood differ, suggesting that to maintain these concentration gradients, an active transport mechanism is required. Because different amino acids have different concentration gradients, different transporters move individual or groups of amino acids. Amino acid transporters are membrane-bound proteins that recognize specific amino acid shapes and chemical properties (e.g., neutral, basic, or anionic). The transporters are divided into sodium-dependent and sodium-independent carriers. Generally the sodium-dependent transporters maintain a larger gradient than the sodium-independent transporters. To date, some transporter proteins have been identified, but many more are yet to be discovered.

Amino Acid Metabolism

The metabolism of most amino acids is linked to the metabolism of other amino acids, and some amino acids can be synthesized from other amino acids. This feature is especially important in conditions of limited dietary protein intake or when metabolic requirements are increased. Some amino acids are essential and are not synthesized in the body, whereas others can be synthesized in the body (nonessential amino acids). (See chapter 1, figure 1.7.)

Amino acids are involved in a wide variety of biochemical and physiological processes, some of which are common to all and some of which are highly specific to certain amino acids. Amino acids are constantly incorporated into proteins (**protein synthesis**), and proteins are constantly broken down (protein breakdown or degradation). These processes are summarized in figure 7.1. The vast majority of the amino acids in the body are incorporated into tissue proteins, but a small pool of free amino acids also exists (about 120 g of free amino acids is present in the skeletal muscle of an adult). Amino acids are constantly extracted from the free amino acid pool for synthesis of various proteins, and breakdown of protein (**protein degradation**) makes amino acids available for the free amino acid pool.

Protein Breakdown

The breakdown of protein serves two main purposes: (1) It provides energy when some of its individual

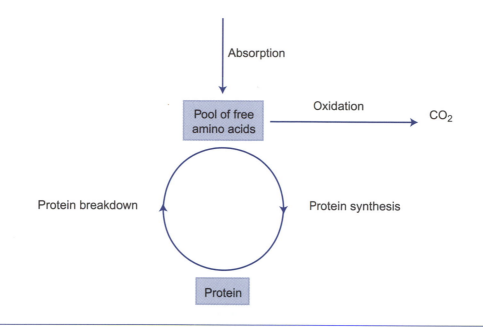

Figure 7.1 Protein metabolism. Amino acids enter the free amino acid pool from the diet (absorption) or from breakdown of protein. Amino acids leave the free amino acid pool for protein synthesis or oxidation to CO_2.

amino acids are converted into acetyl-CoA or TCA-cycle intermediates and are oxidized in the mitochondria. (2) Individual amino acids can be used for the synthesis of other compounds, including neurotransmitters (e.g., **serotonin**), hormones (e.g., epinephrine), and other peptides and proteins. This breakdown of protein and incorporation of the amino acids into a new protein links protein degradation with protein synthesis. Amino acids can also be incorporated into compounds that are not proteins. In this case, the body loses protein. For example, some amino acids are converted into glucose (gluconeogenesis) or fat (lipogenesis) and subsequently stored in adipose tissue.

Before amino acids can be oxidized, the amino group must be removed. Removal of the amino group can be achieved for some amino acids by transferring it to another molecule called a keto-acid, which results in the formation of a different amino acid. This process is called **transamination** and is catalyzed by enzymes called aminotransferases. A good example is the transfer of the amino group from the amino acid leucine to the keto-acid α-ketoglutarate forming α-ketoisocaproate (which can be further metabolized to form acetyl-CoA) and **glutamate,** respectively. Alternatively, the amino group can be removed from the amino acid to form free **ammonia** (NH_3), in a process called oxidative **deamination.** One example is the breakdown of asparagine to form aspartate and NH_3. Because free ammonia is a toxic substance, it is either used to form **glutamine** from glutamate within the muscle or is transported to the liver, where it is converted to urea

and is eventually excreted by the kidneys. Both ammonia and urea can be excreted in urine and sweat.

After the removal of the amino group from an amino acid, the remaining carbon skeleton (the keto-acid) is eventually oxidized to CO_2 in the TCA cycle. The carbon skeleton of amino acids can enter the TCA cycle in several ways. Some can be converted to acetyl-CoA and enter the TCA cycle just like acetyl-CoA from carbohydrate or fat. They can also enter the TCA cycle as α-ketoglutarate or oxaloacetate as metabolites of glutamate and aspartate, respectively (see figure 7.2).

The amino acids that can be converted into α-ketoglutarate, oxaloacetate, or pyruvate can also be used for the synthesis of glucose in the liver (gluconeogenesis). Amino acids or keto-acids that are eventually broken down to acetyl-CoA can also be used in the synthesis of FAs. Acetyl-CoA units can be used in an elongation process to form "longer" FAs by adding on to the hydrocarbon chain of the 16-carbon FA, palmitate. The following are examples of some common aminotransferase reactions:

$$\text{L-glutamate} + \text{oxaloacetate} \rightarrow$$
$$\alpha\text{-ketoglutarate} + \text{L-aspartate}$$

$$\text{L-alanine} + \alpha\text{-ketoglutarate} \rightarrow \text{pyruvate} + \text{L-glutamate}$$

Several amino acids undergo reversible transamination. These amino acids include alanine, aspartate, glutamate, and the BCAAs: leucine, isoleucine, and valine. The BCAAs are the only **essential amino acids** that can undergo transamination. Transamination is

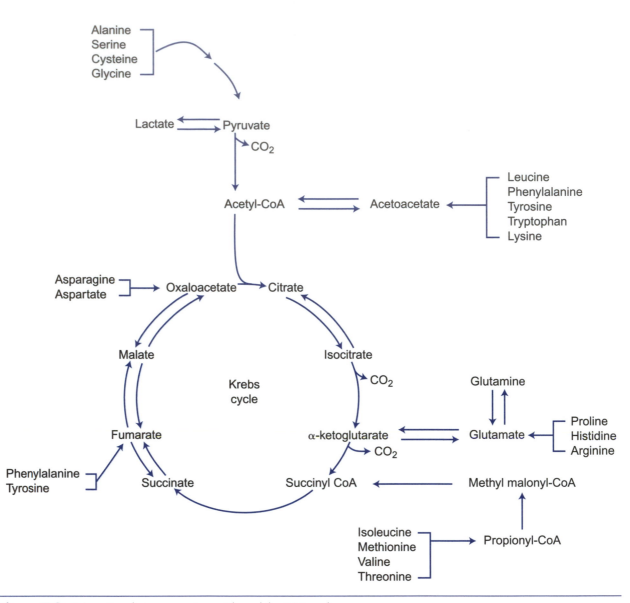

Figure 7.2 Interactions between amino acids and the TCA cycle.

usually rapid, and the main limiting factor is the fact that these processes sometimes take place in different tissues. Amino acids, thus, have to be transported via the circulation. Glutamate serves a central role in these transamination reactions because several amino acids can undergo transamination with glutamate.

Leucine
Valine
Isoleucine
Alanine
Aspartate
Glutamine
NH$_3$ + α-ketoglutarate

} Glutamate

Most of the nitrogen from amino acid degradation is transferred to α-ketoglutarate to form glutamate and subsequently glutamine; these two amino acids are the most abundant free amino acids in muscle. Only 6 of the available 20 amino acids in protein are oxidized in significant amounts by muscle: asparagine, aspartate, glutamate, isoleucine, leucine, and valine. An outline of the pathways involved in degradation of the various amino acids is provided in table 7.1.

Amino Acid Synthesis

The discussion of synthesis of amino acids is by definition limited to the nonessential amino acids because the essential amino acids cannot be synthesized in

Table 7.1 Pathways of Amino Acid Degradation

Metabolic pathway	Important enzymes	Nitrogen end product	Carbon end product
Amino acids converted to other amino acids			
Asparagine	Asparaginase	Aspartate+NH_3	
Glutamine	Glutaminase	Glutamate+NH_3	
Arginine	Arginase	Ornithine+Urea	
Phenylalanine	Phenylalanine hydroxylase	Tyrosine	
Proline		Glutamate	
Cysteine		Taurine	
Transamination to form glutamate			
Alanine		Glutamate	Pyruvate
Aspartate		Glutamate	Oxaloacetate
Leucine		Glutamate	Ketones
Isoleucine		Glutamate	Succinate
Valine		Glutamate	Succinate
Ornithine		2 Glutamates	α-ketoglutarate
Tyrosine		Glutamate	Ketone + fumarate
Cysteine		Glutamate	Ketone + SO_4^-
Other pathways			
Serine	Serine dehydratase	NH_3	Pyruvate
Threonine	Theorine dehydratase	NH_3	Ketobutyrate
Histidine	Histidase	NH_3	Urocanate
Tryptophan		NH_3	Kynurenine
Glycine		NH_3	CO_2
Methionine		NH_3	Ketobutyrate
Lysine		2 Glutamates	Acetate

Adapted from D.E. Matthews, 1999.

the body. In figure 7.3, a summary of the synthetic pathways of nonessential amino acids is given. Again, glutamate plays a central role. Glutamate serves as the donor of nitrogen in the synthesis of many amino acids, which occurs by transferring NH_3 to a carbon skeleton precursor (keto-acid) from the TCA cycle, from another nonessential amino acid, or from an essential amino acid.

Synthesis of amino acids by the transfer of NH_3 to a carbon skeleton precursor from the TCA cycle is rarely limited because of the ample availability of the substrates (carbon skeleton precursors and NH_3). On the other hand, synthesis of amino acids from other amino acids can sometimes be limited because of limited dietary supply. Cysteine and tyrosine are special cases because they are synthesized from essential amino acids and are therefore indirectly dependent on amino acid intake.

Incorporation of Amino Acids Into Protein

Different proteins are synthesized and degraded at different rates. Generally, the proteins that have a regulatory function (such as enzymes) or that act as signals (hormones) have a relatively rapid turnover

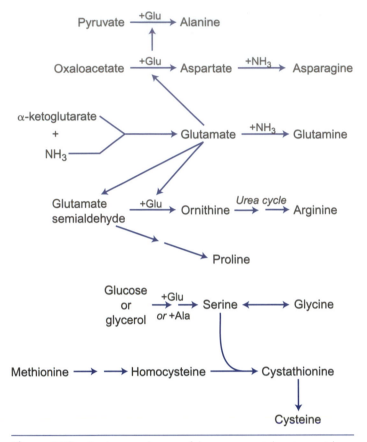

Figure 7.3 Synthetic pathways of the nonessential amino acids.
Adapted from D.E. Matthews, 1998.

Incorporation of Amino Acids Into Other Compounds

Amino acids are used for the synthesis of amino acid–like compounds. A list of the most important products is provided in table 7.2. Amino acids glutamate, tyrosine, and tryptophan, for example, are precursors of neurotransmitters. Glutamate is a special amino acid in this respect because it is not only a precursor of neurotransmitters but is also a neurotransmitter itself. Tyrosine is the precursor of catecholamines (dopamine, ephinephrine, and norepinephrine) and tryptophan is the precursor of serotonin (5-hydroxytryptamine). The roles of amino acids as precursors of creatine and carnitine synthesis are discussed in more detail in chapter 10.

Techniques to Study Protein and Amino Acid Metabolism

The following is a list of currently available techniques to study protein metabolism. These techniques range from very simple techniques, such as the measurement of urea in urine, to very complex techniques involving expensive and very sophisticated equipment in combination with more invasive techniques.

- Urea concentration in urine and sweat
- 3-methylhistidine in urine (indication of myofibrillar protein breakdown)
- Nitrogen balance (nitrogen intake minus nitrogen excretion in sweat and urine)
- Arteriovenous measurements of amino acids across a tissue bed
- Radiolabeled isotopes
- Stable isotopes
- Tracer incorporation into a specific protein (protein synthesis)
- Tracer release from a specific protein (protein breakdown)
- Fractional synthetic rate (FSR)
- Fractional breakdown rates (FBR)

An overview of these techniques, including their strengths and weaknesses, is given in table 7.3.

(hours or days). The structural proteins, such as collagen and contractile proteins (actin and myosin), have a relatively slow turnover (days, weeks, or months). In humans who are weight stable, the overall synthesis and degradation must be in balance, which means that the nitrogen consumed equals the nitrogen excreted in urine, feces, and other routes.

Protein turnover is several times greater than the protein intake, as is illustrated in figure 7.4 for a healthy 70-kg (154-lb) person. A normal daily protein intake is approximately 90 g. In this example, the intake of protein, therefore, provides only about 25% of the amino acids that enter the free amino acid pool each day (340 g). Most of the amino acids that appear in and disappear from the free amino acid pool are derived from proteins in the gut, kidneys, and liver. Even though this protein is a relatively small portion of the total mass of protein, it represents about two-thirds of the total protein turnover because of the very rapid turnover in these tissues. Muscle has a relatively slow protein turnover and provides most of the remainder. Various techniques are used to study protein metabolism and nitrogen balance. These techniques are reviewed later in this chapter.

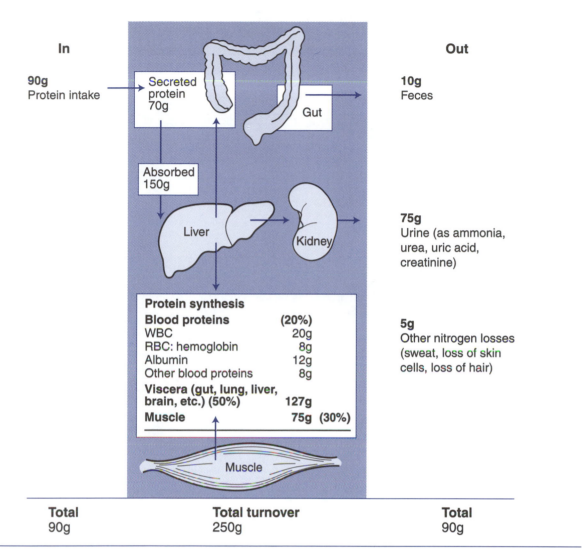

Figure 7.4 Daily protein balance in humans. RBC = red blood cells, WBC = white blood cells.

Adapted from D.E. Matthews, 1998, Proteins and amino acids. In *Modern Nutrition in Health and Disease*, edited by N.E. Shils, J.A. Olson, M. Shike, and A.C. Ross (Philadelphia: Lippincott Williams and Wilkins).

Table 7.2 Products Synthesized from Amino Acids

Product	Synthesized from	Product	Synthesized from
Creatine	Arginine Glycine Methionine	Pyrimidines	Aspartate Glutamine
Glutathione	Cysteine Taurine Glutamine	Histamine	Histidine
		Carnitine	Lysine
Neurotransmitters	Glutamate Tyrosine Tryptophan	Choline Serine	Methionine
Purines	Aspartate Glutamine Glycine	T3, T4 Epinephrine	Tyrosine

Table 7.3 Methods for Estimating Protein Metabolism

Method	Advantages	Disadvantages/Limitations
Urea concentration in urine and sweat	Easy; relatively cheap	Only rough estimate; heavily affected by diet (protein intake)
3-methylhistidine in urine	Simple measure of myofibrillar protein breakdown	Only rough estimate of myofibrillar protein breakdown; requires strict control of meat intake; does not provide information about actual changes in muscle mass
Nitrogen balance (nitrogen intake – nitrogen excretion in sweat and urine)	Accurate method when used over relatively long periods of time	Difficult and time consuming; tends to overestimate nitrogen retention; usually ignores nitrogen loss in sweat; highly dependent on subject compliance; gives no insight into metabolic pathways
Arteriovenous measurements of amino acids across a tissue bed	Gives information about net exchange of amino acids across a tissue; net uptake of essential amino acids related to rate of protein synthesis	Invasive; can have high variability, depending on blood flow measurement
Radiolabeled isotopes	Relatively cheap; relatively easy to measure; small amounts of tracer needed	Potential health risk
Stable isotopes	No health risk	Relatively expensive; sophisticated equipment needed for analyses
Tracer incorporation into a specific protein (protein synthesis)	Gives direct information about protein synthesis in a tissue	Invasive (tissue biopsies needed); relatively expensive; sophisticated equipment needed for analyses
Fractional synthetic rate (FSR) and fractional breakdown rate (FBR)	Uses stable isotopes so no health risk	Short-term measurement; does not provide information about actual changes in muscle mass; relatively expensive; sophisticated equipment needed for analyses

Urea Concentration in Urine

The amount of urea excreted in urine is an indication of whole-body protein breakdown but does not provide detailed information and only gives a very rough indication of protein breakdown. The urinary urea concentration depends on many disturbing factors, such as the level of hydration and the diet (protein intake). When urine is collected over 24 hours, the results become slightly more meaningful because total daily urea excretion can be determined, but the results are still highly dependent on protein intake.

Nitrogen Balance

Most experts in various countries have used nitrogen balance studies to determine the recommended dietary intakes for protein. Subjects are fed a diet with a certain level of protein intake, and for a time (3 days to 14 days), urine and feces are collected over 24-hour periods. The nitrogen intake (protein intake) and nitrogen excretion are measured as accurately as possible. A week or more may be required before collection reflects the adaptations to a particular diet.

Nitrogen excretion can be measured from urine, feces, and sweat. Nitrogen is detectable in feces because not all protein is completely absorbed, and some of the nitrogen secreted into the gastrointestinal tract is not reabsorbed. When nitrogen balance is measured in exercising subjects, nitrogen excretion in sweat is substantial and must be included in the measurements. Nitrogen is excreted mainly in the form of urea (about 90%) but also in creatinine, ammonia, uric acid, and other nitrogen-containing compounds. Often urinary nitrogen is the only measure taken, but nitrogen excretion is underestimated when using this measure alone.

When nitrogen intake exceeds excretion, a person is in positive nitrogen balance. When nitrogen excretion exceeds nitrogen intake, a person is in negative nitrogen balance. The latter situation cannot continue for a long time. The body uses protein, and because it does not contain large stores of protein, the breakdown and atrophy of tissues and organs will occur.

Only when nitrogen intake matches nitrogen excretion is a person in nitrogen balance.

Although the estimation of nitrogen balance is a technique that is often used, it is not easy to apply and it has been criticized for numerous reasons: It is very time consuming and involves several 24-hour periods of urine collection. It is labor intensive for the investigators. Its success is highly dependent on subject compliance. This technique also tends to underestimate nitrogen excretion and thus overestimate nitrogen retention, and it only gives a measure of the net nitrogen balance. Because of its "black box" nature, this technique does not provide any insight into the metabolic pathways involved in changes in protein metabolism.

3-Methylhistidine Excretion

Another method of estimating protein metabolism is the measurement 3-methylhistidine or N-methylhistidine excretion in the urine. When proteins are degraded, 3-methylhistidine cannot be recycled within the muscle and is excreted in the urine. The amount of 3-methylhistidine in urine is, therefore, a measure of contractile protein breakdown. The results of this relatively simple technique can be confounded by the diet. Meat and fish contain a relatively large amount of 3-methylhistidine and could cause erroneous results. The measurement of 3-methylhistidine is, therefore, only meaningful when the diet is strictly controlled. The urinary 3-methylhistidine is also highly dependent on the renal clearance rate. Thus, 3-methylhistidine excretion is often expressed relative to creatinine excretion to allow corrections for renal clearance and individual differences in muscle mass. The technique has several limitations but is regarded as a relatively easy and noninvasive way to get a rough idea of muscle protein breakdown.

Arteriovenous Differences

Nitrogen balance can also be determined across a specific organ. When arterial and venous blood across a certain tissue is sampled, the differences in the amino acid concentration gives information about the net exchange of specific amino acids. The arterial blood delivers amino acids to a tissue, and some of these amino acids are taken up and used for protein synthesis. The venous blood contains amino acids from protein breakdown. Depending on the tissue of interest, measuring arteriovenous differences (AV-differences) can be more or less invasive. For example, AV-differences from tissues like the gut, liver, and brain are very difficult to obtain. On the other hand, AV-differences across an arm or leg muscle are relatively easy to obtain. Recently, techniques have been developed to sample across adipose tissue. Independent of the tissue sampled, measurements of AV-differences always require a medically qualified person with good skills.

The AV-difference provides a measure of net uptake and release of amino acids by a tissue. The most valuable information is obtained from amino acids that are not metabolized. For example, the AV-difference of tyrosine and lysine (which are not metabolized in the muscle) reflect the difference between net amino acid uptake from protein synthesis and the release of amino acids from muscle protein breakdown. This method does not provide an insight into the various metabolic pathways in that tissue. Also, all metabolites of amino acids must be measured to get a true balance. Adding a tracer improves the value of the measurement and allows for more firm conclusions about metabolic pathways that play a role in the tissue. AV-differences of 3-methylhistidine across a muscle may be used as a specific marker of contractile protein breakdown.

Tracer Methods

Labeled tracers are used to follow amino acids in the body. These tracers have identical properties as the amino acid or metabolite they are meant to trace. They are, however, distinguishable because they either emit radiation (radioactive isotopes) or are slightly heavier (stable isotopes). Radioactive labeled tracers such as ^{3}H (hydrogen) and ^{14}C (carbon) have been used most often, but many laboratories now use stable isotopic tracers because, unlike radioisotopes, they do not pose a health risk. Stable isotopes have a different number of neutrons and, therefore, a different molecular mass. The difference in mass can be detected with mass spectrometry.

Stable isotopes occur naturally, and most elements have one abundant mass and up to three less abundant masses. For example, the abundant mass for hydrogen is ^{1}H and the less abundant mass is ^{2}H. For carbon the abundant and less abundant isotopes are ^{12}C and ^{13}C, respectively. Figure 7.5 lists some common stable isotopes and their abundance.

Common stable	Rare stable	Radioactive
^{1}H	^{2}H (0.02%)	^{3}H
^{12}C	^{13}C (1.1%)	^{14}C
^{14}N	^{15}N (0.37%)	^{13}N*
^{16}O	^{18}O (0.04%)	^{17}O*

Figure 7.5 Common stable, rare stable, and radioactive isotopes. The asterisk (*) indicates no long-lived radioisotopes for these elements.

Most tracer techniques are based on the principle of dilution. A tracer is infused, and the dilution of the tracer gives information about endogenous production of the amino acid of interest. This principle can be illustrated by a simple analogy. If you want to know the amount of water in a bucket, you can add a known amount of dye. After mixing the dye with the water, a sample of the mixture can be taken and the concentration of the dye can be determined. From the dilution of the dye, the amount of water in the bucket can be calculated. This calculation is, of course, only accurate if the exact amount of dye is known, mixing with the water is complete, and the concentration of the dye can be determined after mixing. Similar measurements can be made in a dynamic system if the dye is infused at a known constant rate. For example, a dye could be used to calculate the flow of water through a stream. The same principle can be applied by infusing a tracer into the human circulation. Several variations to this technique exist, to study whole-body protein metabolism or the metabolism of specific amino acids. Here we only discuss the principles. The interested reader should refer to other literature to learn more about stable and radioactive tracers (Wolfe 1992; Matthews 1999).

Methods have been developed to calculate the fractional synthetic rate (FSR) and fractional breakdown rate (FBR). These techniques, which use isotopic tracers, calculate the relative rate of protein breakdown and synthesis. Most of the information on protein metabolism currently available is from animal studies. Although the techniques to study protein metabolism in humans are constantly being improved, all methods have their limitations and no agreement has been reached on what method is best to use. Nevertheless, the available information allows us to draw some conclusions about exercise and protein requirements.

Protein Requirements for Exercise

Acute endurance exercise results in increased leucine oxidation. Because leucine is an essential amino acid and cannot be synthesized within the body, the implication is that dietary protein requirements are increased. Studies using a nitrogen balance technique confirm that the dietary protein requirements for athletes involved in prolonged endurance training are higher than those for sedentary individuals. However, these results have been questioned by scientists who have not found differences or even improved nitrogen and leucine balance in more active individuals.

During exercise, the uptake of glutamate and BCAA from the blood is increased. At the same time, the production and the release of alanine and glutamine by the muscle increases almost linearly with increasing exercise intensity. At exercise intensities below 70% $\dot{V}O_2$max, little or no change occurs in the concentration of amino acids in the muscle. At intensities above 70% $\dot{V}O_2$max, a sharp decrease in the intramuscular glutamate and glutamine concentrations is observed. The release of glutamine and alanine by the muscle is thought to remove ammonia from the muscle and transport it to the liver, where these amino acids can be deaminated and the ammonia is converted to urea and subsequently excreted.

In prolonged exercise or very-high-intensity exercise, the net negative protein balance that is normally observed in the hours after eating is increased. Accumulation of amino acids that are not metabolized in the muscle (for example lysine and threonine) increases. Whether this is the result of increased protein breakdown, decreased protein synthesis, or both is still unclear.

After resistance exercise, muscle protein turnover is increased because of an acceleration of both protein synthesis and degradation. Muscle protein breakdown is increased after resistance training but to a smaller degree than muscle protein synthesis (Biolo et al. 1995, 1999; Phillips et al. 1997, 1999). The elevations in protein degradation and synthesis are transient but are still present at 3 hours and 24 hours after exercise, although protein turnover returns to baseline levels after 48 hours. These results seem to apply to resistance exercise or dynamic exercise at a relatively high intensity. Low-intensity to moderate-intensity dynamic endurance exercise does not seem to have the same effects on muscle protein turnover, although studies have shown that endurance exercise may result in increased protein oxidation, especially during the later stages of very prolonged exercise and in conditions of glycogen depletion.

Protein is estimated to contribute about 5% to 15% to energy expenditure in resting conditions. During exercise, this relative contribution is likely to decrease because of an increasing importance of carbohydrate and fat as fuels. During very prolonged exercise, when carbohydrate availability becomes limited, the contribution of protein to energy expenditure may increase up to about 10% of total energy expenditure. Thus, although total protein oxidation is increased during endurance exercise, the relative contribution of protein to energy expenditure remains small. Furthermore, the oxidized amino acids do not appear to be derived from degradation of myofibrillar proteins (Kasperek and Snider 1989). In fact, only 6 of the 20 available amino acids are oxidized by muscle.

Protein Requirements for Endurance Athletes

Even though most researchers agree that exercise increases protein oxidation to some extent and this oxidation increase is accompanied by increased nitrogen losses, controversy persists over whether athletes have to eat more protein than less active individuals. Several research groups claim that evidence supports the contention that athletes should eat more protein, whereas others believes that the evidence is insufficient to make such a statement. One interesting observation is that training seems to have a protein-sparing effect. The better trained a person is, the lower the protein breakdown and oxidation during exercise. The research groups that advocate an increased protein intake for endurance athletes usually recommend an intake of 1.2 g/kg b.w. to 1.8 g/kg b.w. of protein (as opposed to the recommended intake of 0.8 g/kg b.w. of protein for the average population).

Even if protein requirements are increased, in practice athletes have no problem meeting these needs. As an extreme example, we can look at the Tour de France. Cyclists in this event compete for 3 hours to 7 hours a day, and maintaining energy balance is often problematic (Saris et al. 1989; Jeukendrup, Craig, and Hawley 2000). Nevertheless, in this situation, they seem to have no problems in maintaining nitrogen balance (Brouns et al. 1989a). With increasing food intake, the intake of protein automatically increases because many food products contain at least some protein. A study by van Erp-Baart et al. (1989a) showed a linear relationship between energy intake and protein intake. Tour de France cyclists consumed 12% of their daily energy intake (26 MJ, or 6,500 kcal) in the form of protein, and they easily met the suggested increased requirements (~2.5 g/kg b.w./day). These results suggest that provided the energy intake matches energy expenditure on a daily basis, endurance athletes do not need to supplement their diets with protein.

Protein Requirements for Strength Athletes

Unlike endurance exercise, resistance exercise does not increase the rate of leucine oxidation to any major degree. The suggested increased dietary protein requirements are related to increased muscle bulk (hypertrophy).

The question of whether strength athletes have increased protein requirements is controversial, and the nitrogen balance studies that have been done have been criticized because they generally have been of short duration and a steady-state situation may not be established (Rennie and Tipton 2000). Gontzea, Sutzeescu, and Dumitrache (1975) showed that the negative nitrogen balance used by many to indicate increased protein needs, disappears after approximately 12 days of training (see figure 7.6). The protein requirements may, therefore, only be temporarily elevated. However, with a further increase in training load, the protein requirement is likely

Figure 7.6 Nitrogen balance in response to exercise training.

Adapted from I. Gontzea, R. Sutzeescu, and S. Dumitrache, 1975, "The influence of adaptation to physical effort on nitrogen balance in man," *Nutrition Report International* 11(3): 231-236.

to increase again. The recommendation for protein intake for strength athletes is often 1.6 g/kg b.w./day to 1.7 g/kg b.w./day. Again, this requirement seems to be met easily with a normal diet, and no extra protein intake is needed. Protein supplements are often used but are not necessary to meet the recommended protein intake.

Protein Intake by Athletes and Athletes at Risk

The literature contains several reports of protein intake by athletes in a variety of sports. These intakes are usually self-reported but generally give a good indication of nutritional habits and can reveal whether the athlete is achieving the recommended protein intake. In the van Erp-Baart et al. study (1989a), protein intake in a variety of elite athletes was investigated. The lowest recorded intake was in a group of field hockey players, but their intake was still over 1.0 g/kg b.w./day. The highest intakes were recorded for endurance cyclists who consumed almost 3 g/kg b.w./day and bodybuilders who consumed 2.5 g/kg b.w./day. The majority of athletes therefore consume far more than the RDA for protein (0.8 g/kg b.w./day).

However, some individuals may suffer from protein deficiency, which can result in a compromise of function and ultimately to loss of body protein (atrophy). Four groups of athletes are recognized as being at risk from protein and energy deficiency: amenorrheic female runners, male wrestlers, male and female gymnasts, and female dancers. Energy intake can be very low for these groups and as a result protein intake may be low as well. Although protein intake for these groups may be adequate on average, certain individuals within these groups may have protein intakes well below the RDA.

Another group that has been suggested to be at risk is vegetarian athletes. Plant food sources typically contain lower-quality proteins, which often contain low levels of one or more essential amino acids. In addition, the digestibility of plant protein can be low compared with animal protein. Although some concern exists that vegetarian athletes may struggle to meet the protein requirements, the evidence for this is lacking, and adequate protein intake seems possible through a balanced vegetarian diet.

Training and Protein Metabolism

Training can have profound effects on muscle morphology and function. Different types of training seem to have very distinct effects. For example, strength training results in muscle hypertrophy and increased muscle mass (Jones and Rutherford 1987). Endurance training has no effect on muscle mass, but the mitochondrial density inside the muscle fibers increases dramatically (Holloszy and Coyle 1984). However, dynamic exercise training possibly results in increased muscle strength, but this increase depends on the relative intensity and the strength required to complete the training sessions.

Hypertrophy from strength training must be caused by increased protein synthesis. This protein synthesis must occur in the recovery phase between training sessions. Studies have shown that the body adapts to training by becoming more efficient with protein. Protein turnover decreases after training, and less net protein degradation occurs. In other words, after training, athletes become more efficient and "waste" less protein (Butterfield and Calloway 1984). BCAA oxidation at the same relative workload is the same in untrained and trained individuals (Lamont, McCullough, and Kalhan 1999). So although initially the protein requirement may increase, after adaptation to the training this increase seems to disappear.

Effect of Protein Intake on Protein Synthesis

Nutrition always plays a very important role in the establishment of training adaptations. In the hours after exercise, protein synthesis may exceed protein degradation but only after feeding. If feeding is delayed by 24 hours to 48 hours, net protein balance remains negative and no muscle hypertrophy occurs (Rennie and Tipton 2000). Feeding a mixed diet not only provides substrates but also results in a favorable hormonal milieu for protein synthesis. In resting conditions, higher amino acid concentrations in plasma have a stimulatory effect on protein synthesis (Bennet et al. 1990; Bennet and Rennie 1991). Increased availability of glucose and amino acids also results in increased plasma insulin concentrations, which, in turn, may cause a reduction of protein breakdown and a small increase in protein synthesis (Biolo et al. 1995; Bennet and Rennie 1991). Increased availability of amino acids immediately after exercise has a larger effect on protein synthesis compared with resting conditions (Biolo et al. 1995). Amino acids and exercise, thus, seem to have an additive effect on net protein synthesis. However, in these studies, amino acids were infused, and plasma amino acid concentrations were elevated to very high levels.

Intravenous infusion is not a practical method for athletes, and infused amino acids bypass the liver.

The liver normally extracts 20% to 90% of all amino acids after absorption in the gut (first-pass splanchnic extraction). Therefore, whether similar effects are to be expected after oral ingestion of amino acids is not clear. A follow-up study investigated this question (Tipton et al. 1999). In this study, a relatively large amount of amino acids was ingested after resistance exercise. Postexercise muscle protein balance was negative after placebo ingestion, but when amino acids were ingested, the net balance was positive mainly because of an increased muscle protein synthesis. From this study and a limited number of other studies, one can conclude that ingestion of amino acids after exercise enhances net protein synthesis.

Carbohydrate ingestion per se may not have an effect on protein synthesis. However, carbohydrate ingestion elevates plasma insulin concentrations and thereby may reduce the breakdown of protein. The combined ingestion of protein and carbohydrate seems to be preferred after exercise. The protein delivers the substrate (amino acids), and carbohydrate further increases the anabolic hormonal milieu required for net protein synthesis.

Some evidence in support of this hypothesis was recently provided by a study by Rasmussen et al. (2000). After a strenuous bout of resistance exercise, subjects were fed 6 g of essential amino acids plus 35 g of sucrose. Plasma amino acid levels increased threefold, and insulin concentrations increased 10-fold. Muscle protein synthesis increased 3.5-fold, but no increase occurred in protein breakdown (see figure 7.7). In the control condition, a net protein breakdown was observed. These results suggest that the ingestion of a relatively small amount of amino acids with a larger amount of carbohydrate can increase net muscle protein synthesis.

In the past, the amino acid needs of the body were primarily met by ingestion of whole proteins in the diet. However, over the past few years, the supplementation of individual amino acids has become

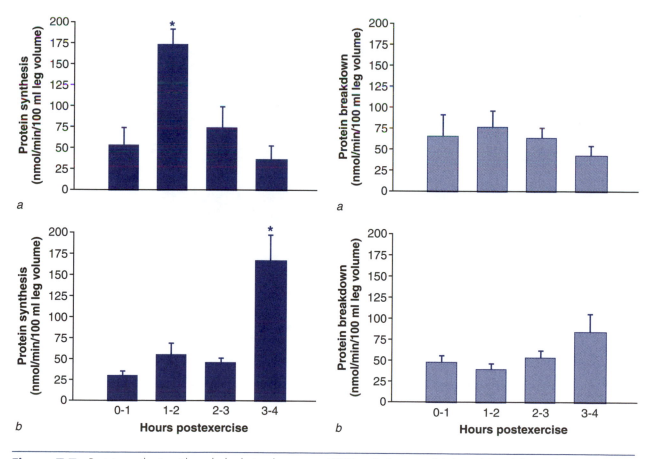

Figure 7.7 Protein synthesis with carbohydrate plus protein (CHO + Pro) ingested 1 hour (a) or 3 hours (b) post-exercise. Protein synthesis (in dark blue) was increased 1 hour to 2 hours after exercise when CHO + Pro was ingested 1 hour after exercise. When CHO + Pro ingestion was delayed, the increase in protein synthesis occurred much later. No major changes occurred in protein breakdown.

Adapted, by permission, from B.B. Rasmussen et al., 2000, "An oral essential amino acid-carbohydrate supplement enhances muscle protein anabolism after resistance exercise," *Journal of Applied Physiology* 88(2): 386-392.

increasingly popular. Technological advances have made it possible to manufacture food-grade ultrapure amino acids. The individual amino acids, called free-form amino acids, are mostly produced by bacterial fermentation.

Scientific studies are focusing on the pharmacologic and metabolic interactions of free-form amino acids. Considerable progress has been made in the area of clinical nutrition, where individual amino acids are used to reduce nitrogen losses and improve organ functions in traumatized and critically ill patients. Individual amino acids also are marketed as supplements for athletes and healthy individuals. Intake of separate amino acids are often claimed to improve exercise performance, stimulate hormone release, and improve immune function among a variety of other positive effects. The following section reviews the facts and fallacies of these claims.

Amino Acids As Ergogenic Aids

Amino acid supplements have become increasingly available and popular in certain athletic circles. Among others, weightlifters and bodybuilders consume various amino acids in attempts to stimulate the release of growth hormone from the pituitary gland, hoping that the growth hormone will, in turn, stimulate muscle development. Amino acids are also used to stimulate the release of insulin from the pancreas. Insulin is considered an anabolic hormone because it facilitates the uptake of amino acids as well as glucose by muscle cells and increases protein and glycogen synthesis. In addition to these effects on protein synthesis, certain amino acids are claimed to provide extra fuel to the muscle and prevent fatigue by changing the concentrations of brain neurotransmitters. Other amino acids have been used in attempts to reduce immunosuppression during strenuous training, to increase ATP and PCr levels in the muscle, and to help athletes lose body weight. An overview of common claims is provided in table 7.4. Such claims are often not based on scientific evidence, and sometimes they are not even based on a sound scientific rationale.

Ingestion of amino acids can have profound physiological effects. However, amino acid metabolism is very complex. One amino acid can be converted into another, and amino acids may influence nerve impulse transmission as well as hormone secretion. Consumption of specific amino acids or even high-protein diets may lead to nutritional imbalances because overload of one amino acid may reduce the absorption of others. The following section discusses the latest scientific findings with regard to the intake of individual amino acids or combinations of amino acids.

Arginine

Infusion of some amino acids into the blood can stimulate the release of growth hormone from the pitu-

Table 7.4 Manufacturers' Claims for Amino Acids

Amino acid	Claim
Arginine	Improves immune function, increases tissue creatine levels, increases release of insulin and growth hormone, leads to fewer gastrointestinal problems, improves performance
Aspartate	Improves energy metabolism in muscle, reduces amount of fatigue causing metabolites, improves endurance performance
Glutamine	Improves immune function (fewer colds), hastens recovery after exercise, improves performance, leads to fewer gastrointestinal problems
Ornithine	Increases growth hormone and insulin release, stimulates protein synthesis and reduces protein breakdown, improves performance
BCAA	Provides fuel for working muscle, reduces fatigue, improves endurance, reduces muscle protein breakdown
Tyrosine	Increases blood concentration of catecholamines, improves fuel mobilization and metabolism during exercise
Tryptophan	Increases the release of growth hormone, improves sleep, decreases sensations of pain, improves performance
Taurine	Delays fatigue, improves performance, facilitates faster recovery, leads to less muscle damage and pain, leads to fewer gastrointestinal problems, scavenges free radicals
Glycine	Increases phosphocreatine synthesis, increases sprint performance, improves strength

itary gland. Arginine is not the only amino acid that can have such an effect. Other amino acids that may stimulate the release of hormones from endocrine glands include lysine and ornithine. The intravenous administration of arginine to adults in a dose of 30 g in 30 minutes caused a marked increase in the secretion of human pituitary growth hormone (Knopf et al. 1966; Merimee, Lillicrap, and Rabinowitz 1965). Intravenous and oral arginine administration also resulted in a marked insulin release from the α-cells of the pancreas (Dupre et al. 1968; Floyd et al. 1966). The finding that arginine increases the secretion of anabolic hormones such as human growth hormone and insulin has made arginine a very popular supplement among bodybuilders and strength athletes. However, the amounts of arginine present in sport nutritional supplements are often rather small (between 1 g/day and 2 g/day) in comparison with the intravenous doses that have been shown to have potent secretagogue actions (30 g/30 min). Well-controlled studies (double-blind, crossover) (Fogelholm et al. 1993; Lambert et al. 1993) failed to show an effect of oral L-arginine supplementation taken in low quantities on the plasma concentrations of growth hormone and insulin (measured over a 24-hour period) in male competitive weight lifters and bodybuilders. It also should be noted that the growth hormone responses that can be obtained by ingesting relatively large amounts of arginine are still smaller than those that can be obtained by 60 min of moderate intensity exercise. Furthermore, the oral ingestion of larger doses of arginine can cause severe gastrointestinal discomfort (Wagenmakers 1999a).

Although arginine infused in large quantities can have anabolic properties, oral ingestion of tolerable doses (i.e., amounts that do not cause gastrointestinal problems) do not result in increased secretion of human growth hormone and insulin. Large increases in insulin secretion can be obtained by ingestion of carbohydrate, and much larger increases in plasma growth hormone are observed during exercise than with even large doses of arginine and other individual amino acids.

Aspartate

Aspartate is often claimed to improve aerobic exercise performance. Aspartate is a precursor of the TCA-cycle intermediates and reduces plasma ammonia accumulation during exercise. Because ammonia formation is associated with fatigue, aspartate supplementation could theoretically be ergogenic.

In a study by Maughan and Sadler (1983), eight subjects cycled to exhaustion at 75% to 80% $\dot{V}O_2$max

after ingestion of 6 g of aspartate (as magnesium and potassium salts) or placebo over 24 hours. No effect of aspartate supplementation was observed on plasma ammonia concentration or exercise time to exhaustion.

Branched-Chain Amino Acids

The three BCAAs, leucine, isoleucine, and valine, are not synthesized in the body. Yet they are oxidized during exercise, and they must, therefore, be replenished by the diet. In the late 1970s, BCAAs were suggested to be the third fuel for skeletal muscle after carbohydrate and fat (Goldberg and Chang 1978). BCAAs are sometimes supplied to athletes in energy drinks to provide extra fuel. Claims have also been made that BCAA supplementation can reduce net protein breakdown in muscle during exercise and reduce fatigue and enhance performance via effects on the brain.

BCAA As Fuel

As mentioned earlier, a study by Goldberg and Chang (1978) suggested that BCAAs can act as a fuel during exercise in addition to carbohydrate and fat. More recently, however, the activities of the enzymes involved in the oxidation of BCAAs were shown to be too low to allow a major contribution of BCAAs to energy expenditure (Wagenmakers et al. 1989, 1991). Detailed studies with a ^{13}C-labeled BCAA (^{13}C-leucine) showed that the oxidation of BCAAs only increases 2-fold to 3-fold during exercise, whereas the oxidation of carbohydrate and fat increases 10-fold to 20-fold (Wolfe et al. 1982; Knapik et al. 1991). Also, carbohydrate ingestion during exercise can prevent the increase in BCAA oxidation. BCAAs, therefore, do not seem to play an important role as a fuel during exercise, and from this point of view, the supplementation of BCAAs during exercise is unnecessary (Wagenmakers 1999a).

BCAA and Protein Breakdown

The claims that BCAAs reduce protein breakdown are mainly based on early in vitro studies, which showed that adding BCAAs to an incubation or perfusion medium stimulated tissue protein synthesis and inhibited protein degradation. Several in vivo studies in healthy individuals (Nair et al. 1992; Frexes-Steed et al. 1992; Louard, Barrett, and Gelfand 1990) failed to confirm the positive effect on protein balance that had been observed in vitro. No BCAA supplementation studies to date have demonstrated an improved nitrogen balance during or after exercise. Therefore, no valid scientific evidence supports the commercial claims that orally ingested BCAAs have an anticatabolic effect during and after exercise or that BCAA supplements may accelerate the repair of muscle damage after exercise (Wagenmakers 1999b).

Central Fatigue Hypothesis

The central fatigue hypothesis, which is illustrated in figure 7.8, was proposed in 1987 as an important mechanism contributing to the development of fatigue during prolonged exercise (Newsholme, Acworth, and Blomstrand 1987). This hypothesis predicts that during exercise, FAs are mobilized from adipose tissue and are transported via the blood to the muscles to serve as fuel. Because the rate of mobilization is greater than the rate of uptake by the muscle, the blood FA concentration increases. Both FAs and the amino acid tryptophan bind to albumin and compete for the same binding sites. Tryptophan is prevented from binding to albumin by the increasing FA concentration, and, therefore, the free tryptophan (fTRP) concentration and the fTRP:BCAA ratio in the blood rises. Experimental studies in humans have confirmed that these events occur. The central fatigue hypothesis predicts that the increase in the fTRP:BCAA ratio results in an increased fTRP transport across the blood-brain barrier, because BCAA and fTRP compete for carrier-mediated entry into the central nervous system by the large neutral amino acid (LNAA) transporter (Chaouloff et al. 1986; Hargreaves and Pardridge 1988). Once taken up, the conversion of tryptophan to serotonin occurs and leads to a local increase of this neurotransmitter (Hargreaves and Pardridge 1988).

Serotonin plays a role in the onset of sleep and is a determinant of mood and aggression. Therefore, the increase in serotoninergic activity might subsequently lead to central fatigue, forcing athletes to stop exercise or reduce the exercise intensity. Of course, the assumption that increased fTRP uptake leads to increased serotonin synthesis and activity of serotoninergic pathways (i.e., increased synaptic serotonin release) is a rather large leap of faith.

The central fatigue hypothesis also predicts that ingestion of BCAA will raise the plasma BCAA concentration and, hence, reduce transport of fTRP into the brain. Subsequent reduced formation of serotonin may alleviate sensations of fatigue and, in turn, improve endurance exercise performance. If the central fatigue hypothesis is correct and the ingestion of BCAAs reduces the exercise-induced increase of brain fTRP uptake and thereby delays fatigue, the opposite must also be true; that is, inges-

Figure 7.8 Central fatigue hypothesis.

tion of tryptophan before exercise should reduce the time to exhaustion. A few studies have included supplemental tryptophan in human subjects before or during exercise, and from these studies the conclusion must be drawn that tryptophan has no effects on exercise performance.

The effect of BCAA ingestion on physical performance was investigated for the first time in a field test by Blomstrand et al. (1991). One hundred and ninety-three male subjects were studied during a marathon in Stockholm. The subjects were randomly divided into an experimental group receiving BCAA in plain water and a placebo group receiving flavored water. The subjects also had free access to carbohydrate-containing drinks. No difference was observed in the marathon time of the 2 groups. However, when the original subject group was divided into fast and slower runners, a small significant reduction in marathon time was observed in subjects given BCAAs in the slower runners only. This study has since been criticized for its design and statistical analysis. Later studies, with various exercise and treatment designs and several forms of administration of BCAA (infusion, oral, and with and without carbohydrates), failed to find a performance effect (Varnier et al. 1994; Blomstrand et al. 1995,1997; Van Hall et al. 1995; Madsen et al. 1996). Van Hall et al. (1995) studied time-trial performance in trained cyclists consuming carbohydrate during exercise with and without BCAAs. A high and a low dose of BCAA was given, but no differences were seen in time-trial performance (see figure 7.9).

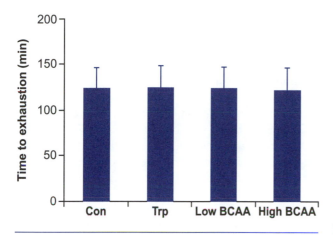

Figure 7.9 Time to exhaustion during cycling at 75% to 80% $\dot{V}O_2$max. No effect is seen with tryptophan, a small dose of branched-chain amino acids (BCAAs), or a large dose of BCAAs.

Reprinted, by permission, from G. Van Hall et al., 1995, "Ingestion of branched-chain amino acids and tryptophan during sustained exercise in man: Failure to affect performance," *Journal of Physiology* 486: 789-794.

Despite the lack of strong evidence for the efficacy of BCAA supplements, athletes continue to use them. However, normal food alternatives are available and are almost certainly cheaper. For example, a typical BCAA supplement sold in tablet form contains 100 mg valine, 50 mg of isoleucine, and 100 mg of leucine. A chicken breast (100 g) contains approximately 470 mg valine, 375 mg of isoleucine, and 656 mg leucine, the equivalent of about 7 BCAA tablets. One-fourth cup of peanuts (60 g) contains even more BCAA and is equivalent to 11 tablets.

Glutamine

Glutamine is a naturally occurring nonessential amino acid; that is, it can be synthesized in the body. It is important as a constituent of proteins and as a means of nitrogen transport between tissues. It is also important in acid-base regulation and as a precursor of the antioxidant glutathione. Glutamine is the most abundant free amino acid in human muscle and plasma. Its alleged effects can be classified as anabolic and immunostimulatory. Based somewhat

on an uncritical evaluation of the scientific literature, glutamine supplements are claimed by various manufacturers and suppliers to have the following beneficial effects:

- More rapid water absorption from the gut
- Improved intracellular fluid retention (i.e., a "volumizing" effect)
- Improved gut barrier function and reduced risk of endotoxemia
- Nutritional support for immune system and prevention of infection
- Stimulation of muscle protein synthesis and muscle tissue growth
- Stimulation of muscle glycogen resynthesis
- Reduction in muscle soreness and improved muscle tissue repair
- Enhanced buffering capacity and improved high-intensity exercise performance

The normal daily intake of glutamine from dietary protein is about 3 g/day to 6 g/day (assuming a daily protein intake of 0.8 g/kg b.m. to 1.6 g/kg b.m. of protein for a 70-kg individual). Researchers examining the effects of glutamine on the postexercise decline in plasma glutamine concentration report that a dose of about 0.1 g/kg b.w. of glutamine has to be given every 30 minutes over a 2-hour to 3-hour period to prevent the fall in the plasma glutamine concentration (Nieman and Pedersen 2000).

Glutamine is utilized at high rates by white blood cells (particularly lymphocytes) to provide energy and optimal conditions for nucleotide biosynthesis and, hence, cell proliferation (Ardawi and Newsholme 1994). Indeed, glutamine is considered important, if not essential, to lymphocytes and other rapidly dividing cell, including the gut mucosa and bone marrow stem cells. Prolonged exercise is associated with a fall in the intramuscular and plasma concentration of glutamine, and this decrease in glutamine availability has been hypothesized to impair immune function (Parry-Billings et al. 1992). Periods of very heavy training are associated with a chronic reduction in plasma glutamine levels, and this reduction may be partly responsible for the immunosuppression apparent in many endurance athletes (Parry-Billings et al. 1992). The intramuscular concentration of glutamine is related to the rate of net protein synthesis (Rennie et al. 1989), and some evidence also indicates a role for glutamine in promoting glycogen synthesis (Bowtell et al. 1999). However, the mechanisms underlying these alleged anabolic effects of glutamine remain to be elucidated.

Glutamine and Fluid Absorption

Water transport from the gut into the circulation is promoted by the presence of glucose and sodium in drinks. Water movement is determined by osmotic gradients, and the cotransport of sodium and glucose into the gut epithelial cells is accompanied by the osmotic movement of water molecules in the same direction. Glutamine is transported into gut epithelial cells by both sodium-dependent and sodium-independent mechanisms, and the addition of glutamine to oral rehydration solutions increases the rate of fluid absorption above that of ingested water alone (Silva et al. 1998). However, the potential benefits of adding glutamine to commercially available sports drinks have not be adequately tested, and any additional benefit in terms of increased rate of fluid absorption and retention is likely to be very small. Placebo-controlled studies that have investigated the effects of glutamine supplementation on extracellular buffering capacity and high-intensity exercise performance have not found any beneficial effect. Glutamine is not included in commercial sports drinks, mainly because of its relative instability in solution.

Glutamine and Muscle Protein Breakdown

Muscle protein breakdown occurs in the fasted state. Research indicates that resistance exercise reduces the extent of this protein catabolism, but an anabolic (muscle growth) response requires an intake of essential amino acids (dietary protein) in the recovery period after exercise (Rasmussen, Tipton, et al. 2000). This intake of essential amino acids promotes amino acid uptake into muscle and increases the tissue protein synthesis rate without affecting the rate of protein breakdown. Provided that ingested protein contains the eight essential amino acids, taking supplements of individual nonessential amino acids at this time is unlikely to provide any additional benefit. Protein synthesis in the tissues of the body requires the simultaneous presence of all 20 amino acids. Some evidence exists for an effect of glutamine supplements in promoting glycogen synthesis in the first few hours of recovery after exercise (Bowtell et al. 1999), but further work using optimal amounts of carbohydrate feeding after exercise needs to be done to substantiate this finding and give it practical relevance. Thus, a postexercise meal consisting of predominantly carbohydrate with some protein would seem to be the best strategy to promote both glycogen and protein synthesis in muscle after exercise (see the discussion on glycogen resynthesis in chapter 5).

Glutamine and the Immune System

Several scientists have suggested that exogenous provision of glutamine supplements may prevent muscle damage and muscle soreness and the impairment of immune function after endurance exercise. However, eccentric exercise-induced muscle damage does not affect the plasma glutamine concentration (Walsh et al. 1998), and no scientific evidence supports a beneficial effect of oral glutamine supplementation on muscle repair after exercise-induced damage, and no evidence supports reduced muscle soreness when glutamine is consumed compared with placebo. Prolonged exercise at 50% to 70% $\dot{V}O_2$max causes a 10% to 30% fall in plasma glutamine concentration that may last for several hours during recovery (Parry-Billings et al. 1992; Walsh et al. 1998; Castell and Newsholme 1997). This fall in plasma glutamine coincides with the window of opportunity for infection after prolonged exercise when an athlete is more susceptible to infections (Walsh et al. 1998).

One study showed that an oral glutamine supplement (5 g in 330 ml water) consumed immediately after and 2 hours after a marathon reduced the incidence of upper respiratory tract infection in the 7 days after the race (Castell, Poortmans, and Newsholme 1996). However, the dose given in that study was unlikely sufficient to prevent the postexercise fall in the plasma glutamine concentration. Furthermore, several recent studies (reviewed in Nieman and Pedersen [2000] and Gleeson and Bishop [2000a]) that investigated the effect of glutamine supplementation during exercise on various indices of immune function failed to find any beneficial effect.

A larger dose of glutamine (0.1 g/kg b.w.) than that given by Castell et al. (1996) ingested at 0 minutes, 30 minutes, 60 minutes, and 90 minutes after a marathon race prevented the fall in the plasma glutamine concentration but did not prevent the fall in mitogen-induced lymphocyte proliferation and lymphocyte-activated killer cell activity (Nieman and Pedersen 2000; Gleeson and Bishop 2000a). Similarly, maintaining the plasma glutamine concentration by consuming glutamine in drinks taken both during and after a prolonged bout of cycling did not affect leukocyte subset trafficking or prevent the exercise-induced fall in neutrophil function, lymphocyte proliferative response, natural killer cell activity, or salivary IgA secretion rate (Nieman and Pedersen 2000; Gleeson and Bishop 2000a). Unlike the feeding of carbohydrate during exercise, glutamine supplements seem not to affect the immune function perturbations that have been examined to date (see chapter 13 for further details).

Glutamine is thought to be relatively safe and well tolerated by most people, although administration to people with kidney disorders is not recommended. No adverse reactions to short-term glutamine supplementation have been reported, and no information is available on long-term use exceeding 1 g/day. Excessive doses may cause gastrointestinal problems.

Glycine

Glycine is a nonessential amino acid that is involved in the synthesis of phosphocreatine. Therefore, it has been theorized to have ergogenic properties. Early studies indicated improvements in strength after glycine (or gelatin that contains about 25% glycine) supplementation. However, these studies were poorly designed. Thus, the effects of glycine remain unresolved.

Ornithine

Ornithine has been suggested to stimulate growth hormone release from the pituitary gland (Evain-Brion et al. 1982) and insulin release from the pancreas. Growth hormone release after infusion of ornithine was even higher than that observed after arginine infusion. However, most ornithine supplements contain 1 g to 2 g of ornithine and this dosage does not affect the 24-hour hormone profile (Fogelholm et al. 1993). Therefore, ornithine does not seem to increase growth hormone release or increase muscle mass or strength. Although ornithine is often claimed to increase the secretion of insulin from the pancreas, a study in bodybuilders in which the effects of ornithine supplementation on insulin release was investigated failed to show any effect (Bucci et al. 1992).

Taurine

Taurine is a nonprotein amino acid and a derivative of cysteine. Taurine has recently become a popular ingredient of many sports drinks. The concentrations of taurine in the brain, heart, and muscle are high, but its role is poorly understood. It has been suggested to act as a membrane stabilizer, an antioxidant, and a neuromodulator. Taurine plays an undefined role in calcium currents in cells, influences ionic conductance in excitable membranes, and plays a role in the regulation of cell volume. Its value as a nutrition supplement is unclear.

Tyrosine

Oral doses of tyrosine (5 g to 10 g) result in increases in circulating concentrations of epinephrine, norepi-nephrine, and dopamine, hormones that are heavily involved in the regulation of body function during physical stress and exercise. Tyrosine supplements are used especially by strength athletes because of their supposed effect of activating metabolic pathways. However, no controlled studies show an effect of tyrosine supplementation on exercise performance. Most tyrosine supplements use a very low dosage (mg), whereas probably large doses are required to alter hormone levels. Regular supplementation of large amounts (5 g to 10 g) may have adverse health effects in the long term because it affects sympathetic nervous system activity.

Tryptophan

Tryptophan was suggested to stimulate the release of growth hormone. The most common proposed ergogenic effect, however, is based on another function. Tryptophan is the precursor of serotonin, a neurotransmitter in the brain that may induce sleepiness, decrease aggression, and elicit a mellow mood. Serotonin has also been suggested to decrease the perception of pain. Segura and Ventura (1988) hypothesized that tryptophan supplementation increases serotonin levels and the tolerance of pain and thereby improves exercise performance. They studied 12 subjects during running to exhaustion at 80% $\dot{V}O_2$max, with ingestion of tryptophan or placebo. Tryptophan was supplemented in four doses of 300 mg in the 24 hours before the endurance test, with the last doses ingested 1 hour before the test (total tryptophan ingestion, 1,200 mg). The investigators observed a 49% improvement in endurance capacity and decreased ratings of perceived exertion after tryptophan ingestion. Because a 49% performance improvement seemed somewhat unrealistic, several other investigators have challenged the results of this study (Stensrud et al. 1992; Van Hall et al. 1995).

In a study by Stensrud et al. (1992), 49 well-trained male runners were exercised to exhaustion at 100% $\dot{V}O_2$max, and no significant effect of tryptophan supplementation on endurance time was found. A very-well-controlled study by Van Hall et al. (1995) included eight cyclists given tryptophan supplements and found no effect on time to exhaustion at 70% $\dot{V}O_2$max (see figure 7.9).

Both tryptophan and BCAAs have been suggested as supplements to reduce central fatigue. Yet, the BCAAs and tryptophan have opposite effects. Whereas some claim that tryptophan reduces central fatigue (Segura and Ventura 1988), others have associated it with the development of central fatigue

(Newsholme, Blomstrand, and Ekblom 1992). Tryptophan could also exert some negative effects, including a blocking of gluconeogenesis and decreased mental alertness. Based on these studies, tryptophan does not seem to be ergogenic and may even be ergolytic in prolonged exercise.

Protein Intake and Health Risks

Excessive protein intake (more than 3 g/kg b.w./day) may have various negative effects, including kidney damage, increased blood lipoprotein levels (which has been associated with arteriosclerosis), and dehydration. The latter may occur as a result of increased nitrogen excretion in urine, which results in increased urinary volume and dehydration. Athletes consuming a high-protein diet must, therefore, increase their fluid intake to prevent dehydration. The recommended protein intakes for athletes (1.2 g/kg b.w./day to 1.8 g/kg b.w./day) and up to approximately 2 g/kg b.w./day do not seem to be harmful.

Intake of individual amino acids has no added nutritional value compared with the intake of proteins containing these amino acids. A possible advantage of the intake of individual amino acids is that larger amounts can be ingested. Purified amino acids were developed for clinical use in intravenous infusion of patients for adequate protein nutrition (particularly when oral consumption is compromised). Individual amino acids are also used as food additives to enhance the protein balance in case the diet is deficient in certain amino acids. Because individual amino acids are often ingested in pharmacological doses and the effects of such large doses are largely unknown, amino acids supplements should be treated as drugs.

In 1989, an epidemic in the United States of the eosinophilia-myalgia syndrome (EMS), a neuromuscular disorder characterized by weakness, fever, edema, rashes, bone pain, and various other symptoms was attributed to the excessive intake of L-tryptophan. L-tryptophan has been classified as neurotoxic and was banned for a while in the United States.

Key Points

- Amino acids are constantly incorporated into proteins (protein synthesis), and proteins are constantly broken down (protein breakdown or degradation) to amino acids. Some amino acids are essential and are not synthesized in the body, whereas others can be synthesized in the body (nonessential amino acids).

- Muscle contains 40% of the total protein in a human body and accounts for 25% to 35% of all protein turnover in the body. The contractile proteins actin and myosin are the most abundant proteins in muscle, together accounting for 80% to 90% of all muscle protein.

- Training has marked effects on body proteins. Both the structural proteins that make up the myofibrillar proteins and the proteins that act as enzymes within a muscle cell change as an adaptation to exercise training. Muscle mass, muscle protein composition, and muscle protein content all change in response to training.

- Methods of studying protein metabolism include nitrogen excretion, nitrogen balance, arteriovenous balance studies, and tracer methods. All methods available to measure protein turnover in humans have their limitations, and no method has been identified as the best one to use.

- Amino acids can be used to synthesize other amino acids, can be incorporated into proteins or other compounds (i.e., FAs and glucose), or can be oxidized in the TCA cycle.

- The BCAAs are the most abundant amino acids in skeletal muscle, together accounting for 20% of all amino acids in muscle. Glutamine is the most abundant free amino acid in muscle and plasma.

- Protein has been estimated to contribute up to about 15% to energy expenditure in resting conditions. During exercise, this relative contribution likely decreases because

(continued)

(continued)

of an increasing importance of carbohydrate and fat as fuels. During very prolonged exercise, when carbohydrate availability becomes limited, the contribution of protein to energy expenditure may increase up to about 10% of total energy expenditure.

■ In the hours after exercise, protein synthesis may exceed protein degradation but only after feeding. If feeding is delayed by 24 hours to 48 hours, net protein balance remains negative and no muscle hypertrophy occurs.

■ The recommended protein intake for strength athletes is generally 1.6 g/kg b.w./day to 1.7 g/kg b.w./day, about twice the value for the general population. The recommended protein intake for endurance athletes is usually 1.2 g/kg b.w./day to 1.8 g/kg b.w. of protein, although in extreme situations, the amount may rise to as much as 2.5 g/kg b.w./day.

■ With increasing food intake, the intake of protein automatically increases because many food products contain at least some protein. The relationship between energy intake and protein intake is linear.

■ Excessive protein intake (more than 3 g/kg b.w./day) may have various negative effects, including kidney damage, increased blood lipoprotein levels (which has been associated with arteriosclerosis), and dehydration.

■ Arginine infused in large quantities can have anabolic properties in patients, but oral ingestion of tolerable amounts do not result in increased secretion of human growth hormone and insulin.

■ BCAAs are among the most popular nutrition supplements. However, the evidence for claims of reduced net protein breakdown and reduced fatigue and enhanced performance via central nervous system mechanisms are not convincing.

Key Terms

ammonia (NH_3) 149

branched-chain amino acid (BCAA) 148

deamination 149

essential amino acids 149

glutamate 149

glutamine 149

nitrogen balance 148

protein degradation 148

protein synthesis 148

serotonin 149

transamination 149

Recommended Readings

McNurlan, M.A., and P.J. Garlick. 2000. Protein synthesis and degradation. In *Biochemical and Physiological Aspects of Human Nutrition*, ed. M.H. Stipanuk. Saunders: Philadelphia.

Rennie, M.J. 1996. Influence of exercise on protein and amino acid metabolism. In *Handbook of Physiology, Section 12: Exercise: Regulation and Integration of Multiple Systems*, ed. J.B. Rowell and J.T. Shepherd. Oxford University Press: New York.

Rennie, M.J., and K.D. Tipton. 2000. Protein and amino acid metabolism during and after exercise and the effects of nutrition. *Annual Review of Nutrition* 20:457-483.

Tarnopolsky, M.A. 1999. Protein and physical performance. *Current Opinion in Clinical Nutrition Metabolic Care* 2:533-537.

Wagenmakers, A.J. 1998. Protein and amino acid metabolism in human muscle. *Advances in Experimental Medicine and Biology* 441:307-319.

Wagenmakers, A.J. 1999. Amino acid supplements to improve athletic performance. *Current Opinion in Clinical Nutrition Metabolic Care* 2(6):539-544.

Chapter 8

Water Requirements and Fluid Balance

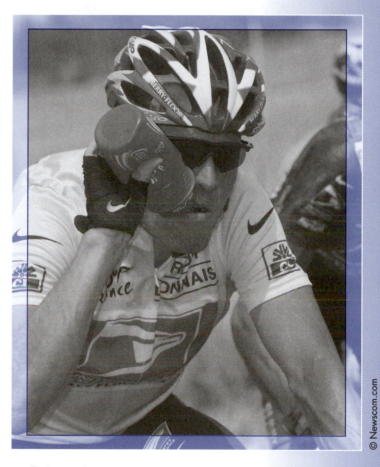

© Newscom.com

Objectives

After studying this chapter, you should be able to do the following:

- Describe how body temperature is regulated at rest and during exercise

- Describe the effect of dehydration on exercise performance

- Describe the effects of fluid intake before and during exercise on exercise performance

- Describe fluid intake strategies that help to ensure that the fluid requirements of athletes are met

- Describe the composition of drinks that are suitable for consumption by athletes during exercise and after exercise

Most athletes and coaches are aware that a reduction in the body's water content (**dehydration**) impairs exercise performance. However, appropriate strategies to prevent or limit dehydration during training and competition are not always followed. The hydration status of the body is determined by the balance between water intake and water loss. As with all the other nutrients, a regular and sufficient water intake is required to maintain health and physical performance. A lack of water intake causes deficiency symptoms, and failure to drink water for more than a few days can result in death. Symptoms associated with overconsumption of water can also be observed.

In most people, water accounts for 50% to 60% of the body mass. Lean body tissues (e.g., muscle, heart, and liver) contain about 75% water by mass, whereas adipose tissue contains only about 5% water by mass, as the bulk of the adipocytes are filled with triacylglycerol fat. The fat content of the body, therefore, largely determines the normal body-water content. For a healthy, lean young male weighing 70 kg (154 lb), the body water amounts to about 42 L (i.e., 60% of body weight). A healthy, lean young female weighing 70 kg has a total body-water volume of about 35 L, equivalent to 50% of her body weight (see table 8.1). The water content of the female body is less than that of the male because (1) the female body is lighter than that of the male and (2) the female body contains a higher proportion of fat (see table 8.1). Thus, for a typical female weighing 60 kg (132 lb), the body-water content is about 30 kg. The total body water is distributed among different body fluid compartments, as illustrated in table 8.2.

An important route of water (and electrolyte) loss from the body is through sweating, which is the

Table 8.1 Fat Content and Volumes of Body Fluid Compartments in Adults and Infants

Body fluid	Infants*	Adult men*	Adult women*
Plasma	4	5	4
Interstitial fluid	26	15	11
Intracellular fluid	45	40	35
Total	75	60	50
Fat	5	18	25

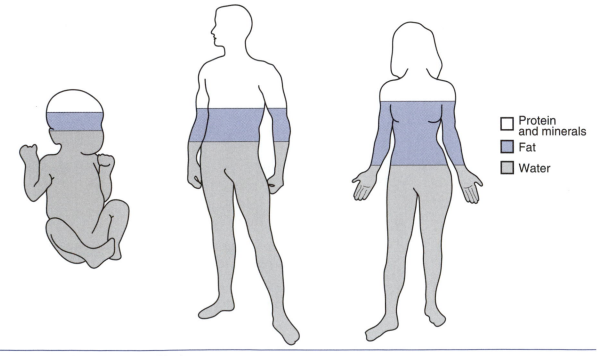

☐ Protein and minerals
☐ Fat
☐ Water

*Values are expressed as a percentage of body mass.

170

Table 8.2 Distribution of Body Water[a] in a Young 70-kg (154-lb) Man

	Volume (L)	Body mass (%)	Total-body water (%)
Intracellular fluid	28	40	62.5
Extracellular fluid	14	20	37.5
Interstitial fluid	10.5	15	30
Blood plasma	3.5	5	7.5

[a]Total-body water volume = 42 L or 60% of body mass.

body's principal means of preventing excessive rises in body temperature (**hyperthermia**) during exercise in the heat. Some understanding of the regulation of body temperature is, therefore, fundamental to the discussion of fluid balance in the body and the formulation of drinks intended for consumption both during and after exercise. Hence, this chapter begins with a brief overview of heat production and **thermoregulation** during exercise, followed by a consideration of the effects of dehydration on exercise performance, before discussing the need for water and electrolyte consumption by athletes.

Thermoregulation and Exercise in the Heat

Increased muscular activity during exercise causes an increase in heat production in the body because of the inefficiency of the metabolic reactions that provide energy for muscle force development. Thermoregulation concerns the mechanisms that prevent excessive rises in body temperature.

Heat Production During Exercise

For every liter of oxygen consumed during exercise such as cycling or running, approximately 16 kJ (4 kcal) of heat is produced and only about 4 kJ (1 kcal) is actually used to perform mechanical work (to be precise, 1.0 kcal = 4.186 kJ; see chapter 3 where this work efficiency is explained in more detail). Thus, for an athlete consuming oxygen at a rate of 4 L/min during exercise, the rate of heat production in the body is about $16,000 \times 4/60 = 800$ J/s, or watts (W), or $16 \times 4 \times 60/1,000 = 3.84$ MJ/h (917 kcal/h). Only a small proportion of the heat produced in active skeletal muscle is lost from the overlying skin. Rather, most of the heat is passed to the body core via the convective flow of venous blood returning to the heart. The rate of temperature increase in the belly of the quadriceps muscle group is close to 1°

C/min (1.8° F/min) during the initial moments of high-intensity cycling (Saltin et al. 1968). This rate of heat storage cannot persist, because the muscle contractile proteins and enzymes would be inactivated by heat-induced denaturation within 10 minutes. Thus, most of the heat generated in the muscle is transferred to the body core and increases in body core temperature are sensed by thermoreceptors located in the hypothalamus. This area of the brain also receives sensory input from skin thermoreceptors and integrates this information to produce appropriate reflex effector responses—increasing blood flow to the skin and initiating sweating—to increase heat loss and limit further rises in body temperature.

Heat Storage During Exercise

During exercise at a constant work rate, heat production increases in a square-wave fashion. The set point of the hypothalamic thermostat does not change during exercise, but some heat storage does occur. When heat loss from the body equals heat production, the rise in body temperature plateaus. However, during high-intensity exercise, particularly in an environment with a high ambient temperature and high humidity, core temperature continues to rise.

During exercise at an intensity equivalent to about 80% to 90% $\dot{V}O_2$max, heat production in a fit individual may exceed 1,000 W (resting heat production is about 70 W), which could potentially increase body temperature by 1° C (1.8° F) every 4 minutes to 5 minutes if no changes occur in the body's heat-dissipating mechanisms. This estimate is based on the specific heat capacity of human tissues, which is 3.47 kJ/kg/°C (0.46 kcal/kg/°F) for lean tissue and 1.73 kJ/kg/°C (0.23 kcal/kg/°F) for fat. For a man weighing 70 kg (154 lb) with 15% body fat, the specific heat capacity of the body is $(3.47 \times 0.85) + (1.73 \times 0.15) = 3.21$ kJ/kg/°C (0.43 kcal/kg/°F). Using this value, you can calculate that at a rate of body heat production of 1,000 W, in 1 minute 1,000 J/s × 60 s = 60,000 J or 60 kJ (14.3 kcal) of heat energy is produced, which raises the body temperature of this 70 kg man by 60 kJ ÷ (70 kg × 3.21 kJ/kg/°C) = 0.27° C (0.49° F). Thus, within 12 to 15 minutes, core body temperature could approach dangerous levels or exercise is terminated because of the symptoms of fatigue that occur from this degree of hyperthermia.

Problems of hyperthermia and heat injury are not restricted to prolonged exercise in a hot environment. Heat production is directly proportional to exercise intensity, so very strenuous exercise, even in a cool environment, can cause a substantial rise in body temperature.

The absolute body temperature at the end of exercise depends on the starting body temperature. A vigorous warm up causes a rise in body temperature and results in a higher final body temperature. When body temperature rises to about 39.5° C (103° F), central fatigue (i.e., in the brain rather than in the working muscles) ensues, and so a high starting temperature is undesirable for athletes exercising in a hot environment. Such large increases in body temperature during exercise tend not to occur in unfit individuals (e.g., the types who jog through a marathon in 4 hours to 6 hours) but are common in highly motivated athletes.

A body temperature of 36° to 38°C (96.8° to 100.4° F) is the normal range at rest and may rise to 38° to 40° C (100.4° to 104° F) during exercise. Further increases are commonly associated with heat exhaustion and occasionally with heatstroke, a life-threatening disorder characterized by a lack of consciousness after exertion and by clinical symptoms of damage to the brain, liver, and kidneys (Gleeson 1998; Sutton and Bar-Or 1980). The elevated core temperature associated with exercise is not regulated at its elevated level (i.e., it is not caused by a resetting of the hypothalamic thermostat). Rather, the elevated temperature is caused by the temporary imbalance between the rates of heat production and dissipation during the early stages of exercise and the rapidity with which the heat-dissipating mechanisms respond to an increase in core temperature.

Environmental Heat Stress and Heat Loss by Evaporation of Sweat

Environmental heat stress is determined by the ambient temperature, relative humidity, wind velocity, and solar radiation (both directly from the sun and reflected from the ground) (see figure 8.1). During exercise, the working muscles produce heat at a high rate and the body temperature rises. If the skin is hotter than the surroundings, heat is lost from the skin by physical transfer (evaporation of sweat, convection, and conduction) to the environment. If the environment is hotter than the skin, heat is gained by convection and conduction. If the environment is saturated with water vapor (i.e., relative humidity = 100%), evaporation of sweat does not occur and heat is not lost from the body. The relative humidity is very important because a high humidity severely compromises the evaporative loss of sweat, and sweat must evaporate from the body surface to exert a cooling effect.

Evaporation of 1 L of water from the skin will remove 2.4 MJ (573 kcal) of heat from the body. The sweat rate during exercise has to be at least 1.6 L/hour if all the heat produced is to be dissipated by evaporative loss alone. In fact, the sweat rate probably has to be nearer 2 L/hour, because at such high sweat rates, some of the sweat rolls off the skin, which has virtually no cooling effect. A reduction in skin blood flow and sweat rate as the body becomes progressively dehydrated or a high humidity limiting evaporative loss of sweat leads to further rises in core temperature, resulting in fatigue and possible heat injury to body tissues. The latter is potentially fatal.

A useful index of environmental heat stress is the wet bulb globe temperature (WBGT), which is calculated as follows:

$$WBGT = 0.7\ T_{wb} + 0.2\ T_{bg} + 0.1\ T_{db}$$

where T_{wb} is the temperature (in °C) of a wet-bulb thermometer, T_{db} is the temperature of a dry-bulb thermometer, and T_{bg} is the temperature of a black-globe thermometer. Note the 70% bias toward the T_{wb}, which recognizes the greater relative importance of the environmental humidity. Some typical environmental scenarios and physiological responses to exercise in different environmental conditions are illustrated in table 8.3.

Heat loss via the evaporation of sweat is largely determined by the water vapor pressure (humidity) of the air close to the body surface. The local humidity may be high if inappropriate, poorly ventilated clothing is worn, reducing the convective flow of air over the skin surface. Sweat drips off the skin, rather than evaporates, and heat loss via this route is severely restricted. If exercise continues at the same intensity, body core temperature rises further, a higher sweat rate is induced, and the athlete dehydrates more rapidly. This dehydration poses further problems for the athlete because progressive dehydration impairs the ability to sweat and, consequently, to thermoregulate. At any given exercise intensity, body temperature rises faster in the dehydrated state, and this condition is commonly accompanied by a higher heart rate

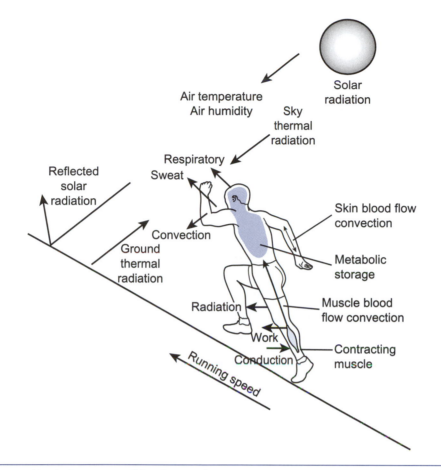

Figure 8.1 Sources of body heat-gain and heat-loss mechanisms.

Table 8.3 Sweat Loss and Heart Rates After 60 Minutes of Exercise

Ambient temperature (°C/°F)	Humidity (%)	Sweat loss (L)	Core temperature (°C/°F)	Heart rate (beats/min)
13 (55)	7	0.8	38.0 (100.4)	140
18 (64)	50	1.2	38.3 (100.9)	143
25 (77)	50	1.4	38.7 (101.6)	145
30 (86)	30	2.1	39.3 (102.7)	148
30 (86)	90	2.8	39.5 (103.1)	150
35 (95)	30	3.0	39.9 (103.8)	153

Exercise performed at about 60% to 70% V̇O$_2$max under different environmental conditions.

during exercise, as shown in figure 8.2. Dehydration equivalent to the loss of only 2% body mass (i.e., the loss of about 1.5 L of water for a typical 70 kg [154 lb] male athlete) is sufficient to significantly impair exercise performance (Armstrong et al. 1985; Craig and Cummings 1966; Maughan 1991; Sawka and Pandolf 1990).

Heat Loss by Radiation and Convection

The other crucial effector mechanism in thermoregulation during exercise in the heat is the increased blood flow through the skin capillaries. This mechanism allows increased heat loss from the body core to the

Figure 8.2 Effect of dehydration on heart rate and rectal temperature during 2 hours of cycling.

environment by radiation and convection. Radiation is the transfer of energy waves by emission from one object and absorption by another. Convection is the exchange of heat between a solid medium (e.g., the human body) and one that moves (e.g., air or water). The rate of heat transfer away from the body core is the product of the skin blood flow and the temperature difference between the core and the skin.

A high skin blood flow alone may not be sufficient to remove heat from the body core during exercise in hot, humid conditions when the skin temperature rises because of the inability to evaporate sweat. The effectiveness of this route of heat loss also largely dependent on the amount of body surface available for heat exchange and the temperature gradient between the body surface and the surrounding atmosphere. When ambient temperature is close to body temperature, heat loss via the skin blood flow is minimal. The body is then almost entirely dependent on evaporative cooling. Inappropriate clothing impairs convection and radiation of heat from the body surface, so total heat dissipation will be reduced to a critically low level.

Regulation of Body Temperature

Sensory information about body temperature is input to the central controller via nerves emanating from both deep-body and peripheral thermoreceptors. The latter, located in the skin, provide advance warning of environmental heat input. Central thermoreceptors, located in the hypothalamus, are sensitive to changes in internal core temperature and effectively monitor the temperature of blood flowing to the brain. Input from these receptors is more important than input from the peripheral receptors in eliciting appropriate effector responses designed to limit increases in body temperature. The central thermal controller, or "thermostat," located in the preoptic anterior hypothalamus also receives nonthermal sensory inputs that are capable of modulating the homeostatic regulation of body temperature.

These other inputs include nervous signals from osmoreceptors and pressure receptors, so changes in plasma osmolarity and blood volume are capable of affecting sweating and cutaneous vasodilation responses to rises in core temperature. These effects are summarized in figure 8.3. Some hormones (e.g., estrogen) and cytokines (e.g., interleukin-1 and interleukin-6) are also capable of influencing thermoregulatory responses. Interleukin-6, also known as endogenous pyrogen, is secreted from macrophages and is responsible for raising the set-point temperature of the hypothalamic "thermostat," causing the rise in core temperature during fever. The influence of other sensory inputs also appears to take place at the level of the hypothalamic neurons and is mediated by neurotransmitters, including dopamine, 5-hydroxytryptamine (5-HT or serotonin), norepinephrine (noradrenaline), and acetylcholine.

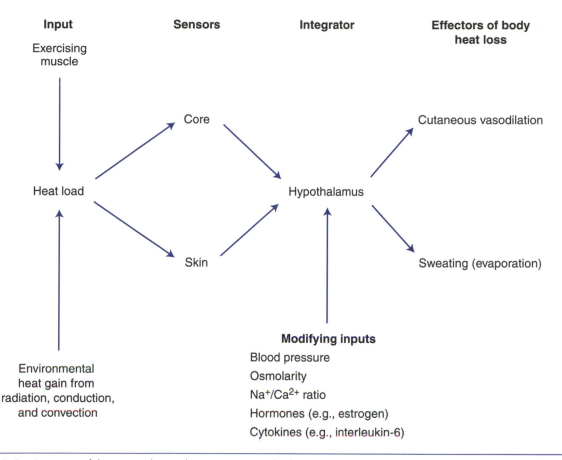

Figure 8.3 Summary of thermoregulation during exercise in the heat.

Exercise Training, Acclimitization, and Temperature Regulation

Exercise training improves temperature regulation during exercise at the same absolute work rate. To obtain thermoregulatory benefits from training, individuals must adequately stimulate thermoregulatory effector responses (viz. sweating and increased skin blood flow). In other words, they must exercise at a sufficiently high intensity. Improvements in thermoregulatory responses to exercise have consistently been seen in studies in which subjects exercised at 70% to 100% $\dot{V}O_2$max and increased their body temperature above 39° C (102.2° F). Studies in which subjects exercised at lower intensities (typically 35% to 60% $\dot{V}O_2$max) have commonly shown little or no thermoregulatory benefit in response to training.

Most serious athletes regularly exercise at intensities above 70% $\dot{V}O_2$max; such training allows individuals to achieve thermal equilibrium during exercise at 25% to 35% $\dot{V}O_2$max in desert heat conditions, but of course this exercise intensity is not race pace. However, appropriate training increases tolerance of exercise in hot conditions, and acclimation to warm environments (achieved by exercising in a hot environment, not just resting exposure to that environment) confers further benefits in terms of the ability to regulate body temperature during exercise in the heat at higher exercise intensities (Greenleaf 1979).

Marathon runners exhibit a lower resting body temperature and have a lower sweating (and shivering) threshold. Thus, set-point temperature seems to decrease as a result of training in endurance athletes. These individuals have also been reported to have a lower resting metabolic rate in thermoneutral conditions and a lower skin temperature. This effect appears to mimic the "insulative hypothermia" reported in Australian aborigines who sleep in the cold desert night: both skin and core temperature drop, reducing the temperature gradient between the body surface and the environment, which reduces heat loss and conserves energy. Heat and cold **acclimatization** are not mutually exclusive and can occur simultaneously in the same individual.

Exercise training improves thermoregulation in the heat by an earlier onset of sweat secretion and by increasing the total amount of sweat that can be produced. Thus, training increases the sensitivity of the sweat rate/core temperature relationship, as well as decreases the internal temperature threshold for sweating. Sweat rates can vary markedly between individuals (up to a maximum of about 3 L/h), even at the same relative exercise intensity, (Maughan 1991), but evidence suggests that individuals characterized as heavy sweaters have larger sweat glands than light sweaters. Training appears to induce a hypertrophy (enlarging) of existing sweat glands, without increasing the total number.

Other adaptations to training include an increase in total blood volume and maximal cardiac output. As a result, blood flow in muscle and skin, with its heat flux, is better preserved during strenuous exercise in the heat. The body does not adapt to dehydration, so exercising in the heat without fluid intake does not confer an additional adaptation in thermoregulation. In fact, progressive dehydration during exercise in the heat reduces the sensitivity of the sweat rate/ core temperature relationship as shown in figure 8.4 and, thus, results in a relative hyperthermia and an earlier onset of fatigue (Nadel et al. 1980; Sawka, Young, Francescone, et al. 1985). In practical terms, the athlete is less able to maintain training loads, so the physiological adaptation to training is not as great. Exercising for prolonged periods in the heat without fluid intake also increases the risk of cramps and heat illness.

Effects of Dehydration on Exercise Performance

Fatigue toward the end of a prolonged sporting event may result as much from dehydration as from fuel substrate depletion. Exercise performance is impaired when an individual is dehydrated by as little as 2% of body weight. Losses in excess of 5% of body weight can decrease the capacity for work by about 30% (see figure 8.5) (Armstrong et al. 1985; Craig and Cummings 1966; Maughan 1991; Sawka and Pandolf 1990).

Sprint athletes are generally less concerned about the effects of dehydration than are endurance athletes. However, the capacity to perform high-intensity exercise, which results in exhaustion within a few minutes, is reduced by as much as 45% by prior dehydration corresponding to a loss of only 2.5% of body weight (Sawka, Young, Cadarette, et al. 1985). Although sprint events offer little opportunity for sweat loss, athletes who travel to compete in hot climates are likely to experience acute dehydration, which persists for several days and may be serious enough to have a detrimental effect on performance in competition.

Even in cool laboratory conditions, maximal aerobic power ($\dot{V}O_2$max) decreases by about 5% when persons experience fluid losses equivalent to 3% of body mass or more, as is shown in figure 8.6 (Pinchan et al. 1988). In hot conditions, similar water deficits can cause a larger decrease in $\dot{V}O_2$max. The endurance capacity during incremental exercise is decreased by marginal dehydration (fluid loss of 1% to 2% of body weight), even if water deficits do not actually result in a decrease in $\dot{V}O_2$max. Endurance capacity is impaired much more in hot environments than in cool conditions, which implies that impaired thermoregulation is an important causal factor in the reduced exercise performance associated with a body-water deficit. Dehydration also impairs endur-

Figure 8.4 Relationship between body core temperature and (a) local sweating rate and (b) forearm skin blood flow (FBF) for euhydrated men (circles) and men dehydrated by 5% of body weight loss (BWL, squares) during exercise in the heat.

Adapted with permissions by the *American Journal of Clinical Nutrition* © Am J Clin Nutr. American Society for Clinical Nutrition.

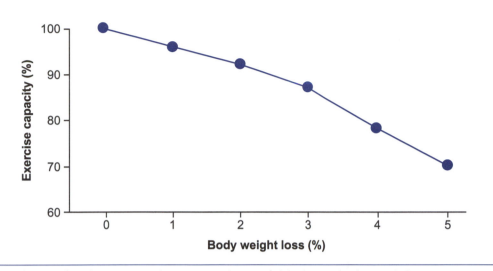

Figure 8.5 Reduction of work capacity with increasing degree of dehydration (body weight loss).

ance exercise performance. Fluid loss equivalent to 2% of body mass induced by a diuretic drug (furosemide) caused running performance at 1,500, 5,000, and 10,000 m distances to be impaired (Armstrong et al. 1985). Running performance was impaired more at the longer distances (by approximately 5% at 5,000 and 10,000 m) compared with the shortest distance (approximately 3% at 1,500 m).

A study investigated the capacity of eight subjects to perform treadmill walking (at 25% $\dot{V}O_2$max with a target time of 140 minutes) in very hot, dry conditions (49° C [120° F], 20% relative humidity) when they were euhydrated and when they were dehydrated by a 3%, 5%, or 7% loss of body mass (Sawka, Young, Francescone, et al. 1985). All eight subjects were able to

complete 140 minutes walking when euhydrated and 3% dehydrated. Seven subjects completed the walk when 5% dehydrated, but when dehydrated by 7%, six subjects stopped walking after an average of only 64 minutes. Thus, even for relatively low-intensity exercise, dehydration clearly increases the incidence of exhaustion from heat strain. Sawka et al. (1992) had subjects walk to exhaustion at 47% $\dot{V}O_2$max in the same environmental conditions as their previous study. Subjects were euhydrated and dehydrated to a loss of 8% of each individual's total-body water. Dehydration reduced exercise endurance time from 121 minutes to 55 minutes. Dehydration also appeared to reduce the core temperature a person could tolerate, as core temperature at exhaustion was about 0.4° C

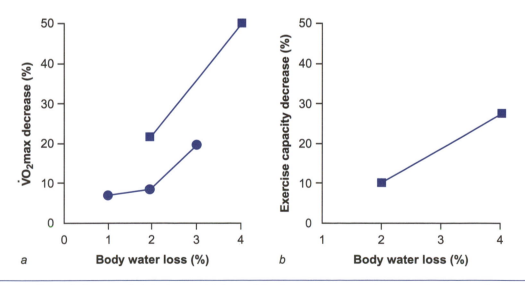

Figure 8.6 Effect of degree of dehydration (% loss of body water) on (a) decrement in maximal oxygen uptake ($\dot{V}O_2$max) and (b) reduction in physical work capacity during heat exposure.

Data from E.N. Craig and E.G. Cummings, 1966 and G. Pinchan et al., 1988.

(0.7° F) lower in the dehydrated state. The main reasons dehydration has an adverse effect on exercise performance can be summarized as follows:

- Reduction in blood volume
- Decreased skin blood flow
- Decreased sweat rate
- Decreased heat dissipation
- Increased core temperature
- Increased rate of muscle glycogen use

A reduced maximal cardiac output (i.e., the highest pumping capacity of the heart that can be achieved during exercise) is the most likely physiologic mechanism whereby dehydration decreases a person's $\dot{V}O_2$max and impairs work capacity in fatiguing exercise of an incremental nature. Dehydration causes a fall in plasma volume both at rest and during exercise, and a decreased blood volume increases blood thickness (viscosity), lowers central venous pressure, and reduces venous return of blood to the heart. During maximal exercise, these changes can decrease the filling of the heart during diastole (the phase of the cardiac cycle when the heart is relaxed and is filling with blood before the next contraction), hence, reducing stroke volume and cardiac output. Also, during exercise in the heat, the opening up of the skin blood vessels reduces the proportion of the cardiac output available to the working muscles.

Even for normally hydrated (euhydrated) individuals, climatic heat stress alone decreases $\dot{V}O_2$max by about 7%. Thus, both environmental heat stress and dehydration can act independently to limit cardiac output and blood delivery to the active muscles during high-intensity exercise. Dehydration also impairs the body's ability to lose heat. Both sweat rate and skin blood flow are lower at the same core temperature for the dehydrated compared with the euhydrated state (see figure 8.4) (Nadel et al. 1979 1980; Sawka and Wenger 1988). Body temperature rises faster during exercise when the body is dehydrated. The reduced sweating response in the dehydrated state is probably mediated through the effects of both a fall in blood volume (hypovolemia) and elevated plasma osmolarity (i.e., dissolved salt concentration) (see figure 8.7) on hypothalamic neurons. As explained previously, as core temperature rises towards about 39.5° C (103° F), sensations of fatigue ensue. This critical temperature is reached more quickly in the dehydrated state.

Dehydration not only elevates core temperature responses but also negates the thermoregulatory advantages conferred by high aerobic fitness and heat acclimatization. The effects of dehydration (5%

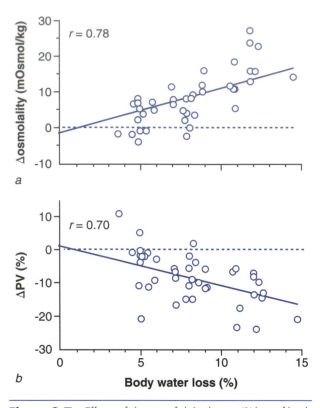

a

b

Figure 8.7 Effects of degree of dehydration (% loss of body water) on *(a)* plasma osmolality and *(b)* plasma volume in heat-acclimated persons.

Adapted with permissions by the *American Journal of Clinical Nutrition*. © Am J Clin Nutr. American Society for Clinical Nutrition.

loss of body weight) on core temperature responses in the same persons when unacclimated and when acclimated to heat are shown in figure 8.8. Heat acclimation lowered core temperature responses when subjects were euhydrated. However, when they were dehydrated, similar core temperature responses were observed for both unacclimated and acclimated states (Pinchan et al. 1988).

A person's ability to tolerate heat strain appears to be impaired when dehydrated, so the critical temperature for experiencing central fatigue is likely to be nearer 39.0° C (102.2° F) when dehydrated by more than about 5% of body mass (Sawka et al. 1992). The larger rise in core temperature during exercise in the dehydrated state is associated with a bigger catecholamine response, and these effects may lead to increased rates of glycogen breakdown in the exercising muscle, which, in turn, may contribute to earlier onset of fatigue in prolonged exercise.

Dehydration is associated with a reduced gastric emptying rate of ingested fluids during exercise in the heat. For example, one study reported a 20% to 25% reduction in gastric emptying when subjects were dehydrated by 5% of body mass (Neufer et al. 1989).

Figure 8.8 Core temperature responses during exercise in the heat in euhydrated or dehydrated (5% loss of body weight) persons both before (unacclimated, UA) and after becoming heat acclimated (HA).

Adapted with permissions by the American Journal of Clinical Nutrition. © Am J Clin Nutr. American Society for Clinical Nutrition.

Fluid consumption should begin during the early stages of exercise in the heat, not only to minimize the degree of dehydration but also to maximize the bioavailability of ingested fluids. Dehydration poses a serious health risk in that it increases the risk of cramps, heat exhaustion, and life-threatening heat stroke (Sutton and Bar-Or 1980).

Mechanisms of Heat Illness

Heat injury is most common during exhaustive exercise in a hot, humid environment, particularly if the athlete is dehydrated. These problems affect not only highly trained athletes but also less well-trained sport participants. In fact, less well-trained individuals have less-effective thermoregulation during exercise, work less economically, use more carbohydrate for muscular work, and take longer to recover from exhausting exercise than do highly trained individuals.

During the initial stages of exercise in a hot environment, sweating begins and the skin blood vessels dilate, effecting increased heat loss from the body. However, as central blood volume and pressure fall, sympathetic nervous activity increases and the skin blood vessels constrict. A more powerful constriction of the blood vessels supplying the abdominal organs leads to cellular hypoxia in the region of the gastrointestinal tract, liver, and kidneys. Cellular hypoxia leads to the production of reactive oxygen species (ROS), including superoxide anion, hydrogen peroxide, hydroxyl radical, peroxynitrite, and nitric oxide (NO). The latter is a potent blood vessel dila-

tor, and although its production can be viewed as protective (i.e., helping to conserve some blood flow through the capillary beds of the abdominal organs), ultimately the ROS may cause damage through their actions on membranes. The ROS cause peroxidation of lipids in cellular membranes, making them leaky. In the gastrointestinal tract, this action allows the passage of bacterial toxins (endotoxins) from the gut into the systemic circulation, leading to endotoxemia (blood poisoning) and a drastic fall in blood pressure (hypotension). Increased levels of NO probably contribute to the development of hypotension. The consequences for the athlete can be heat syncope (fainting) and organ injury (see figure 8.9).

Animal studies have shown a disappearance of manganese-superoxide dismutase (Mn-SOD), an important antioxidant enzyme that deactivates ROS, after 2 hours of heat exposure and a later induction of Mn-SOD in the liver cells of animals exposed to elevated core temperatures (41° C [106° F]) over a 24-hour period. Increased levels of hemoglobin-NO, semiquinone radical (a marker of mitochondrial oxidative stress), and ceruloplasmin (a copper-binding protein with antioxidant properties) have also been found in the hepatic portal vein after exposure to heat stress.

A doubling of hepatic portal blood endotoxin levels has also been reported within 24 hours of the onset of heat exposure. Thus, ROS generation appears to increase within abdominal tissues during heat exposure. Antioxidant status is compromised within the first few hours but gradually recovers and is enhanced after 24 hours of heat exposure.

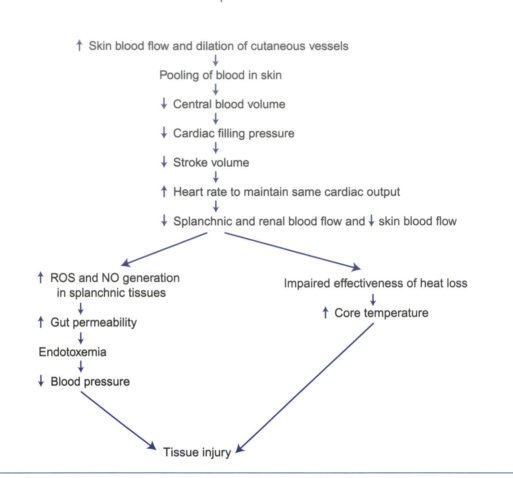

Figure 8.9 Potential mechanisms of heat-stress injury.

ROS generation probably increases most in areas of high metabolic activity and greatest potential for a reduction in blood flow.

This ischemia/reperfusion mechanism involving the gastrointestinal tract may play a role in the vascular dysfunction and tissue injury associated with heat stress. Further studies are warranted on the possible benefits of antioxidant supplementation in people who regularly experience very high body temperatures such as athletes who train and compete in hot, humid climates.

Effects of Fluid Intake on Exercise Performance

Oral fluid ingestion during exercise helps restore plasma volume to near pre-exercise levels and prevents the adverse effects of dehydration on muscle strength, endurance, and coordination. Elevating blood volume just before exercise by various **hyperhydration** strategies has been suggested to be effective in enhancing exercise performance, but only a few studies have directly investigated this possibility.

Pre-Exercise Hyperhydration

Because even mild dehydration has debilitating effects on exercise performance, hyperhydration (greater than normal body water content) has been hypothesized to improve thermoregulation by expanding blood volume and reducing plasma osmolarity, thereby improving heat dissipation and exercise performance. Although some studies report higher sweating rates, lower core temperatures, and lower heart rates during exercise after hyperhydration, several of these studies used control conditions that represented dehydration rather than euhydration, making results questionable. However, the findings generally support the notion that hyperhydration reduces the thermal and cardiovascular strain of exercise. Relatively few studies have directly investigated the effects of hyperhydration on exercise performance, but one well-controlled study reported that expansion of blood volume by 450 to 500 ml improved cycling time trial performance by 10% (81 minutes compared with 90 minutes).

Temporary hyperhydration is induced in test subjects by having them drink large volumes of water or water-electrolyte solutions for 1 hour to 3 hours before exercise. However, much of the fluid overload is rapidly excreted, and so expansion of the body water and blood volume is only transient. Studies in which the blood volume was directly expanded by infusion reported decreased cardiovascular strain during exercise but yielded conflicting results on sweat loss, heat dissipation, and exercise performance. Some studies that limited the rise in plasma osmolarity during exercise reported improved heat dissipation but did not address the question of whether it actually affects exercise performance.

Greater fluid retention is achieved if glycerol is added to fluids consumed before exercise. One study has reported a higher sweating rate and lower core temperature when subjects exercised in the heat after hyperhydrating with glycerol (1 g/kg b.w.) and water (21.4 ml/kg b.w.) compared with an equal volume of water alone (Lyons et al 1990). However, other studies report no thermoregulatory advantage during exercise after glycerol solution–induced hyperhydration (Inder et al. 1998; Latzka et al. 1997, 1998). In these studies, the volume of water consumed (500 ml) may have been too small. In a study by Murray et al. (1991), no indications of hyperhydration were found. Generally, however, the ingestion of 1 g/kg b.w. of glycerol with 1 to 2 liters of water seems to protect against heat stress and thus may have some health benefits when exercising in hot conditions. A recent study examined the effect of ingestion of a large bolus of water (20 ml/kg b.w.) with or without added glycerol (1 g/kg b.w.) 2 hours before 90 minutes of submaximal cycling (98% of lactate threshold) in dry, hot conditions (35° C [95° F], relative humidity = 30%) followed by a 15-minute time trial (Anderson et al. 2001). Although pre-exercise glycerol ingestion did not affect skin temperature, muscle temperature, circulating catecholamine, or muscle metabolic responses to the steady state exercise, heart and core temperature were lower than with the ingestion of water alone. Furthermore, time-trial performance (total work performed) was improved significantly by 5%. In subsequent studies, this finding could not be confirmed, even though those studies reported indications of improved thermoregulation. Thus, whether glycerol improves endurance performance in the heat remains unclear. (For more information on glycerol, see chapter 10.)

Fluid Intake During Exercise

During exercise, especially in a hot environment, dehydration can only be avoided by matching fluid consumption with sweat loss. However, this effort is difficult for a number of reasons:

- Sweat rates during strenuous exercise in the heat can be around 2 to 3 L/h. A volume of ingested fluid in the stomach of more than about 1 L feels uncomfortable for most people when exercising, so achieving fluid intakes that match sweat losses during exercise is often not practical.

- Sweat rates vary widely among different individuals under the same ambient conditions. (Figure 8.10 shows the sweat rates of individuals competing in marathon race in Scotland [Maughan 1985].) Hence, to accurately prescribe the amounts that should be drunk is difficult without knowing the athlete's sweat rate under the prevailing climatic conditions.

- Thirst is not a good indicator of body-water requirements or the degree of dehydration. In general, the sensation of thirst is not perceived until a person has lost at least 2% of body weight through sweating. As already mentioned, even this mild degree of dehydration is sufficient to impair exercise performance. Numerous studies show that ad libitum intake of water during exercise in the heat results in incomplete replacement of body-water losses (observed values of fluid intakes and losses are shown in table 8.4).

- The rules or practicalities of specific sports may limit the opportunities for drinking during competition.

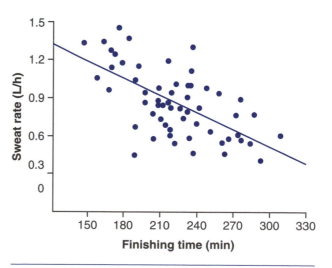

Figure 8.10 *Sweat rates for subjects who competed in a marathon race held in cool (about 12° C [54° F]) conditions. The sweat rate was related to the running speed, but a large variation existed between individuals, even those running at the same speed.*

Data from R.J. Maughan, 1985.

Table 8.4 Fluid Losses and Intakes of Athletes

Sport	Ambient temperature (°C/°F)	Sweat loss (mL/h)	Fluid intake (mL/h)
Marathon running	15–20 (59–68)	800–1,200	500
Soccer	10 (50) 25 (77)	1,000 1,200	350 500
Basketball	20–25 (68–77)	1,600	1,080
Rowing	10 (50) 30 (86)	1,165 1,980	580 960
Cycling	30 (86)	2,000	800

Because endurance exercise capacity is impaired even by mild dehydration and small decreases in plasma volume, athletes should try to minimize the extent of dehydration by ingesting fluids during exercise. Regular water intake during prolonged exercise is effective in improving both exercise capacity (time to exhaustion [see figures 8.11 and 8.12]) and exercise performance (time to complete a given amount of work [see figure 8.13]) (Fallowfield et al. 1996; Maughan et al. 1987).

Fluid intake during prolonged exercise offers the opportunity to ingest some fuel as well. The addition of carbohydrate to some drinks consumed during exercise has an additional independent effect in improving exercise performance (see figures 8.12 and 8.13) (Below et al. 1995). Further details can found in chapter 5. Too much added carbohydrate in a sports drink, although providing more fuel for the working muscles, however, decreases the amount of water that can be absorbed. In this situation, water is actually drawn out of the interstitial fluid and plasma into the lumen of the small intestine by osmosis. This effect is demonstrated in figure 8.14, which shows that the ingestion of a concentrated glucose solution, hypertonic with respect to plasma, delays the restoration of plasma volume during exercise compared with the ingestion of a hypotonic glucose-electrolyte drink (Maughan et al. 1987).

As long as the fluid remains hypotonic with respect to plasma, the uptake of water from the small intestine is not adversely affected. In fact, the presence of small amounts of glucose and sodium tend to slightly increase the rate of water absorption compared with pure water (Maughan and Murray 2000). Rather than to replace electrolytes lost through sweating, sodium and other electrolytes are added to sports drinks to

- increase palatability,
- maintain thirst (and therefore promote drinking),
- prevent hyponatremia (low serum sodium concentration, which can occur when individuals ingest far more water than their requirements),

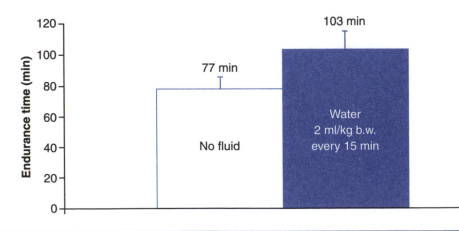

Figure 8.11 Effect of water intake on endurance capacity.

From J.L. Fallowfield, C. Williams et al., 1996, "Effect of water ingestion on endurance capacity during prolonged running," *Journal of Sports Sciences* 14: 497-502. Reprinted, with permission, from Taylor and Francis Ltd., http://www.tandf.co.uk/journals/titles/02640414.html.

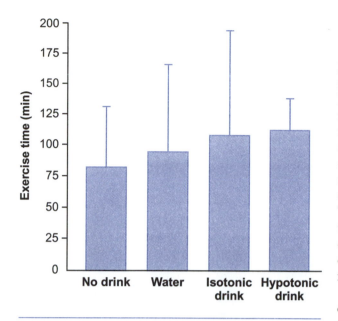

Figure 8.12 Effects of ingestion of different drinks on exercise capacity during a cycle ergometer test to exhaustion at 70% V̇O₂max. Ingestion of water resulted in a longer time to exhaustion than in the no-drink trial, but ingestion of the two dilute carbohydrate-electrolyte drinks resulted in the longest endurance times.

From Galloway and Maughan, 2000, "The effects of substrate and fluid provision on thermoregulatory and metabolic responses to prolonged exercise in a hot environment," *Journal of Sports Sciences* 18(5): 339-351. Reprinted, with permission, from Taylor and Francis Ltd., http://www.tandf.co.uk/journals/titles/02640414.html.

- increase the rate of water uptake, and
- increase the retention of fluid.

Replacement of the electrolytes lost in sweat can normally wait until the postexercise recovery period. Fluid intake during strenuous exercise of less than 30 minutes duration offers no advantage. Gastric emptying is inhibited at high work rates, and insignificant amounts of fluid are absorbed during exercise of such short duration. For exercise lasting more than 1 hour or exercise in hot or humid conditions, consumption of carbohydrate-electrolyte sports drink is warranted. These drinks supply fluid together with carbohydrate that helps maintain blood glucose and high levels of carbohydrate oxidation. The electrolyte (sodium) content partly offsets salt losses in sweat but, perhaps more importantly, maintains the desire to drink.

Sweat-loss rates during exercise depend on exercise intensity, duration, and environmental conditions but also vary considerably among different individuals. Some people may lose up to 3 L/h of sweat during strenuous activity in a warm environment (see figure 8.15) (Sawka and Pandolf 1990), and even at low ambient temperatures of about 12° C (54° F), sweat loss can exceed 1 L/h (see figure 8.10) (Maughan 1985). Because the electrolyte composition of sweat is hypotonic to plasma (in other words, the total concentration of dissolved anions and cations is considerably lower in sweat than in plasma; see table

Figure 8.13 Effect of carbohydrate and fluid ingestion on a cycling time trial performed at the end of a prolonged exercise test at 31° C (88° F) in which either a small (200 ml) or large (1,330 ml) fluid volume with either zero carbohydrate or a large amount (79 g) of carbohydrate was given. Ingestion of water and carbohydrate has independent and additive effects in improving exercise performance.

Data from P. Below et al., 1995.

Figure 8.14 Plasma volume changes during exercise with consumption of a hypertonic or hypotonic glucose–containing beverage. Because of the faster gastric emptying and faster intestinal absorption of water, ingestion of dilute carbohydrate-electrolyte solutions (open squares) is more effective in restoring plasma volume during exercise compared with the ingestion of an equal volume of a concentrated glucose solution (closed squares).

European Journal of Applied Physiology, Metabolic and circulatory responses to the ingestion of glucose polymer and gluclose/electrolyte solutions during exercise in man, R.J. Maughan et al., 45: 356-362, 1987, © Springer-Verlag.

Figure 8.15 Approximate hourly sweating rates as a function of environmental conditions and running speed.

Adapted from M.N. Sawka and S.J. Mountain, 2000.

8.5), the replacement of water rather than electrolytes is the priority during exercise. Plasma volume falls by up to 20% during exercise, the magnitude of the fall being related to the relative exercise intensity. Typically, at work rates equivalent to 60% to 80% of the maximal oxygen uptake, plasma volume falls acutely by about 10% to 15% because of the increased capillary hydrostatic pressure and osmotic uptake of water into active skeletal muscle tissue. Without fluid intake, particularly in a warm, humid environment, further falls in plasma volume and increases in plasma osmolarity occur because of the loss of hypotonic sweat, as exercise proceeds.

As mentioned previously, the decrease in plasma volume that accompanies dehydration may be of particular importance in influencing work capacity. Blood flow to the muscles must be maintained at a high level to supply oxygen and fuel substrates (glucose and fatty acids), but a high blood flow to the skin is also necessary to convect heat to the body surface, where it can be dissipated. When the ambient temperature is high and plasma volume is decreased by sweat loss during prolonged exercise (as shown in figure 8.16), skin blood flow is likely to be compromised (Costill and Fink 1974), allowing central venous pressure and blood flow to the working muscle to be maintained but reducing heat loss and causing body temperature to rise to dangerous levels. To prevent dehydration, water must be replaced at a faster rate. Metabolic water production increases during exercise but not enough to compensate for water loss through sweating. Oral fluid ingestion during exercise helps restore plasma volume to near pre-exercise levels (see figure 8.16) and prevents the adverse effects of dehydration

on thermal and cardiovascular strain, muscle strength, endurance, and coordination.

A study compared time to exhaustion during cycling at 60% $\dot{V}O_2$max in warm ambient conditions (30° C [86° F]) when six subjects were given either (a) no drink, (b) 500 ml of a 15% carbohydrate-electrolyte drink immediately before exercise and 125 ml of the same drink every 10 minutes throughout exercise, or (c) 500 ml of a 2% carbohydrate-electrolyte drink immediately before exercise and 250 ml of the same drink every 10 minutes throughout exercise (Galloway and Maughan 2000). As shown in figure 8.17, with no drink, subjects fatigued after 71 minutes (median range 39 minutes to 97 minutes). With the 15% carbohydrate-electrolyte drink, they could continue for longer times (median 84 minutes, range 63 minutes to 145 minutes). However, the best performance was achieved with the 2% carbohydrate-electrolyte drink (median 118 minutes, range 83 minutes to 168 minutes). Interestingly, the median core temperature at exhaustion was the same in all 3 trials (39.5° C [103° F]). A significant fall in plasma volume occurred within the first 15 minutes of exercise on all trials. Subsequently, plasma volume remained below resting values on the no-drink and the 15% carbohydrate-electrolyte trials, but on the 2% carbohydrate-electrolyte trial, plasma volume was gradually restored during exercise.

Gonzalez-Alonso et al. (1998) showed that exercising-limb perfusion may be reduced during prolonged exercise combined with heat stress and dehydration. The maintenance of plasma volume on the 2% carbohydrate-electrolyte trial may have resulted in better perfusion of active muscles during exercise and

Table 8.5 Concentrations of Electrolytes in Sweat, Plasma, and Intracellular Water

Electrolyte	Sweat (mmol/L)	Plasma (mmol/L)	Intracellular water (mmol/L)
Cations			
Sodium	20–80	130–155	10
Potassium	4–8	3.2–5.5	150
Calcium	0.1–1.0	2.1–2.9	0.01
Magnesium	0.1–0.2	0.7–1.5	15
Anions			
Chloride	20–60	96–110	8
Bicarbonate	1–35	23–28	10
Phosphate	0.1–0.2	0.7–1.6	65
Sulphate	0.1–2.0	0.3–0.9	10

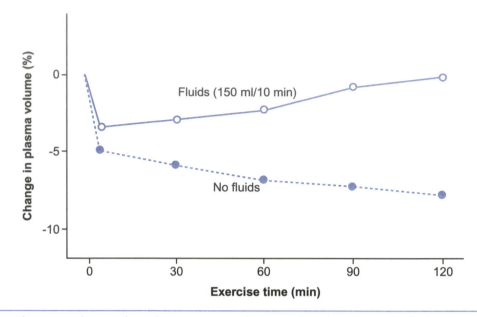

Figure 8.16 Changes in plasma volume during exercise in the heat with and without regular fluid ingestion.

Reprinted, by permission, from D.L. Costill, and W.J. Fink, 1974, "Plasma volume changes following exercise and thermal dehydration," *Journal of Applied Physiology* 37: 521-525.

Figure 8.17 Time to exhaustion (median and range) during cycling at 60% $\dot{V}O_2$max at an ambient temperature of 31° C (88° F). Six subjects received *(a)* no drink, *(b)* 500 ml of a 15% carbohydrate-electrolyte drink (CHO-E) immediately pre-exercise and 125 ml of the same drink every 10 minutes throughout exercise, or *(c)* 500 ml of a 2% CHO-E drink immediately before exercise and 250 ml of the same drink every 10 minutes throughout exercise. The three treatments were significantly different from each other in terms of endurance performance.

From Galloway and Maughan, 2000, "The effects of substrate and fluid provision on thermoregulatory and metabolic responses to proloned exercise in a hot environment," *Journal of Sports Sciences* 18: 339-351. Reprinted by permission from Taylor and Francis Ltd. http://www.tandf.co.uk/journals/titles/02640414.html.

may have resulted in better maintenance of cellular hydration.

Ingestion of relatively cool fluid may have an additional small benefit during exercise in the heat because the additional volume of fluid in the body after drinking adds to the body's heat-storage capacity. The improvement in heat-storage capacity can be calculated based on the specific heat capacity of water, which is 4.184 kJ/kg/°C (0.555 kcal/kg/°F). For example, the ingestion of 2 L of fluid at 10° C

(50° F) increases heat-storage capacity by $4.184 \times 2 \times (37 - 10)$ kJ = 225 kJ (54 kcal).

In the study by Galloway and Maughan (2000), subjects ingested fluids cooled to 14° C (57° F), and these investigators calculated that the extra fluid consumed on the 2% carbohydrate-electrolyte treatment (2.3 L) could have produced an 8-minute improvement in performance because of its effect in increasing body heat-storage capacity compared with the no-drink treatment.

Daily Water Balance

The typical daily water balance for a sedentary individual living in a cool or temperate climate (ambient temperature 10° to 20° C [50° to 68° F]) is shown in figure 8.18. Variable amounts of water are lost from the body through sweating in response to the requirement for thermoregulation, but for a sedentary individual in cool conditions, evaporative loss of water through the skin only amounts to about 600 ml/day. Additional water is lost in the feces (about 100 ml/day) and urine. Normally, about 800 ml to 1,600 ml of urine is produced each day. The kidneys are able to regulate the amount of water lost in urine, although even in severe dehydration, some urine is still produced to maintain fluid flow through the kidney tubules (nephrons) and excrete toxic nitrogenous wastes such as ammonia and urea. Urinary water loss is not usually less than 800 ml/day.

Environmental conditions affect a person's water requirements by altering the losses that occur by the various routes. Water losses may be 2 to 3 times greater for a sedentary individual living in a hot climate compared with a sedentary individual living in a temperate climate. These higher rates of water loss are not exclusively caused by increased sweating, but may also be incurred by a marked increase in transcutaneous and respiratory water losses. These routes of water loss are heavily influenced by the humidity of the ambient air, which may be a more important factor than the ambient temperature. Respiratory water losses are greater when the relative humidity (RH) of the ambient air is low because air breathed out of the body is fully saturated with water vapor (RH = 100%). Although these losses are quite small for a sedentary individual in a moist, warm environment (about 200 ml/day), they may be increased approximately twofold in low-humidity conditions (RH = 0% to 20%) and may rise up to 1,500 ml/day during periods of hard training in cold, dry air at altitude.

Water intake comes from drinks and food; some foods (especially plant material) have a high water content. Water in food, in fact, makes a major contribution to total water intake. Water is also produced internally (metabolic water) from the catabolism of carbohydrates, fat, and protein. For example, in the complete oxidation of 1 molecule of glucose, 6 molecules of carbon dioxide, and 6 molecules of water are produced. In a sedentary individual, metabolic water production will amount to about 300 ml/day, although most of this water is lost in expired gas, as oxidizing fuel in the body generates carbon dioxide, which stimulates breathing and, hence, increases respiratory water loss. Although an athlete increases his or her metabolic water production because of the increased rate of fuel catabolism

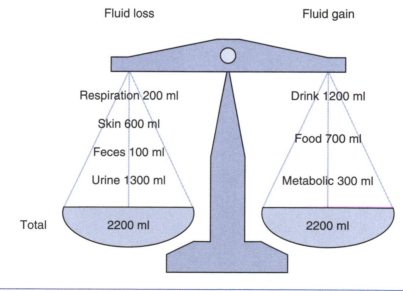

Figure 8.18 Daily water balance for a sedentary adult individual.

during exercise, this increase, again, is offset by the obligatory increase in lung ventilation and respiratory evaporative water loss.

The body's water balance is under tight regulation involving nervous and hormonal factors that respond to a number of different inputs. The osmolarity of the blood plasma is maintained within tight limits around 290 mOsmol/L. A rise or fall in the plasma osmolarity is sufficient to alter kidney function from maximum water conservation to maximum water excretion. Because sodium is the major electrolyte in the extracellular fluids (it accounts for 50% of plasma osmolarity), the maintenance of osmotic balance is closely coupled to the intake and excretion of sodium and water. Even small reductions in the plasma osmolarity invoke a marked increase in urine output (diuresis), and this increase is normally sufficient to prevent fluid overload when large volumes of water or low-electrolyte drinks such as beer are consumed. However, some cases of **hyponatremia** (low plasma sodium concentration) have been reported, usually in individuals who have ingested excessively large volumes of plain water or low-electrolyte drinks in a relatively short time.

The subjective sensation of thirst initiates the desire to drink and is therefore a key factor in the regulation of fluid intake. Although the kidneys can quite effectively conserve water or electrolytes by reducing the rate of loss, they cannot restore a fluid deficit. Only consumption of fluid can correct this imbalance. The sensation of thirst is mainly evoked by the detection of elevated plasma osmolarity (and to a lesser extent, by reductions in blood volume and pressure) by osmoreceptors located in the hypothalamus of the brain. The thirst sensation results in a profound desire to drink and an increase in the secretion of antidiuretic hormone (ADH) from the posterior pituitary gland, which acts on the kidneys to reduce urine excretion. Other factors that promote thirst are learned responses such as dryness of the mouth or throat, salty tastes, and feeling hot. Thirst is quickly alleviated by drinking fluid, and alleviation can occur before a significant amount of the fluid is absorbed in the gut. This effect suggests a role for sensory receptors in the mouth and stomach. Distension of the stomach wall appears to reduce the perception of thirst and may result in fluid ingestion being stopped prematurely. Thus, the absence of the sensation of thirst cannot be used as an indicator that fluid balance (euhydration) is established; often the perception of thirst is not present until a significant degree of dehydration has occurred.

An electrolyte imbalance commonly called "water intoxication," which results from hyponatremia (low plasma sodium) caused by excessive water consumption, is occasionally reported in endurance athletes. This condition appears to be most common among slow runners in marathon and ultramarathon races and probably arises because of the loss of sodium in sweat coupled with very high intakes (8 L to 10 L) of water (Noakes et al. 1985). The symptoms of hyponatremia are similar to those of dehydration and include mental confusion, weakness, and fainting. Therefore, this condition can be misdiagnosed when it occurs in individuals participating in endurance races. The usual treatment for dehydration is administration of fluid intravenously and orally. If this treatment is given to a hyponatremic individual, the consequences can be fatal.

Fluid Requirements for Athletes

Athletes must be fully hydrated before they train or compete because the body cannot adapt to dehydration. Training quality will suffer if an athlete becomes dehydrated during training, as will performance quality if an athlete becomes dehydrated during competition.

Ensuring Adequate Hydration Before Exercise

An adequately hydrated state can be assured by a high fluid intake in the last few days before competition. A useful check is to observe the color of the urine. It should be pale in color, although this simple test cannot be reliably used if the athlete is taking vitamin supplements, as some of the excreted water-soluble B vitamins add a yellowish hue to the urine. A clearer indication of hydration status is obtained by measuring urine osmolality. (Note that the units of osmolality are Osmol/kg, whereas osmolarity is expressed as Osmol/L.) This measurement can be done quickly and simply using a portable osmometer. A urine osmolality of over 900 mOsmol/kg definitely indicates that the athlete is relatively dehydrated; values of 100 mOsmol/kg to 300 mOsmol/kg indicate that the athlete is well hydrated. Measuring the athlete's body weight after rising and voiding each morning may also prove useful. A sudden drop in body mass on any given day is likely to indicate dehydration. Approximate fluid intake requirements in liters per day in hot, dry conditions are shown in figure 8.19. The fluid intake requirement (to maintain water balance, or euhydration) increases as ambient temperature increases and as daily energy expenditure increases.

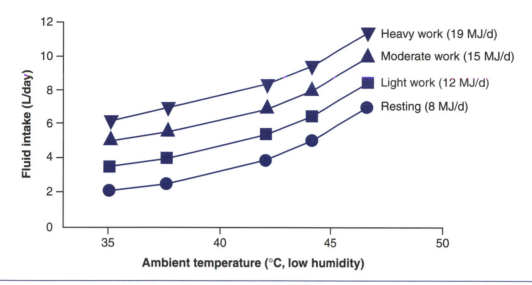

Figure 8.19 Approximate daily fluid intake requirements for individuals at rest or performing different amounts of physical work while living at different ambient temperatures.

Adapted from M.N. Sawka and S.J. Montain, 2000.

Ensuring Hydration During Exercise

Relying on feeling thirsty as the signal to drink is unreliable because a considerable degree of dehydration (certainly sufficient to impair athletic performance) can occur before the desire for fluid intake is evident. Ideally, athletes should consume enough fluids during activity to make body weight remain fairly constant before and after exercise. Guidelines for the amounts of fluid to be consumed before, during, and after exercise can only be very general because of the large interindividual sweating responses. However, the American and Canadian Dietetic Associations recommend that approximately 500 ml of fluid be consumed 2 hours before exertion, followed by another 500 ml about 15 minutes before prolonged exercise. In hot and humid environments, frequent consumption (every 15 to 20 minutes) of small volumes (120 to 180 ml) of fluid are recommended throughout exertion. Athletes should become accustomed to consuming fluid at regular intervals (with or without thirst) during training sessions so they do not experience discomfort during competition. For most persons exercising for 30 minutes to 60 minutes in moderate temperature conditions, an appropriate beverage is cool water.

Composition of Sport Drinks During Exercise

Fluid ingestion during exercise also supplies exogenous fuel substrate (usually carbohydrate) as well as helps maintain plasma volume and prevents dehydration. However, the availability of ingested fluids may be limited by the rate of gastric emptying or intestinal absorption. Gastric emptying of fluids is slowed by the addition of carbohydrate or other macronutrients that increase the osmolarity of the solution ingested. Hence, with increasing glucose concentration in the fluid ingested, the rate of fluid volume delivery to the small intestine is decreased, although the rate of glucose delivery is increased.

Water absorption in the small intestine is by osmosis and is promoted by the coupled transport of glucose and sodium. Hence, the composition of fluids to be used during exercise depends on the relative needs to replace water and provide fuel substrate. Where rehydration is the main priority (e.g., for prolonged exercise in the heat), the solution should contain some carbohydrate as glucose or glucose polymers (20 g/L to 60 g/L) and sodium (20 mmol/L to 60 mmol/L) and should not exceed isotonicity (290 mOsmol/L). Most commercially available sports drinks contain 60 g/L to 80 g/L of carbohydrate (predominantly as glucose, glucose polymers, or both, although some drinks may also contain fructose or sucrose) and 20 mmol/L to 25 mmol/L of sodium. Table 8.6 compares the compositions of several commercially available drinks that are commonly consumed by athletes during training or competition. In cool environments, where substrate provision to maintain endurance performance is more important, a more concentrated solution incorporating large amounts of glucose polymers in concentrations of 550 mmol/L to 800 mmol/L glucosyl units (100 g/L to 150 g/L) is recommended. To minimize the limitation imposed by the rate of gastric emptying, the osmolarity of the beverage should be minimized

Table 8.6 Compositions of Commonly Consumed Sport Drinks

Drink	Carbohydrate (g/L)	Sodium (mmol/L)	Potassium (mmol/L)	Osmolality (mOsmol/kg)
Coca-Cola	105	3	0	650
Allsport	80	10	6	516
Gatorade	60	18	3	349
Isostar	65	24	4	296
Lucozade Sport	64	23	4	280
Lucozade	180	0	0	658
Powerade (U.K.)	60	24	4	285
Powerade (U.S.)	80	5	4	381

by providing the glucose in the form of glucose polymers, and the volume of fluid in the stomach should be kept as high as is comfortable by frequent ingestion of small amounts of fluid.

The importance of practicing drinking during training is often neglected. This practice will accustom athletes to the feeling of exercising with fluid in the stomach. It also provides the opportunity to experiment with different volumes and flavorings to determine how much fluid intake athletes can tolerate and which formulations suit them best. Measuring fluid consumption and body mass changes before and after training gives an idea of the athlete's sweat rate under different environmental conditions. This information will help determine an individual athlete's requirements for fluid intake during competition.

The ideal drink for fluid replacement during exercise is one that tastes good to the athlete, does not cause gastrointestinal discomfort when consumed in large volumes (this rules out all fizzy carbonated drinks), promotes rapid gastric emptying and fluid absorption to help maintain extracellular fluid volume, and provides some energy in the form of carbohydrate for the working muscles. Cool, pleasantly flavored, sweetened beverages are preferred by exercising subjects, and the presence of sodium in the drinks seems to promote their consumption, probably by maintaining thirst.

Rehydration After Exercise

Replacement of water and electrolytes in the postexercise recovery period may be of crucial importance where repeated bouts of exercise must be performed and rehydration must be maximized in the time available. As previously mentioned, dehydration is associated with impaired thermoregulation and

increased cardiovascular strain and with the loss of the thermoregulatory advantages conferred by heat acclimation and high aerobic fitness. With progressive dehydration, losses of intracellular as well as extracellular fluid volume occurs. Loss of intracellular volume may have important implications for recovery from exercise given the emerging evidence of a role for cell volume in the regulation of cell metabolism. A reduced intracellular volume reduces rates of glycogen and protein synthesis, whereas a high cell volume stimulates these processes.

The main factors influencing the effectiveness of postexercise rehydration are the volume and composition of the fluid consumed. Plain water is not the ideal rehydration beverage when rapid and complete restoration of body fluid balance is necessary and when all intake is in liquid form. Ingestion of water alone causes a rapid fall in the plasma sodium concentration and in the plasma osmolarity. These changes reduce the stimulation to drink (thirst) and increase the urine output, both of which delay the rehydration process. Plasma volume is more rapidly and completely restored if some sodium chloride (77 mmol/L, or 0.45 g/L) is added to the water consumed (Nose et al. 1988). This sodium concentration is similar to the upper limit of the sodium concentration found in sweat but is considerably higher than the sodium concentration of many commercially available sports drinks, which usually contain 10 mmol/L to 25 mmol/L (see table 8.6). Optimal rehydration after exercise can only be achieved if the sodium lost in sweat is replaced along with the water.

Shirreffs et al. (1996) showed that, provided that an adequate volume of fluid is consumed, euhydration is achieved when sodium intake is greater than sodium loss (see figure 8.20). Ingesting a beverage containing sodium not only promotes rapid fluid absorption in

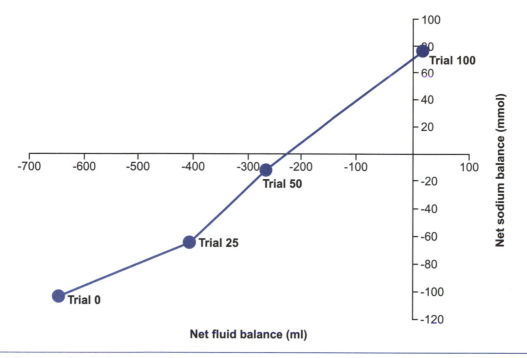

Figure 8.20 Net sodium balance plotted against net fluid balance, 6 hours after the end of a rehydration period, during which subjects ingested different drinks in a volume equivalent to 150% of sweat loss. The drinks containing sodium at a concentration of 0 mmol/L, 25 mmol/L, 50 mmol/L, or 100 mmol/L (trials 0, 25, 50, and 100, respectively) were ingested after exercise. At the end of the 6-hour rehydration period, water balance was only achieved when the sodium intake was greater than the sweat sodium loss.

Reprinted, by permission, from S.M. Shirreffs and R.J. Maughan, 2000, "Rehydration and recovery of fluid balance after exercise," *Exercise and Sport Sciences Reviews* 28(1): 27-32.

the small intestine but also allows the plasma sodium concentration to remain elevated during the rehydration period and helps maintain thirst while delaying stimulation of urine production. Sodium is the major cation in the extracellular fluid. The inclusion of potassium in the beverage consumed after exercise would be expected to enhance the replacement of intracellular water and thus promote rehydration, but currently little experimental evidence supports this expectation. The rehydration drink should also contain carbohydrate (glucose or glucose polymers) because the presence of some glucose also stimulates fluid absorption in the gut and improves beverage taste. After exercise, the uptake of glucose into the muscle for glycogen resynthesis should also promote intracellular rehydration.

Fluid Consumption After Exercise

Until recently, athletes were generally encouraged to consume a volume of fluid equivalent to their sweat loss incurred during exercise to adequately rehydrate in the postexercise recovery period. In other words, they were to consume about 1 L of fluid for every kg lost during an exercise session. This amount is insufficient because it does not take into account the obligatory urine losses that are incurred after beverage consumption over a period of hours. Existing data indicate that ingestion of 150% or more of weight loss (i.e., 1.5 L of fluid consumed during recovery for every kg of weight lost during exercise) may be required to achieve normal hydration within 6 hours after exercise (Shirreffs et al. 1996; Shirreffs and Maughan 1998, 2000 [see figure 8.21]). Current (1996) American College of Sports Medicine (ACSM) guidelines on fluid ingestion before, during, and after exercise are shown in figure 8.22.

Intake of caffeine and alcohol in the postexercise recovery period is generally discouraged because of their diuretic actions. However, the diuretic effect of alcohol appears to be blunted when consumed by persons who are moderately dehydrated after exercise in a warm environment (Shirreffs and Maughan 1997). If shandy (a mixture of beer and lemonade) is consumed in the postexercise period, then (as expected) the urinary output increases with increasing alcohol intake. However, this increase only approaches statistical significance (compared with lemonade alone) when alcohol content is around 4% w/v. This concentration of alcohol in the rehydration

Figure 8.21 Net fluid balance plotted against time after dehydration (loss of 1,500 ml body water) induced by mild exercise in a hot environment. Zero net fluid balance represents euhydration. Drink volume ingested was half of (50%), equal to (100%), one-and-a-half times (150%), and twice (200%) the sweat loss. The drink sodium concentration was either (a) 23 mmol/L or (b) 61 mmol/L. Mild dehydration was present 6 hours after rehydration when a large volume of the low-sodium drink (23 mmol/L) was consumed, but with the same volume, hyperhydration was achieved with the high-sodium drink (61 mmol/L).

Reprinted, by permission, from S.M. Shirreffs et al., 1996, "Post-exercise rehydration in man: Effects of volume consumed and drink sodium content," Medicine and Science in Sport Exercise 28: 1260-1271..

Adequate fluid replacement helps maintain hydration and therefore promotes the health, safety, and optimal physical performance of individuals participating in regular physical activity. The following are general recommendations on the amount and composition of fluids that should be ingested in preparation for, during, and after exercise or athletic competition.

1. Individuals should consume a nutritionally balanced diet and drink adequate fluids during the 24-hour period before an event, especially during the period that includes the meal before exercise, to promote proper hydration before exercise or competition.

2. Individuals should drink about 500 ml (about 17 fl oz) of fluid about 2 hours before exercise to promote adequate hydration and allow time for excretion of excess ingested water.

3. During exercise, athletes should start drinking early and at regular intervals in an attempt to consume fluids at a rate sufficient to replace all the water lost through sweating (i.e., body weight loss), or they should consume the maximal amount that can be tolerated.

4. Ingested fluids should be cooler than ambient temperature (between 15° and 22° C [59° and 72° F]) and flavored to enhance palatability and promote fluid replacement. Fluid should be readily available and served in containers that allow adequate volumes to be ingested with ease and with minimal interruption of exercise.

5. Addition of proper amounts of carbohydrates or electrolytes to a fluid replacement solution is recommended for exercise events of duration greater than 1 hour because

such additives do not significantly impair water delivery to the body and may enhance performance. For exercise of less than 1 hour, little evidence exists of physiological or physical performance differences as a result of consuming a carbohydrate-electrolyte drink and plain water.

6. During intense exercise lasting longer than 1 hour, carbohydrates should be ingested at a rate of 30 g/h to 60 g/h to maintain oxidation of carbohydrate and delay fatigue. This rate of carbohydrate delivery can be achieved without compromising fluid delivery by drinking 600 ml/h to 1,200 ml/h of solutions containing 4% to 8% carbohydrates (g/100 ml). The carbohydrates can be sugars (glucose or sucrose) or starch (e.g., maltodextrins).

7. Inclusion of sodium (0.5 g/L to 0.7 g/L of water) in the rehydration solution ingested during exercise lasting longer than 1 hour is recommended because it may enhance palatability, promote fluid retention, and possibly prevent hyponatremia in certain individuals who drink excessive quantities of fluid. Little physiological evidence suggests the need for sodium in an oral rehydration solution for enhancing intestinal water absorption as long as sodium is sufficiently available from the previous meal.

Figure 8.22 American College of Sports Medicine Guidelines on fluid intake for exercise.

Figure 8.23 Percentage change in plasma volume with dehydration equivalent to 2% of body weight, followed by rehydration with drinks containing 0%, 1%, 2%, and 4% (w/v) alcohol in a volume equivalent to one-and-a-half times the sweat loss. Note that plasma volume restoration was delayed with the 4% alcohol drink.

Reprinted, by permission, from S.M. Shirreffs and R.J. Maughan, 1997, "Restoration of fluid balance after exercise-induced dehydration: Effect of alcohol consumption," *Journal of Applied Physiology* 83: 1152-1157.

drink is also associated with a slower rate of recovery of plasma volume, as shown in figure 8.23, whereas drinks containing 1% and 2% alcohol seem just as effective as lemonade alone.

In most circumstances, athletes should consume solid food as well as drink between exercise bouts, unless food intake is likely to result in gastrointestinal disturbances. In one study, the same fluid volume consumed as a meal-plus-water combination compared with a sports-drink alone resulted in a smaller volume of urine produced and hence greater fluid retention (Maughan, Leiper, and Shirreffs 1996). The greater efficacy of the meal-plus-water treatment in restoring whole-body fluid balance was probably a consequence of its greater total sodium and potassium content. In exercise situations where sweat losses are large, the total sodium and chloride losses are high. For example, the loss of 10 L of sweat, with a sodium concentration of 50 mmol/L, amounts to a loss of about 29 g of sodium chloride.

Obviously, food intake can be important in restoring these salt losses because most commercial sports drinks do not contain more than about 25 mmol/L sodium. Rehydration after exercise can only be achieved if sweat electrolyte losses as well as water are replaced. One problem is that drinks with high-sodium content (i.e., 40 to 80 mmol/L) are unpalatable to some people, which results in reduced consumption. On the other hand, drinks with low-sodium content (e.g., most soft drinks) are much less effective for rehydration, and they also reduce the stimulus to drink.

Key Points

- High rates of sweat secretion are necessary during hard exercise to limit the rise in body temperature that would otherwise occur. If the exercise is prolonged, body-temperature increase leads to progressive dehydration and loss of electrolytes.

- Body temperatures of 36° to 38° C (96.8° to 100.4° F) are considered as the normal range at rest and may increase to 38° to 40° C (100.4° to 104° F) during exercise. When body temperature rises toward 39.5° C (103° F), central fatigue ensues. Further increases are commonly associated with heat exhaustion and occasionally with life-threatening heat

(continued)

Sport Nutrition

(continued)

stroke, characterized by a lack of consciousness after exertion and by clinical symptoms of organ damage.

■ Some people may lose up to 2 to 3 L/h of sweat during strenuous activity in a hot environment. Even at low ambient temperatures of about 10° C (50° F), sweat loss can exceed 1 L/h.

■ Because the electrolyte composition of sweat is hypotonic to plasma, the replacement of water rather than electrolytes is the priority during exercise.

■ Fatigue towards the end of a prolonged event may result as much from the effects of dehydration as from substrate depletion. Exercise performance is impaired when an individual is dehydrated by as little as 2% of body weight, and losses in excess of 5% of body weight can decrease the capacity for work by about 30%.

■ Oral fluid ingestion during exercise helps restore plasma volume to near pre-exercise levels and prevents the adverse effects of dehydration on muscle strength, endurance, and coordination. Dehydration also poses a serious health risk in that it increases the risk of cramps, heat exhaustion, and life-threatening heat stroke.

■ Relying on feeling thirsty as the signal to drink is unreliable because a considerable degree of dehydration (certainly sufficient to impair athletic performance) can occur before the desire for fluid intake is evident. Ideally, athletes should consume adequate fluids during activity so that body weight remains fairly constant before and after exercise.

■ The composition of drinks to be taken during exercise should suit individual circumstances. Where rehydration is the main priority (e.g., for prolonged exercise in the heat), the solution should contain some carbohydrate as glucose or glucose polymers (20 to 60 g/L) and sodium (20 to 60 mmol/L) and should not exceed isotonicity (290 mOsmol/L).

■ Optimal rehydration after exercise can only be achieved if the sodium lost in sweat is replaced along with the water. Plasma volume is more rapidly and completely restored in the postexercise period if some sodium chloride is added to the water consumed. A volume equivalent to at least one-and-a-half times the sweat loss must be consumed to ensure that complete rehydration is achieved at the end of a 6-hour recovery period after exercise.

Key Terms

acclimatization 175
conduction 172
convection 172
dehydration 170

euhydration 178
evaporation 172
hyperhydration 180
hyperthermia 171

hypertonic 182
hyponatremia 188
hypotonic 182
hypovolemia 178

osmosis 182
radiation 172
thermoregulation 171

Recommended Readings

Armstrong, L.E. 2000. *Performing in Extreme Environments*. Human Kinetics: Champaign, IL.

Maughan, R.J. 2000. Water and electrolyte loss and replacement in exercise. In *Nutrition in Sport*, ed. R.J. Maughan, 226-240. Blackwell Science: Oxford.

Maughan, R.J., and L.M. Burke. 2002. Sport nutrition. *Handbook of Sports Medicine and Sciences*. Blackwell Science: Oxford.

Maughan, R.J., and R. Murray. (eds). 2000. *Sports Drinks: Basic Science and Practical Aspects*. CRC Press: Boca Raton, FL.

Maughan, R.J., and E.R. Nadel. 2000. Temperature regulation and fluid and electrolyte balance. In *Nutrition in Sport*, ed. R. J. Maughan, 203-215. Blackwell Science: Oxford.

Sawka, M.N., W.A. Latzka, and S.J. Montain. 2000. Effects of dehydration and rehydration on performance. In *Nutrition in Sport*, ed. R.J. Maughan, 216-225. Blackwell Science: Oxford.

Shirreffs, S.M. 2000. Rehydration and recovery after exercise. In *Nutrition in Sport*, ed. R.J. Maughan, 256-265. Blackwell Science: Oxford.

Shirreffs, S.M., and R.J. Maughan. 2000. Rehydration and recovery of fluid balance after exercise. *Exercise and Sport Sciences Reviews* 28:27-32.

Chapter 9

The Micronutrients: Vitamins and Minerals

© Michael Zito/SportsChrome USA

Objectives

After studying this chapter, you should be able to do the following:

- Describe the vitamins and minerals that are required to maintain a healthy body

- Describe some of the major dietary sources of essential micronutrients

- Describe the role of micronutrients in growth and repair of body tissues, in metabolism as cofactors for enzymes, in oxygen transport, in immune function, and in defense against free radicals

- Describe the effects of exercise training on micronutrient requirements

- Describe particular groups of athletes who may be at risk for micronutrient deficiencies

- Describe some of the consequences of micronutrient deficiency and excess

In addition to the macronutrient (i.e., carbohydrate, fat, and protein), humans must consume relatively small amounts of certain micronutrients (i.e., organic vitamins and inorganic minerals) in the diet to maintain health. In addition to being found in foods, micronutrients are also available individually or in a variety of combined preparations referred to as supplements. Many top athletes consume large quantities of vitamin and mineral supplements in the mistaken belief that they will help prevent infection or injury, speed recovery, or improve athletic performance. Some minerals are likely to do more harm than good. Although vitamin and mineral supplementation may improve the nutritional status of individuals consuming marginal amounts of micronutrients from food and may improve performance in athletes with deficiencies, no evidence indicates that doses in excess of the RDA improve performance.

This chapter deals with the micronutrient requirements of athletes and the problems associated with inadequate or excessive intakes. Emphasis is on those vitamins and minerals that are important for athletic performance. Rather than dealing with the role and requirement for each individual vitamin and mineral, this chapter describes some of the important roles for which various vitamins and minerals are needed (e.g., in forming the building blocks of body tissues, as cofactors in enzyme catalyzed metabolic reactions, for oxygen transport and oxidative metabolism, and as **antioxidants**). This approach should help the reader understand (1) why micronutrients are an essential component of the diet, (2) why the requirement for some micronutrients may be increased in athletes, (3) which groups of athletes are most at risk for inadequate micronutrient intake, and (4) the scientific basis of advice given to athletes regarding their intake of vitamin and mineral supplements. Any sustained deficiency of an essential vitamin or mineral results in ill health, and an unhealthy athlete is extremely unlikely to perform to the best of his or her potential. Several micronutrients are important for the maintenance of immune function, and this important role is discussed in greater detail in chapter 13.

Water-Soluble and Fat-Soluble Vitamins

Vitamins are organic compounds that are needed in very small quantities in the diet. They are essential for specific metabolic reactions in the body and for promoting normal growth and development. With the exception of vitamin D, which can be synthesized in the presence of sunlight, vitamin K, and small quanti-

ties of selected B vitamins, which can be produced by the bacterial microflora of the gastrointestinal tract, vitamins are not produced by the human body and must be consumed in the diet.

Although vitamins do not directly contribute to the energy supply, they play an important role in energy metabolism as reusable coenzymes in many metabolic reactions. Many vitamins, particularly from the B group, are cofactors in the pathways of energy metabolism, including glycolysis, the β-oxidation of FAs, the tricarboxylic acid cycle, and the electron-transport chain. A deficiency of some of the B group vitamins that act as cofactors of enzymes in carbohydrate (e.g., thiamin [vitamin B_1], niacin [vitamin B_3], and pyridoxine [vitamin B_6]), fat (e.g., riboflavin [vitamin B_2], thiamin, pantothenic acid, and biotin), and protein (e.g., pyridoxine) metabolism, causes premature fatigue and inability to maintain a heavy training program.

Other vitamins play a role in heme synthesis and red and white blood cell production (e.g., folic acid, and cobalamin [vitamin B_{12}]) or assist in the formation of bones, connective tissue, and cartilage (e.g., vitamins C and D). Several vitamins, including A, C, and E act as antioxidants and help protect the body tissues against the potentially damaging effects of **free radicals.**

Thirteen different compounds are now considered vitamins, and they are classified either as water-soluble or fat-soluble. The water-soluble vitamins, C (ascorbic acid), B_1 (thiamin), B_2 (riboflavin), B_3 (niacin), B_6 (pyridoxine), pantothenic acid, and biotin, are involved in mitochondrial energy metabolism. Folic acid and vitamin B_{12} (cobalamin) are mainly involved in nucleic acid synthesis and, hence, are important for maintaining healthy populations of rapidly dividing cells in the body (e.g., red blood cells, immune cells, and the gut mucosa). Of the fat-soluble vitamins, A (retinol), D (calciferol), E (tocopherol), and K (menadione), only vitamin E has a probable role in energy metabolism. Vitamins A, C, and E have antioxidant properties. Vitamin K is required for the addition of sugar residues to proteins to form glycoproteins, such as the blood-clotting factors. Tables 9.1 and 9.2 summarize the major roles of the vitamins and the main effects of dietary deficiency or excess.

Vitamin deficiencies reduce body function and impair health. Indeed, most of the vitamins were first recognized by the deficiency symptoms and illnesses that arose when their intake was inadequate (e.g., scurvy in vitamin C–deficient sailors; rickets in vitamin D–deficient children). Although marginal deficiencies of vitamins may have only a

Table 9.1 The Major Functions of Fat-Soluble Vitamins and the Effects of Dietary Deficiency or Excess

Vitamin	Major roles in body	Effect of deficiency	Effect of excess
A (retinol)	Maintains epithelial tissues in skin, mucous membranes, and visual pigments of eye; promotes bone development and immune function	Night blindness, infections, impaired growth, and impaired wound healing	Nausea, headache, fatigue, liver damage, joint pains, peeling skin, and abnormal fetal development in pregnancy
D (calciferol)	Increases calcium absorption in gut and promotes bone formation	Weak bones (rickets in children and osteomalacia in adults)	Nausea, loss of appetite, irritability, joint pains, and calcification of soft tissues (e.g., kidneys)
E (α-tocopherol)	Defends against free radicals; protects cell membranes	Hemolysis and anemia	Headache, fatigue, and diarrhea
K (menadione)	Forms blood-clotting factors	Bleeding and hemorrhage	Thrombosis and vomiting

Table 9.2 The Major Functions of Water-Soluble Vitamins and the Effects of Dietary Deficiency or Excess

Vitamin	Major roles in body	Effect of deficiency	Effect of excess
B$_1$ (thiamin)	Forms coenzyme with thiamine pyrophosphate; promotes carbohydrate metabolism and central nervous system function	Loss of appetite, apathy, depression, beriberi, and pain in calf muscles	No toxic effects
B$_2$ (riboflavin)	Forms coenzymes with FAD and FMN; promotes carbohydrate and fat oxidation; maintains healthy skin	Dermatitis, lip and tongue sores, and damage to cornea of eyes	No toxic effects
B$_3$ (niacin)	Forms coenzymes with NAD and NADP; promotes anaerobic glycolysis, carbohydrate and fat oxidation, and fat synthesis; maintains healthy skin	Weakness, loss of appetite, skin lesions, gut and skin problems, and pellegra	Headache, nausea, skin irritation, liver damage, and inhibition of lipolysis
B$_6$ (pyridoxine)	Forms coenzyme with pyridoxal phosphate; promotes protein metabolism, formation of hemoglobin and red blood cells, glycogenolysis, and gluconeogenesis	Irritability, convulsions, anemia, dermatitis, and tongue sores	Loss of nerve sensation and abnormal gait
B$_{12}$ (cobalamin)	Forms coenzyme for DNA and RNA; promotes formation of red and white blood cells; maintains nerve, gut, and skin tissue	Pernicious anemia, fatigue, nerve damage, paralysis, and infections	No toxic effects
Folic acid	Forms coenzyme for DNA and RNA; promotes formation of hemoglobin and red and white blood cells; maintains gut	Anemia, fatigue, diarrhea, gut disorders, and infections	No toxic effects
Biotin	Forms coenzyme for CO$_2$ transfer; promotes carbohydrate, fat, and protein metabolism	Nausea, fatigue, and skin rashes	No toxic effects
Pantothenic acid	Forms coenzyme A for energy metabolism; promotes carbohydrate and fat oxidation and fat synthesis	Nausea, fatigue, depression, and loss of appetite	No toxic effects
C (ascorbic acid)	Antioxidant; promotes collagen formation, development of connective tissue, catecholamine and steroid synthesis, and iron absorption	Weakness, slow wound healing, infections, bleeding gums, anemia, scurvy	No toxic effects in smaller doses (<1,000 mg/day); diarrhea, kidney stones, and iron overload in larger doses

FMN = flavin mononucleotide.

small impact on otherwise healthy young sedentary individuals, such deficiencies may crucially affect athletic performance in elite athletes. The margins between winning and coming second can be very small in many sports, and something that impairs performance by only 1% could easily affect the outcome of a competitive event. Tables 9.3 and 9.4 show the amounts of vitamins normally required in adults' diet (recommended daily allowances [RDA] or adequate intakes [AI]) and the major food sources from which they are obtained.

Effect of Exercise on Vitamin Requirements

Various experimental vitamin depletion studies have determined that inadequate vitamin status is associated with impaired exercise performance, particularly when more than one vitamin is deficient in the diet. Athletes are generally assumed to need an increased vitamin intake because exercise increases the vitamin requirements. Theoretically, exercise can induce a marginal vitamin status (defi-

Table 9.3 The Major Sources of Fat-Soluble Vitamins

Vitamin	Sources	RDA or AI*
A (retinol)	Liver, fish, dairy products[a], eggs, margarine; formed in body from provitamin A (carotenoids) found in carrots, dark-green leafy vegetables, tomatoes, and oranges	0.9 mg (M)[b] 0.7 mg (F)
D (calciferol)	Liver, fish, eggs, fortified dairy products, oils, and margarine; formed by action of sunlight on the skin	5 μg* (M, F)
E (tocopherol)	Liver, eggs, whole-grain cereal products, vegetable oils, seed oils, margarine, and butter	15 mg (M, F)
K (menadione)	Liver, eggs, green leafy vegetables, cheese, and butter; formed in large intestine by bacteria	120 μg* (M) 90 μg* (F)

RDA = recommended daily allowance; AI* = adequate intake. M = males; F = females.
[a]Dairy products include milk, cream, butter, and cheese
[b]RDA for vitamin A is 0.9 mg of retinol or 5.4 mg of β-carotene for males; 80% of these values for females.

Table 9.4 The Major Sources of Water-Soluble Vitamins

Vitamin	Sources	RDA or AI*
B₁ (thiamin)	Whole-grain cereal products, fortified bread, pulses, potatoes, legumes, nuts, pork, ham, and liver	1.2 mg (M) 1.1 mg (F)
B₂ (riboflavin)	Dairy products[a], meat, liver, eggs, green leafy vegetables, and beans	1.3 mg (M) 1.1 mg (F)
B₃ (niacin)	Meat, liver, poultry, fish, whole-grain cereal products, lentils, and nuts; formed in the body from essential amino acid tryptophan	16 mg (M) 14 mg (F)
B₆ (pyridoxine)	Meat, liver, poultry, fish, whole-grain cereal products, potatoes, legumes, green leafy vegetables, dairy products[a], bananas, and nuts	1.3 mg (M, F)
B₁₂ (cobalamin)	Meat, fish, shellfish, poultry, liver, eggs, dairy products[a], and fortified breakfast cereals	2.4 μg (M, F)
Folic acid	Meat, liver, green leafy vegetables, whole-grain cereal products, potatoes, legumes, nuts, and fruit	400 μg (M, F)
Biotin	Meat, milk, egg yolk, whole grain cereal products, legumes, most vegetables	30 μg* (M, F)
Pantothenic acid	Liver, meat, dairy products[a], eggs, whole-grain cereal products, legumes, and most vegetables	5 mg* (M, F)
C (ascorbic acid)	Citrus fruits, green leafy vegetables, broccoli, potatoes, peppers, and strawberries	90 mg (M) 75 mg (F)

RDA = recommended daily allowance; AI* = adequate intake. M = males; F = females.
[a]Dairy products include milk, cream, butter, and cheese.

ciency) by causing decreased absorption from the digestive tract; increased excretion in sweat, urine, and feces; increased turnover (degradation); and increased requirement (retention) because of biochemical adaptation to training (e.g., increased mitochondrial density in skeletal muscle with endurance training and muscle hypertrophy with strength training).

Assessing Vitamin Status

Vitamin (and mineral) status can be estimated directly from biopsy samples of body tissues (e.g., skeletal muscle), from blood cells or plasma, or indirectly from analysis of the diet. The vitamin status of an individual however, is difficult to determine accurately. A diagnosis of vitamin deficiency is best made by considering a variety of sources of information, including blood analysis, an assessment of dietary intake, and clinical symptoms. Most studies that have used blood analysis (either by direct measurement of the plasma concentration of the vitamin or by indirect measurement of vitamin-requiring enzyme activities) have not revealed any distinct differences between athletic populations and sedentary people. Furthermore, very little evidence suggests that the vitamin intakes of athletes in general are inadequate, based on the **recommended dietary allowances** (RDAs), except in those athletes with extremely low dietary energy intakes or in athletes who fail to consume a well-balanced diet.

Recommended Intakes of Vitamins

Each vitamin has a minimal requirement that covers only the basic needs and is just sufficient to prevent clinical deficiency and ensuing disease symptoms. The estimated average requirement (EAR) is higher, and it ensures a safety margin. As discussed in chapter 1, the EAR represents the amount of a nutrient deemed sufficient to meet the needs of the average individual in a certain age and gender group. The recommended daily intake (RDI) or recommended dietary allowances (RDA) of any particular vitamin is defined as the intake required to meet the known nutritional needs of more than 97% of healthy persons. For some vitamins, including biotin, pantothenic acid, and vitamin D, there is currently insufficient scientific evidence to estimate an EAR, and in these cases an adequate intake (AI) has been set. Individuals should use the AI as a goal for intake where no RDAs exist.

This EAR is normally distributed, and the RDA recommendation is set so that it covers 97.5% of all healthy individuals with an ordinary (normal) diet.

This coverage is achieved by adding two standard deviations to the average daily requirement. Thus, individuals who consume less than the RDA of a nutrient are not necessarily deficient in that nutrient, but the more the actual intake lies below the RDA, the greater the risk of a deficiency state that is detrimental to the health of the individual (see figure 1.10). However, the data used to determine the RDAs often did not include athletes, or the activity levels of the subjects were not reported. Therefore, the RDAs may not be an accurate means of evaluating the nutritional needs of individuals engaged in regular strenuous exercise. The RDAs are calculated from population-based data. Metabolic, environmental, and genetic factors as well as age, gender, and body mass can make individual nutrient requirements differ from these estimated needs.

Although physical activity may increase the requirement for some vitamins (e.g., vitamins C, B_2, and possibly B_6, A, and E), this increased requirement typically can be met by consuming a balanced high-carbohydrate, moderate-protein, low-fat diet. As shown for vitamin B_1 (thiamin) and vitamin C in figure 9.1, vitamin intakes in athletes are correlated with energy intakes up to 20 MJ/day (4,800 kcal/day). Thus, provided that energy intake matches the energy requirement, and athletes consume a reasonably balanced diet, they get all the vitamins they need from food, without any need for supplements.

Individuals at risk for low vitamin intake are those who consume a low-energy or an unbalanced diet. When the energy intake is very high (>20 MJ/day [>4,800 kcal/day]), athletes tend to consume a large number of "in between meals" and high-energy sports drinks, often composed mainly of refined carbohydrate and low in protein and micronutrients; consequently, the nutrient density for vitamins drops. Vegetarian athletes obviously have problems obtaining sufficient intakes of some vitamins, particularly vitamin B_{12} [cobalamin], whose only natural dietary source is from meat. Fortunately, in Western countries, milk and several breakfast cereals are fortified with vitamin B_{12}, so this potential problem can be overcome by appropriate food selection and vitamin supplementation.

Vitamin losses in sweat are negligible and no increased vitamin excretion in urine and feces of athletes is evident. Temporary increases in the plasma concentrations of some vitamins (e.g., vitamin C [as can be seen in figure 9.2], vitamin E, and vitamin B_6, as pyridoxal 5'-phosphate) have been reported after an acute bout of exercise, which may reflect a

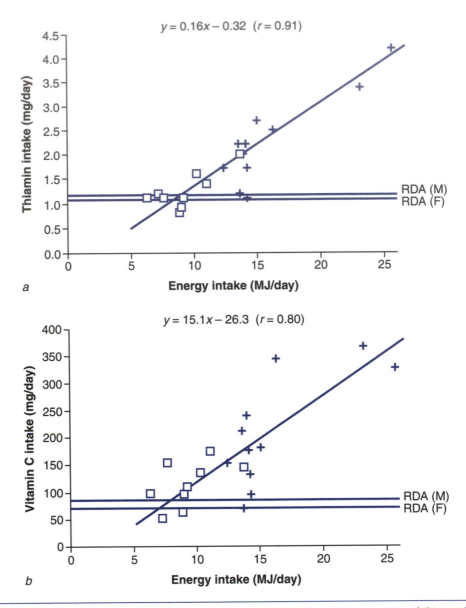

Figure 9.1 The relationship between mean intake of dietary energy and *(a)* thiamin (vitamin B₁) and *(b)* ascorbic acid (vitamin C) intake in male (crosses) and female (open squares) athletes. Each point represents a mean value for a group.
Data from Erp-Baart et al., 1989; Fogelholm, 1994.

redistribution of labile pools of these vitamins. However, in general, vitamin turnover seems to be remarkably unaffected by exercise.

Physical training may increase the vitamin B$_2$ (riboflavin) and vitamin B$_6$ (pyridoxine) requirement, which may be a consequence of increased retention of these vitamins in skeletal muscle. Adaptations to regular prolonged exercise include an increased number of mitochondria in skeletal muscles and increased oxidative enzyme activity, which might explain the increased retention of vitamins that are cofactors in energy metabolism within the muscle. Because of the increased free-radical production

during exercise compared with the resting state, an increased intake of antioxidant vitamins (A, C, and E) may be desirable for individuals engaged in regular physical activity. A free radical is an atom or molecule that possess at least one unpaired electron in its outer orbit. The free radicals produced by oxidation in the mitochondria include the superoxide ($\cdot O_2^-$), hydroxyl ($\cdot OH$), and nitric oxide ($\cdot NO$). These radical species are highly reactive and directly target lipid membrane structures by lipid peroxidation, causing membrane instability and increased permeability. Free radicals can also cause oxidative damage to proteins, including enzymes and DNA.

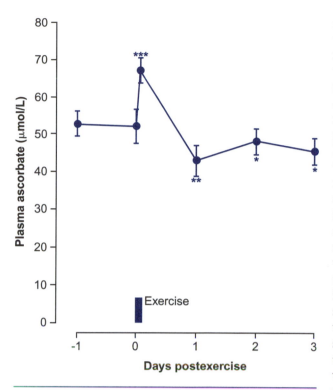

Figure 9.2 The effect of running a 21-kilometer road race on the plasma concentration of vitamin C. Data are means ± SEM from nine subjects. Statistical significance of differences of means compared with the immediately pre-exercise value on day 0: P<0.05, ** P<0.01, *** P<0.001.

Reproduced, with permission, from M. Gleeson, J.D. Robertson, and R.J. Maughan, 1987, *Clinical Science* 73, 501-505. Copyright © the Biochemical Society and the Medical Research Society.

Dietary Surveys of Vitamin Intakes in Elite Athletes

Ideally athletes should obtain all their nutrients from food. A well-balanced diet, including foods from each of the five food groups (meat, dairy, cereal, fruit, and vegetables) should provide adequate amounts of all 13 essential vitamins. Arguably, because total-energy intake of most athletes exceeds that of sedentary non-athletes, a greater amount and variety of vitamins should be available to the athlete through their dietary intake. Unfortunately, surveys of the dietary habits of elite athletes indicate that such individuals do not always consume a well-balanced diet. Elite athletes are at risk for nutrient deficiencies because of the fatiguing and time-consuming demands of training. A combination of increased vitamin turnover, additional loss of some nutrients, poor food selection, and limited time for food preparation are contributing factors.

The first two comprehensive reports on the actual dietary intakes of athletes published in 1981 revealed inappropriate macronutrient composition of the diets, with fat and protein components being too high, and in one study (Barry et al 1981), this inadequate diet was coupled with suboptimal intakes of thiamin, niacin, and folic acid. Intakes of these vitamins among female athletes were well below the recommended daily requirements. Some dietary surveys performed on elite endurance athletes have reported low (<85% of the RDA) or excessively high (>200% of the RDA) intakes of vitamins. However, apart from reports of low vitamin D intake in South African runners (Peters and Goetzsche 1997) and low vitamin A intake in Dutch elite strength athletes (van Erp-Baart et al. 1989b), deficient as well as excess intakes are reported fairly consistently only for the water-soluble vitamins. Low intakes of vitamins A and D are likely to be attributable to the restriction of dietary fat intake in weight-conscious athletes. In a national dietary survey of Dutch athletes (van Erp-Baart et al. 1989b) who participated in endurance, strength, or team sports, intakes of vitamins B_2, B_6, and C appeared to be more than adequate in endurance athletes, but were marginal in some strength athletes and team games players (see figure 9.3). This difference was attributed to the higher total dietary energy intakes in the endurance athletes. Several groups of athletes in this study consumed vitamin supplements well in excess of the RDA.

In contrast, the groups most at risk for inadequate intake of vitamins (B-vitamins in particular) are female adolescent athletes and athletes who are attempting to maintain low body weights (e.g., wrestlers, gymnasts, ballet dancers) by restricting their total-energy intake. Clearly, foods have to be chosen very carefully, or vitamin supplements should be taken by these groups of athletes.

Macrominerals and Microminerals

A mineral is an inorganic compound found in nature, and the term is usually reserved for those compounds that are solid. In nutrition, the term mineral usually refers to those dietary constituents essential to life processes. Minerals are classified as **macrominerals** or **microminerals** (trace elements), based upon the extent of their occurrence in the body and the amounts that are needed in the diet. The seven macrominerals are potassium, sodium, chloride, calcium, magnesium, phosphorus, and sulfur, and each constitutes at least 0.01% of total body mass (see table 9.5).

Inadequate mineral nutrition has been associated with a variety of human diseases, including **anemia,** cancer, diabetes, hypertension, **osteoporosis,** and

Figure 9.3 Daily intakes of *(a)* vitamin C, *(b)* vitamin B₂, and *(c)* vitamin B₆ in athletes from different sports. Open columns represent intake from food sources; filled columns indicate intake from supplements. M = males; F = females. Endurance: 1 = Tour de France M; 2 = Tour de l'Avenir M; 3 = triathlon M; 4 = cycling M; 5 = marathon speedskating M; 6 = swimming M; 7 = rowing M; 8 = running M; 9 = rowing F; 10 = cycling F; 11 = running F; 12 = sub-top swimming F. Strength: 1 = body building M; 2 = judo M; 3 = weightlifting M; 4 = judo M; 5 = top gymnastics F; 6 = subtop gymnastics F; 7 = body building F. Team sport: 1 = water polo M; 2 = soccer M; 3 = field hockey M; 4 = volleyball F; 5 = field hockey F; 6 = handball F. * = Note that these are based on the RDAs in 1989. These have now changed (see appendix C).

International Journal of Sports Medicine: From A.M.J. Erp van-Baart et al., "Nationwide survey on nutritional habits in elite athletes. PartII: Mineral and vitamin intake," 1989; 10 (suppl 1): S11-S16. Reprinted by permission.

tooth decay. Thus, appropriate dietary intake of essential minerals is necessary for optimal health and physical performance (see tables 9.6 and 9.7). Some minerals (e.g., calcium and phosphorus) are the building blocks for body tissues, including bones and teeth. A number of minerals (e.g., magnesium, copper, and zinc) are essential for the normal function of enzymes that are involved in the regulation of metabolism, and some minerals (e.g., iron, and zinc) have an essential role in the functioning of immune cells. Several other minerals (e.g., sodium, potassium, and chloride) exist as ions or **electrolytes** dissolved in the intracellular and extracellular fluids. Like the vitamins, minerals cannot be used as a source of energy.

Figure 9.3 (continued)

Table 9.5 Adult Total-Body Content and Body Fluid Concentrations of Macrominerals

Macromineral	Symbol	Atomic weight	Total amount in body (mg)	Body fluid concentration (mg/L)		
				Plasma	Sweat	Urine
Calcium	Ca	40	1,500,000	85–15	0–40	100–180
Chlorine	Cl	35.5	75,000	3,400–3,900	700–2,100	5,000–7,500
Magnesium	Mg	24	25,000	16–30	4–15	60–100
Potassium	K	39	180,000	130–220	160–320	800–3,200
Phosphorus	P	31	850,000	20–50	3–6	20–1,100
Sodium	Na	23	65,000	3,000–3,500	460–1,840	2,500–5,000

Electrolyte concentrations in interstitial fluid are virtually identical to those in plasma.

Recommended Intake of Minerals

At least 20 mineral elements are known to be essential for humans, and 14 trace elements have been identified as essential for maintenance of health. In addition to those listed in table 9.7, trace amounts of arsenic, nickel, silicon, tin, and vanadium may also be essential, but deficiencies or excesses (because of dietary sources) for these micronutrients are extremely rare. Deficiencies of one or more of the trace elements result in symptoms of disease, and many deficiencies are also associated with immune dysfunction and increased incidence of infection (see table 9.7).

The RDA has been established for seven minerals and the AI is available for 5 others (see tables 9.8 and 9.9). An estimated mineral requirement has been proposed for potassium, sodium, and chlorine. The trace elements (e.g., iron, zinc, copper, chromium, and selenium) each constitutes less than 0.01% of total body mass (see table 9.10) and are needed in quantities of less than 100 mg/day.

Effect of Exercise on Mineral Requirements

A temporary depression of the free (unbound) plasma concentration of some trace elements (e.g., iron, zinc,

Table 9.6 The Major Functions of Macrominerals and the Effects of Dietary Deficiency or Excess

Macromineral	Major roles in the body	Effect of deficiency	Effect of excess
Calcium	Promotes bone and teeth formation, muscle contraction, membrane potentials, and nerve impulse transmission; regulates enzyme activity	Osteoporosis, brittle bones, impaired muscle contraction, muscle cramps	Impaired trace metal absorption, cardiac arrhythmia, constipation, kidney stones, and calcification of soft tissue
Chlorine	Promotes nerve impulse conduction and hydrochloric acid formation in the stomach	Convulsions	Hypertension[a]
Magnesium	Promotes protein synthesis and metalloenzyme, ATPases, and 2,3-DPG formation; bone component	Muscle weakness, fatigue, apathy, muscle tremor, and cramps	Nausea, vomiting, and diarrhea
Potassium	Promotes membrane potential, nerve impulse generation, muscle contraction, and acid-base balance	Hypokalemia, muscle cramps, apathy, loss of appetite, and irregular heart beat	Hyperkalemia, cardiac arrhythmia, and cardiac failure
Phosphorus	Promotes bone formation; buffer in muscle contraction; component of ATP, PCr, NADP, DNA, RNA, and cell membranes	Osteoporosis, brittle bones, muscle weakness, and muscle cramps	Impaired iron, zinc, and copper absorption; impaired calcium metabolism
Sodium	Promotes blood volume homeostasis, nerve impulse generation, muscle contraction, acid-base balance	Hyponatremia, dizziness, coma, muscle cramps, nausea, vomiting, loss of appetite, and seizures	Hypertension and nausea
Sulfur	Acid-base balance; liver function	Unknown and very unlikely to occur	Unknown

In rare instances chlorine deficiency can be caused by excess vomiting.

[a]In conjunction with excess sodium.

Table 9.7 The Major Functions of Microminerals (Trace Elements) and the Effects of Dietary Deficiency or Excess

Micromineral	Major roles in body	Effect of deficiency	Effect of excess
Chromium	Augments insulin action	Glucose intolerance, and impaired lipid metabolism	Rare toxic effects
Cobalt	Forms component of vitamin B_{12} needed for red blood cell development	Pernicious anemia	Nausea, vomiting, and death
Copper	Promotes normal iron absorption, oxidative metabolism, connective tissue formation, and hemoglobin synthesis; forms cofactor with superoxide dismutase	Anemia, impaired immune function, and bone demineralization	Nausea and vomiting
Fluorine	Promotes bone and teeth formation	Dental caries	Discolored teeth, inhibited glycolysis in high doses
Iodine	Forms component of thyroid hormones T3 and T4	Goiter and reduced metabolic rate	Depressed thyroid gland activity
Iron	Transports oxygen as hemoglobin and myoglobin; forms cytochromes and metalloenzymes; promotes immune function	Anemia, fatigue, and increased infections	Hemochromatosis, liver cirrhosis, heart disease, and increased infections

(continued)

Table 9.7 (continued)

Micromineral	Major roles in body	Effect of deficiency	Effect of excess
Manganese	Forms cofactor with energy metabolism enzymes; promotes bone formation and fat synthesis	Poor growth	Weakness and confusion
Molybdenum	Forms cofactor with riboflavin in carbohydrate and fat metabolism enzymes	No deficiency effects	Rare toxic effects
Selenium	Forms cofactor with glutathione peroxidase	Cardiomyopathy, cancer, heart disease, impaired immune function, and erythrocyte fragility	Nausea, vomiting, fatigue, and hair loss
Zinc	Forms metalloenzymes; promotes protein synthesis, immune function, tissue repair, energy metabolism, and antioxidant activity	Impaired growth, impaired healing, increased infections, and anorexia	Impaired absorption of Fe and Cu, increased HDL cholesterol/LDL cholesterol ratio, anemia, nausea, vomiting, and impaired immunity

Table 9.8 Sources and Recommended Daily Allowances or Adequate Intakes of Macrominerals for Adults 19 to 50 Years of Age

Macromineral	Sources	RDA or AI*	Percent absorbed
Calcium	Dairy products, egg yolk, beans and peas, dark-green vegetables, and cauliflower	1,000 mg* (M, F)	30–40
Chlorine	Meat, fish, bread, canned foods, table salt, beans, and milk	750 mg** (M, F)	90–99
Magnesium	Seafood, nuts, green leafy vegetables, fruits, whole-grain products, milk, and yogurt	420 mg (M); 320 mg (F)	25–60
Potassium	Meat, fish, milk, yogurt, fruit, vegetables, and bread	2,000 mg** (M, F)	90–99
Phosphorus	Meat, eggs, fish, milk, cheese, beans, peas, whole-grain products, soft drinks	700 mg (M, F)	80–90
Sodium	Meat, fish, bread, canned foods, table salt, sauces, and pickles	420 mg** (M) 320 mg** (F)	90–99

RDA = Recommended Daily Allowance; AI* = Adequate Intake. AI** = Estimated requirement. M= males; F = females.

Also shown is the proportion of the ingested amount that is absorbed; the remainder is excreted in the feces.

Table 9.9 Sources and Recommended Daily Allowances or Adequate Intakes of Microminerals for Adults 19 to 50 Years of Age

Micromineral	Sources	RDA or AI*	Percent absorbed
Chromium	Liver, kidney, meat, oysters, cheese, whole-grain products, beer, asparagus, mushrooms, nuts, and stainless steel cookware	35 µg* (M) 25 µg* (F)	<1
Cobalt	Meat, liver, and milk	As part of vitamin B_{12}	

(continued)

Table 9.9 (continued)

Micromineral	Sources	RDA or AI*	Percent absorbed
Copper	Liver, kidney, shellfish, meat, fish, poultry, eggs, bran cereals, nuts, legumes, broccoli, banana, avocado, and chocolate	0.9 mg (M, F)	20–50
Fluorine	Milk, egg yolk, seafood, and drinking water	4 mg* (M) 3 mg* (F)	
Iodine	Iodized salt, seafood, and vegetables	150 µg (M, F)	
Iron	Liver, kidney, eggs, red meats, seafood, oysters, bread, flour, molasses, dried legumes, nuts, leafy green vegetables, broccoli, figs, raisins, and cocoa	8 mg (M) 18 mg (F)	10–30 (heme iron) 2–10 (nonheme iron)
Manganese	Whole grains, peas and beans, leafy vegetables, and bananas	2.3 mg* (M) 1.8 mg*(F)	
Molybdenum	Liver, kidney, whole-grain products, beans, and peas	45 µg (M, F)	
Selenium	Meat, liver, kidney, poultry, fish, dairy produce, seafood, whole grains, and nuts from selenium-rich soil	55 µg (M, F)	
Zinc	Oysters, shellfish, beef, liver, poultry, dairy products, whole grains, vegetables, asparagus, and spinach	11 mg (M) 8 mg (F)	20–50

RDA = Recommended daily allowance; AI* = adequate intake. M = males; F = females.

Also shown (where known) is the proportion of the ingested amount that is absorbed; the remainder is excreted in the feces.

Table 9.10 Adult Total-Body Content and Body Fluid Concentrations of Microminerals (Trace Elements)

Micromineral	Symbol	Atomic weight	Total amount in body (mg)	Body fluid concentration (mg/L)ᵃ		
				Plasma	Sweat	Urine
Chromium	Cr	52	6			
Cobalt	Co	59	<1			
Copper	Cu	64	100	0.7–1.7	0.2–0.6	0.03–0.04
Fluorine	F	19	2,500			
Iodine	I	127	11			
Iron	Fe	56	5,000	0.4–1.4	0.3–0.4	0.1–0.15
Manganese	Mn	55	12			
Molybdenum	Mo	96	9			
Selenium	Se	79	13			
Zinc	Zn	65	2,000	0.7–1.3	0.7–1.3	0.2–0.5

* Electrolyte concentrations in interstitial fluid are virtually identical to those in plasma.

ᵃValues only shown where concentration of mineral is greater than 0.1 mg/L.

copper) may occur after prolonged exercise, mainly because of a redistribution of the mineral to other tissue compartments (e.g., erythrocytes and leukocytes) or because of the release of proteins from liver and neutrophils that chelate (bind) the mineral as part of the acute-phase response to inflammation (see figure 9.4). Regular exercise, particularly in a hot environment, incurs increased losses of several minerals in sweat and urine, which means that the daily requirement for most minerals is increased in

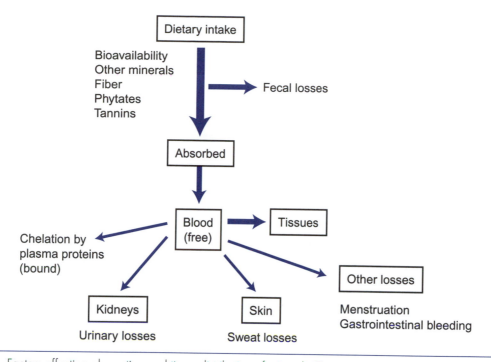

Figure 9.4 Factors affecting absorption and tissue distribution of minerals. Exercise may increase losses of minerals in urine and sweat, and several other components of the diet may interfere with mineral absorption.

athletes engaged in heavy training. However, with the exception of iron and zinc, isolated mineral deficiencies are rare.

Iron losses in sweat may be as high as 0.3 mg iron/ L of sweat (see table 9.10). When an athlete exercises hard in a hot environment, sweat production could well be about 2 L/h. If the athlete exercises for 2 hours a day in such conditions, the additional daily sweat loss is 4 L, which incurs a loss of 1.2 mg of iron. Because, on average, only about 10% of dietary iron can be absorbed in the gut, to replace this additional loss of iron, about 12 mg of extra iron must be consumed in food. The RDA for iron for men is 8 mg (18 mg for females), so the sweat losses under these conditions approximately doubles the dietary requirement for iron.

However, controversy exists regarding iron losses in sweat and whether athletes can lose enough iron in sweat to cause iron deficiency. In a careful study that minimized iron loss in shedded skin cells and iron contamination of skin, a much lower iron concentration in sweat (averaging only 23 µg /L) was reported (Brune et al. 1986). The most recent study of exercising athletes (Waller and Haymes 1996) also suggests that losses of iron in sweat are modest and, furthermore, that the concentration of iron in sweat declines over time (at least during the first hour of exercise). These authors estimated that about 6% to 11% of the iron typically absorbed each day is lost in sweat during an hour of exercise and that losses

for men are approximately twice those for women because of the higher sweat rate in men.

Exercise may further increase the requirement for iron because of the adaptive increase in muscle myoglobin concentration and red cell mass in response to endurance training (Eichner 2000). Some athletes are susceptible to gastrointestinal bleeding during prolonged strenuous exercise. About 20% of recreational runners are estimated to experience occult fecal blood after distance races. Bleeding may arise because of irritation of the stomach lining or superficial hemorrhage of the colon caused by ischemic insult (i.e., restricted blood supply because of constriction of blood vessels supplying the tissue). During strenuous exercise, blood is diverted to the working muscles, and when exercise is prolonged (and particularly when accompanied by dehydration and hyperthermia), the restriction of blood flow to the colon may cause inflammation and blood vessel damage, a condition called segmental hemorrhagic colitis (Eichner 2000). Measurement of fecal iron loss in elite male distance runners showed that during training and racing, gastrointestinal blood loss amounted to about 6 ml/day (Nachtigall et al. 1996).

Substantial amounts of magnesium are lost in sweat (see table 9.5), and increased urinary losses of both magnesium and zinc have been reported in athletes engaged in high-intensity exercise. These additional losses, if not matched by increased dietary intakes could cause magnesium and zinc deficiency with chronic training. Several studies report lower resting serum concentrations of magnesium and zinc in athletes compared with sedentary control subjects, but serum levels of these minerals for athletes were still within the accepted normal ranges.

Dietary Surveys of Mineral Intakes in Elite Athletes

The interpretation of dietary records for adequacy of mineral (particularly, trace element) intake should be done with some caution. This assessment is difficult because of the differences in the bioavailability of trace elements in various foods and because not all foods have been analyzed for their mineral composition. Furthermore, assessment of a person's mineral status based on a chemical analysis of blood or biopsy samples is not always possible. In many cases, the plasma concentration of a particular mineral does not give an accurate reflection of the body stores of the mineral. Given those limitations, information based on dietary surveys of athletes and their blood chemistry suggests that iron, zinc, calcium, and magnesium status may be of some concern, especially for young athletes and women athletes of all ages.

Several groups of athletes may have low iron stores, including middle-distance and long-distance runners, female endurance athletes, and adolescent athletes. However, the proportion of athletes with low iron stores is no greater than that found in the general United States population, where the incidence of iron depletion (a serum ferritin level of less than 12 µg/L) is 21% of women and 25% of adolescent girls. The incidence of iron depletion in male athletes may be higher than for sedentary males, in whom iron deficiency is low (less than 2% of the male population in the United States). Males generally meet the RDA for calcium, but females, especially adolescents, do not. Young female athletes concerned with maintaining low body weights and low body fat, such as gymnasts, dancers, and runners, have low calcium intakes (Aulin 2000). The story is similar for zinc and magnesium: most male athletes appear to meet the RDA for these minerals, but many groups of female athletes do not. Limited information is available for other minerals, but reports of isolated trace element deficiencies in athletes, apart from iron and zinc, are extremely rare.

Micronutrients Form the Building Blocks of Tissues

Although vitamins are not structural components in body tissues, several minerals, including calcium, phosphorus, and fluorine are, particularly in bones and teeth. Vitamin D is required for the normal absorption of dietary calcium, and deficiency of this vitamin is associated with brittle bones. Vitamin C is required for normal production of collagen and, hence, is important for the maintenance of healthy connective tissue and cartilage.

The mineral in bone is calcium phosphate crystalline salts in the form of hydroxyapatite. Bone matrix is a mixture of collagen fibers, which resist pulling forces, and solid hydroxyapatite crystals, which resist compression. Bone tissue is not metabolically inert. Even in adults, bone undergoes continuous turnover and remodeling of the matrix with simultaneous release and uptake of calcium. The cells involved in bone formation are osteoblasts, and the cells responsible for breakdown (demineralization) are osteoclasts (see figure 9.5). When the rate of demineralization exceeds the rate of bone formation, osteoporosis, a weakening of the bone structure, occurs.

The hormones calcitonin and parathyroid hormone (PTH) are principally involved in the regulation of calcium metabolism in bone tissue, and their main actions are shown in figure 9.5. PTH stimulates bone demineralization when calcium levels in blood are low. PTH and ultraviolet radiation from sunlight also stimulate production in the skin of the active form of vitamin D, which promotes the uptake of calcium in the small intestine. Calcitonin is released from the thyroid gland and stimulates bone formation when the plasma concentration of calcium rises.

Calcium intake influences the development of osteoporosis. Among different groups of athletes, calcium intakes are closely related to total-energy intakes (see figure 9.6). Other factors that influence the development of osteoporosis are estrogen levels, alcohol and caffeine intake, family history, female gender, and the amount and type of physical activity (Aulin 2000). Emphasis in the prevention of osteoporosis should be on maximizing the body's stores of calcium at an early age and minimizing calcium loss. A calcium intake of 1,000 mg/day to 1,300 mg/day is recommended to protect against the development of osteoporosis. The performance of regular weight-bearing activity promotes the deposition of calcium in bone.

Several groups of athletes can be identified as possibly having insufficient calcium intake (see table 9.11) and, hence, having an increased risk of osteoporosis. The absence of menstruation (amenorrhea) or infrequent menstruation (oligomenorrhea), which are commonly associated with low levels of body fat, low energy intakes, and high physical activity (especially gymnastics, swimming, and long-distance running) is associated with a high risk of early osteoporosis

Figure 9.5 Bone formation and demineralization in calcium homeostasis.

Figure 9.6 The relationship between mean intake of dietary energy and calcium intake in male (crosses) and female (open squares) athletes. Each point represents a mean value for a group.

From A.M. Van Erp-Baart, W.H. Saris, R.A. Binkhorst, J.A. Vos, and J.W. Elvers, "Nationwide survey on nutritional habits in elite athletes," 1989, *International Journal of Sports Medicine* Vol. 10: S3-S10. Reprinted by permission.

because of the chronically low plasma estrogen levels (Aulin 2000). This condition, which forms part of the "female athlete triad" syndrome and can be precipitated by eating disorders, is dealt with in more detail in chapter 12. The steroid hormone estrogen promotes bone formation in females; in males, the hormone testosterone assumes this role. In young female athletes, amenorrhea may hinder bone growth at a time when bone should be forming at its maximum rate. Side effects, such as the increased risk of stress fractures,

could hinder athletic performance as well as cause potentially debilitating problems later in life. When amenorrhea is present, increasing the consumption of calcium to 120% of the RDA appears to help bones to maintain density and develop properly.

Such nutrition guidance should be given to low-body-weight amenorrheic women. Weight conscious athletes (e.g., gymnasts) may markedly reduce their consumption of dairy products to decrease their intake of dietary fat. However, because the main

Table 9.11 Risk Factors for Marginal Mineral Nutrition in Athletes

Conditions and causes	Sports
Low body weight—chronically low energy intakes to achieve low body weight	Gymnastics, jockeys, ballet, ice dancing, and dancing
Making competition weight—drastic weight-loss regimens to achieve desired weight category	Weight class sports (rowing, wrestling, boxing, and judo)
Low fat—drastic weight-loss regimens to achieve low body fat	Bodybuilding
Vegetarian diets	Endurance events
Training in hot humid climate	Endurance events

sources of calcium are milk, butter, and cheese, their intake of calcium may fall considerably below the RDA. Most low-fat dairy products (e.g., skimmed milk) contain similar amounts of calcium as the full-fat dairy product, so athletes should be encouraged to include low-fat dairy products in their diet to preserve calcium intake.

Phosphorus, in the form of phosphate salts, is the other major inorganic constituent of bones and teeth. The adult male body contains about 850 g of phosphorus, of which 80% is found in bone. Phosphorus is also found as a component of nucleic acids (DNA and RNA) and phospholipids, which form the lipid bilayer of cell membranes. The RDA for adolescents and young adults (aged 9 years to 18 years) is 1,250 mg of phosphorus; for persons older than 19 years, the requirement is 700 mg. Phosphorus deficiency is very rare because many food items contain substantial amounts of it.

Fluorine is necessary for the normal formation of healthy bones and teeth, and it protects against dental caries (tooth decay by oral bacteria). Frequent intakes of soft drinks and carbohydrates—particularly sugars—depress the pH in the mouth and cause a net demineralization of the teeth. Sugars in the mouth are metabolized to organic acids by bacteria in plaque. Given the relatively high intake of sugary foods and sports drinks by athletes, good oral hygiene and plaque control are very important. The RDA for fluorine is 3 mg/day to 4 mg/day, and this trace element is found in milk, egg yolk, and seafood. Several toothpastes and mouth rinses contain fluorine (as sodium fluoride), and in some countries, including the United States, fluoride is added to drinking water. Excess intake of fluoride is poisonous because of its inhibitory effects on a number of enzymes, including some of the enzymes of glycolysis.

Several other trace elements have been suggested to be capable of increasing lean-body mass. Boron

supplementation has been reported to increase the serum estrogen and testosterone concentrations in postmenopausal women; subsequent studies found no effect on serum testosterone, lean-body mass, or muscle strength in male athletes who took boron supplements. Chromium is also claimed to increase lean-body mass, through potentiating insulin action. Insulin promotes glucose and amino acid uptake into muscle and stimulates muscle protein synthesis. However, the majority of studies show that chromium supplements are not effective in increasing lean-body mass, and chromium supplementation is accompanied by increased urinary excretion of chromium. Chromium stores are unlikely to be inadequate in individuals consuming a well-balanced diet, because chromium is widely available in fruits, vegetables, cereals, and organ meats.

Vanadium appears to increase tissue sensitivity to insulin in individuals suffering from type II (non–insulin-dependent) diabetes, but to date, no studies have established whether vanadium compounds exhibit insulinlike actions, such as promoting muscle protein and glycogen synthesis. A study showed no effect of vanadium on insulin sensitivity in healthy individuals assessed by an oral glucose tolerance test (Jentjens and Jeukendrup 2002). (See chapter 10 for details of studies that have investigated the effects of boron, chromium, and vanadium supplementation.)

Micronutrients As Antioxidants

Antioxidants prevent or limit the actions of free radicals, usually by removing their unpaired electron and, thus, converting them into something far less reactive. Vitamins with antioxidant properties (including vitamins C, E, and β-carotene [provitamin

A]) may be required in increased quantities in athletes to inactivate the products of exercise-induced increased free-radical formation and **lipid peroxidation.** Free radicals damage membranes, proteins, and DNA. Damage to DNA could result in mutations that cause cancer. Several minerals (including selenium, copper, and manganese) are components of antioxidant enzymes involved in the defense against free radicals. Increased intakes of antioxidant vitamins and other antioxidant compounds have been suggested to reduce the extent of exercise-induced muscle damage, although present evidence is not convincing, so more studies of the effects of antioxidants on exercise-induced muscle soreness and damage are needed.

Antioxidant Protection Against Exercise-Induced Skeletal Muscle Damage

Unaccustomed exercise or muscle activity that involves eccentric actions (lengthening of the muscle during activation) can damage some of the myofibers. Such exercises include downhill running, bench stepping, and lowering of weights. The consequences of exercise-induced muscle damage include muscle pain, soreness, and stiffness; reduced range of motion; higher than normal blood lactate concentration and perceived exertion during exercise; and loss of strength and reduced maximal dynamic power output that can last 5 days to 10 days. Exercise-induced muscle damage also impairs the restoration of muscle glycogen stores. Damaged muscle has an impaired ability to take up glucose from the blood, which is required to resynthesize glycogen in the muscle. This condition results in decreased endurance performance in subsequent exercise bouts.

A practical index of muscle damage in athletes performing heavy training is elevated muscle proteins (e.g., myoglobin, creatine kinase [CK], or lactate dehydrogenase) in the blood plasma. The damaged muscle tissue causes an initial activation of the immune system, as white blood cells are attracted to the damaged muscles to begin breakdown of damaged fibers and initiate the repair process. This process involves the production of free radical **reactive oxygen species** (ROS) by the invading leukocytes. Growing evidence indicates that ROS is an underlying cause of disrupted muscle homeostasis, muscle soreness, and elevated CK activity in eccentric type exercise. ROS can also cause oxidative damage to DNA and proteins, including enzymes.

Reactive Oxygen Species and Other Free Radicals

In normal cellular metabolism, ROS are produced during the aerobic process by which humans and animals derive energy from the mitochondria. In the electron-transport chain, located on the inner mitochondrial membrane, 95% to 97% of all the oxygen consumed by cells is reduced via cytochrome oxidase to yield water (and energy that is used to resynthesize ATP from ADP and Pi). The remaining 3% to 5% of oxygen consumed at rest can be used in an alternate pathway for the univalent reduction of oxygen, and, thus, ROS are produced. One free-radical molecule can start a destructive process by removing electrons from stable compounds, such as polyunsaturated FAs, and forming large numbers of ROS, thereby transforming stable compounds into highly reactive free radicals.

Additional sources of ROS and other free radicals are ultraviolet light, alcohol, cigarette smoke, high-fat diets, and the respiratory burst of white blood cells, such as neutrophils and monocytes, that are capable of ingesting foreign material, including bacteria. The generation of ROS by the neutrophil respiratory burst is an essential mechanism of the host defense mechanism of the immune system for killing bacteria and clearing away damaged tissue. However, these ROS can also initiate damaging chain reactions, such as lipid peroxidation, and the subsequent release of large numbers of ROS. In addition to the mitochondria respiratory chain producing free radicals during whole-body eccentric exercise, invading neutrophils and monocytes are thought to be important sources of oxidative stress. Several inflammatory diseases have been associated with increased generation of ROS by monocytes. Migration of neutrophils into damaged muscle tissue occurs within the first hour after eccentric exercise and is followed by infiltration of monocytes and macrophages, reaching a maximum at 24 hours to 72 hours after exercise.

Increases in the free iron concentration of body fluids (caused, for example, by hemolysis or ischemia-reperfusion) may amplify ROS toxicity by increasing the generation of the highly reactive hydroxyl radical. Ferric iron (Fe^{3+}) ions can stimulate free-radical reactions by breaking down lipid peroxides to chain-breaking alkoxyl radicals, and ferrous (Fe^{2+}) ions can react with H_2O_2 to give $\cdot OH$ and other highly reactive species in what is called a Fenton reaction:

$$Fe^{2+} + H_2O_2 \rightarrow Fe^{3+} + \cdot OH + OH^-$$

The hydroxyl radical can also be formed through the Haber-Weiss reaction:

$$Fe^{2+} + H_2O_2 + \cdot O_2^- \rightarrow Fe^{3+} + \cdot OH + OH^- + O_2$$

This potential is one of the reasons why iron supplements should not be recommended indiscriminately. Individuals with higher than normal iron stores seem to be at increased risk for cancer, stroke, and coronary heart disease. Because free radicals have been implicated in the etiology of these diseases, an excess of iron could potentiate their adverse effects.

Antioxidant Mechanisms

An antioxidant is a compound that protects biological systems against the harmful effects or reactions that create excessive oxidants. Dietary antioxidants significantly decrease the adverse effects of ROS. Enzymatic and nonenzymatic antioxidants prevent oxidation initiated by ROS by

- preventing ROS formation,
- intercepting ROS attack by scavenging the reactive metabolites and converting them to less-reactive molecules,
- binding transition metal ion catalysts, such as copper and iron, to prevent initiation of free-radical reactions,
- reacting with chain-propagating radicals, such as the peroxyl and alkoyl species, to prevent continued hydrogen abstraction from FA side chains, and
- providing a favorable environment for the effective functioning of other antioxidants or

acting to regenerate the nonenzymatic antioxidant molecules.

Antioxidant enzymes can affect free-radical generation at both the initiation and propagation stage. The antioxidant enzymes superoxide dismutase (SOD) and catalase can inhibit the initial phase by inactivating precursor molecules of ROS production (see figure 9.7). At the propagation stage, glutathione peroxidase—another antioxidant enzyme—can scavenge $\cdot OH$ and lipid peroxides as described earlier. The trace elements copper and manganese are required as cofactors of SOD, and selenium is also a component of antioxidant defense because it is a cofactor of glutathione peroxidase/reductase and, thus, influences the quenching of ROS. The effects of exercise on manganese and selenium status are presently unknown, but training is associated with an increase in levels of antioxidant enzymes, suggesting that there may be an increased requirement for these trace elements during periods of increased training. As with other minerals, losses of manganese and selenium in urine and sweat are likely higher in athletes than in nonathletes. However, any supplements should be taken with caution. Selenium supplements of amounts up to the RDA appear nontoxic, yet the safety of larger doses has not been confirmed, and intakes of 25 mg (approximately $40 \times$ RDA) have been associated with vomiting, abdominal pain, hair loss, and fatigue.

In addition to the enzyme defense system, some low-molecular-weight substances act as scavengers

Figure 9.7 The antioxidant action cascade.

of radicals. These substances include vitamins A, C, and E; carotenoids such as β-carotene; and compounds such as plant **polyphenols**. Fat-soluble vitamin E is a chain-breaking free-radical scavenger and is particularly effective at preventing initiation and propagation of lipid peroxidation in cellular membranes and, thus, maintaining membrane stability. Water-soluble vitamin C is capable of regenerating vitamin E in the antioxidant cascade as illustrated in figure 9.7.

Polyphenol compounds scavenge peroxyl, superoxide, and nitric oxide radicals. Rich sources of polyphenols include tea, wine (particularly red wine), fruits, and vegetables. Flavonoids, a subclass of polyphenols that includes the flavonols, flavonones, and anthocyanidins contain a number of phenolic hydroxyl (-OH) groups attached to ring structures that confer their antioxidant activity. Differences in the antioxidant power of individual flavonoids result from the variation in the number and arrangement of the hydroxyl groups, as well as extent and nature of the glycolation of these groups. Flavonoids are reported to inhibit the enzyme lipoxygenase and to inhibit oxidant generation by neutrophils in a manner similar to vitamin E. As with vitamin E, the antioxidant power of the flavonoids results from donating a hydrogen atom from a hydroxyl moiety. However, studies in chemical systems show flavonoids to be 3 to 10 times more effective than vitamin E in their scavenging abilities. In addition they may have anti-inflammatory effects. Flavonoids are used clinically to decrease inflammation and endothelial damage in diseases in which free radicals play a major role.

FREE RADICALS AND ANTIOXIDANT STUDIES

Several studies have attempted to determine whether pretreatment with antioxidants can reduce or alter the time course of eccentric exercise-induced muscle damage. In an animal study, mice treated with superoxide dismutase (SOD), the antioxidant enzyme involved in the elimination of the superoxide radical, showed smaller reductions in muscle force output 3 days after eccentric exercise (Zerba et al. 1990). The finding that SOD reduced loss of muscle function supports the role of free radicals in eccentric contraction–induced damage. However, muscle levels of SOD and free-radical activity were not measured in this study. Furthermore, force reduction in mice given SOD supplements was only found in older mice. Endogenous levels of protective antioxidant enzymes decline with age (Meydani et al. 1993). These studies suggest that older humans and animals have an increased susceptibility to muscle damage with increasing age. Similarly, Cannon et al. (1990) compared the effect of an antioxidant supplement with a placebo treatment in two age groups (younger than 30 years and older than 55 years) using downhill running as the muscle-damaging exercise protocol. The authors found that vitamin E supplementation eliminated the differences between the two age groups.

Maughan et al. (1989) measured serum lipid peroxide concentration as total thiobarituric acid-reactive substances (TBARS) and found that subjects with the greatest increase in serum CK showed the highest TBARS concentrations, suggesting that free-radical reactions and subsequent loss of membrane integrity could be responsible for the release of muscle-derived enzymes into the circulation. However, although TBARS may be a useful indicator of free-radical damage, methodological difficulties mean that care should be taken when interpreting results of such studies. One of the problems of free-radical research has been the difficulty in directly measuring free-radical activity, particularly in vivo (see Duthie [1999] for a review). However, these indirect measures of free-radical activity suggest that free radicals are formed during exercise.

Although free radicals are difficult to detect directly, electron spin resonance (ESR) has been used to try and measure increased free-radical production. Davies et al. (1982) observed a 2-fold to 3-fold increase in ROS concentration in the muscles and liver after exercise to exhaustion in rats. More recent studies support these findings. Fielding et al. (1993) demonstrated a relationship between neutrophil infiltration, ultrastructural damage, and increased muscle membrane permeability after downhill running in humans. Postexercise muscle infiltration and in vitro neutrophil superoxide generation were closely related to the time course of release of CK into the circulation and muscle ultrastructural damage. These events may be causally related to other symptoms of muscle damage, such as loss of muscle strength and muscle soreness.

(continued)

(continued)

A study by Jackson (2000) reported that dietary vitamin E deficiency in rats increased the susceptibility of skeletal muscles to contractile damage as indicated by CK release, but rats supplemented with 240 mg/kg/day of vitamin E exhibited lower CK release after a downhill run. Moreover, the peak CK activity in serum was significantly correlated to neutrophil superoxide release. In contrast, Van Der Meulen et al. (1997) found that 5 days to 8 days of intravenous injections in mice increased vitamin E content threefold but did not alter the extent of eccentric exercise-induced muscle damage in situ. Moreover, vitamin E did not alter the force deficit or change the percentage of muscle fibers damaged. However, in the same study, postexercise CK levels were significantly reduced with vitamin E injections, suggesting that vitamin E may help to reduce membrane damage related to enzyme efflux but may not alter other indices of muscle damage induced by eccentric contractions. However, neither antioxidant capacity nor ROS production was measured in these studies.

Warren et al. (1992) investigated rat muscle susceptibility to oxidative stress and observed lower CK release in a group given vitamin E supplements compared with a control group. Although force loss was similar in both groups, the susceptibility of the muscles to oxidant stress was decreased after supplementation. The authors concluded that vitamin E supplementation may be useful in reducing free-radical damage, but muscle-fiber damage caused by eccentric exercise does not appear to be altered by vitamin E supplementation.

Several human studies have also shown contrasting findings. Cannon et al. (1990) reported that vitamin E (400 IU/day) for 48 days increased the amount of CK in the plasma of subjects older than 55 years. Moreover, plasma CK activity correlated with superoxide release from neutrophils at the time of peak CK levels; however, significant increases in plasma lipid peroxides were not observed. Cannon et al. (1990) concluded that free radicals are involved with the delayed increase in muscle-membrane permeability after damaging exercise but are not involved in the initial injury.

Meydani et al. (1993) studied the effects of a 45-minute run at 75% of maximal heart rate. The subjects were given either a placebo or vitamin E (800 IU) for 48 days before the exercise. Those given the vitamin E supplement decreased production of urinary TBARS after eccentric exercise, which suggested that vitamin E reduced free radical–mediated damage. However, the reliability of TBARS as a measure of lipid peroxidation has been questioned. Kaminiski and Boal (1992) studied the effect of vitamin C supplementation for 7 days after exercise in a double-blind crossover trial. Although this study noted that vitamin C treatment reduced muscle damage, as indicated by muscle soreness, it did not measure any biochemical markers of muscle damage, and a carryover effect from the previous bout of exercise was likely.

Because of the inconsistent and often contradictory findings, whether antioxidant vitamins are helpful in reducing free radical–mediated damage is not clear. These conflicts may be the result of different indices of muscle damage being measured, variations in mode and intensity of exercise, previous training, the dose and the length of time of supplementation, and the ages of the subjects. However, antioxidants react with free radicals and deactivate them, lowering the amount of ROS produced and, therefore, may reduce or prevent muscle damage. By reducing the initial damage, reducing the later infiltration of neutrophils and macrophages could be possible.

Flavonoids and Free Radicals

Some flavonoids are excellent scavengers of free radicals such as $\cdot O_2^-$ and $\cdot OH$. All subgroups of flavonoids decrease oxidant-induced lipid peroxidation and membrane permeability to potassium ions in isolated human erythrocytes (Meydani et al. 1993). Therefore, the ability of these compounds to chelate metal ions and prevent free-radical formation suggests that they may play an important protective role. In addition, flavonoids are also scavengers of the $\cdot NO$ radical.

The $\cdot NO$ radical generated by inflammatory cells is reported to be toxic after reaction with the $\cdot O_2^-$ radical. Scavenging $\cdot NO$ radicals could therefore contribute to the proposed beneficial effect of the flavonoids.

Arteriosclerosis begins in a process in which $\cdot NO$ radicals play an unfavorable role, which adds additional weight to the possibility that flavonoids reduce the risk of coronary heart disease (CHD) (Acker et al. 1995). Further support for this possibility was provided by the Dutch Zutphen Elderly study, which showed an inverse correlation between intakes of flavonoids and incidence of CHD (Hertog et al. 1993). Moreover, a higher flavonoid intake from red wine may explain why the French have a lower mortality from CHD compared with the British, despite the fact that the consumption of saturated fat in France is greater than that in the UK.

However, the in vivo evidence for a protective effect of increased flavonoid intake is limited. The antioxidant capacity of plasma is increased in response to the oral ingestion of phenol-rich beverages, such as red wine and teas. Polyphenols are rapidly absorbed, and peak plasma concentrations are reached within 1 hour of consuming nonalcoholic red wine. In vitro studies have demonstrated that alcohol-free red wine displays a stronger antioxidant activity than does alcohol-free white wine, and the only consistent chemical difference between the two wines is the phenol content, which is 20 times higher in red wine than in white wine. The higher phenol content results from the incorporation of the grape skins into the fermented grape juice during production of red wine. White wine production does not use the grape skins, only the fermented grape juice. The biological actions of phenols may add significantly to the suggested protective effects of increased consumption of fruits and vegetables, such as the reduced risk of various cancers and CHD. Indeed, red wine inhibits LDL oxidation in vitro and reduces the susceptibility of plasma components to lipid peroxidation.

Possible Risks of High-Dose Antioxidant Supplementation

Antioxidants obviously provide some defense against the damaging effects of free radicals. This information, together with recent media attention on the effects of dietary and supplemental vitamins C, E, and carotenoids in preventing CHD and some forms of cancer, has prompted many individuals to take large doses of these vitamins. However, excessive antioxidant ingestion may not be uniformly helpful. For example, in heavy smokers, increased intake of vitamin E and β-carotene actually increases the incidence of lung cancer (Blot 1997; De Luca and Ross 1996). One possible reason for this effect is that antioxidants may interfere with important processes needed to kill cancer cells. Administration of antioxidants inhibits apoptosis (cell death), an important defense mechanism that inhibits tumor development by eliminating new mutated cells. ROS are intermediate messengers in several apoptosis signaling pathways. So excess antioxidants may effectively "shoot the messengers." Thus, in situations where individuals have damaged their DNA (e.g., by heavy smoking or by exercise)

the administration of antioxidants may prevent the effective removal of damaged cells.

Some side effects are associated with consuming excessive amounts of individual antioxidant vitamins. Very large doses of vitamin C are associated with urinary stone formation and impaired copper absorption. Excess intakes of vitamin A by pregnant women can cause birth defects. Large intakes of vitamin E can impair absorption of vitamins A and K. Thus, more is not always better.

The controversy continues as to whether physically active individuals should consume large amounts of antioxidant compounds. At present, the data are insufficient to strongly recommend antioxidant supplements for athletes. Further research is needed to fully document the efficacy and safety of long-term antioxidant use. Some facts may help athletes come to a decision on whether or not to supplement with antioxidants:

- Numerous studies indicate that the body's natural antioxidant defense system is upregulated as an adaptation to exercise training.
- Antioxidant supplementation does not improve exercise performance.
- People who exercise regularly have a lower incidence of CHD, obesity, diabetes, and some (though not all) types of cancer compared with sedentary individuals, suggesting that the benefits of regular physical exercise outweigh the risks of free radical–mediated damage.
- Megadoses of antioxidant vitamins can have undesirable side effects in some individuals.
- Athletes should consume a natural diet that is rich in antioxidants.

Essential Functions of the Micronutrients

Micronutrients perform or are associated with a variety of functions essential to the maintenance of life and health, including oxygen transport, enzyme-catalyzed reactions, immunity, and electrolytes.

Oxygen Transport

Iron, as a component of hemoglobin, myoglobin, and cytochromes, is essential for oxidative metabolism. Hemoglobin is the protein in red blood cells that transports oxygen. Myoglobin is the respiratory pigment found inside the muscle fibers. The cytochromes are components of the electron-transport chain located on the inner mitochondrial membrane.

Thus, iron is essential for both oxygen transport and utilization. In addition to the iron in the "functional compartment"—mainly in hemoglobin and myoglobin—about one-fourth, or 1,000 mg, of the total-body iron content in adult males is in storage. In contrast, iron stores are typically lower in adult women (300 mg to 500 mg), even lower in 18-year-old to 21-year-old women (<200 mg), and virtually absent in adolescents and young children. Unlike most adult male athletes, female and adolescent athletes need a regular supply of dietary iron to maintain iron balance and avoid anemia.

The gradual depletion of iron from the body when dietary intake is inadequate is commonly referred to as "iron drain." This condition is thought to progress through a number of stages with different functional and diagnostic criteria, as described in table 9.12. Iron is stored in the body complexed with ferritin, a protein found mostly found in the liver, spleen, and bone marrow. Soluble ferritin is released from cells into the blood plasma in direct proportion to cellular ferritin content. Hence, the plasma, or serum, ferritin concentration can be used to indicate the status of the body's iron stores.

Iron depletion (low iron stores as evidenced by a serum ferritin concentration less than 12 μg/L) is common in female athletes (with a lesser incidence in male athletes), but whether this deficiency affects athletic performance in the absence of anemia remains controversial. Researchers have reported that depletion of the body's iron stores without anemia can be associated with increased lactate production during maximal exercise, indicative of a reduced oxygen utilization by working muscle, and can also be associated with an increased subjective feeling of exercise overload in elite athletes. A few studies indicate that some performance benefits may be obtained from iron supplementation in iron-depleted female athletes who are not anemic (Brownlie et al. 2002; Brutsaert et al. 2003). Furthermore, adaptations to endurance training, including improvements in maximal oxygen uptake and endurance performance, are enhanced by iron supplementation in iron-depleted, nonanemic women (Brownlie et al. 2002; Hinton et al. 2000).

Other studies have shown that $\dot{V}O_2$max, endurance performance, and muscle oxidative enzyme activity can be maintained even when the body iron stores are severely depleted. What seems certain is that if the condition should progress to a state of iron deficiency resulting in anemia (low blood hemoglobin concentration [see table 9.12]), athletic performance is negatively affected. At this stage, not enough iron is available in the bone marrow to manufacture normal amounts of hemoglobin and red blood cells, leading to the production of small, pale red blood cells.

Anemia lowers the oxygen-carrying capacity of the blood and reduces exercise performance. In severe cases of anemia, affected individuals report

Table 9.12 Stages of Iron Drain From Normal Iron Status Through to Iron Deficiency Anemia

Stage	Characteristics	Blood hemoglobin (g/L)	Serum ferritin (μg/L)	Serum transferrin saturation (%)
		Diagnostic criteria		
Normal iron status	Normal iron status measurements and normal appearance of RBCs	>120 (F) >140 (M)	>30 (F) >110 (M)	20–40 (M, F)
Iron depletion	Normal hematocrit and hemoglobin but low serum ferritin with normal to high transferrin saturation	>120 (F) >140 (M)	<30 (M, F)	20–40 (M, F)
Iron deficiency	Normal hemoglobin but low serum ferritin, iron, and transferrin; low transferrin saturation	>120 (F) >140 (M)	<12 (M, F)	<16 (M, F)
Iron deficiency anemia	Low hematocrit and hemoglobin; low serum ferritin, iron, and transferrin saturation; small and pale RBCs	<120 (F) <140 (M)	<10 (M, F)	<16 (M, F)

M = males; F = females. RBCs = red blood cells (erythrocytes). Hematocrit = packed cell volume (normal = 38%–45% [F], 42%–48% [M]). Serum iron concentration is normally 0.4 mg/L–1.4 mg/L. Characteristics of each stage and the associated diagnostic criteria are based on blood measures.

Adapted from V. Deakin, 2000, Iron depletion in athletes. In Clinical sports nutrition, edited by L. Burke and V. Deakin (McGraw-Hill Companies), 273-311.

sensations of breathlessness on mild exertion and generally feel so lethargic that they can no longer carry out everyday activities. Impaired functioning of several enzymes that require iron as a cofactor may result in mental dysfunction, impaired temperature control, and weakened immunity, which exacerbate the symptoms of reduced exercise tolerance.

Iron deficiency is reported to be the most widespread micronutrient deficiency in the world, and field studies consistently associate iron deficiency with increased morbidity from infectious disease. The incidence of iron-deficiency anemia is rare and is similar among athletes and the general population. The cause of anemia in athletes may be low energy intakes, insufficient iron intakes to maintain iron stores (see figure 9.8), or low meat intake (which provides the most readily available dietary source of iron).

Exercise may cause some hemolysis of red blood cells, alterations of iron metabolism, and increased losses in sweat and urine. In some susceptible individuals, additional losses caused by gastrointestinal bleeding may be incurred during prolonged strenuous exercise. The body adapts to endurance training by increasing the red blood cell mass and the myoglobin content of skeletal muscle. Altitude exposure causes an additional increase in red blood cell production. Hence, regular exercise increases the dietary requirement for iron.

The periodic screening of serum ferritin levels in athletes is recommended, as changes in the storage and transport of iron typically precede decreases in functional iron (hemoglobin) levels. During training, some athletes experience a transient fall in hemoglobin concentration and hematocrit, which is probably caused mostly by the increase in plasma volume that is commonly associated with the initiation of training or a sudden increase in the training load. This condition is sometimes called "sports anemia," and this form of hemodilutional iron deficiency has no apparent effect on exercise performance.

About 60% of iron in animal tissues is in the heme form; that is, iron associated with hemoglobin and myoglobin and thus is only found in animal foods. Nonheme iron is found in both animal and plant foods. Heme iron is absorbed better than nonheme iron. About 10% to 30% of ingested heme iron is absorbed in the gut, whereas only about 2% to 10% of nonheme iron is absorbed. The bioavailability of iron (and many minerals) is influenced by the form in which it is consumed.

Some substances found in foods may promote or inhibit absorption of minerals. For example, vitamin C prevents the oxidation of ferrous iron (Fe^{2+}) to ferric (Fe^{3+}). Because ferrous iron is more readily absorbed, vitamin C facilitates nonheme iron absorption but has no effect on heme iron absorption. Thus, drinking a glass of fresh orange juice improves the absorption of iron from bread or cereals. Some natural substances found in foods such as tannins (e.g., in tea), phosphates, phytates, oxalates, and excessive fiber may decrease the bioavailability of nonheme iron. Iron absorption is also a function of storage: the larger the stores, the poorer the absorption, and vice versa.

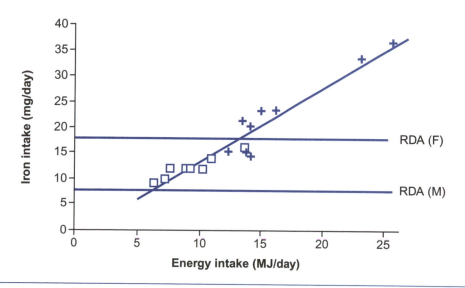

Figure 9.8 The relationship between mean intake of dietary energy and iron intake in male (crosses) and female (open squares) athletes. Each point represents a mean value for a group.

From A.M. Van Erp-Baart, W.H. Saris, R.A. Binkhorst, J.A. Vos, and J.W. Elvers, "Nationwide survey on nutritional habits in elite athletes," 1989, *International Journal of Sports Medicine* Vol. 10: S3-S10. Reprinted by permission.

Thus, individuals with inadequate stores have better absorption, regardless of the diet.

The low bioavailability of iron in vegetarian diets possibly contributes to lower serum ferritin levels in athletes consuming a modified vegetarian diet, and iron may also be short in a lactovegetarian diet because of the absence of heme iron. However, a number of studies have failed to find that exercise per se decreased iron status, although this failure may be attributed to the relatively low training volumes employed. The general consensus is that all athletes should include heme iron–rich foods such as lean red meat, poultry, and fish in their daily diets.

Because the losses of iron in feces, urine, and sweat are increased by prolonged bouts of exercise, most athletes need more iron in their diet than sedentary individuals. Weaver and Rajaram (1992) noted that iron losses may be around 70% higher in athletes compared with the reference value for sedentary people. However, iron intakes equivalent to twice the RDA can be achieved through consumption of a well-balanced diet sufficient to meet daily energy requirements. Studies on different groups of athletes have shown that iron intake is proportional to energy intake (see figure 9.8), such that athletes consuming in excess of 10 MJ/day (2400 kcal/day) from a varied food base will obtain the RDA of iron. Thus, endurance athletes who match their energy intake (from varied food sources) to their energy expenditure are likely to obtain more than enough iron. Those at risk for poor iron status are those athletes consuming low energy intakes or avoiding food sources rich in heme iron. Vegetarian athletes should ensure that plant food choices are iron-dense (e.g., green leafy vegetables). Breakfast cereals are usually fortified with iron and are a good source.

Megadoses of iron are not advised, and routine oral iron supplements should not be taken without medical supervision. Only after laboratory confirmation of very low iron status or iron-deficiency anemia should iron supplements be used. Prolonged consumption of large amounts of iron can cause a disturbance in iron metabolism in susceptible individuals, with an accumulation of iron in the liver. Hepatic iron accumulates as a compound called hemosiderin, which in excess can cause cell damage in the 0.3% of the population who are genetically predisposed. This condition causes cirrhosis and can be fatal. Excess intake of iron may also reduce absorption of other divalent cations, particularly zinc and copper. Groups at risk for insufficient iron intake who may be suitable candidates for iron supplementation include female endurance athletes, gymnasts, vegetarians, and those undergoing restricted energy intakes.

Anemia can also arise from deficiencies of vitamin B_6, vitamin B_{12}, folic acid, and copper. Vitamin B_6 is required for the synthesis of the porphyrin ring component of hemoglobin and myoglobin. Vitamin B_{12}, which contains the trace element cobalt, is required for the synthesis of nucleic acids, which are essential for the proliferation of stem cells that develop into red and white blood cells in the bone marrow. For the same reason, folic acid is also required for normal blood cell production. Deficiencies of these micronutrients are associated with megaloblastic or pernicious anemia, reduced blood leukocyte count, and impaired lymphocyte proliferation. Major food sources of vitamin B_{12} are meat, liver, and milk. Hence, athletes who avoid animal foods are at risk for cobalt/vitamin B_{12} deficiency. Some food products, notably breakfast cereals and milk, are fortified with vitamin B_{12}. For example, in the UK, 120 g of cornflakes, or alternatively, 40 g of cornflakes with 150 ml of pasteurized whole milk provides 1 μg of vitamin B_{12} (67% of the RNI). Copper is a cofactor of many enzymes and plays an important role in the formation of red blood cells.

Phosphorus, in addition to its function as a constituent of bones, teeth, and cell membranes, is also a component of 2,3, diphosphoglycerate (2,3-DPG), which is found predominantly in red blood cells. 2,3-DPG alters the affinity of hemoglobin for oxygen and promotes more effective unloading of oxygen from the erythrocytes in the tissue capillaries, where the partial pressure of oxygen is lower than in the arteries. In response to altitude exposure, the erythrocyte concentration of 2,3-DPG increases.

Cofactors in Enzyme Catalyzed Reactions

Many of the B vitamins are reusable coenzymes in energy metabolism, and some of their roles can be seen in figure 9.9. Niacin (B_3), pyridoxine (B_6), and thiamin (B_1) are involved in carbohydrate metabolism; riboflavin (B_2), thiamin, pantothenic acid, and biotin are involved in fat metabolism; and vitamin B_6 and vitamin K are involved in protein metabolism. Niacin is the precursor of the important coenzymes nicotinamide adenine dinucleotide (NAD) and nicotinamide adenine dinucleotide phosphate (NADP); riboflavin is the precursor of flavin adenine dinucleotide (FAD) and flavin mononucleotide (FMN). These nicotinamide and flavin nucleotides are involved in oxidation/reduction reactions in energy metabolism, including some of the reactions of glycolysis, the TCA cycle, and the electron-transport chain (see figure 9.9). Pantothenic acid is the precursor of coenzyme-A (CoA), which is essential for

Figure 9.9 B vitamins as precursors of coenzymes in energy metabolism. CoA = coenzyme A; FAD = flavin adenine dinucleotide; NAD = nicotinamide adenine dinucleotide; PLP = pyridoxal phosphate; TPP = thiamin pyrophosphate.

the processes involved in both carbohydrate and fat oxidation (see chapter 2). A deficiency of these vitamins can result in premature fatigue and inability to maintain a heavy training program.

Zinc serves either a structural or a catalytic role in more than 200 human enzymes. It is a cofactor of several enzymes involved in energy metabolism and is also required for normal cell replication, immune function, and wound healing. Some zinc-containing enzymes, such as carbonic anhydrase and lactate dehydrogenase, are involved in intermediary metabolism during exercise.

Studies have indicated that the intake of zinc among some groups of athletes (wrestlers, female endurance runners, and gymnasts) is considerably less than the RDA (11 mg/day and 8 mg/day for males and females, respectively). Prolonged exercise may cause significant losses of zinc and magnesium in sweat. Losses of these minerals in urine is also increased as a result of intensive training. The total amount of zinc in the human body is about 2 g, and most of it is in muscle (60%) and bone (30%). Hence, measurements of zinc concentrations in blood may not be very meaningful. Although losses of zinc in sweat and urine are increased in physically active individuals, no evidence indicates that these losses are sufficient to cause concern. Small amounts of zinc are present in many foods of both animal and plant origin, and no benefit of additional zinc supplements for health or performance has been established.

Magnesium is an essential cofactor for more than 300 enzymes involved in biosynthetic processes and energy metabolism. It is essential for the normal functioning of ATPases, including myosin ATPase involved in muscle contraction, and it is involved in glycogen breakdown, protein synthesis, and fat oxidation. Magnesium is also required for the maintenance of electrical potentials in muscles and nerves and so is important for normal neuromuscular coordination. The total body content of magnesium is about 25 g (see table 9.5). The RDA for magnesium is 420 mg/day for men and 320 mg/day for women; hence, magnesium is a macromineral rather than a trace element. The main dietary sources of magnesium are listed in table 9.8. Several studies have reported low serum magnesium concentrations in athletes, and prolonged strenuous exercise is associated with increased losses of magnesium in urine and sweat. Although, as with zinc and iron, a single bout of exercise is extremely unlikely to induce substantial magnesium losses, a state of mild magnesium deficiency could be induced during a period of heavy training, particularly in a warm environment where sweat losses are high.

Magnesium deficiency in both humans and animals is associated with neuromuscular abnormalities, including muscle weakness, cramps, and structural damage of muscle fibers and organelles. The abnormalities may be caused by an impairment of calcium homeostasis secondary to an oxygen free radical–induced alteration in the integrity of the membrane of the sarcoplasmic reticulum. A lack of magnesium may also be associated with a depletion of selenium and reduced glutathione peroxidase activity, which would be expected to increase the susceptibility to damage by free radicals. Hence, magnesium deficiency possibly potentiates exercise-induced muscle damage and stress responses, but direct evidence for activity this is lacking. Magnesium deficiency exacerbates the inflammatory state after ischemic insult to the myocardium, which may be caused by a substance P–mediated increase in the secretion of proinflammatory cytokines in the magnesium-deficient state.

Copper is a cofactor of many enzymes, including several oxidases, and appears to be needed for the proper use of iron. Copper plays an important role in energy metabolism and the synthesis of hemoglobin, catecholamines, and some peptide hormones. Copper is also required for the normal formation of erythrocytes and the development of connective tissue. The RDA for copper for adult men and women is 0.9 mg/day. Intakes up to 10 mg/day are safe, and toxicity from dietary copper ingestion is extremely rare. The main dietary sources of copper are shown in table 9.9. Even though copper deficiency is rare in humans, athletes who take zinc supplements may compromise the gastrointestinal absorption of copper because of the similar physicochemical properties of these 2 minerals. Athletes should also be aware that large doses of vitamin C can limit copper absorption.

The results of changes in copper status caused by exercise and training are controversial and perhaps reflect the inadequacy of measuring techniques or redistribution of copper between body compartments, although athletes have been reported to lose copper in sweat. Compared with sedentary control subjects, several groups of athletes have similar or higher resting blood levels of copper. Thus, the copper status of athletes seems to be normal. After an acute bout of prolonged exercise, the plasma copper concentration may rise or remain unchanged. One study reported a substantial increase in plasma copper concentration during the first 8 days of a 20-day running road race, and this elevation persisted for the remainder of the race. This increase was attributed to a rise in the production of ceruloplasmin by the liver as part of the acute-phase response. Ceruloplasmin is a gly-

coprotein that binds copper and is thought to exert a protective effect against cellular damage caused by free radicals. As explained previously, manganese and selenium are cofactors of the antioxidant enzymes superoxide dismutase and glutathione reductase/peroxidase, respectively.

Micronutrients in Immune Function and Resistance to Infection

Both heavy exercise and nutrition exert separate influences on immune function; these influences appear to be greater when exercise stress and poor nutrition act synergistically. The poor nutritional status of some athletes very likely predisposes them to immunodepression. Several vitamins, including vitamin B_{12} and folic acid, are needed for the normal production of white blood cells that defend the body against invading pathogens. Other vitamins, including A, C, and E are needed for normal functioning of these cells. Several minerals, including zinc, iron, copper, and selenium are also essential for optimal immune function. The role of both micronutrients and macronutrients in immune function and resistance to infection is dealt with in detail in chapter 13.

Electrolytes in Body Fluids

An electrolyte conducts an electric current when dissolved in water. Electrolytes, which include acids, bases, and salts, usually dissociate into ions carrying either a positive charge (cation) or a negative charge (anion). The major electrolytes in the body fluids are sodium, potassium, chloride, bicarbonate, phosphate, sulfate, magnesium, and calcium. Of these, sodium, potassium, and chloride are found in the highest concentrations, although their distribution differs between the intracellular and extracellular fluid.

Sodium and chloride are found in higher concentrations in the extracellular fluid, whereas potassium is found in higher concentration inside cells. These concentration differences arise because of active transport mechanisms in cell membranes. The sodium-potassium ATPase actively pumps 3 sodium ions out of the cell for every 2 potassium ions pumped into the cell, which sets up an electrical potential (charge) difference across the cell membrane, with the interior of the cell being slightly electrically negative compared with the outside. This electrical potential difference can be measured as a voltage difference and amounts, in most cells, to about 70 millivolts. This resting membrane potential can be reversed by a sudden influx of positive ions into the cell, which is the basis of the action potential generated in nerve and muscle fibers when sodium channels in the membranes of these cells are temporarily opened.

Sodium, as the principal cation in the extracellular fluids (see table 9.5), serves primarily to maintain normal body fluid balance, osmotic pressure, and blood pressure. The role of excess sodium intake in the etiology of high blood pressure (hypertension) is discussed in chapter 1. Normal body fluid levels of sodium are critical for nerve impulse transmission and muscle contraction. The body has effective hormonal control mechanisms for dealing with wide variations in dietary sodium intake.

If the plasma concentration of sodium falls, aldosterone secretion from the adrenal glands is increased, and this steroid hormone stimulates the kidney to reabsorb more sodium so that less is excreted in the urine. When the plasma concentration of sodium rises, aldosterone production falls, allowing increased urinary excretion of sodium. Other hormones, notably vasopressin or antidiuretic hormone (ADH), via its effect on water reabsorption by the kidney, help to maintain normal sodium concentration in the body fluids. During prolonged moderate exercise or shorter durations of high-intensity exercise, the plasma sodium concentration increases, which helps maintain blood volume. Exercise also leads to an increased secretion of both aldosterone and ADH, which results in the conservation of body sodium and water.

The estimated minimum daily requirement for sodium in adults is 0.5 g (amount contained in 1.25 g of table salt), and the upper recommended intake of sodium is 2.4 g/day. Sodium is in rather small amounts in most natural foods, but many processed foods have substantial amounts of salt added. For example, a 180 g (5 oz) serving of cooked fresh beans contains 25 mg of sodium, whereas and equal portion of canned beans contains 750 mg of sodium. Because of health concerns, food manufacturers have, in recent years, reduced the salt content of processed foods. Even so, the average consumption of sodium by individuals in the United States is reported to be about 4.5 g/day. About one-third of this amount is from natural foods, one-half is from processed foods, and the rest is from table salt.

The typical sodium content of several foods is shown in table 9.13. Fresh meats, fruits, and vegetables generally contain relatively small amounts of sodium, whereas several processed foods such as sauces, pickles, chips, "ready meals," and processed meats (e.g., sausages and burgers) contain much greater amounts of sodium.

Deficiency of sodium is rare, partly because of the widespread availability of sodium in many food products and partly because humans have a natural appetite for salt. However, substantial losses of sodium and chloride from the body can result from prolonged sweating. Although sweat composition is quite variable, the average amount of sodium and chloride lost in sweat is around 1.2 g/L and 1.4 g/L, respectively. Because most persons sweat at a rate of 1 L/h to 2 L/h during strenuous exercise, even in ambient temperatures around 20° C (68° F), salt losses can be considerable. Thus, for the athlete exercising in the heat, short-term deficiencies of sodium and chloride may be incurred, which, if not corrected in the recovery period, can have debilitating effects on subsequent exercise performance.

Low blood sodium levels (hyponatremia) can also occur with drinking excessive volumes of water over a period of several hours, which can lead to potentially fatal water intoxication (see chapter 8). Chloride is the major anion in the extracellular fluids (see table 9.5) and, like sodium, is involved in the regulation of body fluid balance and electrical potentials across cell membranes. Chloride ions are also a component in the formation of hydrochloric acid in the stomach, which promotes the denaturation and digestion of dietary proteins. The estimated minimum daily requirement for chloride in adults is 0.75 g. The dietary intake of chloride, as might be expected, parallels that of sodium.

Potassium is the major cation found inside cells. The intracellular concentration is about 150 mmol/L compared with around 4 mmol/L in the extracellular fluids. Potassium is also involved in body fluid homeostasis and in the generation of electrical impulses in nerves, skeletal muscle, and the heart. Potassium excretion in the urine is, like that of sodium, regulated by aldosterone. A rise in the plasma potassium concentration stimulates the secretion of aldosterone, leading to an increased urinary excretion of potassium. Conversely, a fall in the plasma potassium concentration causes a reduction in aldosterone secretion from the adrenal cortex and, hence, greater potassium retention by the kidneys. The estimated minimum daily requirement for potassium in adults is 2.0 g. Potassium is found in most foods and is particularly abundant in bananas, citrus fruits, vegetables, and milk (see table 9.14). Because potassium balance is tightly regulated in the body, long-term deficiencies or excesses are extremely rare. However, short-term imbalances may occur in certain circumstances. For example, low blood potassium levels (hypokalemia) have been reported in persons suffering from diarrhea, during prolonged fasting, and after diuretic drug administration.

Table 9.13 Sodium Content of Common Food Items

Food item	Amount	Sodium content (mg)
Meat		
Luncheon meat	1 oz (28 g)	450
Beef	1 oz (28 g)	25
Chicken	1 oz (28 g)	13
White fish	1 oz (28 g)	33
Tuna (in oil)	1 oz (28 g)	270
Salmon (canned)	1 oz (28 g)	140
Pork sausage	1 oz (28 g)	70
Cereal and starch products		
Bread	1 slice	130
Corn flakes	1 oz (28 g)	280
Pretzels	1 oz (28 g)	890
Chips/crisps (plain, salted)	1 oz (28 g)	195
Chips/crisps (salt and vinegar)	1 oz (28 g)	335
Vegetables and fruits		
Beans (fresh, cooked)	1 oz (28 g)	5
Baked beans (canned)	1 oz (28 g)	150
Red kidney beans (canned)	1 oz (28 g)	85
Peas (canned)	1 oz (28 g)	55
Pickled onions	1 oz (28 g)	225
Potato (baked)	1 medium size	6
Banana	1 medium size	1
Orange	1 medium size	1
Dairy products		
Milk (semiskimmed)	100 ml	120
Butter	1 teaspoon (5 g)	50
Cheese	1 oz (28 g)	445
Cottage cheese	1 oz (28 g)	20
Other common products		
Margarine	1 teaspoon (5 g)	50
Spaghetti sauces	1 oz (28 g)	340
Soups	100 ml	500
Tomato ketchup	1 tablespoon (15 g)	100
Soy sauce	1 tablespoon (15 g)	1,020
Bolognese sauce	1 oz (28 g)	140
Gravy powder	1 oz (28 g)	1,620
Cakes and tarts	1 oz (28 g)	85
Isotonic sports drinks	100 ml	46
Table salt	1 teaspoon (5 g)	5,000

Table 9.14 Potassium Content of Common Food Items

Food item	Amount	Potassium content (mg)
Meat		
Beef	1 oz (28 g)	100
Chicken	1 oz (28 g)	70
White fish	1 oz (28 g)	160
Cereal and starch products		
Bread	1 slice	65
Corn flakes	1 oz (28 g)	100
Vegetables and fruits		
Potato (baked)	1 medium size	780
Carrot	1 medium size	275
Broccoli	1 medium size stalk	270
Banana	1 medium size	460
Orange	1 medium size	260
Apple	1 medium size	35
Dairy products		
Milk (semiskimmed)	100 ml	180
Butter	1 teaspoon (5 g)	10
Cheddar cheese	1 oz (28 g)	28
Yogurt	100 g	450

Low plasma potassium concentrations can lead to muscle weakness and fatal cardiac arrest. A higher than normal blood level of potassium (hyperkalemia) is also potentially very dangerous because this condition, too, can cause cardiac arrhythmias, resulting in death. For this reason, individuals should not take large doses of potassium supplements. During high-intensity exercise, active skeletal muscle releases potassium ions that enter the circulation and cause a temporary rise in the plasma potassium concentration. However, under normal circumstances, normal potassium levels are rapidly restored during the recovery period. Some potassium is excreted in sweat, but these losses are relatively small (160 mg/L to 320 mg/L) compared with the losses of sodium and chloride, so potassium status can easily be restored with the ingestion of a postexercise meal.

Other Tissue Functions

Calcium, in addition to being an important structural component of bone, is involved in nerve conduction and muscle excitation and contraction. In the sarco-plasm (cytosol) of resting muscle, the concentration of free calcium ions (Ca^{2+}) is low (about 10 nM), whereas in the extracellular fluid and sarcoplasmic reticulum (SR), the concentration is much higher; the blood plasma concentration of free calcium, for example, is about 1 mM (100,000 times higher than in the muscle sarcoplasm). Release of calcium from the SR in response to membrane depolarization after the arrival of an action potential allows the myosin and actin filaments to interact, bringing about muscle contraction (see chapter 2). Calcium is then pumped back into the SR by an active transport mechanism, which restores the low cytosolic calcium ion concentration, allowing relaxation of the muscle.

Calcium is also required for the activation of numerous enzymes involved in energy metabolism. For example, the activity of phosphorylase, the key enzyme involved in muscle glycogen breakdown, is stimulated by an increased cytosolic calcium ion concentration. Several enzymes of glycolysis are also activated by increased levels of intracellular calcium, which neatly links the provision of energy to the same process that allows the muscle to perform work.

Calcium and vitamin K (menadione) are required for normal blood clotting. Vitamin K is required for the synthesis of blood-clotting factors. This vitamin is a coenzyme in the posttranslational modification of protein structure, specifically the addition of sugar moieties to form glycoproteins.

Zinc seems to have a role in appetite regulation. Oral zinc supplementation has been shown to be effective in restoring normal eating behavior and body weight in patients suffering from the eating disorder anorexia nervosa (see chapter 12). Zinc has been suggested to be involved in the pathogenesis of this eating disorder. Among female athletes, gymnasts and dancers have a particularly high incidence of eating disorders, and several dietary surveys indicate that these groups consume inadequate amounts of zinc. Indeed, in a study of female adolescent dancers and gymnasts, 75% were found to consume less than two-thirds of the RDA for zinc. Thus, athletes who attempt to maintain low body weights should be concerned that adequate amounts of zinc are consumed.

In addition to being coenzymes in energy metabolism, several of the B-complex vitamins are also required for normal neuromuscular function. For example, vitamin B_6 is needed for the synthesis and metabolism of many neurotransmitters, including norepinephrine and dopamine.

Vitamin A (retinol), as well as being an antioxidant, forms the visual pigments of the eye and is, therefore, important for normal vision, particularly in fading light.

Effects of Vitamins on Exercise Performance

A number of papers have been written about the effects of vitamin supplementation on exercise performance. Older studies have suggested a potential ergogenic role of vitamins, based on the argument that the RDAs may not represent optimal intakes. However, many of the early studies that claimed to show beneficial effects of vitamin supplementation on exercise performance were poorly designed, often with no control (placebo) group against which to compare the effects of supplementation or no information about current vitamin status in the test subjects. After more recent, double-blind placebo-controlled studies, the notion that excess vitamin intake improves exercise performance has been discredited. Even so, many athletes consume relatively large amounts of vitamin and mineral supplements as a kind of "insurance policy," so that they feel satisfied

in their own minds that they are not at risk for any vitamin deficiency.

Severe or prolonged vitamin deficiencies are, of course, deleterious to health and would, therefore, be expected to impair athletic performance. Vitamin and mineral supplementation may improve the nutritional status of individuals consuming marginal amounts of nutrients from food and may improve performance in those with deficiencies. However, athletes should not rely on tablets to supply them with the necessary micronutrients. In addition to the established vitamins, many other compounds present in small quantities in fresh fruit and vegetables are probably needed for optimal health.

Short-term inadequacy of vitamin intake is characterized by lowered vitamin concentrations in body tissues and fluids and decreased activities of certain enzymes. However, functional disturbances, including a decreased $\dot{V}O_2$max or physical performance capacity may not appear until weeks or months later. In the opposite scenario, very large intakes of vitamins increase the body's vitamin stores (particularly fat-soluble vitamins) and will increase the activity of some enzymes but will not necessarily improve physical work capacity. Furthermore, excessive intakes of the fat-soluble vitamins (A, D, E, and K) for prolonged periods are possibly harmful.

Ergogenic Effect of Mineral Supplementation

Some minerals are specifically promoted as potential ergogenic aids to performance. These supplements, often consumed in bulk quantities a few hours before competition, include phosphates and sodium bicarbonate. Phosphate salts are suggested as a potential ergogenic aid because these ions are an important intracellular buffer. Phosphate groups are a component of the body's energy currency, namely ATP. So phosphate loading might increase the resynthesis rate of ATP from ADP and phosphate. Another possible ergogenic mechanism could be improving oxygen extraction from the blood by muscle fibers via an elevated erythrocyte 2,3-DPG concentration. However, at present, experimental evidence for these claims is lacking.

Bicarbonate is an important extracellular buffer. Reliable evidence indicates that bicarbonate ingestion (most commonly consumed as sodium bicarbonate, although sodium itself has no independent effects in acid-base regulation) can improve performance in events in which lactic acid accumulation in the muscle is a major cause of fatigue, such as 400-meter to 1,500-

meter running (see chapter 10). However, consumption of the amount of sodium bicarbonate necessary to alter blood acid-base balance sufficiently to influence performance (approximately 20 g) can cause gastrointestinal discomfort and diarrhea. Because of these unpleasant side effects, bicarbonate loading can temporarily result in inadequate absorption of essential micronutrients and carbohydrate, and so can delay the restoration of muscle glycogen stores after exercise. The side effects and their consequences are important factors to consider for sports events involving competition on successive days. Further details of phosphate and bicarbonate loading are found in chapter 10.

Recommendations for Micronutrient Intake in Athletes

In general, supplementation with individual vitamins, including the consumption of large doses of simple antioxidant mixtures is not recommended. Consuming megadoses of individual vitamins (common among athletes) is likely to do more harm than good. Because most vitamins function mainly as coenzymes in the body, once these enzyme systems are saturated, the vitamin in free form can become toxic. For example, very large doses of vitamin C are associated with urinary stone formation and impaired copper absorption, and megadoses of vitamin B_6 can cause sensory neuropathy. Excess intakes of vitamin A by pregnant women can cause birth defects. Athletes should obtain complex mixtures of antioxidant compounds from increased consumption of fruits and vegetables.

Vitamin supplements are not necessary for athletes eating a well-balanced diet. Many athletes are, however, concerned about ensuring adequate intakes of vitamins, without the risks of oversupplementation. A daily intake of a low-dose vitamin preparation, supplying not more than the RDA, provides an adequate and safe level of vitamin intake, especially during periods of intensive training and carbohydrate loading before competition. Similarly, most athletes do not require mineral supplements, because their diet is already more than adequate to meet any increased requirements resulting from the effects of regular intensive exercise.

However, particular groups of athletes are at risk for marginal mineral intake. These athletes compete in sports events in which a low body weight is essential for success (e.g., gymnasts and dancers) or compete within certain body-weight categories (e.g., boxers, wrestlers, and weight lifters). Participants in such sports often train frequently and intensively but consume low-energy diets or undergo drastic weight-loss regimens to maintain or lose body weight before competition. The low-energy intakes (<8 MJ/day [<1900 kcal/day]) in these situations are likely to lead to an inadequate intake of essential minerals (and vitamins). Because many athletes are very young and still in a period of body growth and development, they can be detrimentally affected by micronutrient deficiencies. Specific recommendations can be given to athletes to ensure an adequate calcium intake when on an energy-restricted diet:

- Include three servings a day of low-fat dairy foods.
- Include these dairy foods in high-carbohydrate meals (e.g., skimmed milk on cereal).
- Eat fish with bones (e.g., sardines).
- Include calcium-enriched soy products.
- Eat leafy green vegetables (e.g., cabbage, broccoli, spinach).

Dietary recommendations can also be given to athletes to increase available iron intake on a high-carbohydrate diet:

- Eat foods rich in heme iron at least 4 times a week (e.g., liver or lean red meat).
- Eat iron-fortified foods (e.g., breakfast cereal).
- Include non–heme iron food sources (e.g., dried fruit, legumes, and green leafy vegetables).
- Combine nonheme-iron foods with meat or vitamin C–rich food (e.g., orange juice) to increase iron absorption.
- Avoid drinking tea at meals.

Other athletes who are at risk for marginal mineral intake are those who abstain from normal diets (i.e., consume extremely unbalanced diets with a low micronutrient density) and vegetarian athletes. Hence, micronutrient supplementation is recommended for such athletes.

Amenorrheic female athletes should certainly take calcium supplements, and other female athletes should consider taking calcium supplements, to ensure adequate calcium status and maintain healthy bones. Moderately elevated intakes of calcium do not appear to be harmful, possibly because the blood calcium concentration is under tight hormonal regulation, and moderate excesses can be excreted in the urine.

Athletes who train and compete in hot environments should also consider increasing their intake of minerals (particularly iron, zinc, and magnesium) because mineral losses in sweat can be considerable. Even so, daily supplements of these minerals should not exceed 1 to 2 times the RDA. As with vitamins, excessive intakes of minerals can be toxic and can impair the absorption of other essential trace elements.

Poor diets are the main reason for any micronutrient deficiencies found in athletes, although, in certain cases, regular strenuous exercise contributes to the deficiency. With the possible exceptions of iron and calcium, micronutrient deficiencies can easily be corrected by eating a well-balanced diet. An inadequate knowledge of proper dietary practices, lack of time for food preparation, misleading advertisements for micronutrient supplements, and a lack of qualified dietary advice are possible reasons for suboptimal micronutrient intakes in athletes. Few studies have definitively documented beneficial effects of mineral or vitamin supplementation on exercise performance, except where supplementation was needed to correct an existing deficiency. Athletes who take micronutrient supplements are, for the most part, taking them to ensure good health, not to enhance sports performance. However, an unhealthy athlete is unlikely to perform to the best of his or her potential.

Key Points

- Although vitamin and mineral supplementation may improve the nutritional status of athletes consuming marginal amounts of micronutrients from food and may improve performance in athletes with deficiencies, there is no convincing evidence to indicate that doses in excess of the RDA improve performance.

- Vitamins and minerals are needed in the body for several important processes, including the growth and repair of body tissues, as cofactors in enzyme catalyzed metabolic reactions, for oxygen transport and oxidative metabolism, for immune function, and as antioxidants. Any sustained deficiency of an essential vitamin or mineral will cause ill health and an unhealthy athlete is extremely unlikely to perform to the best of his or her potential.

- Vitamins are organic compounds that are needed in very small quantities in the diet. They are essential for specific metabolic reactions in the body and to promote normal growth and development. With the exception of vitamin D, which can be synthesized in the presence of sunlight, and vitamin K and some B-vitamins, which can be produced by the bacterial microflora of the gastrointestinal tract, vitamins are not produced by the human body and must be consumed in the diet.

- Although vitamins do not directly contribute to energy supply, they play an important role in regulating metabolism, acting as reusable coenzymes in intermediary metabolism. A deficiency of some of the B-group vitamins, which act as cofactors of enzymes in carbohydrate (e.g., niacin, pyridoxine [B_6], and thiamin [B_1]), fat (e.g., riboflavin [B_2], thiamin, pantothenic acid, and biotin), and protein (pyridoxine) metabolism, results in premature fatigue and inability to maintain a heavy training program. Other vitamins play a role in red and white blood cell production (folic acid and cobalamin [B_{12}]) or assist in the formation of bones, connective tissue, and cartilage (e.g., vitamins C and D).

- The water-soluble vitamins, C (ascorbic acid), thiamin, riboflavin, pyridoxine, niacin, pantothenic acid, and biotin are involved in mitochondrial energy metabolism. Folic acid and vitamin B_{12} are mainly involved in nucleic acid synthesis and, hence, are important for maintaining healthy populations of rapidly dividing cells in the body (e.g., red blood cells, immune cells, and the gut mucosa). Vitamin C is also an antioxidant.

- The fat-soluble vitamins are A (retinol), D (calciferol), E (tocopherol), and K (menadione). Of these vitamins, only vitamin E has a probable role in energy metabolism. In

(continued)

(continued)

addition, vitamins A and E have antioxidant properties. Vitamin K is required for the addition of sugar residues to proteins to form glycoproteins.

■ Although physical activity may increase the requirement for some vitamins (e.g., vitamin C, riboflavin, and possibly pyridoxine, vitamin A, and vitamin E), this increased requirement typically is met by consuming a balanced high-carbohydrate, moderate-protein, low-fat diet. Vitamin and mineral intakes in athletes are correlated with energy intakes up to 20 MJ/day (4,800 kcal/day), so, provided that energy intake matches the energy requirement, athletes get all the micronutrients they need from food, without any need for supplements.

■ Evidence suggests that antioxidants provide an important defense mechanism in the body against the damaging effects of free radicals. Many athletes consume large doses of antioxidant vitamins (vitamins A, C, and E). However, excessive antioxidant ingestion may not be uniformly helpful. The controversy continues as to whether physically active individuals should consume antioxidant compounds in amounts above RDA values. At present, the data are insufficient to strongly recommend antioxidant supplements for athletes.

■ Most athletes do not require micronutrient supplements, because their diets are already more than adequate to meet any increased requirements resulting from the effects of regular intensive exercise. However, particular groups of athletes are at risk for marginal mineral and vitamin intake. These athletes compete in sports events in which a low body weight is essential for success (e.g., gymnasts and dancers) or compete within certain body-weight categories (e.g., boxers, wrestlers, and weight lifters). Participants in these sports are often training frequently and intensively but consume low-energy diets or undergo drastic weight-loss regimens to maintain or lose body weight before competition.

■ Amenorrheic female athletes should certainly take calcium supplements, and other female athletes should consider taking calcium supplements, to ensure adequate calcium status and maintain healthy bones. Athletes who train and compete in hot environments should also consider increasing their mineral intake (particularly iron, zinc, and magnesium) because mineral losses in sweat can be considerable. Even so, daily supplements of these minerals should not exceed 1 to 2 times the RDA. As with vitamins, excessive intakes of minerals can be toxic and can impair the absorption of other essential trace elements.

■ Poor diets are the main reason for any micronutrient deficiencies among athletes, regular strenuous exercise can contribute to deficiency. With the possible exceptions of iron and calcium, these deficiencies could easily be corrected by eating a well-balanced diet. An inadequate knowledge of proper dietary practices, lack of time for food preparation, misleading advertisements for micronutrient supplements, and a lack of qualified dietary advice are possible reasons for suboptimal micronutrient intakes by athletes.

Key Terms

anemia 203
antioxidant 198
electrolyte 204
free radical 198

lipid peroxidation 213
macromineral 203
micromineral (or trace element) 203
osteoporosis 203

polyphenols 215
recommended dietary allowance (RDA) 201
reactive oxygen species (ROS) 213

Recommended Readings

Chen, J. 2000. Vitamins: Effects of exercise on requirements. In *Nutrition in Sport*, ed. R. J. Maughan, 282-291. Blackwell Science: Oxford.

Clarkson, P.M. 1991. Minerals: Exercise performance and supplementation in athletes. *Journal of Sports Sciences* 9: 91-116.

Clarkson, P.M. 2000. Trace Minerals. In *Nutrition in Sport*, ed. R. J. Maughan, 339-355. Blackwell Science: Oxford.

Fogelholm, M. 2000. Vitamins: Metabolic functions. In *Nutrition in Sport*, ed. R. J. Maughan, 266-280. Blackwell Science: Oxford.

Haymes, E.M. 1991. Vitamin and mineral supplementation to athletes. *International Journal of Sport nutrition* 1: 146-169.

Ji, L.L. 1995. Oxidative Stress During Exercise: Implications of antioxidant nutrients. *Free Radical Biology & Medicine* 18:1079-1086.

Sen, C.K., S. Roy, and L. Packer. 2000. Exercise-induced oxidative stress and antioxidant nutrients. In *Nutrition in Sport*, ed. R. J. Maughan, 292-317. Blackwell Science: Oxford.

van der Beek, E.J. 1991. Vitamin supplementation and physical exercise performance. *Journal of Sports Sciences* 9: 77-89.

Chapter 10

Nutrition Supplements

© Sport The Library

Objectives

After studying this chapter, you should be able to do the following:

- Describe various categories of nutrition supplements

- Discuss the nutrition supplements that have ergogenic properties

- Discuss the potential hazards and risks of nutrition supplements

- Understand critical analyses of research findings and reports and the importance of them

The use of **ergogenic** aids or nutrition supplements is not new. As long ago as 500 to 400 B.C., dietary fads were being used to enhance performance (Applegate and Grivetti 1997). Many athletes today are still hopeful of finding a special beverage or pill that will improve performance.

Beyond genetic endowment and training, many athletes turn to ergogenic aids (Applegate 1999). For many modern athletes, sport nutrition has become synonymous with nutrition supplements, and the ideas athletes have about nutrition supplements are heavily influenced by the manufacturers and sellers of these supplements who claim their products increase muscle mass, improve stamina, and so on.

Weight loss and muscle gain are important concerns for many athletes as well as for individuals not involved in athletic training. Because achieving those goals is very difficult with the conventional methods (reducing energy intake and increasing energy expenditure through physical activity), these supplements may sound very attractive to many. Nutritional supplements are used by 40% to 100% of all athletes in one form or another (Burke and Read 1993), and evidence suggests that athletes use several nutrition supplements at the same time and in very high doses. In this chapter, we review the claims and the experimental evidence for a selection of common supplements. Because more than 600 nutrition supplements are now on the market (see figure 10.1), we cannot review them all. Instead, we will focus on the most common ones.

Nonregulation of Nutrition Supplements

An abundance of information can be found in advertising and on the Internet about nutritional supplements. However, most claims are not backed up by scientific studies, and many of them are unrealistic or even impossible. Often claims are based on studies in non–peer-reviewed journals or results from studies are inappropriately extrapolated. The claims that manufacturers make about nutrition supplements are apparently difficult to regulate.

In contrast to prescription drugs, which are carefully regulated, nutrition supplements receive very little governmental oversight, and retailers have enormous freedom in making marketing claims. For instance, the United States Food and Drug Administration (FDA) strictly regulates the clinical testing, the advertising, and the promotion of prescription drugs, which makes unproven claims impossible. Nutrition supplements are under no such regulation. Drugs are extensively tested for safety before they can be sold, but nutrition supplements are not tested. The Dietary Supplement Health and Education Act of 1994 created a new category of product called dietary supplements. These dietary supplements are treated as nutrition and are defined as "vitamins, minerals, herbs and botanicals, amino acids, and other dietary substances intended to supplement the diet by increasing the total dietary intake, or as any concentrate, metabolite, constituent or combination of these ingredients." Although manufacturers must submit

Acetylcholine	Conjugated linoleic acids	Phosphatidylserine
Androstenedione	Creatine (monohydrate)	Octacosanol
Arginine	Dessicated liver	Omega-3 fatty acids
Bee pollen	Ephedra	Royal jelly
Boron	Gamma oryzanol	Smilax
Branched-chain amino acids	Ginseng	Sodium bicarbonate
Caffeine	Glandulars	Sodium citrate
Carnitine	Glucosamine	Sodium phosphate
Choline	Glucose polymers	Spirulina
Chondroitin	Glutamine	Succinate
Citrulline	Inosine	Vanadium
Chromium picolinate	MCT	Wheat germ oil
Coenzyme Q10	Pangamic acid*	

Figure 10.1 A listing of some nutrition supplements available on the market. Asterisk (*) indicates not available for sale.

information of new products (including the claims) to the FDA, this information is for notification rather than authorization (Ross 2000).

Critical Evaluation of Nutrition Supplements Studies

Athletes and others must critically examine claims made by the dietary supplements industry, including the "scientific evidence" that supports the claims. Following are some factors that should be considered when evaluating reports of scientific studies.

- Does the study have a clear hypothesis? A well-designed study has a clear hypothesis and a strong theoretical basis for the expected outcome. Some studies, however, are designed with a "shotgun" approach. A supplement is given, and many variables are measured. The more variables that are examined, the greater the chance that some of them will change. The application of study results should have a sound scientific rationale. For example, sodium bicarbonate may improve buffering capacity, which could result in improved 800-meter running performance. However, by no rationale can sodium bicarbonate be expected to improve Ironman triathlon performance, an event lasting 8 hours to 14 hours.

- Was the study on cells, muscle, animals, or humans? Often results are extrapolated from findings in cell cultures. These in vitro experiments greatly help our understanding of metabolism and molecular interactions. However, in vivo situations may be very different. For instance, test tube samples are not exposed to hormonal changes that exist in living organisms. Also, muscle cells in the body may behave differently than isolated muscle cell preparations. Even if living animals are tested, the metabolism of animals may be very different from the metabolism of humans. Rats have relatively large stores of muscle glycogen and very small stores of intramuscular triacylglycerol compared with humans. High-fat diets in rats clearly improve exercise capacity (see chapter 6). However no evidence indicates that high-fat diets improve performance in humans. Thus, results from different types of studies cannot simply be extrapolated to the human athlete.

- Was the population for which claims are made comparable to the population in the study? Coenzyme Q10 supplementation improves

$\dot{V}O_2$max and exercise capacity in cardiac patients but has no effect on $\dot{V}O_2$max or exercise capacity in healthy individuals. Vanadium supplementation increases insulin sensitivity (reduces insulin resistance) in patients with type II diabetes but does not seem to be effective in healthy individuals with normal insulin sensitivity. These examples show how outcomes can differ in a target group that has different ages, sexes, body compositions, or fitness levels than the study group.

- Were external variables controlled? In an ideal study, all variables and conditions are identical, so that the only difference between the trials is the treatment each group receives. Then, all observed changes can be attributed with great certainty to the treatment. For example, if the effect of caffeine on exercise performance is examined, and the environmental conditions were different in the caffeine and control trial, the observed effects might be related to environmental conditions as much as to caffeine.

- Was the study placebo controlled? If subjects have prior knowledge or expectations with respect to a treatment or supplement, their performance could be affected. The proper choice of a placebo avoids this kind of performance bias. However, with some nutrition interventions matching placebos are very difficult to find. For example branched-chain amino acids (BCAA) have a very bitter taste, and it is very difficult to have a placebo with a similar (horrible) taste. In this case, subjects may be aware of what they receive and this knowledge could influence the outcome.

- Were adequate techniques used? Endurance capacity (time to exhaustion) has a large day-to-day variability (Jeukendrup et al. 1996). Methods used to measure this variability may not detect small differences in performance. Similarly, some measures of body composition have a relatively large error and, thus, will not be able to detect small changes in fat or fat-free mass. If a treatment (supplement) is said to have no effect, perhaps the particular method used in the study was not sensitive enough to pick up small differences (Hopkins et al. 1999). A small change in performance (<3%) that is undetectable in a laboratory setting may determine success or failure in a sports event.

- Were the trials randomized? Randomization reduces the confounding effects of variables that were not controlled or could not be controlled.

233

When a small number of subjects are tested, a so-called counterbalanced design it is preferred. If trials are randomized, 8 subjects may end up in the treatment group in the first trial and only 2 in the control group. A counterbalanced design prevents this imbalance by appointing equal numbers of the control and treatment group to the first trial. Thus, half of the subjects will take the supplement first; the other half will take the placebo first. Failure to randomize treatments in a study may confound the outcome and hence make any conclusions untrustworthy.

- Was a crossover design used? In a crossover study design the same subjects perform both the treatment trial and the placebo trial, allowing comparisons to be made within the same person. Although this type of study design can cause complications, particularly if a test substance that exerts effects in the body for a long time is given before the placebo, it is considered the ideal study design. Failure to use a cross-over design may not necessarily affect the trustworthiness of the conclusions, but it is very likely that variation between subjects in the measured variables will be greater than that within the same subjects. Hence, if a crossover design is not used, many more subjects will have to be studied to obtain the same degree of confidence that the conclusions are valid.

- Was it a random assignment or was self-selection used? If subjects are allowed to self-select their trial group, a significant bias may be introduced. For example, in a study of the effects of chromium on weight loss, subjects most motivated to lose weight would likely choose to be in the chromium group and not the placebo group.

- Do other studies confirm the findings? If one study reports an ergogenic effect of a supplement, it may be true. However, if several studies come to the same conclusion, the supplement most likely does have an ergogenic effect. The more studies that have been conducted, the larger the variety of subjects tested, and the more varied the dosages of the supplement used, the more generalizable the conclusion.

- Was the study peer reviewed? Papers sent for publication to peer-reviewed journals undergo a rigorous process whereby usually 2 or 3 referees, who are experts in the area, evaluate the paper based on specific criteria. Quality research withstands the critical review and evaluation by colleagues. Articles published in popular magazines or on consumer-oriented Web sites do not undergo this extensive review process and are, therefore, often full of errors and untruthful claims.

A Detailed Look at Nutrition Supplements

The most important supplements are discussed in this section. Table 10.1 contains a list of selected supplements, along with claims and scientific evidence for those claims. Supplements discussed in previous chapters, such as carbohydrate-electrolyte drinks (see chapter 5) and individual amino acids (see chapter 7) are not discussed.

Androstenedione

Androstenedione is one of the most popular nutrition supplements in the United States. It is believed to stimulate the endogenous synthesis of testosterone

Table 10.1 Selected Nutrition Supplements, Product Claims, and Supporting Scientific Evidence

Ergogenic aids	Description	Claim	Scientific Evidence
Androstenedione	Synthetic product to stimulate testosterone synthesis	Increases testosterone, increases muscle mass, and improves recovery	Does not increase testosterone; has no effect on strength
Bee pollen	Mixture of bee saliva, plant nectar, and pollen	Increases energy levels, enhances physical fitness, improves endurance, and boosts immune function	No supporting evidence
Beta-hydroxy beta methylbutyrate (HMB)	Metabolite of the essential amino acid leucine	Decreases protein breakdown, improves muscle mass, and increases strength	Possible small effects on lean-body mass and strength

(continued)

Table 10.1 *(continued)*

Ergogenic aids	Description	Claim	Scientific Evidence
Boron	Trace element present in vegetables and noncitrus fruits	Improves bone density, muscle mass, and strength	Improves bone mineral density in postmenopausal women; no effect on bone density, muscle mass, or strength in men
Caffeine	Substance in coffee and chocolate	Increases performance and alertness	Improves performance in most events, except very short high-intensity exercise; increases cognitive functioning during exercise
Carnitine	Vitamin-like substance important for FA transport	Improves fat oxidation, helps weight loss, and improves $\dot{V}O_2max$	Not taken up by muscle and, therefore, not effective
Choline	Precursor of the neurotransmitter acetylcholine	Improves performance and decreases fatigue	No supporting evidence
Chromium picolinate	Trace element that potentiates insulin action	Builds muscle and helps weight loss	No supporting evidence
Coenzyme Q10	Part of the electron-transport chain in the mitochondria	Improves $\dot{V}O_2max$, improves performance, reduces fatigue	No supporting evidence
Creatine	High-energy phosphate carrier important for direct energy	Improves strength, reduces fatigue, and increases protein synthesis	Improves performance in single and repeated sprint bouts; improves recovery between bouts; anabolic properties unclear
DHEA	A precursor of testosterone and estradiol	Improves immune function, increases life span, protects against cardiovascular diseases, increases lean-body mass, and increases well-being	Some evidence in humans
Dihydroxyacetone	An intermediate of carbohydrate metabolism used in combination with pyruvate	Facilitates carbohydrate and fat metabolism and improves performance	Limited supporting evidence
Fish oil	Polyunsaturated fatty acids	Increases $\dot{V}O_2max$	No supporting evidence
Ginseng	Root of the *Araliaceous* plant	Improves strength, performance, stamina, and cognitive functioning; reduces fatigue	No supporting evidence, but studies poorly designed
Glutamine	An amino acid	Improves immune function, muscle glycogen resynthesis, recovery, and endurance	Does not affect immune function; possibly affects muscle glycogen resynthesis
Glandulars	Extracts of animal glands	Improves strength, performance, stamina	No supporting evidence
Glycerol	Backbone of a triacylglycerol molecule	Induces hyperhydration, decreases heat stress, and improves performance	Induces hyperhydration and decreases heat stress during exercise; effects on performance unclear
Inosine	Nucleoside	Increases ATP stores, improves strength, training quality, and performance	No supporting evidence

(continued)

Table 10.1 (continued)

Lecithin	Phosphatidylcholine	Increases $\dot{V}O_2$max and performance	No supporting evidence
Medium-chain triacylglycerols (MCT)	Synthesized from coconut oil	Supplies energy, reduces muscle glycogen breakdown, and improves performance	No supporting evidence
Pangamic acid (vitamin B_{15})	Varied composition depending on supplier	Increases oxygen delivery	No supporting evidence
Phosphate salts	Mineral	Increases ATP, provides energy, and buffers lactic acid	Possible ergogenic effects; improves performance in events 1 hour or shorter
Phosphatidylserine	Structural component of cell membranes	Reduces stress responses and improves recovery	Very little supporting evidence
Polylactate	Polymer of lactate	Provides energy	No effects on performance
Pyruvate	An intermediate of carbohydrate metabolism	Improves endurance capacity, insulin sensitivity, and recovery; increases glycogen storage	Limited supporting evidence
Sodium bicarbonate	Buffer present in blood	Buffers lactic acid and improves high-intensity exercise performance	Improves high-intensity exercise performance
Sodium citrate	Buffer	Buffers lactic acid and improves high-intensity exercise performance	Larger doses can improve performance
Vanadium	Trace element	Helps weight loss; improves insulin sensitivity and recovery	Increases insulin sensitivity in patients with insulin resistance; studies in healthy individuals lacking
Yohimbine	α_2-adrenoceptor blocker	Increases testosterone, increases fat-free mass, and improves strength	No supporting evidence
Wheat germ oil	Extracted from embryo of wheat	Improves endurance	No supporting evidence

and, thereby, increase protein synthesis, build muscle mass, and improve recovery. Androstenedione was first developed in the former East Germany to enhance the performance of athletes. The regulations in the Dietary Supplement Health and Education Act of 1994 allow it to be sold as a food supplement, and it is available over the counter in almost any drug store or pharmacy in the United States.

If androstenedione functions as an anabolic steroid, it also has the side effects of an anabolic steroid, including acne, growth of facial and body hair, growth of the prostate, and impaired testicular function. The evidence that androstenedione has anabolic properties, however, is far from convincing. Although only a few studies have investigated the effects of androstenedione on serum testosterone concentrations and muscle strength, some conclusions can be drawn from them.

A study determined effects of short-term and long-term (8 weeks) oral androstenedione supplementation (300 mg/day) on serum testosterone and estrogen concentrations and skeletal muscle fiber size and strength in a group of individuals in a strength-training program (King et al. 1999). The group of 20 was randomly divided into a placebo group and an androstenedione group. Interestingly, no changes were observed in serum testosterone concentrations, but serum estradiol concentrations increased after androstenedione administration. Strength training resulted in increased strength, increased lean-body mass, and increased cross-sectional area of type II muscle fibers after 8 weeks, but the androstenedione group and the placebo group showed no differences. A lack of effect on serum testosterone concentrations was also reported by 3 other studies in which 100 mg/day to 200 mg/day were ingested for 2 days to 12 weeks (Ballantyne et al.

2000; Rasmussen, Volpin, et al. 2000; Wallace et al. 1999). Rasmussen. Tipton, et al. (2000) did not find effects on protein synthesis and breakdown or phenylalanine balance across the leg. Therefore, the conclusions that androstenedione has no effect on the plasma testosterone concentration, does not change protein metabolism, has no anabolic effect, and does not alter the adaptations to resistance training seem appropriate.

However, androstenedione may have negative health effects. A study reported a decrease in serum HDL cholesterol, a lack of which has been associated with increased risk of cardiovascular disease. Ethical issues are also involved. Androstenedione is a substance banned by the International Olympic Committee (IOC), and athletes have been disqualified and banned from their sport for using it.

Bee Pollen

Pollen is a fine, powdery substance produced by the anthers of seed-bearing plants. Bees collect it from the plants and store it in their hives. It has a rich mixture of vitamins, minerals, and amino acids and is, therefore, believed to be "healthy," even more so because it is a natural product, as opposed to some of the multivitamin and mineral supplements. Pollen is often referred to as the "perfect food" or "complete food," and manufacturers claim that it improves endurance, reduces free-radical damage, helps weight control, increases longevity, and prevents asthma. However, no reliable information exists to prove its effectiveness as an ergogenic aid. On the basis of the available information on supplementation with vitamins, minerals, and amino acids (see chapters 7 and 9), ergogenic effects would not be expected. One study (Chandler and Hawkins 1984) in which the effect of bee pollen supplementation was investigated showed no influence on maximal oxygen uptake, exercise performance, or metabolism. Bee pollen can be harmful for people who are allergic to specific pollens.

Beta-Hydroxy Beta Methylbutyrate

Beta-hydroxy beta methylbutyrate (HMB) is a metabolite of the essential amino acid leucine (see figure 10.2) and is synthesized in the body at an estimated rate of about 0.2 g/day to 0.4 g/day (Nissen et al. 1996). Its use as a supplement has increased dramatically in the past few years, especially among bodybuilders. HMB is claimed to increase lean-body mass and strength and improve recovery. It is also said to improve immune function, lower blood cholesterol, protect against stress, and reduce body fat.

The first studies of HMB were performed in rats, and the studies demonstrated that supplementing

Transaminase   KIC-dioxygenase

Leucine ⟶ α-keto isocaproate (KIC) ⟶ HMB

Figure 10.2 Sythsis of HMB from the amino acid leucine.

the amino acid leucine can be anticatabolic, possibly through the actions of its metabolite HMB. Later studies investigated HMB as a potential anticatabolic agent in farm animals. No effect of HMB supplementation on protein metabolism was observed in growing lambs (Papet et al. 1997). Subsequently, HMB was hypothesized to reduce protein breakdown in humans, resulting in increased muscle mass and strength. In addition, subjects given HMB supplements were believed to have a decreased stress-induced muscle glycogen breakdown. HMB, thus, was claimed to benefit both strength and endurance athletes.

Information about the effects of HMB in humans is scarce. Nissen et al. (1996) studied 41 untrained male volunteers who participated in a resistance-training program for 3 weeks. The program consisted of three 90-minute weight-lifting sessions a week. Participants were divided into three groups, and each group received a different dose of HMB. The first group received placebo, the second group received 1.5 g/day of HMB, and the third group received 3.0 g/day of HMB. Lean tissue (determined by total-body electrical conductance, a technique with a similar principle as bioelectrical impedance analysis [BIA]) tended to increase more in the HMB groups, and this occurred in a dose-dependent matter (see figure 10.3). Total upper-body and lower-body strength also increased more in with the higher doses of HMB (see figure 10.4).

Figure 10.3 The effect of HMB supplementation on body composition.

Reprinted, by permission, from S. Nissen, 1996, "Effect of Leucine Metabolite Beta-Hydroxy-Beta-Methylbutyrate on muscle metabolism during resistance-exercise training," *Journal of Applied Physiology* 81(5): 2095-2104.

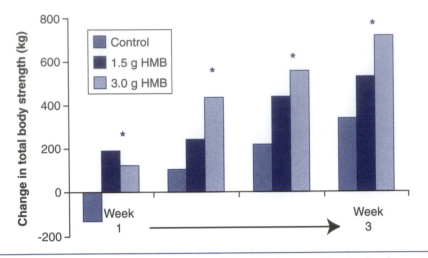

Figure 10.4 Change in body strength (total upper-body and lower-body strength) with placebo or HMB. * = indicates significant linear effect of HMB supplementation.

Reprinted, by permission, from S. Nissen, 1996, "Effect of Leucine Metabolite Beta-Hydroxy-Beta-Methylbutyrate on muscle metabolism during resistance-exercise training," *Journal of Applied Physiology* 81(5): 2095-2104.

However, the group that had the largest increase in lean-body mass (3.0 g/day of HMB) was also the group with the lowest lean-body mass and muscle strength to begin with. Therefore, this group would be expected to gain more than the placebo group, who already had a larger lean-body mass. Also, this study had no diet control, so the leucine intake is not known.

In part 2 of the study by Nissen et al. (1996), subjects trained for 7 weeks, 6 days a week, and they were given 3.0 g/day of HMB or placebo. This study showed an increase in fat-free mass in the HMB group after 14 days, but after 39 days, no differences were observed. Strength was also measured in this second study, but no differences were found in the strength measurements except for bench press. A small improvement in bench press strength occurred with HMB supplementation (2.6 kg after 7 weeks of training with HMB versus 1.1 kg with placebo). A point of criticism again is that the diet was not controlled. Since then, a number of studies have provided mixed results. Some have found an increase in lean-body mass or muscle strength (Jowko et al. 2001; Nissen et al. 2000; Panton et al. 2000), whereas others have found no effect on body composition and strength (Slater et al. 2001) or signs of muscle damage after eccentric exercise (Paddon-Jones et al. 2001). In a recent meta-analysis, HMB was found to increase net lean mass gains by 0.28% a week and strength gains by 1.4% a week (Nissen and Sharp 2003).

Nissen et al. (2000) collected data in 9 studies ranging from 3 to 8 weeks duration. No negative effects of 3.0 g/day of HMB were noted on organ and tissue function, emotional perception, or gastrointestinal tolerance. The authors concluded that 3.0 g/day is a safe

dose. Some evidence suggests that HMB can result in increased lean-body mass and muscle strength. However, the findings are mostly by one laboratory and need to be confirmed by others. From a practical point of view, potential users should keep in mind that most of the studies have used 3 g/day of HMB, whereas most recovery products currently on the market contain extremely small amounts of HMB.

Boron

The trace element Boron influences calcium and magnesium metabolism (Volpe et al. 1993), steroid hormone metabolism, and membrane function. It is present in noncitrus fruits, leafy vegetables, nuts, and legumes. Although no RDA has been established for boron, the recommended daily intake is often 1 mg/day (Nielsen 1996). For humans boron is not an essential trace element.

Boron has been studied in relation to osteoporosis. One of these studies found that boron supplementation for 48 days increased the serum estrogen and testosterone levels of postmenopausal women. It also reduced calcium, phosphorus, and magnesium excretion in urine and is, therefore, suggested to possibly contribute to improved bone mineral density (Nielsen et al. 1987).

The finding that boron increased testosterone levels in postmenopausal women has been extrapolated to the claim that it may improve muscle growth and strength in strength athletes. However, the women in this study had been deprived of boron for 4 months. Continued supplementation did not further elevate testosterone levels, and boron supplementation in men did not affect testosterone levels at all. Another placebo-controlled study investigated the effects of boron supplementation (2.5 mg/day of boron for 7 weeks) on serum testosterone, lean-body mass, and strength in bodybuilders. Besides elevated plasma boron levels, no effect was found (Green and Ferrando 1994). Therefore, although interactions are shown between boron and calcium and magnesium metabolism (Volpe et al. 1993), boron does not appear to be an ergogenic aid.

Caffeine

The use of **caffeine** dates back to Paleolithic times. The raw fruit of the coffee plant (*Coffea arabica*) was used to brew a drink with stimulant properties. This strongly caffeinated beverage was later replaced by a beverage prepared from roasted coffee beans. Caffeine remains the most widely consumed drug in Europe and America (Curatolo and Robertson 1983), and it has long been used by athletes in the belief that it improves performance.

Caffeine was only recently (January 1, 2004) taken off the list of banned substances by the International Olympic Committee (IOC). Before January 2004, caffeine was one of the few compounds for which the IOC had set a tolerance limit. This limit was defined at a caffeine concentration in urine of 12 µg/ml. Because caffeine is a substance that can influence exercise performance, its use is a question of sports ethics. (For further readings and details on caffeine metabolism and the ergogenic effects of caffeine, see Armstrong [2002], Graham et al. [1994], and Spriet [1995b].)

Caffeine originates naturally in 63 species of plants as several types of methylated xanthines. Caffeine and caffeine-like substances can be found in a variety of foods and drinks, but the main sources for these substances are coffee beans, tea leaves, cocoa beans,

Figure 10.5 Chemical structure of caffeine and caffeine-like compounds.

Reprinted, by permission, from W.J. Pasman et al., 1995, "The effect of varied dosages of caffeine on endurance performance time," *International Journal of Sports Medicine* 16(4): 225-230.

and cola nuts (see figure 10.5. and table 10.2). Coffee accounts for 75% of all caffeine consumption.

Caffeine is readily absorbed after ingestion. Blood levels rise and peak after approximately 60 minutes. The half-life is reported to be between 2 hours and 10 hours. Caffeine is primarily degraded in the liver, with the resulting single methyl group xanthines and methyluric acids eliminated in urine. About 0.5% to 3.5% of ingested caffeine is excreted unchanged in urine. A study showed that significant amounts of caffeine are also excreted via sweat (Kovacs et al. 1998).

Effects of Caffeine in Endurance Exercise

Costill et al. (1977), Essig et al. (1980), and Ivy et al. (1979) showed that caffeine ingested 1 hour before the start of an exercise bout increased plasma FA concentrations and improved performance. The improvement in performance was explained by the increased availability of FAs, which lead to a suppression of carbohydrate metabolism and consequently to a decreased glycogen utilization. However, the results of studies investigating the ergogenic effects of caffeine and the possible role of FAs are contradictory. Several studies showed increased plasma FA concentrations but did not show any effect on fat oxidation (Knapik et al. 1983; Tarnopolsky et al. 1992). A few studies observed changes in plasma FA concentration but not on performance (Erickson et al. 1987; Powers et al. 1983; Tarnopolsky et al. 1989). Other studies did not observe any effect on either fat metabolism or performance (Bond et al. 1987; Toner et al. 1982; Winder 1986).

Although not all studies show effects of caffeine on endurance performance, quite a few well-conducted studies show improved endurance capacity after ingesting caffeine at a dose of 3 mg/kg b.w. to 9 mg/kg b.w. (Costill et al. 1978; Graham et al. 1987; Graham and Spriet 1991; Pasman et al. 1995; Spriet et al. 1992). At exercise intensities around 85% $\dot{V}O_2$max, improvements of 10% to 20% are typically found in time to exhaustion. In most of these studies, caffeine also decreased perceived ratings of exertion. The same exercise, thus, feels easier with caffeine. The fact that not all studies found that caffeine has a performance enhancing effect might be related to various factors, including the dosage of caffeine, the fitness level of the subjects, habitual caffeine consumption, and, maybe most importantly, the type and duration of exercise.

Effects of Caffeine in Maximal Exercise

A few studies investigated the effects of caffeine ingestion on high-intensity exercise (around 100% $\dot{V}O_2$max and lasting 3 to 8 minutes). Some, but not all, studies

Table 10.2 Caffeine Content in Food, Beverages, and Medications

Item	Caffeine content (mg)	Item	Caffeine content (mg)
Coffee		**Pain relievers (per tablet)**	
Drip method 150 ml (5 oz)	110–150	Anacin	32
Percolated 150 ml (5 oz)	64–124	Excedrin	65
Instant 150 ml (5 oz)	40–108	Midol	32
Decaffeinated 150 ml (5 oz)	2–5	Plain aspirin	0
Starbucks grande 480 ml (16 oz)	550	Vanquish	33
Starbucks tall 360 ml (12 oz)	375	**Diuretics**	
Starbucks short 240 ml (8 oz)	250	Aqua Ban	200
Starbucks tall latte 360 ml (12 oz)	70	Pre-mens forte	100
Tea		**Cold Remedies**	
1 min brew 150 ml (5 oz)	9–33	Coryban-D	30
3 min brew 150 ml (5 oz)	20–46	Dristan	0
5 min brew 150 ml (5 oz)	20–50	Triamincin	30
Instant tea 150 ml (5 oz)	12–28	**Weight-control aids**	
Iced tea 360 ml (12 oz)	22–36	Dexatrim	200
Chocolate		Prolamine	140
Made from mix	6	**Stimulants**	
Milk chocolate (1 oz)	6	Pro-plus	50
Baking chocolate	35	NoDoz	100
Chocolate bar (100g)	12–15	**Prescription pain relievers**	
Soft drinks (can)		Cafergot	100
Mountain Dew	55	Darvon compound	32
Mello Yello	52	Fiorinal	40
Coca Cola	46	Migramal	1
Diet Coke	46		
Pepsi Cola	38		
Diet Pepsi	36		
Dr Pepper	40		
Red Bull 250 ml (8.3 oz)	80		

(Falk et al. 1989; Sasaki et al. 1987) demonstrated a positive effect of caffeine on exercise performance at these high intensities. Jackman et al. (1996) found that ingestion of 6 mg/kg b.w. of caffeine increased time to exhaustion at 100% $\dot{V}O_2$max. However, muscle glycogen concentrations were still relatively high at exhaustion, and, therefore, the authors concluded that the mechanism was not through glycogen sparing. Caffeine (150 mg to 200 mg) also improved 1,500-meter time in well-trained runners (4:46.0 minutes versus 4:50.2 minutes) (Wiles et al. 1992).

Generally, caffeine seems to improve performance during exercise around 100% $\dot{V}O_2$max and lasting approximately 5 minutes. The mechanism for this improvement is unknown but has been suggested to be an effect of caffeine on the neuromuscular pathways that facilitate recruitment of muscle fibers or increase the number of fibers recruited. Also, caffeine possibly has direct effects on muscle ion handling or enhanced anaerobic energy production or an effect on the brain that decreases sensations of effort (Spriet 1995b).

Effects of Caffeine in Supramaximal Exercise

The effects of caffeine on short-term supramaximal exercise performance are uncertain. Williams et al. (1988) reported no effect on power output or muscular endurance during 15-second sprints after caffeine ingestion. Similar findings were reported by Collomp et al. (1991), who found that ingestion of 5 mg/kg b.w. of caffeine did not affect 30-second Wingate test performance. A study investigated the effects of caffeine ingestion on repeated Wingate exercise tests (Greer et al. 1998), and found that caffeine had no effect on the first two Wingate tests but decreased power output during the third and fourth tests. Caffeine, therefore, seems to have no positive effect on sprint performance. However, given the limited number of studies, this conclusion cannot be reached definitively.

Effects of Caffeine on Cognitive Functioning

Caffeine has an effect on cognitive functioning. In a study by Hogervorst et al. (1999), caffeine was added to a carbohydrate-electrolyte drink, which was consumed before and during exercise. Cognitive functioning (attention, psychomotor skills, and memory) was measured immediately after a time trial (approximately 1 hour of all-out exercise). Caffeine improved all measures of cognitive functioning, and these effects were evident for the ingestion of 2 mg /kg b.w. and 3 mg/kg b.w. of caffeine. Some studies have also reported improved concentration with caffeine.

Effects of Caffeine Dosage

A few studies have investigated the effects of different dosage of caffeine on exercise performance (or endurance capacity). In a study by Pasman et al. (1995) cyclists received three different dosages of caffeine or placebo 1 hour before a ride to exhaustion at about 80% $\dot{V}O_2$max. The dosages were 0 mg/kg b.w., 5 mg/kg b.w., 9 mg/kg b.w., and 13 mg/kg b.w. With the lowest dose (5 mg/kg b.w.), endurance capacity was improved by 20%, but an increase in dosage had no further effect on performance (see figure 10.6). In runners, ingestion of 3 mg/kg b.w. and 6 mg/kg b.w. of caffeine had positive effects, whereas the improvement in time to exhaustion with 9 mg/kg b.w. of caffeine did not reach statistical significance (Graham and Spriet 1995).

Kovacs et al. (1998) studied the effect of adding relatively small amounts of caffeine (2 mg/kg b.w.,

Figure 10.6 Effect of ingesting different amounts of caffeine 1 hour pre-exercise on time to exhaustion at about 80% $\dot{V}O_2$max.

Data reproduced with permission from Pasman et al. 1995.

3 mg/kg b.w., or 4.5 mg/kg b.w.) to a carbohydrate-electrolyte solution. Time-trial cycling performance was improved with the lowest dosage of 2 mg/kg b.w. and was more improved with 3 mg/kg b.w., but a higher dose did not further affect performance. These results suggest that a caffeine intake of 3 mg/kg b.w. of caffeine exerts an ergogenic effect, but higher intakes will not result in an increased benefit.

Effects of Caffeine in Habitual Users

Studies have tried to address the question of whether habitual consumers of caffeine have an altered response during exercise. Although habitual caffeine users may have markedly different metabolic responses to caffeine (e.g., blunted FA response and blunted catecholamine excretion) (Dodd et al. 1991; Van Soeren et al. 1993), no studies show that changes in performance are different.

Interestingly, withdrawal from caffeine for 2 days to 4 days had no effect on the observed performance effect of caffeine (Van Soeren and Graham 1998). Although caffeine (6 mg/kg b.w.) improved performance compared with placebo, performance was not altered after 2 days or 4 days of withdrawal. This study also suggests that the mechanisms by which caffeine works is not related to availability of substrate or catecholamines. No evidence suggests that habitual caffeine intake or withdrawal influences the performance effects of caffeine.

Mechanisms of Caffeine Action

Several theories of how caffeine could exert its effects have been proposed (see figure 10.7). The

Caffeine increases lipolysis and spares muscle glycogen

1. Caffeine increases circulating epinephrine levels, which stimulates lipolysis
2. Caffeine antagonizes adenosine receptors that normally inhibit hormone-sensitive lipase and FA oxidation (only shown in vitro)
3. Caffeine inhibits phosphodiesterase leading to an increased concentration of 3',5'-cyclic monophosphate (cAMP) (only shown in vitro)

Caffeine increases excitability of the muscle fibers

1. Caffeine has a direct effect on key regulatory enzymes such as phosphorylase
2. Caffeine increases influx of calcium from the extracellular space
3. Caffeine increases release of calcium from the sarcoplasmic reticulum
4. Caffeine increases the sensitivity of the myofilaments to calcium

Caffeine influences signal transduction from the brain to the motor neuron

1. Caffeine stimulates catecholamine release and the release of neurotransmitters (dopamine, β-endorphins), possibly resulting in decreased perception of effort
2. Caffeine may lower the excitation threshold for motor neuron recruitment
3. Caffeine alters excitation/contraction coupling
4. Caffeine increases ion transport within the muscle
5. Caffeine facilitates transmission of nervous signals

Figure 10.7 Suggested mechanisms by which caffeine exerts its ergogenic effect.

precise mechanisms behind the ergogenic effect of caffeine are still unclear, but are unlikely to be related to changes in metabolism (increased fat metabolism and decreased muscle glycogen breakdown). The most likely explanation seems to be changes in central drive, in muscle fiber recruitment, and in perceived exertion caused by central nervous system effects of caffeine.

Below are some of the mechanisms that have been suggested:

- The traditional hypothesis for the ergogenic effect of caffeine is that caffeine stimulates lipolysis, increases fat oxidation, and, thereby, spares muscle glycogen, which is generally believed to improve endurance performance. Caffeine indeed stimulates lipolysis and the mobilization of FAs. These actions might occur indirectly by increasing the circulating epinephrine levels or directly by antagonizing adenosine receptors that normally inhibit hormone-sensitive lipase and FA oxidation.

- Another possible mechanism is a direct effect of caffeine or one of its metabolites on skeletal muscle. Possibilities include the handling of ions, inhibition of phosphodiesterase leading to an increased concentration of 3',5'-cyclic adenosine monophosphate (cAMP), and direct effect on key regulatory enzymes such as phos-

phorylase. Most of these hypotheses are derived from in vitro studies in which unphysiologically high concentrations of caffeine were used, and whether similar effects would have been found with more physiological concentrations is unclear.

- A third possibility, which is used to explain some of the suggested influences of caffeine on high-intensity exercise, is an increased influx of calcium from the extracellular space, increased release of calcium from the sarcoplasmic reticulum, and increased sensitivity of the myofilament to calcium, all resulting in an increased excitability of the muscle fibers.

- A fourth possible mechanism is the stimulating effect of caffeine on the central nervous system, which affects the perception of effort or affects the signal transduction from the brain to the neuromuscular junction. The cellular actions responsible for this central nervous system activation are not clear, but may be related to catecholamine release and, more likely, the release of neurotransmitters.

Side Effects of Caffeine

Caffeine use has side effects. Individuals who normally avoid caffeine may experience gastrointestinal distress, headaches, tachycardia, restlessness, irritability, tremor, elevated blood pressure, psychomotor agitations, and premature left ventricular contractions, all caused by the effect of caffeine on the central nervous system. Caffeine is also a diuretic and, therefore, should not be consumed in the hours before exercise when hydration is required. During exercise, the diuretic effect of caffeine is counteracted by catecholamines (Wemple et al. 1997), causing constriction of renal arterioles and reducing glomerular filtration rates. The catecholamines possibly increase sodium and chloride reabsorption rates in the proximal and distal tubules by affecting aldosterone, an antidiuretic hormone, resulting in greater water retention. Caffeine has no effect on sweat rates. Thus, caffeine is a diuretic in resting conditions but not during exercise. Very high intakes of caffeine have been associated with peptic ulcer, seizures, coma, and even death.

Table 10.3 Sources of Dietary Carnitine

Source	Total L-carnitine content (mg/100g)
Sheep	210
Lamb	78
Beef	64
Pork	30
Rabbit	21
Chicken	7.5
Milk	2.0
Egg	0.8
Peanut	0.1

L-Carnitine

L-carnitine (**carnitine**) a substance present in relatively high quantities in meat (the Latin word *caro-carnis* means meat or muscle), has received a lot of attention the past 20 years. As a supplement, it has been very popular among athletes and it has been the focus of many studies. Carnitine became especially popular after rumors circulated that it helped the Italian national soccer team to become world champions in 1982.

Carnitine supplementation is said to increase $\dot{V}O_2$max and reduce lactate production during maximal and supramaximal exercise. However, the most important claim is that carnitine improves fat metabolism, reduces fat mass, and increases muscle mass. It is generally advertised as a "fat burner." Therefore, carnitine is often used to lose weight, reduce body fat, and improve "sharpness". Endurance athletes use carnitine to increase the oxidation of fat and spare muscle glycogen.

Carnitine in the Body

L-carnitine is derived from red meats and dairy products in the diet (see table 10.3) and from endogenous production in the body. Even when dietary sources are insufficient, healthy humans produce enough from methionine and lysine to maintain functional body stores. For this reason, carnitine is not regarded as a vitamin, but as a vitamin-like substance.

Carnitine is synthesized in the liver and kidney, which together contain only 1.6% of the whole-body carnitine store (about 27 g). About 98% of the carnitine of the human body is pres-

ent in skeletal and heart muscle. Skeletal muscle and the heart are dependent upon transport of carnitine through the circulation, which contains about 0.5 % of whole-body carnitine.

Muscle takes carnitine up against a very large (~1000-fold) concentration gradient (plasma carnitine is 40 μmol/L to 60 μmol/L, and muscle carnitine and 4 mmol/L to 5 mmol/L) by a saturable active transport process (see figure 10.8). Carnitine is an end product of human metabolism and is only lost from the body via excretion in urine and stool. Daily losses are minimal (<60 mg/day) and are reduced to less than 20 mg/day on meat-free and carnitine-free diets (Bremer 1983). These minimal losses imply that the rate of endogenous biosynthesis, which is needed to maintain functional body stores, is also only about 20 mg/day. The amounts lost in stool can usually be ignored except after ingestion of oral supplements.

Carnitine 40-60 μmol/L

Blood

Muscle

Carnitine 4000-5000 μmol/L

Figure 10.8 Transport of carnitine into the muscle sarcoplasm occurs against a large concentration gradient.

Carnitine in Fat Metabolism

L-carnitine plays an important role in fat metabolism. In the overnight fasted state and during exercise of low to moderate intensity, long-chain FAs are the main energy sources used by most tissues, including skeletal muscle. The primary function of L-carnitine is to transport long-chain FAs across the mitochondrial inner membrane, as the inner membrane is impermeable both to long-chain FAs and to fatty acyl-CoA esters (Bremer 1983) (see figure 6.6). Once inside the mitochondria, FAs can be degraded to acetyl-CoA through β-oxidation. The acetyl-CoA units will then be available for the TCA cycle to provide energy.

Carnitine plays an important role in maintaining the acetyl-CoA/CoA ratio in the cell. During high-intensity exercise a large production of acetyl-CoA occurs, resulting in an increased acetyl-CoA/CoA ratio. This increased ratio, in turn, inhibits the pyruvate dehydrogenase (PDH) complex and reduces flux through the PDH complex and, hence, acetyl-CoA formation, resulting in increased lactate formation. Therefore the acetyl-CoA/CoA ratio should be maintained. Acetyl-CoA reacts with free carnitine to form Acetyl-carnitine and CoA.

$$acetyl\text{-}CoA + carnitine \rightarrow acetyl\text{-}carnitine + CoA$$

In theory, carnitine therefore acts as a sink for excess acetyl-CoA and blunts the accumulation of lactic acid, thereby enhancing high-intensity exercise performance.

Carnitine As a Slimming Agent

The belief that carnitine is a slimming agent is based on the assumption that regular oral ingestion of carnitine increases the muscle carnitine concentration. Another assumption is that if carnitine concentration in the muscle increases, fat oxidation also increases, thus leading to a gradual loss of the body fat stores. Several carefully conducted studies (Barnett et al. 1994; Vukovich et al. 1994) showed clearly that oral carnitine ingestion (up to 6 g/day for 14 days) does not change the muscle carnitine concentration. Also, calculations based on enzyme kinetics indicate that human muscle in resting conditions has more than

enough free carnitine to allow the enzyme carnitine palmitoyl transferase I (CPT I) to function at maximal activity. Claims that carnitine promotes weight loss, therefore, are not only unfounded but also theoretically impossible.

Carnitine in Endurance Exercise

The belief that carnitine is an ergogenic aid for endurance exercise is based on similar assumptions to the weight-loss assumptions (Wagenmakers 1999b): that carnitine concentration in muscle becomes too low to allow CPT I to function at a high velocity and to support the increased rate of fat oxidation during exercise; that oral ingestion of carnitine increases the total carnitine concentration in muscle; and that the increase in muscle carnitine increases the oxidation rate of plasma FAs and intramuscular triacylglycerols during exercise, thereby reducing muscle glycogen breakdown and postponing fatigue.

During high-intensity exercise, the free carnitine concentration in muscle does fall because this free carnitine reacts with acetyl-CoA. During very-high-intensity exercise, the free carnitine concentration falls to very low levels. Studies report values as low as 0.5 mmol/kg w.w. after 3 minutes to 4 minutes at 90% $\dot{V}O_2$max (Constantin-Teodosiu et al. 1991). These values approach the Km (see sidebar) of CPT I for carnitine (250 μM to 450 μM) measured in vitro (Bremer 1983). This decrease in free carnitine has been suggested as one of the mechanisms by which plasma FA and intramuscular triacylglycerol oxidation are reduced during high-intensity exercise (Constantin-Teodosiu et al. 1991; Timmons et al. 1996).

However, as discussed, the second assumption about carnitine as an ergogenic aid is not true because direct measurements in muscle after 14 days on 4 g/day to 6 g/day of carnitine failed to show increases in the muscle carnitine concentration (Barnett et al. 1994; Vukovich et al. 1994). This finding implies that carnitine supplementation cannot increase fat oxidation and improve exercise performance by the proposed mechanism. Indeed, many original investigations, which are summarized in numerous reviews (Heinonen 1996; Wagenmakers 1999b), have confirmed

Km

The Km is the substrate concentration that results in an enzyme-catalyzed reaction proceeding at 50% of the maximum rate. So at carnitine concentrations of 250 μM to 450 μM, the reaction catalyzed by CPT I is proceeding at about 50% of its maximum rate. For further explanation about Km see appendix A.

that carnitine supplementation does not increase fat oxidation and reduce glycogen breakdown and does not improve performance during prolonged cycling and running exercise.

Carnitine in High-Intensity Exercise

As previously indicated, carnitine may increase the availability of free CoA and maintain the acetyl-CoA/CoA ratio (see figure 10.9). This function of carnitine is especially important during maximal and supra-maximal exercise such as competitive sprint and middle-distance running and 50-meter to 400-meter swimming. If carnitine supplementation increases muscle carnitine concentration and, therefore, CoA availability in these conditions, the flux through the PDH complex could increase and less lactic acid would be produced (see figure 10.9). Theoretically, this process could delay fatigue and improve exercise performance. However, all these mechanisms are just theories because carnitine supplementation does not increase the muscle carnitine concentration. Most controlled original investigations have failed to show effects of carnitine supplementation on $\dot{V}O_2$max, high-intensity exercise performance, and lactate accumulation.

Choline

Acetylcholine transmits the electrical potential from the neuron to the muscle cell leading to calcium release from the sarcoplasmatic reticulum and muscle contraction. Experimental studies in animals suggest that depletion of the neuromuscular transmitter acetylcholine contributes to fatigue during sustained electrical stimulation or exercise (Pagala et al. 1984). Whether this transmission defect is at the presynaptic or postsynaptic membrane or across the synapse has not been elucidated.

The precursor of acetylcholine, **choline,** is a normal component of the human diet, most abundant in meat and diary products. It is also an integral part of several phospholipids incorporated into cell membranes, including phosphatidylcholine **(lecithin)**, lysophatidylcholine, and sphingomyelin (Zeisel 1998). Peak serum concentrations of choline occur several hours after ingestion of lecithin (Zeisel et al. 1991). Ingestion of choline or lecithin raises plasma choline levels in a dose-dependent matter. Based on these functions, choline supplements have been hypothesized to affect nerve transmission, increase strength, or facilitate the loss of body fat.

Strenuous exercise decreases plasma choline levels. They were reduced by 40% in participants of the 1985 Boston Marathon (Conlay et al. 1986), and similar findings were reported after the 1986 Boston Marathon (Wurtman and Lewis 1991). Von Allworden et al. (1993) reported a 16.9% average decline in plasma choline concentration after 2 hours of strenuous cycling (35 km/h). Neuromuscular transmission may have been impaired before the end of marathons or during the late stages of other forms of prolonged strenuous exercise, unless choline is supplied by

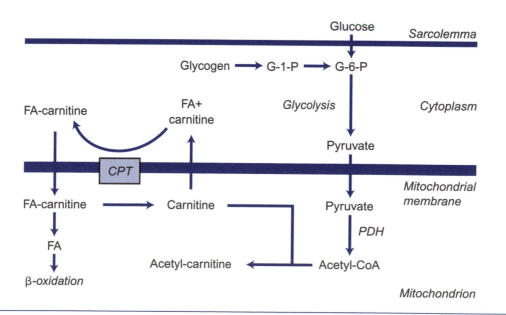

Figure 10.9 A potential link between FA uptake, carnitine, and glucose metabolism. Carnitine acts as a buffer for acetyl-CoA, thereby preventing a buildup of pyruvate and preventing lactate accumulation. This activity may, however, reduce free carnitine availability and, at least in theory, FA transport into the mitochondria.

neuronal or muscular membrane phospholipids or ingestion. Low acetylcholine concentrations have been associated with impaired neuromuscular transmission and fatigue. The acetylcholine concentration in the brain is directly related to the plasma choline concentration. Several studies of choline uptake and distribution after intravenous administration of choline show that plasma choline and acetylcholine in kidney, liver, lung, and heart are directly proportional to the amounts administered. Haubrich et al. (1975) reported that intravenous infusion of choline in guinea pigs led to incorporation of choline into acetylcholine within minutes in a variety of tissues.

Whether this reaction is also the case for skeletal muscle in vivo is still unknown. However, some evidence from in vitro studies indicates that newly synthesized acetylcholine is released during neuromuscular stimulation when choline is added to the perfusion medium (Bierkamper and Goldberg 1980). Gardiner and Gwee (1974) infused choline in rabbits and measured an elevated choline concentration in all tissues, including muscle. Unfortunately, acetylcholine was not measured. Thus, prolonged neuromuscular efforts may conceivably result in depletion of plasma choline, which might lead to fatigue because of insufficient availability of acetylcholine. Increasing plasma choline levels, on the other hand, by ingesting choline might increase acetylcholine availability and thereby reduce fatigue.

One preliminary report showed that ingestion of choline citrate during a 20-mile run prevented the fall in plasma choline concentration, and performance was improved compared with a placebo-treated group (Sandage et al. 1992). Spector et al. (1995) reported no effect on performance after the ingestion of 4.86 g choline bitartrate. During the placebo trial, however, no fall in choline was observed and none of the subjects displayed choline depletion. In such conditions, choline ingestion is unlikely to improve performance. Interestingly, these authors reported a significant negative correlation between the decrease in choline concentration and time to exhaustion, suggesting that choline may play a role in the development of fatigue.

Von Allworden et al. (1993) gave subjects 0.2 g/kg b.w. of lecithin 1 hour before they cycled for 2 hours at 35 km/h. Lecithin ingestion increased plasma choline concentrations by 26.9%, whereas placebo ingestion decreased choline concentrations by 16.9%. Unfortunately, exercise performance was not evaluated in this study. The claims of choline as a supplement are largely based on theory and findings of in vitro studies. Although some interesting observations have been made in humans, the grounds for recommending choline as an ergogenic aid are insufficient.

Chromium

Chromium is a very popular supplement because it is said to be a "muscle builder" and "fat burner," and enormous marketing hype has surrounded this supplement over the past few years. **Chromium** is a trace element that is present in foods such as brewers yeast, American cheese, mushrooms, and wheat germ, and it is considered an essential nutrient. Because of insufficient methods to assess chromium status, the U.S. Food and Nutrition Board could not establish an RDA for chromium. Instead, a range of adequate intake (AI) values is recommended: 25-35 μg per day (Food and Nutrition Board 1989). Anderson and Kozlovski (1985) suggested that many people in the United States are not ingesting even 50 pg/day of chromium. However, the AI was established using less sophisticated equipment than is available today, so the recommended values may be too high (Stoecker 1996).

Chromium potentiates insulin action, and insulin stimulates glucose and amino acid uptake by muscle cells. The stimulated amino acid uptake is thought to increase in protein synthesis and muscle mass gain. In fact, chromium supplements do increase muscle mass and growth in animals (Stoecker 1996). However, the effect of chromium on muscle mass in humans is less clear-cut. Chromium is marketed predominantly in the form of chromium picolinate, although chromium nicotinate and chromium chloride supplements also exist. Picolinic acid is an organic compound that binds to chromium and is thought to enhance the absorption and transport of chromium (Evans 1989).

Evans (1989) was the first to report that ingesting chromium increased lean tissue in exercising humans. In those studies, untrained college students and trained football players were given 200 μg of chromium picolinate or a placebo each day for 40 days to 42 days while they were on a resistance-training program. Those subjects who took chromium supplements gained significantly more lean-body mass compared with the placebo group. However, lean-body mass was only estimated from circumference measures, and the changes observed were small, so measurement error could have influenced the results.

Subsequent studies (Clancy et al. 1994; Hallmark et al. 1996; Hasten et al. 1992; Lukaski et al. 1996) have not confirmed the results of Evans (1989). In these carefully controlled studies, which used more sophisticated techniques to measure body composition, no effects were found in lean-body mass.

Thus, the majority of the studies show that chromium supplements are not effective in increasing lean-body mass. Based upon laboratory studies of cultured cells, chromium picolinate was suggested to accumulate in cells and cause chromosome damage (Stearns et al. 1995). Although this finding has not been confirmed in human studies (McCarty 1996), caution must be exercised in the use of chromium supplements.

Coenzyme Q10

Coenzyme Q10 (CoQ10), or ubiquinone is an integral part of the electron transport chain of the mitochondria. CoQ10, therefore, plays an important role in oxidative phosphorylation. In heart muscle, it has been used therapeutically to treat cardiovascular disease and promote recovery from cardiac surgery. CoQ10 supplementation in patients with those conditions improves oxidative metabolism and exercise capacity (Khatta et al. 2000), and it also functions as an antioxidant, promoting the scavenging of free radicals. Manufacturers extrapolated the results of improved $\dot{V}O_2$max in cardiac patients to healthy and trained athletes. CoQ10 is claimed to increase $\dot{V}O_2$max and increase "stamina" and "energy."

A few studies have investigated the effects of CoQ10 supplementation in athletes. Although most of these studies report elevated plasma CoQ10 levels, no changes were observed in $\dot{V}O_2$max, performance, or blood lactate at submaximal workloads. Ingestion of 120 mg/day of CoQ10 for 20 days was reported to result in marked increases in plasma CoQ10 concentrations, but the muscle CoQ10 concentration was unaltered (Svensson et al. 1999). Of course, if CoQ10 supplementation does not alter muscle CoQ10 concentration, it cannot be expected to have any effects on any of the performance-related variables.

CoQ10 may even have some negative effects. It possibly augments free-radical production during high-intensity exercise when an abundance of hydrogen ions are present in the cells (Malm et al. 1997). Paradoxically, this effect is the opposite of what CoQ10 is claimed to do.

Creatine

Creatine became a popular supplement after the 1992 Olympics in Barcelona. Gold medal winners Linford Christie in the men's 100-meter dash and Sally Gunnell in the women's 400-meter hurdles supposedly used creatine supplements. By the Olympic Games in Atlanta in 1996, approximately 80% of all athletes used creatine (Williams et al. 1999). The worldwide creatine consumption by athletes is now estimated to be around 3,000,000 kg/year. This section discusses the efficacy of creatine in different sports and the supposed

mechanisms of action. For more detail on the role of creatine in metabolism and performance, see Casey and Greenhaff (2000), Greenhaff (1998), and Terjung et al. (2000). A good and complete source of information is a book by Williams, Kreider, and Branch (1999).

Creatine in the Body

Creatine, or methylguanidine-acetic acid, is a naturally occurring compound present mostly in muscle tissue. It is not an essential nutrient, because it can be synthesized within the human body. In normal, healthy individuals, diet and oral ingestion together provide approximately 2 g/day of creatine. At the same time and at approximately the same rate (2 g/day), creatine is broken down to creatinine and excreted in the urine.

The primary dietary sources of creatine are fish and red meat (see table 10.4). Strict vegetarians and vegans have negligible creatine intake because plants contain only trace amounts. They are, therefore, dependent on endogenous synthesis of creatine. Oral ingestion of creatine suppresses the biosynthesis. When a creatine-deficient diet is consumed, the urinary excretion of creatine and creatinine is reduced.

Creatine synthesis in the human body is a 2-step reaction. First, the guanidino group of arginine is transferred to glycine forming guanidinoacetate. Second, creatine is formed via transfer of a methylgroup from S-adenosylmethionine to guanidinoacetate. The majority of creatine synthesis in humans occurs in the liver and kidneys (see figure 10.10).

Table 10.4	Sources of Dietary Creatine	
Food type	**Creatine content (g/100mg)**
Fish	
Shrimp	Trace
Cod	0.3
Herring	0.65–0.1
Plaice	0.2
Salmon	0.45
Tuna	0.4
Meat	
Beef	0.45
Pork	0.4
Other	
Milk	0.01
Cranberries	0.002

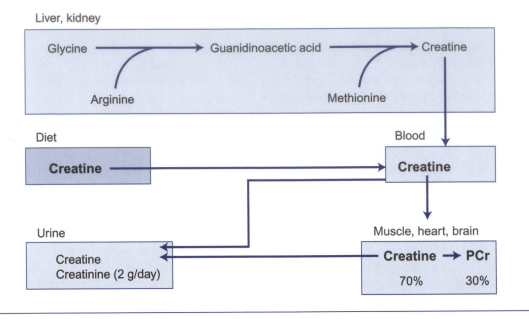

Figure 10.10 Creatine synthesis and transport in the body.

In a 70-kg (154-lb) man, the total-body creatine pool is approximately 120 g, 95% of which is in muscle (skeletal, heart, and smooth muscle). The remaining 5% is in brain, liver, kidneys, and testes. Creatine synthesized in liver and kidney and absorbed from the diet is transported via the blood to the muscle. Muscle takes up creatine against a concentration gradient by a sodium-dependent saturable active transport process. In the muscle cell, creatine is phosphorylated, after which it is trapped within the muscle. This process helps to create a very high total-creatine gradient (30 mmol/kg w.w. to 40 mmol/kg w.w. or 120 mmol/kg d.w. to 160 mmol/kg d.w. in skeletal muscle, with 60% to 70% in the form of phosphocreatine) (Wyss et al. 2000). Type I and type II muscle fibers have differing creatine content; type II fibers having about 30% more creatine than type I fibers.

Creatine in the Metabolic Process

The role of creatine and phosphocreatine is discussed in chapter 2 but will be briefly repeated here. As muscle contracts, adenosine triphosphate (ATP) is degraded to adenosine diphosphate (ADP) and inorganic phosphate (Pi) to provide the energy:

$$ATP \rightarrow ADP + Pi + energy$$

During intense maximal exercise, the ATP stores can only provide energy for about 1 second to 2 seconds. When the whole-muscle ATP concentration falls by about 30%, the muscle fatigues (Hultman et al. 1991; Karlsson and Saltin 1970). To prevent fatigue, regeneration of ATP must occur at a rate similar to that of

ATP hydrolysis to maintain ATP concentration close to resting levels.

An important function of phosphocreatine in muscle is to provide the high-energy phosphate group for ATP regeneration during the first seconds of high-intensity exercise, thus allowing time for glycogen breakdown and glycolysis (the other main process generating cytosolic ATP during high-intensity exercise) to speed up to the required rate. Transfer of the phosphate group from phosphocreatine to adenosine diphosphate (ADP) is catalyzed by the enzyme creatine kinase, resulting in regeneration of ATP and release of free creatine:

$$\text{Phosphocreatine (PCr) + ADP} \\ \text{+ } H^+ \rightarrow \text{Creatine (Cr) + ATP}$$

PCr is present in resting muscle in a concentration that is 3 to 4 times that of ATP (see appendix A). During the 100-meter sprint, 22 g of ATP is estimated to be broken down per second, or about 50% of the ATP content per kg of active muscle. Because fatigue occurs in human muscle when the whole-muscle ATP concentration falls by about 30%, the need for rephosphorylation of the ADP formed during contraction is obvious.

Anaerobic degradation of PCr and glycogen is responsible for a significant rate of ATP resynthesis during the first seconds of high-intensity exercise (Hultman et al. 1991; Karlsson and Saltin 1970). However, the PCr store in muscle is limited and is depleted within 5 seconds of supramaximal exercise. In this manner, the concentration of skeletal muscle

ATP is maintained to some degree during single bouts or repeated bouts of supramaximal exercise. Anaerobic ATP resynthesis, however, cannot be maintained at the same rate as during the first few seconds of supramaximal exercise, and, consequently, over the course of 30 seconds, ATP turnover rates fall by about 20%. High PCr stores possibly reduce the need for anaerobic glycolysis and lactic acid formation during intense exercise, which might be another potential benefit of creatine supplementation.

A third important function of creatine is its potential buffering capacity for hydrogen ions as these ions are used during ATP regeneration, as shown in the previous equation. A higher creatine concentration in the muscle also implies an increased flux through the creatine kinase reaction, resulting in increased PCr synthesis during recovery from high-intensity exercise. The roles of creatine listed previously suggest that elevating muscle creatine and PCr stores benefit high-intensity exercise performance. What way would be easier to achieve this than simply eating creatine?

Creatine Supplementation

Harris et al. (1992) were the first to state that ingesting creatine monohydrate could increase total-muscle creatine stores (creatine and phosphocreatine). In that study, ingesting 5 g of creatine 4 times to 6 times a day for several days increased the total creatine concentration by an average of 25 mmol/kg d.w., and 30% of the increase in total creatine content was in the form of phosphocreatine. The authors suggested that these increases could improve exercise performance but did not test this suggestion in their study. The first

performance study was conducted by Greenhaff et al. (1993). Subjects ingested 20 g/day of creatine for 5 days, and creatine indeed improved performance by about 6% during repeated bouts of maximal knee extensor exercise. After that study, more studies were performed investigating different modes of exercise (Balsom et al. 1993a, 1993b; Birch et al. 1994; Harris et al. 1992; Volek et al. 1997). In 1999, of the 62 laboratory-based studies performed on creatine supplementation and high-intensity exercise performance, 42 reported positive effects, and the remainder showed no effects (Williams et al. 1999).

Creatine Loading Regimens

Most studies used a creatine loading regimen of 20 g/day in 4 portions of 5 g each given at different times of the day for a 6-day period. This regimen has been shown to increase the muscle creatine concentration, on average, by about 25 mmol/kg d.w. This increase corresponded to about 20% of the basal total-muscle creatine concentration of about 125 mmol per kg d.w. Hultman et al. (1996) found that after an initial loading phase of 20 g/day for 6 days, a subsequent dose of 2 g/day was enough to maintain the high total-creatine concentration for 35 days, whereas stopping of creatine supplementation after 6 days caused a slow gradual decline of the creatine concentration in muscle.

When creatine was ingested at a dose of 3 g/day, the rate of increase in muscle creatine was correspondingly lower, but after 28 days on 3 g/day the total-creatine concentration was similar to the rapid-loading regimen (see figure 10.11). Therefore, a loading dose of 20 g/day for 6 days followed by a maintenance dose of 2 g

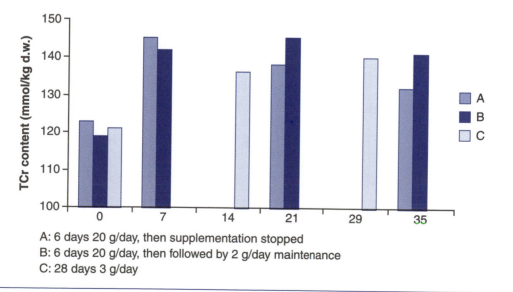

A: 6 days 20 g/day, then supplementation stopped
B: 6 days 20 g/day, then followed by 2 g/day maintenance
C: 28 days 3 g/day

Figure 10.11 Different protocols of creatine loading. TCr = total creatine.

Reprinted, by permission, from E. Hultman et al., 1996, "Muscle creatine loading in men," *Journal of Applied Physiology* 81(1): 232-237.

/day to 3 g/day is advised if athletes want to increase muscle creatine to maximal levels quickly, whereas a continuous dose of 3 g/day leads to the same maximal end level in about 1 month. The increase in muscle PCr concentration was about 40% of the increase in total-creatine concentration with both procedures.

Considerable variation exists among subjects in the initial total-muscle creatine concentration. The reasons for variation are largely unknown, but may at least be partly related to the habitual diet. The largest increase in muscle creatine concentration is observed in individuals with the lowest initial concentration, whereas individuals with already high creatine concentrations benefit only marginally (Harris et al. 1992) (see figure 10.12). A concentration of 160 mmol/kg d.w. appears to be the maximal creatine concentration achievable as a result of creatine supplementation. However, only about 20% of subjects reached this level after creatine supplementation.

Total-muscle creatine can be increased more (mean increase 30 mmol/kg d.w. to 40 mmol/kg d.w.) when creatine (20 g/day for 5 days) is ingested in solution with simple carbohydrates (Green et al. 1995; Green et al. 1996). In a study, the total-muscle creatine con-

centration was increased in most subjects close to the upper limit of 160 mmol/kg d.w. Carbohydrate ingestion is thought to stimulate muscle creatine uptake via an insulin-dependent mechanism. Insulin may stimulate the sodium-potassium pump activity and thereby the sodium-dependent muscle creatine transport.

In a study by Casey et al. (1996) the changes in performance were related to the changes in total-muscle creatine content (see figure 10.13). A strong correlation was observed in that those individuals who displayed the largest increases in total-muscle creatine concentration also exhibited the largest performance benefit. A change in muscle creatine content of about 20 mmol/kg d.w. is said to be necessary before significant changes in performance are observed. About 30% of all individuals do not display such large increases in muscle creatine and, therefore, do not benefit. They are often referred to as nonresponders.

Creatine and Weight Gain

Creatine supplementation (20 g/day for 5 days to 6 days) is generally accompanied by increases in body weight of 0.5 kg to 3.5 kg. (For a complete overview, see Williams et al. [1999]). The average increase in

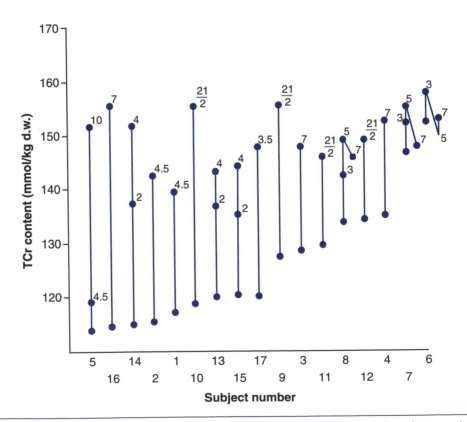

Figure 10.12 Individual responses to creatine loading. Individuals with low creatine stores benefit most, whereas individuals with already high creatine stores have minimal increases in muscle creatine. Numbers in graph are days of supplementation at a rate of 20-30 g/day. 21/2 indicates subjects who ingested creatine on alternate days for 21 days.

Reprinted, by permission, from Hultman et al., 1996, "Muscle creatine loading in men," *Journal of Applied Physiology* 81(1): 232-237.

body mass is about 1 kg. Theoretically, this increase in body mass and possible change in body composition results from increases in intracellular water, stimulation of protein synthesis, or a decrease in protein breakdown. Because the decrease in urine production exactly paralleled the time course of the increase in muscle creatine concentration (see figure 10.13), creatine likely causes water retention

in skeletal muscle cells because of an increase of the intracellular osmolarity of the muscle fibers. Evidence suggests that some of the weight gain may be attributable to the anabolic effect of creatine (Kreider et al. 1998), although in the short term (5 days to 6 days) this effect is not likely to be an important factor.

The increase in body mass may be beneficial or have no effect in some disciplines. However, in sports that involve weight-bearing activities, such as running or gymnastics, the weight gain caused by creatine supplementation could have a negative impact on performance.

Creatine and High-Intensity Exercise

The findings of Greenhaff et al. (1993), who used high-intensity intermittent exercise, have been repeated by various other investigations using cycle ergometry, bench press, or running as the mode of exercise. Most of these studies (about 70% of all studies) found improvements in strength, force production, or torque.

Balsom, Ekblom, et al. (1993) randomly assigned 16 trained subjects to a creatine group (25 g/day for 6 days) and a placebo group. One test these subjects performed was a repeated sprint test, in which they sprinted 10 times for 6 seconds with 30 seconds of recovery between bouts. Although subjects fatigued with both creatine and placebo, after 7 sprints, fatigue was significantly greater in the placebo group. Casey et al. (1996) investigated the effect of acute creatine supplementation (20 g/day for 5 days) on isokinetic cycle performance (2 × 30 seconds with 4 minutes recovery in between). Increases in peak power and total work were already observed in the first of the two bouts after creatine supplementation. The improvements in total work production were positively correlated with the increased concentration of PCr in type II muscle fibers after supplementation (see figure 10.14).

Several studies investigated the effect of creatine supplementation versus placebo on 25-meter, 50-meter, and 100-meter performance in elite swimmers performing their best stroke (Burke et al. 1996; Mujika et al. 1996; Peyrebrune et al. 1998). These studies failed to show an ergogenic effect of creatine supplementation. Two studies, however, showed improvements in 10 × 50 meter or 8 × 45 meter swimming velocity (Leenders et al. 1999; Peyrebrune et al. 1998). Rossiter et al. (1996) observed an ergogenic effect of creatine versus placebo supplementation on the 1,000-meter performance of competitive rowers. Recent findings suggest that creatine also improves high-intensity exercise performance in competitive squash players (Romer et al. 2001). The players fatigued less toward

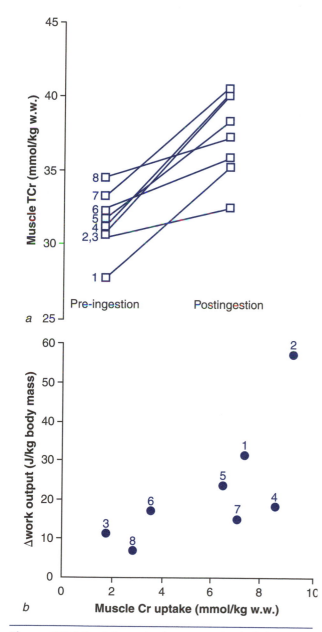

Figure 10.13 Relationship between individual changes in mixed muscle creatine concentration and changes in total work production after creatine loading (4 g/day to 5 g/day for 5 days). Work production was measured during 2 bouts of 30 seconds maximal isokinetic cycling exercises.

Reprinted, by permission, from A. Casey et al., 1996, "Creatine ingestion favorably affects performance and muscle metabolism during maximal exercise in humans," *American Journal of Physiology* 271(1): E31-7.

Figure 10.14 Urinary volume before and after either placebo or creatine ingestion. Creatine was administered as 5 g 4 times a day for 5 days. There was a clear relationship between the decreased urinary output and the increase in body mass after creatine ingestion.

Reprinted, by permission, from E. Hultman et al., 1996, "Muscle creatine loading in men," *Journal of Applied Physiology* 81(1): 232-237.

the end of a game when supplemented with creatine. Thus, creatine supplementation may not always result in a positive effect on performance in competitive situations. Whether creatine has an effect may depend on the initial muscle creatine concentrations, the type of exercise, and the level of the athlete.

Creatine and Endurance Exercise

In endurance exercise, most ATP is resynthesized by oxidative phosphorylation in the mitochondria. Net PCr breakdown and the net contribution of PCr to energy production are minimal. However, creatine and PCr provides a shuttle system for the transfer of high-energy phosphate groups from the ATP production site (the mitochondria) to the ATP consumption site (the contracting myofibrils) (see figure 10.15). A phosphate group of ATP produced in the mitochondria is donated to creatine to form phosphocreatine. From phosphocreatine, the phosphate group is donated to ADP, and ATP is formed and can be used for muscle contraction. Theoretically, creatine could, therefore, facilitate aerobic energy production and enhance performance in prolonged exercise.

Balsom, Harridge, et al. (1993) investigated the effect of creatine supplementation for 6 days on endurance exercise performance in well-trained runners. No effect occurred during a supramaximal treadmill run to exhaustion in the laboratory, but a significant decrease in performance occurred during a 6-kilometer terrain run. Subjects showed an increase in body weight of 0.5 kg to 1.0 kg, which possibly explains the negative result during the terrain run. In another study, 5 days of creatine supplementation (20 g/day) had no influence on oxygen uptake, respiratory gas exchange, and blood-lactate concentration during submaximal incremental treadmill exercise and recovery. These data seem to suggest that the availability of creatine and PCr are not rate limiting for the diffusion of energy-rich phosphate groups through the cytosol and that creatine supplementation, therefore, does not have an effect on muscle metabolism in endurance exercise. The studies that have investigated the effects of creatine supplementation on endurance performance generally have not reported an ergogenic effect.

Creatine in Resistance Training

Vandenberghe et al. (1997) investigated the effect of creatine loading on muscle PCr phosphate concentration, muscle strength, and body composition after a 10-week resistance-training program. Compared with placebo, maximal strength of the trained muscle groups increased 20% to 25% more, maximal intermittent exercise capacity of the arm flexors increased 10% to 25% more, and fat-free mass increased by 60% more with creatine supplementation. This study and others suggest that the combination of creatine ingestion and strength training is more effective than strength

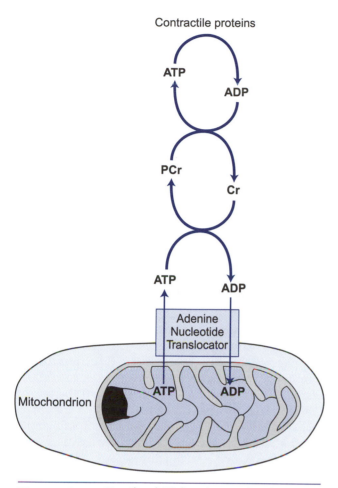

Figure 10.15 Transfer of ATP from the site of synthesis (mitochondria) to the site of usage (contractile proteins). Creatine and phosphocreatine play an important role in this process.
Adapted from A.J.M. Wagenmakers, 1999

training only. In addition, Wagenmakers (1999b) suggested that creatine supplementation allows for more repetitions and, thus, a better quality of training and at the same time may have an anabolic effect.

Creatine causes fluid retention, which may result in muscle cell swelling. Cell swelling acts as a universal anabolic signal, causing an increase of protein synthesis and net protein deposition (Lang et al. 1998). Although several animal and clinical studies suggest that creatine ingestion has anabolic effects, no evidence in healthy individuals indicates that creatine affects protein metabolism.

Mechanisms of Creatine Action

Several mechanisms by which creatine exerts its effect have been proposed:

- The most obvious explanation is increased PCr availability, particularly in type II muscle

fibers (Casey et al. 1996). Evidence indicates that increased PCr stores in the muscle improve contractile function by maintaining ATP turnover.
- Another possible mechanism is the increased rate of PCr resynthesis (Greenhaff et al. 1994), which is particularly important in the short recovery periods during repeated bouts of maximal exercise.
- The increased use of PCr as an energy source could reduce anaerobic glycolysis and lactic acid formation. This activity could theoretically reduce hydrogen ion formation in the muscle and delay fatigue caused by increased muscle acidity.
- Creatine could buffer some of the hydrogen ions produced during high-intensity exercise. This process would delay fatigue in high-intensity exercise that is limited by lactic acid formation.
- As indicated in figure 10.15, creatine plays an important role in shuttling high-energy phosphates from the site of ATP production (mitochondria) to the site of ATP breakdown (myofibrils). This role of creatine was suggested as a potential mechanism for improved performance in endurance type activities. However, these types of activities are not affected by creatine supplementation suggesting that this mechanism may not be important.
- Creatine may have anabolic properties.

Creatine and Safety

No studies have reported detrimental health effects of creatine. However, according to numerous anecdotal reports, creatine supplementation causes ailments; gastrointestinal, cardiovascular, and muscular problems; nausea, vomiting, and diarrhea; alterations in kidney and liver function; muscle cramps; and elevated blood pressure. As pointed out in a round-table discussion by the American College of Sports Medicine, "The evidence is not definitive and/or it is incomplete to indict the practice of creatine supplementation as a health risk; at the same time, our lack of information cannot be taken as an assurance that creatine supplementation is free from health risks. Ignorance provides little comfort of untoward effects yet to be discovered."

Dehydroepiandrosterone

Dehydroepiandrosterone (DHEA) and its sulphated ester (DHEAS) are relatively weak androgen steroid hormones synthesized primarily in early adulthood

253

(20 years to 25 years of age) by the adrenal cortex. It is not present in large quantities in our diet but when taken as a supplement, it becomes a precursor for at least two hormones: testosterone and estradiol. Because DHEA is a precursor for testosterone, it is thought to increase testosterone concentration and thereby increase protein synthesis and muscle mass. DHEA is, therefore, one of the most popular supplements, especially in the United States. Synthetic DHEA is categorized as a nutrition supplement because the substance also occurs naturally. As a result its classification, the Food and Drug administration has no control over what manufacturers say about the product. They call DHEA a "superhormone" that increases lean-body mass, reduces the ageing process, boosts immune function, and protects against heart disease. Because the plasma DHEA concentration decreases with age, many studies have focused on the effects of the supplement in older individuals. Manufacturers abuse the results of this research and claim that restoring the blood DHEA concentrations to "youth" levels slows the ageing process. Little is known about the physiological role of DHEA or the cellular and molecular mechanisms of its action. However DHEA is known to interact with the receptors of the neurotransmitter γ-amino butyric acid (GABA) in the brain.

Early support for DHEA as a supplement comes from animal studies in which the animals were given this hormone. The test animals showed improved immune function and resistance to arteriosclerosis, cancer, viral infections, obesity, and diabetes. Some studies even reported extended life span. Rats, however, normally have extremely low DHEA levels and may respond very differently than humans. Human studies showed a decreased risk of cardiovascular diseases in men with high DHEA levels but an increased risk in women. Subsequent studies reported minimal protective effects of DHEA in men and no effects or negative effects in women (Johannes et al. 1999). In one study, DHEA supplementation resulted in enhanced protection against cardiovascular diseases (Jakubowicz et al. 1995). In general, though, the results of various studies are not consistent, and whether DHEA really protects against cardiovascular disease is difficult to determine (Sirrs and Bebb 1999).

Studies that investigated the effects of DHEA on body composition showed a rise in blood androgen levels after supplementation (100 mg/day to 1600 mg/day of DHEA), but no effects on body weight or lean-body mass were observed. In addition, Welle et al. (1990) did not observe effects on energy or protein metabolism. Nestler et al. (1988) reported a small decrease in fat mass without a change in total-body mass, which suggests that DHEA resulted in an increase in lean-body mass. In a study by Mortola and Yen (1990), 100 mg/day of DHEA for 3 months resulted in a 1% increase in lean-body mass. In that study, fat mass decreased in men but increased in women. A study of obese subjects who received 1,600 mg/day of DHEA for 28 days did not report any changes in body composition. These results, although varied and not convincing, seem to indicate that DHEA has a small effect on muscle mass and immune function. Most of these studies were performed in subjects 40 years to 75 years of age, and little is known about the effects in young adults.

Because so little is known about the possible side effects of DHEA, concern has been expressed by various researchers and institutions. DHEA is an uncontrolled substance and is readily available in pharmacies, in drug stores, and over the Internet. Clinicians fear that elevated plasma DHEA through supplementation might stimulate dormant prostate tumors or cause hypertrophy of the prostate gland itself. Ethical questions also arise about the use of hormones as ergogenic substances. Both the International Olympic Committee and the US Olympic Committee have placed DHEA on the list of banned substances with a zero tolerance.

Dihydroxyacetone

Dihydroxyacetone is an intermediate of glycolysis. Long-term ingestion of this substance in combination with pyruvate is suggested to have positive effects on both carbohydrate and fat metabolism. The studies on dihydroxyacetone and pyruvate are discussed in the section on pyruvate.

Fish Oil

Fish oil is a natural source of long-chain omega-3 FAs, including both docosahexaenoic acid and eicosapentaenoic acid. Guezennec et al. (1989) suggested that increasing the fraction of PUFA in the phospholipids of erythrocyte (red blood cell) membranes improves membrane fluidity and increases red blood cell deformability (flexibility), resulting in improved peripheral oxygen supply. They conducted a study in which 14 male subjects were divided into 2 groups; 1 group received a normal diet and 1 group received a diet rich in fish oil for 6 weeks. The fraction of omega-3 FAs increased in erythrocyte membranes, but no change in red blood cell deformability was seen under resting conditions. During hypobaric exercise, red blood cell deformability decreased less with the fish oil feeding.

Brilla and Landerholm (1990) studied the effects of fish oil feeding and exercise training in 32 sedentary males and found that exercise training resulted in an increased $\dot{V}O_2$max, whereas fish oil supplementation had no effect. Oostenbrug et al. (1997) supplemented trained cyclists for 3 weeks with placebo or fish oil (6 g/day). Fish oil did not alter red blood cell characteristics in this study and had no effect on $\dot{V}O_2$max, maximal power output, or time-trial performance.

Physical training improves red blood cell deformability and changes the FA composition of membranes toward a higher percentage of unsaturated FAs, so the enhanced fluidity under resting conditions could be masked by physical training (Kamada et al. 1993). The enhanced membrane fluidity may be especially important when the uptake of oxygen becomes limiting, as during exercise under hypoxic conditions. However, the physiologic consequences of PUFA are still hypothetical, and further studies are necessary to evaluate the possible effects on hemorrheologic changes during exercise.

Ginseng

Ginseng is the root of the *Araliaceous* plant and is a quite popular supplement among athletes. It is commonly described as an "adaptogen," a substance that helps the body to adapt to stress situations. Ginseng has been used for several thousand years in Asia. Its effects are said to include improved sleep, improved memory, reduced fatigue, and relief of heart pain, headache, and nausea. The known varieties of ginseng are American, Chinese, Korean, Japanese, and Siberian (see figure 10.16), and the three main medicinal species are *Panax ginseng* (Chinese or Korean ginseng), *Panax japonicum* (Japanese ginseng from India, Southern China, and Japan), and *Panax quinquefolium* (American ginseng). Siberian, or Russian, ginseng, although claimed to have a similar stimulant effect, is an entirely different plant, *Eleutherococcus senticosus*. It is used as a cheaper substitute of the *Panax ginseng*.

The main active constituents of the *Panax* species are triterpenoid glycosides, or saponins (also referred to as ginsenosides or panaxosides). The structure and distribution of saponins may vary with species and variety. At least 13 different saponins exist. *Panax ginseng* is believed to be the most potent form of ginseng and has become the standard. Animal studies support some of the claims about ginseng. Running performance in rats improved 132% after acute administration of ginseng and 179% after 7 days of

Russian/Siberian ginseng	*Eleutherococcus senticosus*
Chinese/Korean ginseng	*Panax ginseng*
American ginseng	*Panax quinquefolium*
Japanese ginseng	*Panax japonicum*

Figure 10.16 Different species of ginseng.

administration. The ingestion of ginseng was accompanied by an increase in the basal ACTH and cortisol levels in rats. In humans, the effects are not clear, and several studies show inconsistent results. Most of the human studies did not have an appropriate design and were not placebo controlled or were not randomized. Some of these uncontrolled studies reported improvements in $\dot{V}O_2$max and exercise performance. In one study, 5 subjects ingested 2 g/day of *Panax ginseng* for 4 weeks, and 6 subjects acted as a control group. Measurements included substrate utilization, plasma hormone concentrations, ratings of perceived effort, and endurance capacity. No differences were found in any of these variables between the group given ginseng and the control group. Similar findings were reported by other researchers (Allen et al. 1998; Engels and Wirth 1997). At present, very little or no evidence in the literature supports the claim that ginseng is an ergogenic aid.

Glandulars

Glandulars are extracts from animal glands such as the adrenals, the thymus, the pituitary, and the testes. They are claimed to enhance the function of the equivalent gland in the human body. For example, orchic extract from the testes supposedly enhances testosterone levels (Williams 1993). However, glandular extracts are degraded during the digestive process and are inactive when absorbed. Therefore, they cannot exert a pharmacological effect.

Glycerol

Glycerol was believed to be a substrate for gluconeogenesis and, as such, could provide a fuel during exercise. More recently, a probably more important role of glycerol became apparent—a way to hyperhydrate before exercise in hot environmental conditions. Glycerol is a 3-carbon molecule that normally serves as the backbone of a triacylglycerol molecule. We, therefore, ingest a fairly large amount of glycerol, as part of triacylglycerol, on a daily basis. Glycerol is also released into the bloodstream after lipolysis. Thus, during exercise, when lipolysis is stimulated, plasma glycerol concentrations become elevated.

Glycerol As a Fuel

The studies that investigated the efficacy of glycerol as a fuel found the contribution of glycerol to the overall energy expenditure to be relatively small. Glycerol cannot be oxidized directly in very large amounts in the muscle. Therefore, glycerol must be converted into a glucose molecule in gluconeogenesis in the liver before being used as a fuel. This process is relatively slow, and, hence, the contribution of glycerol to fuel supply during exercise is negligible.

Glycerol As a Hyperhydrating Agent

When ingested with a relatively large volume of water (1 L to 2 L), glycerol improves water absorption (Wapnir et al. 1996) and increases water retention in the extracellular space, especially in plasma (Gleeson et al. 1986; Koenigsberg et al. 1995). This action may occur through either of 2 mechanisms: (1) Glycerol may move to the extracellular space and, via osmosis, draw water into this compartment. In other words, glycerol acts like a sponge. (2) A small increase in the plasma osmolarity may increase ADH secretion from the posterior pituitary gland and, hence, urine production is decreased. Hyperhydration with glycerol before exercise decreases overall heat stress during exercise, as indicated by lower heart rate and body temperature (Lyons et al. 1990). The recommended protocol for the intake of glycerol and water before exercise is given in table 10.5.

Although these studies look promising, quite a few studies found no effect of glycerol on thermoregulation (Inder et al. 1998; Latzka et al. 1997;

Latzka et al. 1998). In these studies, the volume of water consumed (500 ml) may have been too small. In a study by Murray et al. (1991), no indications of hyperhydration were found. Generally, however, the ingestion of 1 g/kg b.w. of glycerol with 1 L to 2 L of water seems to protect against heat stress and may, thus, have some health benefits when exercising in extreme conditions. Some studies showed that reduced cardiovascular stress and decreased body temperature resulted in improved exercise performance. This finding could not be confirmed, even though those studies reported indications of improved thermoregulation. Whether glycerol improves endurance performance remains unclear. Glycerol has significant side effects, including nausea, heartache, blurred vision, headaches, gastrointestinal problems, dizziness, and light-headedness. Also, the large volume of fluid that needs to be consumed with the glycerol makes many users feel bloated.

Inosine

Inosine is a nucleoside, a purine base comparable to adenine, which is one of the structural components of ATP. Inosine is obtained through the diet or synthesized endogenously in the body. Manufacturers claim that inosine increases ATP stores, thereby improving muscle strength, training quality, and performance. In addition, inosine is thought to improve oxygen delivery to the cells and to improve endurance. The latter belief is based on the role inosine plays in the formation of 2,3-diphosphoglycerate, a substance in erythrocytes that facilitates the release of oxygen to the tissues. Other suggested mechanisms for ergogenic effects of inosine include augmenting cardiac contractility, vasodilating activity, and stimulation of insulin release, increasing glucose delivery to the myocardium. The studies that have investigated the effects

Table 10.5 Recommended Protocol for Glycerol and Water Intake to Optimize Pre-Exercise Hydration

Glycerol ingestion starts 2.5 h (150 min) before exercise	
150 min pre-exercise	5 ml/kg glycerol in a 20% solution
120 min pre-exercise	5 ml/kg water
105 min pre-exercise	5 ml/kg water
90 min pre-exercise	5 ml/kg glycerol in a 20% solution + 5 ml/kg water
60 min pre-exercise	5 ml/kg water
0 min	Start exercise

Stated doses are in ml per kg body weight.

of inosine on strength and endurance performance do not provide support for the claims and theories.

- In one carefully conducted study, trained men (n = 4) and women (n = 5) were administered 6 g/day of inosine or placebo for 2 days (Williams et al. 1990). No change occurred in 3-mile treadmill run time, $\dot{V}O_2$max, or perceived exertion, and blood lactate levels were also similar. After a 30-minute break, subjects performed another run, in which speed was kept constant but the gradient gradually increased. Time to fatigue in this run was reduced with inosine (i.e., it had an **ergolytic** effect).

- Another study investigated the effects of 5 g/day of inosine or placebo for 5 days (Starling et al. 1996). No effects were found on performance in a 30-second Wingate test or a 30-minute, self-paced time trial. In addition, a supramaximal constant-load sprint test was performed, and fatigue occurred 10% earlier with inosine compared with placebo, again indicating that inosine can be detrimental to performance. No effects were observed in heart rate or ratings of perceived exertion.

- A study investigated the effects of 10 g/day of inosine supplementation over periods of 5 days and 10 days. Seven trained volunteers performed tests, a 5 times 6-second sprint, a 30-second sprint, and a 20-minute time trial. Performance was not affected by inosine supplementation. In addition, no changes in erythrocyte 2,3-diphosphoglycerate concentrations were observed.

Inosine has adverse effects in that it increases serum uric acid levels. The levels observed by Starling et al. (1996) are often associated with gouty arthritis, particularly pain in the knee and foot joints. Inosine has no ergogenic effects and can even be ergolytic. Inosine supplements should, therefore, be avoided.

Lactate Salts and Polylactate

Lactate is a good fuel for the human heart, and the rate of lactate clearance and oxidation in several studies exceeded those rates achieved by glucose. Most of the lactate that appears in the blood during moderate-intensity exercise is oxidized by the active muscle fibers with a high oxidative capacity. The lactate molecule possibly serves as a shuttle for transport of glucose-derived carbon moieties between various organs and cells (e.g., from the exercising muscle to the heart, from type II fibers in an active muscle to the neighboring type I fibers in the same muscle or to the type I fibers of another active muscle) (Brooks 1986). Lactate ingestion during exercise may provide a good fuel for the muscle.

Lactate Salts

Lactate can be provided as sodium or potassium lactate. However, a solution containing these salts has a very high osmolarity when significant amounts of lactate must be ingested. The amounts of sodium or potassium that would also have to be ingested are very large and are likely to produce severe gastrointestinal problems. Solutions of lactate salts can be taken in maximal bolus amounts of about 10 g without causing gastrointestinal problems. The performance effects of these amounts have not been investigated but are expected to be nonexistent, given the amount of endogenous lactate formed.

Polylactate

This problem of too much lactate salt could theoretically be solved by using polylactate (see the following chemical compositions), a lactate polymer, which would reduce the osmolarity yet provide relatively large amounts of lactate.

$$CH_3\text{-}CH(OH)\text{-}COOH \quad \text{(lactic acid)}$$

$$CH_3\text{-}CH(OH)\text{-}COO^- \quad \text{(lactate ion)}$$

$$CH_3\text{-}CH(OH)\text{-}CO[O\text{-}CH(CH_3\text{-}CO]n\text{-}OCH(CH_3)\text{-}COOH$$
$$\text{(polylactate)}$$

Polylactate is used as a supplement and is included in some sports drinks. It can be produced through controlled chemical synthesis. If polylactate dissolved in water and could be quickly hydrolyzed in the gastrointestinal tract of humans, similarly to glucose polymers, it could be the ideal chemical form to ingest carbohydrate. However, polylactate does not normally occur in food products and does not dissolve very well in water. The human body does not contain enzymes to degrade polylactate. Thus, the bioavailablity and intestinal absorption are very low or even zero (Wagenmakers 1999). Because of its slow biodegradability, polylactate is use by orthopedic and dental surgeons to replace steel plates in the repair of broken bones. Polylactate, in the true chemical sense, cannot function to generate lactate at a high rate and cannot function as a nutritional ergogenic aid during exercise.

Two studies (Fahey et al. 1991; Swensen et al. 1994), nevertheless, claim to have investigated the performance effects of polylactate. A careful reading of the published papers reveals that the authors appear to have investigated the effects of a commercial product called Poly-L-lactate. This supplement contains molecules of lactate bound to amino acids. Because of the much larger molecular mass of the amino acids, the lactate content of this supplement is relatively low (< 50% lactate). One of the amino acids is arginine, which is known to cause gastrointestinal problems when ingested in large amounts. Swensen et al. (1994) indeed observed severe gastrointestinal distress (abdominal cramping, diarrhea, and in some cases vomiting) when Poly-L-lactate was administered in concentrations of 5% (w/v) (~2.5% w/v lactate). To prevent gastric distress, Swensen et al. (1994) added only 0.75% Poly-L-lactate to a 6.25% glucose polymer solution and compared that with a 7% glucose polymer solution. As expected, given the fact that the energy content of the drinks was almost identical, no difference occurred in time to exhaustion during exercise at 70% $\dot{V}O_2$max until exhaustion. Polylactate can, therefore, not be considered as an ergogenic aid. The main problem with lactate supplements (in each of the available forms) is that performance effects can only be expected at ingestion rates that are not tolerated by the gastrointestinal tract.

Lecithin

Lecithin, or phosphatidyl choline, is a phospholipid that occurs naturally in a variety of food items, including beans, eggs, and wheat germ. It contains both choline and phosphorus and is theorized to be an ergogenic aid for those reasons. It is claimed to improve strength and reduce fatigue. A study investigated the effect of lecithin on 15-minute, all-out cycling performance after a 105-minute ride at 70% $\dot{V}O_2$max (Burns et al. 1988). No effects of two dosages of lecithin containing 1.1 g and 1.8 g of choline were observed. The only observed change was a rise in plasma choline concentration. Lecithin, therefore, does not appear to be an ergogenic aid. (See also the sections on choline and phosphorus.)

Medium-Chain Triacylglycerol

Medium-chain triacylglycerol (MCT) is sold as a supplement to replace normal fat because MCT is said not to be stored in the body. Therefore, MCT helps athletes to lose body fat. It is a fairly popular supplement among body builders. It is also used as an extra energy source in various energy bars. MCT is normally present in our diet in very small quantities, and a few natural sources are available. MCT is usually synthesized from coconut oil. After hydrolysis of the oil, the medium-chain and long-chain FAs are separated, and the fraction of medium-chain FAs is subsequently esterified to form an MCT. Medium-chain FAs are used in enteral and parenteral nutrition to provide patients with a rapidly available energy source. Because of this clinical use, a possible role for medium-chain FAs in sport nutrition became the subject of investigation.

Medium-chain FAs contain 8 carbons to 10 carbons, whereas long-chain FAs contain 12 or more carbons. Unlike most long-chain triacylglycerols (LCTs), MCTs are liquid at room temperature, partly because of the small molecular size of MCTs. MCTs are more polar and, therefore, more soluble in water. This greater water solubility and smaller molecular size has consequences at all levels of metabolism. MCTs are more rapidly digested and absorbed in the intestine than LCTs. Furthermore, medium-chain FAs follow the portal venous system and enter the liver directly, whereas long-chain FAs pass into the lacteals and follow the slow lymphatic system (Bach and Babayan 1982; Isselbacher 1968).

MCT may, therefore, be a valuable exogenous energy source during exercise in addition to carbohydrates (Jeukendrup et al. 1995). Also, MCT ingestion may improve exercise performance by elevating plasma FA levels and sparing muscle glycogen (Van Zeyl et al. 1996) because it increases the availability of plasma FAs, reduces the rate of muscle glycogen breakdown, and delays the onset of exhaustion.

MCT added to carbohydrate drinks did not inhibit gastric emptying (Beckers et al. 1992). In fact, the drinks with MCT empty faster from the stomach than isoenergetic carbohydrate drinks. In a subsequent study, the oxidation rates of orally ingested MCT were investigated (Jeukendrup et al. 1995). In a randomized cross-over design, 8 well-trained athletes cycled 180 minutes at 57% $\dot{V}O_2$max. Subjects ingested carbohydrate, carbohydrate+MCT, or MCT. During the 60-minute to 120-minute period, the amount of MCT oxidized was 72% of the amount ingested with carbohydrate +MCT, whereas during the MCT trial, only 33% was oxidized. It was concluded that more MCT is oxidized when ingested in combination with carbohydrate. Data confirmed that oral MCT might serve as an energy source in addition to glucose during exercise, because the metabolic availability of MCT was high during the last hour of exercise, with oxidation rates being as high as 70% of the ingestion rate. However, the maximal amount of oral MCT that is tolerated in the gastrointestinal tract is about 30 g, and this small amount limited the contribution of oral MCT to total energy expenditure to between 3% and 7% (see figure 10.17).

Figure 10.17 Small contribution of MCT to total energy expenditure.

Horowitz et al. (2000) argued that MCT ingestion might be particularly effective in reducing muscle glycogen breakdown in conditions where FA availability may be limiting fat oxidation, such as during high-intensity exercise. During exercise at 85% $\dot{V}O_2$max plasma FAs are reduced to very low levels, which reduces fat oxidation (Romijn et al. 1995). Therefore, Horowitz et al. (2000) fed their subjects 25 g of MCT 1 hour before 30 minutes of exercise at 84% $\dot{V}O_2$max. Plasma β-hydroxybutyrate levels were elevated after MCT ingestion, but plasma FA concentrations remained low during exercise, and, thus, glycogen breakdown was not affected by the MCT feedings. Interestingly, Van Zeyl et al. (1996) reported a reduction in the rate of muscle glycogen oxidation when a larger amount of MCT was ingested (86 g in 2 hours). They also claimed that MCT added to a 10% (w/v) carbohydrate solution improved time-trial performance in trained cyclists compared with a 10% carbohydrate solution alone. The authors did not report gastrointestinal disturbances. The same research group repeated the study with a low dose and a high dose of MCT (27 g and 54 g, respectively, in 2 hours) (Goedecke et al. 1999) but could not reproduce the findings by Van Zeyl et al. (1996). In fact, although MCT ingestion did not affect gastrointestinal symptoms in this study, and plasma FA and β-hydroxybutyrate levels were elevated, fuel oxidation and exercise performance were unchanged. When a large amount of MCT was ingested in a study by Jeukendrup et al. (1998) (86 g in 2 hours), subjects experienced gastrointestinal problems and their performance did not improve. In fact, MCT ingestion caused deterioration in performance compared with

the placebo (water) treatment. Angus et al. (2000) studied the effects of carbohydrate + MCT ingestion on 100-kilometer time-trial performance. Subjects ingested 42 g/hour of MCT during their time trials in combination with carbohydrate, but performance was not affected.

MCT is rapidly emptied from the stomach, absorbed, and oxidized, and the oxidation of exogenous MCT is enhanced when coingested with carbohydrate. Ingestion of 30 g MCT does not affect muscle glycogen breakdown, and the contribution of MCT to energy expenditure is small. Ingestion of larger amounts of MCT results in gastrointestinal distress. Therefore, MCT does not appear to have the positive effects on performance that are often claimed.

Pangamic Acid

Pangamic acid, often referred to as vitamin B_{15}, is surrounded by many unfounded claims. Most of these claims are based on anecdotal reports of athletes (or manufacturers), and they include increased maximal oxygen uptake, reduced lactate formation, and improved performance. Two studies have found no effect of pangamic acid on lactate concentration in the blood or on performance (Girandola et al. 1980; Gray and Titlow 1982). Pangamic acid is not a vitamin, and it is not essential, it has no known function in the human body. In contrast, synthetic pangamic acid has been shown to be harmful (Herbert 1979) and FDA guidelines forbid the sale of pangamic acid as a dietary supplement or as a drug.

Phosphatidylserine

The supplement phosphatidylserine is usually a natural soy-derived glycerophospholipid. It is a typical structural component of cell membranes, and it has been hypothesized to alter the cell membrane phospholipid composition and, hence, the properties of the membrane. Theoretically, when phosphatidylserine is incorporated in cell membranes, it can alter the number and the affinity of various receptors. Phosphatidylserine has been suggested to alter the neuroendocrine response to stress (including exercise stress).

In a study, subjects received 800 mg/day of phosphatidylserine for 10 days (Monteleone et al. 1992). The stress response (as measured by plasma ACTH and cortisol concentration) after three 6-minute intervals of strenuous exercise was smaller than with placebo. These results agreed with earlier observations by the same researchers that phosphatidylserine injection reduced hypothalamic-pituitary-adrenal axis activation in humans (Monteleone et al. 1990).

Phosphatidylserine potentially affects cognitive functioning. It reversed a memory decline that occurred in 25-year-old to 65-year-old healthy humans (Crook et al. 1991). The authors of the study argued that phosphatidylserine is rapidly absorbed by the gut into the bloodstream and transported across the blood-brain barrier. It may also be rapidly incorporated into membranes of the central nervous system, which have a naturally high phosphatidylserine content. This action could help to activate and regulate proteins involved in generation, storage, and reception of nerve impulses. Before definite conclusions can be drawn, however, more studies are needed.

Phosphatidylserine supplements that are for sale are derived from soy beans, whereas the phosphatidylserine in the above studies was bovine derived (cerebral cortex). The possibility cannot be excluded that soy-derived phosphatidylserine has no effects or different effects than those reported in the studies. Also, whether the observed decreases in serum ACTH and cortisol concentrations are a desirable effect is not clear. Although cortisol is generally known as a catabolic hormone, and decreasing cortisol is hypothesized to decrease catabolism, no evidence supports this conclusion.

Phosphorus

The body contains about 850 g of phosphorus (phosphate salts), 80% of which is found in bone. Besides having a structural function in bone and teeth, phosphorus is a component of nucleic acids and cell membranes. Phosphorus is a component of the high-energy phosphates (ATP and PCr) and, thus, plays an important role in energy metabolism. It is also a cofactor or component for many B-vitamins and 2,3-diphosphoglycerate (2,3 DPG) in erythrocytes. Phosphate salts also serve as an important intracellular buffer.

Phosphorus is an essential nutrient and the RDA for males and females is 1,200 mg from 11 years of age to 24 years of age. Persons older than 25 years have somewhat lower requirements (800 mg). Diets usually contain sufficient phosphorus because phosphorus is present in relatively large quantities in many foods.

Ingestion of larger amounts of phosphorus, or "phosphate loading," has been suggested to result in improved performance. The proposed mechanisms include increased ATP synthesis (Chasiotis 1983) and improved oxygen extraction in muscle cells because of elevations of 2,3-DPG in erythrocytes. For these purposes phosphate salts are usually ingested in relative large quantities, typically 4 g/day.

Studies have found different results. An early study observed an increased $\dot{V}O_2$max and decreased lactate concentration at submaximal workload when 8 cyclists ingested 4 g/day of sodium phosphate for 3 days (Cade et al. 1984). The study did not have a crossover design, but the control group, who received a placebo, did not show improvements. Similar findings were reported by three other studies after subjects ingested 3.6 g to 4.0 g of sodium phosphate or tribasic sodium phosphate (Kreider et al. 1990, 1992; Stewart et al. 1990). In addition, improvements in 5-mile run and 40-kilometer time-trial performance were reported. However, quite a few studies did not find differences in $\dot{V}O_2$max, performance, or lactate concentrations (Bredle et al. 1988; Duffy and Conlee 1986; Galloway et al. 1996; Mannix et al. 1990).

The inconsistencies in these findings may be related to the differences in the experimental protocols (the amount of phosphate ingested, the timing of the ingestion, the type of subjects, the exercise mode, and so on). Also, most of these studies used very small numbers of subjects, which can make relatively small changes in exercise performance difficult to detect. At present, little scientific evidence indicates that phosphate loading improves exercise performance, and more studies are needed before we can confidently recommend phosphate as an ergogenic aid (Tremblay et al. 1994).

Pyruvate (and Dihydroxyacetone)

Pyruvate and dihydroxyacetone (DHA) are 3-carbon intermediates of carbohydrate metabolism. They are formed in the glycolytic pathway. Some evidence suggests that supplementation or infusion of these metabolites can influence metabolism. Pyruvate and DHA are claimed to increase fat oxidation during exercise. They are also claimed to increase muscle glycogen storage, improve endurance capacity, and alter body composition (decrease fat mass).

Suggestions from the literature regarding the efficacy of pyruvate are based on long-term supplementation of pyruvate (7 days or more). Although only one study investigated the acute effects of pyruvate and lactate infusion, the results suggest a negative effect on running performance in rats compared with saline or glucose infusion (Bagby et al. 1978). Pyruvate infusion seemed to accelerate carbohydrate metabolism and increase both muscle and liver glycogen breakdown.

When pyruvate was given as a supplement to human subjects for 7 days, improved endurance capacity was observed in two studies from the same research group (Stanko et al. 1990a, 1990b). In the first study, subjects received 100 g/day of pyruvate-

DHA or placebo (maltodextrins) for 7 days and performed arm ergometry to exhaustion before and after the supplementation period (Stanko et al. 1990a). Muscle biopsies taken from the triceps showed that muscle glycogen concentrations at rest were significantly elevated by the pyruvate-DHA supplementation (88 mmol/kg w.w. versus 130 mmol/kg w.w.). Endurance times were increased from 133 minutes after the control diet to 160 minutes after pyruvate-DHA supplementation. In the second study, subjects were fed a high-carbohydrate diet for 7 days or a high-carbohydrate diet supplemented with 75 g of DHA and 25 g of pyruvate (Stanko et al. 1990b). Subjects performed cycling exercise to exhaustion at 70% $\dot{V}O_2$max and, again, the supplement increased endurance time (79 minutes versus 66 minutes).

Morrison et al. (2000) administered a much smaller dose of pyruvate (7 g/day for 7 days) or placebo to 7 trained cyclists in a randomized cross-over trial. Subjects cycled to exhaustion at 74% to 80% $\dot{V}O_2$max. Time to exhaustion was not increased with pyruvate, and with this smaller dose, no changes in blood pyruvate concentration were found.

No explanation is apparent for the improved endurance times reported by Stanko and colleagues (1990). However, they measured fractional extraction of glucose across one leg at rest and during exercise and found that glucose uptake was increased after pyruvate-DHA supplementation. They also observed that carbohydrate oxidation was unaffected, which suggests that subjects used less muscle glycogen when supplemented with pyruvate-DHA. In the first study, muscle glycogen was not measured, and, therefore, this question could not be answered. In the second study, muscle biopsies were taken from the vastus lateralis, but no differences were found between the control diet and the pyruvate-DHA supplemented diet. Inconsistencies between the studies by Stanko et al. (1990) and Morrison et al. (2000) may be related to the different dosages of pyruvate, the different training status of the subjects, or the coingestion of DHA in the study. More studies are needed before definitive conclusions can be drawn about the ergogenic effect of pyruvate.

Sodium Bicarbonate

When maximal exercise is performed for more than 30 seconds, most of the energy is derived from anaerobic glycolysis (see chapter 2). Lactic acid is formed at high rates and the increased acidity of the muscle is an important limiting factor for performance in events lasting 1 minute to 10 minutes. Reducing the muscle acidity and increasing the buffering capacity are theoretically ways of improving performance in

such events, and bicarbonate ingestion has been proposed as one of the ways to achieve these effects. A group of substances with this buffering function is the **alkalinizers** (e.g., sodium bicarbonate and sodium citrate). This section only summarizes the research findings on bicarbonate, but a number of detailed reviews have been published the past few years that are well worth studying (Horswill 1995; Linderman and Gosselink 1994).

Anaerobic Glycolysis

Events of 60 seconds to 10 minutes, such as 400-meter, 800-meter, and 1,500-meter running; track cycling events; and speed skating, rely heavily on anaerobic glycolysis for ATP regeneration. In this process, lactic acid is produced, resulting in a decreased pH in the muscle cell. This increased acidity interferes with the contraction process. As a result, a high acidity causes fatigue. From the moment this high-intensity exercise starts, lactic acid (hydrogen ions and lactate) builds up in the muscle and is transported into the blood. The decrease in muscle pH is, therefore, with some delay, reflected by the blood pH.

The pH of blood is normally 7.4 and after high-intensity exercise may decrease to 7.1 or slightly lower. The pH of the muscle is normally around 7.0 and may decrease to about 6.5. The body has several systems to adjust and regulate the acid-base balance. Chemical buffers provide a very effective and rapid way of normalizing the H^+ concentration. Other systems include excretion of CO_2 via pulmonary ventilation and H^+ excretion via the kidneys.

The primary buffers in the muscle are phosphates and tissue proteins. The most important buffers in the blood are proteins, hemoglobin, and bicarbonate. During intense exercise, the intracellular buffers are insufficient to buffer all the hydrogen ions formed. The efflux of H^+ into the circulation increases, and bicarbonate has a role in buffering these H^+ ions.

$$H^+ + HCO_3^- \rightarrow H_2CO_3 \rightarrow H_2O + CO_2$$

The mechanism by which bicarbonate supposedly exerts its action is through this buffering of H^+ in the blood (not in the muscle as is often claimed). The buffering of H^+ in the blood, however, increases the H^+ gradient and increases efflux of H^+ from the muscle. Numerous studies on the effects of bicarbonate ingestion and exercise performance have yielded equivocal results.

Various studies suggest that a minimal dose of bicarbonate ingestion is needed to improve performance. Meta-analyses from the available literature suggest a dose-response relationship between the amount of bicarbonate ingested and the observed performance effect (Horswill 1995; Matson and Vu Tran 1993) (see figure 10.18). A dose of 200 mg/kg b.w. ingested 1 hour to 2 hours before exercise seems to improve performance in most studies, whereas 300 mg/kg b.w. seems to be the optimum dose (with tolerable side effects for most athletes). Doses of less than 100 mg/kg b.w. do not affect performance. This finding seems to make sense because a minimal amount of bicarbonate is needed to significantly increase the buffering capacity of the blood. Intakes greater than 300 mg/kg b.w. tend to result in gastrointestinal problems (bloating, abdominal discomfort, and diarrhea).

Figure 10.18 Effect of different dosages on exercise performance.

Adapted, by permission, from C.A. Horswill, 1995 "Effects of bicarbonate, citrate, and phosphate loading on performance," *International Journal of Sports Nutrition* 5: S111-S119.

No studies show an effect on exercise performance in high-intensity exercise lasting less than 1 minute. Exercise such as squat, bench press, and jumping are unaffected. Also, exercise of long duration is generally unaffected. Therefore, a window for efficacy of bicarbonate has been identified between approximately 1 minute and 7 minutes. Interestingly, a study by McNaughton, Dalton, and Palmer (1999) showed improved performance in a 1-hour time trial, which was accompanied by a higher blood pH throughout the exercise.

Side Effects

The side effects of sodium bicarbonate intake in such large doses can be quite severe. At doses of 300 mg/kg b.w. many athletes experience diarrhea, gastrointestinal discomfort, bloating, and cramps 1 hour after loading. The effects are dose dependent. The main cause of these problems is the large amount of sodium that is ingested with the bicarbonate, and the

reaction of bicarbonate with the HCl in the stomach, which generates a large volume of CO_2 that distends the stomach wall. Drinking large amounts of water during the loading is likely to alleviate some of the problems.

Sodium Citrate

Sodium citrate works similarly to bicarbonate. It increases the buffering capacity of the extracellular space to increase the efflux of hydrogen ions from the intracellular space. Sodium citrate is effective in limiting the decrease in blood pH and improving high-intensity exercise performance of 2-minute to 4-minute duration (McNaughton and Cedaro 1992; McNaughton 1990). One study also showed improved performance in a 30-kilometer cycling time trial (Potteiger et al. 1996). The typical doses for sodium citrate are 300 mg/kg b.w. to 500 mg/kg b.w. Like sodium bicarbonate, sodium citrate is likely to cause gastrointestinal problems such as diarrhea, cramping, and bloating. Sodium citrate may act as a buffering agent, improving exercise performance in events up to about 10 minutes. It is said to improve high-intensity (~80% $\dot{V}O_2$max) endurance performance, but this claim has not been proved.

Vanadium

Vanadium, a trace element widely distributed in nature and normally present in human tissues, has insulin-like properties. Foods that contain vanadium include cereal and grain products, dietary oils, meat, fish, and poultry. In supplements, vanadium is usually ingested as vanadyl sulphate or bis-maltolato-oxovanadium (BMOV). One of the reasons to ingest vanadium in these compounds is that less-toxic effects have been shown in rats.

The insulin-like effects of vanadium compounds are well documented in vitro and in vivo (Verma et al. 1998). In humans with type II diabetes mellitus (non–insulin dependent diabetes mellitus), an increase in insulin-mediated glucose uptake (Halberstam et al. 1996), glycogen synthase activity, and glycogen synthesis has been demonstrated after vanadium administration (Cohen et al. 1995). These observations in insulin-resistant populations, lead to suggestions that vanadium can help weight loss, improve insulin sensitivity, and increase muscle glycogen storage.

However, no studies in healthy humans without insulin resistance are available that demonstrate insulin-like effects after acute or chronic administration of vanadium (compounds). In fact, a recent study did not show changes in insulin sensitivity measured with an oral glucose tolerance test in non–insulin-resistant subjects after acute or chronic (7 days) vanadyl sulphate administration (Jentjens and Jeukendrup 2002). The amounts required for biological effects of vanadium in humans (1 mg/kg/day to 2 mg/kg/day) obviously greatly exceeds the amounts that can be normally consumed in the diet (<30 µg/day) (Verma et al. 1998).

Neither the short-term nor the long-term toxicity of the agents have been systematically studied in humans. Currently, no human studies are available that describe toxic effects after 2 weeks to 10 weeks of vanadyl sulphate administration at dosages between 100 mg/day and 125 mg/day (Boden et al. 1996; Cohen et al. 1995; Halberstam et al. 1996). Some individuals may experience diarrhea, cramps, and nausea after intake of vanadium compounds. In rats, vanadium in excess amounts is toxic. Although some evidence indicates that vanadium can influence insulin sensitivity in patients with type II diabetes, such does not seem to be the case in healthy individuals. Thus, no evidence supports an ergogenic role of vanadium.

Wheat Germ Oil

Wheat germ oil is extracted from the embryo of wheat. It is high in linoleic acid, vitamin E, and octacosanol, a solid white alcohol that is theorized to have ergogenic effects. Wheat germ oil is advertised to increase endurance, stamina, and vigor. Several theories have been developed about the possible physiological effects of wheat germ oil, including enhanced glycogen metabolism and increased maximal oxygen uptake. Although many studies have focused on the metabolic effects of wheat germ oil, no evidence supports the contention that it is an effective ergogenic aid.

Contamination of Nutrition Supplements

Recently, speculation has arisen that some of the positive drug tests recorded in various sports have resulted from the use of nutrition supplements rather than deliberate use of banned products. Contamination of these supplements has been suggested as the reason for the positive drug tests. The supplements may have been contaminated with small amounts prohormones or other compounds that are on the list of banned substances. The steroid nandrolone has been especially prominent. Some competitive athletes are afraid to take supplements because of uncertainty over which supplements are contaminated and which are clean.

The IOC-accredited laboratory in Cologne in Germany reported that a range of different steroids—including nandrolone and testosterone, as well as their precursor compounds—were found in various dietary supplements. In fact, of the 634 supplements tested, 94 of them (i.e., nearly 15%), contained enough anabolics to cause a positive result on a drug test. None of these products gave any indication on the label that they contained steroid compounds. From the supplements made in the United States, almost one product in five of the 240 tested contained **prohormones.**

The substances listed below are ingredients that have been identified in supplements that are either directly banned by the IOC or that cause a positive doping outcome in some people:

- Ephedrine
- Strychnine
- Androstenedione, androstenediol, dehydroepiandrosterone (DHEA) (may lead to an elevated testosterone/epitestosterone ratio)
- 19-Norandrostenedione, 19-norandrostenediol, and related compounds (may lead to a positive test for metabolites of the steroid nandrolone)

Because athletes sign a code of conduct, they are responsible for what they take, even when it is a supplement that has insufficient quality control or labeling. Caffeine and pseudoephedrine were on this list as well but because these substances have been taken off the list of banned substances and been put on a monitoring program, these substances will no longer cause positive doping tests.

Unfortunately, current legislation does little to protect athletes and other consumers from insufficiently labeled, mislabeled, contaminated, or even unsafe ingredients in dietary supplements. Although regulations vary widely from country to country, food supplements are never subject to the standard of manufacture and quality control that is required of foods and drugs. Also, legislation regarding product claims is less strict. Many manufacturers make claims that have never been proved scientifically. With clever marketing techniques and numerous retail outlets, supplement sellers make their products attractive and easy to obtain for athletes who do not know anything about the source or purity of the ingredients.

Thus, if an athlete decides that the benefits outweigh the risks of taking a supplement, a product from a large, respectable company is probably the best choice. Reputable brands of vitamins, minerals, and other common supplements manufactured by the major food and drug companies are normally manufactured to the highest standards and should be safe. Contamination is especially a problem in some smaller and more exotic companies. Companies that do not sell steroids and prohormones are less likely to have their products contaminated by these substances.

In the end, each athlete must do a cost-benefit analysis. On one side of the equation are the poten-tial benefits of taking a product, which necessitate a thorough evaluation of the evidence to determine if the benefits are real. On the other side is the risk, including the possibility that a seemingly innocent product may result in a positive doping test, with all the consequences that follow.

Key Points

- Nutritional supplements are used by 40% to 100% of all athletes in one form or another.
- From a regulatory point of view, dietary supplements are treated as nutrition and are defined as vitamins, minerals, herbs and botanicals, amino acids, and other dietary substances intended to supplement the diet by increasing the total dietary intake, or as any concentrate, metabolite, constituent, or combination of these ingredients. There is no strict regulation regarding testing, advertising, and the promotion of nutrition supplements.
- Few nutrition supplements have proven benefits in terms of performance, recovery, or effects on body weight or body composition.
- There is some evidence to suggest that HMB can result in increased lean-body mass and muscle strength. However, these findings are mostly by one laboratory and need to be confirmed by others.
- Caffeine (3 mg/kg to 9 mg/kg caffeine) has an ergogenic effect in endurance exercise (1-2 hours) and exercise around 100% $\dot{V}O_2$max lasting approximately 1 to 5 min as well as effects on cognitive functioning. Caffeine also has side effects that can include gastrointestinal distress, headaches, tachycardia, and restlessness.
- Oral creatine supplementation of 20 g/day for 5 days increases the total-muscle cre-atine content in men by about 20% (30% to 40% of the increase is phosphocreatine). A subsequent daily dose of 2 g is enough to maintain this concentration. This allows an increase in the amount of work performed during single and repeated bouts of short-term, high-intensity exercise but may also result in some weight gain.
- A dose of 200 mg/kg b.w. bicarbonate ingested 1 hour to 2 hours before exercise seems to improve performance in most studies, whereas 300 mg/kg d.w. seems to be the opti-mum dose. Side effects are diarrhea, gastrointestinal discomfort, bloating, and cramps 1 hour after loading.

Key Terms

alkalinizer 261

beta-hydroxy beta methylbutyrate (HMB) 237

caffeine 239

carnitine 243

choline 245

chromium 246

coenzyme Q10 247

creatine (Cr) 247

dehydroepiandrosterone (DHEA) 253

dihydroxyacetone 254

ergogenic 232

ergolytic 257

ginseng 255

inosine 256

lecithin (phosphatidylcholine) 245

prohormones 263

Recommended Readings

Bahrke, M.S., and C.E. Yesalis. 2002. *Performance Enhancing Substances in Sport and Exercise.* Human Kinetics: Champaign, IL.

Wagenmakers, A.J. 1999. Amino acid supplements to improve athletic performance. *Current Opinion in Clinical Nutrition and Metabolic Care* 2(6):539-544.

Williams, M.H. 1998. *The Ergogenic Edge.* Human Kinetics: Champaign, IL.

Williams, M.H., R.B. Kreider, and J.D. Branch. 1999. *Creatine the Power Supplement.* Human Kinetics: Champaign, IL.

Chapter 11

Weight Management

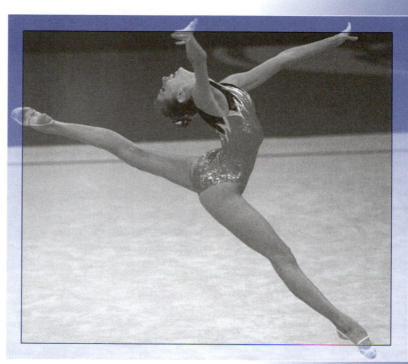

© Empics

Objectives

After studying this chapter, you should be able to do the following:

- Describe the principles of methods available to measure body composition

- Compare different techniques of measuring body composition and discuss their advantages and limitations

- Categorize sports and the importance of body weight or composition

- Describe ways of losing body weight by dieting

- Describe the role of exercise in losing body weight

- Describe the benefits and risks of making weight and discuss the possibilities to minimize the risks

Body weight, or body composition, is an important determinant of performance in many sports. Some athletes try to achieve weight loss, and others try to achieve weight gain. In some sports, reducing body fat is important, whereas in other sports, increasing lean-body mass is important. In most weight-bearing activities, such as running and jumping, extra weight may be a disadvantage, though in some contact sports, such as American football and rugby, extra weight may be an advantage. Every sport has an "optimal physique," and in some sports, a specific discipline or position requires a different body type. For dancing and gymnastics, leanness is important mainly for aesthetic reasons.

The desire to lose or gain weight is not limited to competitive athletes but is also common among recreational athletes and sedentary individuals who wish to change their physical appearance. While obesity is a growing problem, images in the media create continuous pressure to be lean and well proportioned. The stereotypical athlete is particularly lean and toned. Many athletes try to lose weight through either diet or exercise or both. This chapter discusses the relationship between body composition and performance, followed by a discussion of how body composition can be assessed and, finally, the problems associated with weight loss and weight gain and the applications in various categories of sport.

Ideal Body Weight and Composition

Body size, structure, and composition are separate, yet interrelated, aspects of the body that make up the physique. Body size refers to the volume, mass, length, and surface area of the body; body structure refers to the distribution or arrangement of body parts such as the skeleton, muscle, and fat; and body composition refers to the amounts of constituents in the body. Size, structure, and composition all contribute to optimal sports performance. Evidence from sports participants in various age groups demonstrates an inverse relationship between fat mass and performance of physical activities requiring translocation of the body weight either vertically, such as in jumping, or horizontally, as in running. Excess fat is detrimental to performance in these types of activities because it adds mass to the body without additional capacity to produce force. Also, acceleration is directly proportional to force but inversely proportional to mass, so excess fat, at a given level of force application, results in slower changes in velocity and direction. Excess fat also increases the metabolic cost of physical activities that require movement of the total-body mass. Thus, in most performances involving movement of the body mass, a relatively low percentage body fat is advantageous both mechanically and metabolically.

By studying the anthropometry of high-level athletes, we can get an idea about optimum body size, structure, and composition for various sports. In some sports, a low percentage body fat is a requirement. For example, Olympic marathon runners have 3% to 4% body fat. Tour de France cyclists have between 4% and 6% body fat. Linebackers in American football have between 12% and 15% body fat, whereas defensive linemen have 16% body fat or more.

Body mass may also be dramatically different in different sports. Female distance runners may weigh 50 kg to 55 kg (110 lb to 120 lb), whereas female shot putters may weigh 75 kg to 85 kg (165 lb to 185 lb). Ballet dancers may weigh no more than 45 kg (100 lb). These body composition assessments reveal that athletes generally have physique characteristics unique to their specific sport and discipline.

Body Composition

By measuring body composition one can quantify the most important structural components of the body: muscle, bone, and fat. A variety of techniques have been developed to measure body composition (see table 11.1). Such measurements are more meaningful than the traditional weight and height relationship. Height-weight tables, such as the one shown in figure 11.1 provide a normal range of body weights for any given height. Such figures and tables have limitations, especially when applied to an athletic population. For instance, a bodybuilder (180 cm, 100 kg [6 ft, 220 lb]) may have very low body fat but could be classified as overweight. Clearly the "extra" weight is muscle and not body fat, which would lead to erroneous classification and possibly mistaken advice.

Body Mass Index

A rough but better measure than the height-weight tables is the **body mass index (BMI),** also known as Quetelet index. Also derived from body mass and height, BMI is calculated thus:

$$BMI = \text{body mass in kilograms}/(\text{height in meters})^2$$

An individual who is 1.76 m (5 ft, 9 in) and weighs 72 kg (158 lb) has a BMI of $72/(1.76)^2 = 23.2$. The normal range is between 18.5 kg/m² and 25.0 kg/m². Individuals with a BMI higher than 25 kg/m² are classified as "overweight," and individuals with a BMI higher than 30 kg/m² are classified as obese.

Table 11.1 Various Techniques to Measure Body Composition

Method	Description
Anthropometry	Measurements of body segment girths to predict body fat
Skinfold thickness	Measurement of subcutaneous fat with a calliper that gives an estimation of lean-body mass and fat mass
Hydrostatic weighing (underwater weighing or hydrodensitometry)	Underwater weighing based on Archimedes' principle to estimate lean-body mass and fat mass
Air displacement plethysmography (BOD POD)	Measurement of air displacement to estimate lean-body mass and fat mass
Bioelectrical impedance analysis (BIA)	Measurement of resistance to an electrical current to estimate total-body water, lean-body mass, and fat mass
Computed tomography (CT)	Computer-assisted X-ray scan to image body tissues and measure bone mass
Duel energy x-ray absorptiometry (DEXA or DXA)	X-ray scan at two intensities to measure total-body water, lean-body mass, fat mass, and bone-mineral density

Even with this formula, the bodybuilder would be classified as overweight or even obese as the equation does not take into account body composition ($BMI = 100/(1.80)^2 = 30.9$). Two individuals might have the same BMI but completely different body composition. One could achieve his body weight with mainly muscle mass as a result of hard training, whereas the other could achieve his body weight by fat deposition as a result of a sedentary lifestyle. Without information about body composition, they both might be classified as obese. In children and the elderly, the BMI is very difficult to interpret because the muscle and bone weights are changing in relationship to height.

The BMI, however does provide useful information about risks for various diseases and is used in many epidemiological and clinical studies. For example, BMI correlates with the incidence of cardiovascular complications (hypertension and stroke), certain cancers, type II diabetes, gall stones, osteoarthritis, and renal disease (Calleet al. 1999).

Densitometry

Several techniques of **densitometry** have been developed to measure body composition and to distinguish between the most important components: carbohydrate (typically <1% of body mass), minerals (~4%), fat (~15%), protein (~20%), and water (~60%). Each of these components has a different density. Density is mass divided by volume and is usually expressed in grams per cubic centimeter (g/cm^3). The density of bone for instance is 1.3 g/cm^3 to 1.4 g/cm^3, the density of fat is 0.9 g/cm^3 and the density for fat-free (lean) tissue is 1.1 g/cm^3. A lower total-body density value represents a higher fat mass.

The Greek inventor Archimedes (287 B.C.–212 B.C) discovered a fundamental principle to assess human body composition. King Heron II of Syracuse had commissioned a goldsmith to make a crown of pure gold. When the goldsmith delivered the crown, the King noticed that the color of the gold was slightly lighter. Suspecting that some of the gold had been replaced with silver, the King asked Archimedes to invent a way to measure the gold content of the crown without melting it down. Archimedes thought very hard about this problem for several weeks. Then, stepping into a bath filled to the top with water and watching the overflow, he realized he had found a way to measure the density of an object. Archimedes jumped from the bath and ran naked through the streets, shouting his famous words "Eureka, Eureka!" Archimedes had found a way to solve the mystery of the King's crown. He reasoned that a substance must have a volume proportional to its mass, and measuring the volume of an irregularly shaped object would require submersion in water and collecting the overflow. He found that pure gold with the same mass as the crown displaced less water than the crown and that silver displaced more water (see figure 11.2). He concluded that the crown was made

Are you at a healthy weight?

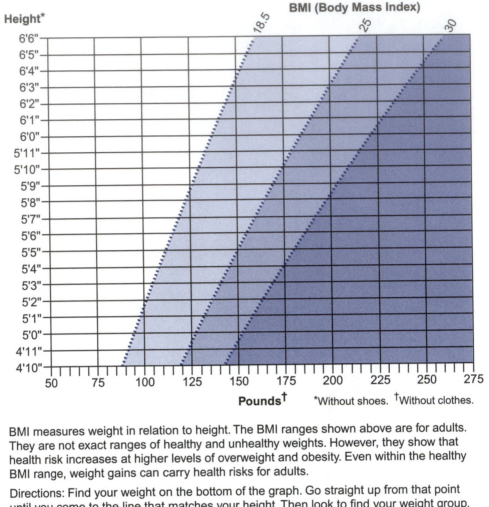

BMI measures weight in relation to height. The BMI ranges shown above are for adults. They are not exact ranges of healthy and unhealthy weights. However, they show that health risk increases at higher levels of overweight and obesity. Even within the healthy BMI range, weight gains can carry health risks for adults.

Directions: Find your weight on the bottom of the graph. Go straight up from that point until you come to the line that matches your height. Then look to find your weight group.

☐ Healthy Weight BMI from 18.5 up to 25 refers to healthy weight.

☐ Overweight BMI from 25 up to 30 refers to overweight.

☐ Obese BMI 30 or higher refers to obesity. Obese persons are also overweight.

Figure 11.1 Relationship between height, weight, and body mass index (BMI) and criteria for overweight and obesity.
Adapted from *Dietary Guidelines for Americans* 2000. Available from http://.ars.usda.gov/dgac/.

of a mixture of gold and silver and confirmed the king's suspicions.

Assume a 1,000-g crown that is an alloy of 70% gold and 30% silver. Because its volume is 64.6 cm³, it displaces 64.6 g of water (water has a density of 1.00 g/cm³). The crown's apparent mass in water is, thus, 1,000 g minus 64.6 g, or 935.4 g. The 1,000 g of pure gold has a volume of 51.8 cm³, and so its apparent mass in water is 1,000 minus 51.8 g, or 948.2 g. Thus, when both ends of the scale are immersed in water, there is an apparent mass of 935.4 g at one end and an apparent mass of 948.2 g at the other end, an imbal-

ance of 12.8 g. Scales from Archimedes' time could easily detect such an imbalance in mass.

The same principle can be used to distinguish between fat mass and fat-free mass in the human body (see figure 11.3). With this technique, called underwater weighing or hydrostatic weighing, a person is submerged in water and the body weight is accurately measured before and after submersion. Assume a 75-kg (165-lb) person is submerged in water and weighs 3 kg (6.6 lb) in water. According to the Archimedes' principle the loss of weight in water of 72 kg (158.4 lb) equals the weight of the displaced

270

Figure 11.2 Archimedes' principle of determining the volume of an irregularly shaped object by submerging it in water and collecting the overflow. From this measurement and the weight of the object in air, the density (weight/volume) can be calculated.

water. The volume of the water displaced must be corrected for the temperature of the water at the time of weighing because the water density changes with temperature. The density is 1.00 g/cm³ at 4° C (39.2° F), but measurements are usually performed in warmer water temperatures. Without correction, the body density in our example would be 75,000/72,000 = 1.0417 g/cm³.

Siri (1956) developed a method to estimate the percentage of body fat from these measurements. The method assumes a density of 0.90 g/cm³ for the density of fat and 1.10 g/cm³ for the density of fat-free tissues. The equation for calculating the percentage body fat, often referred to as the Siri equation, is

% body fat = (495/body density) − 450

Using the same example of a 75-kg (165-lb) person, the percentage body fat is (495/1.0417)−450 = 25.2%. Fat mass (FM) can then be calculated as 25.2% × 75 kg = 18.9 kg and fat-free mass (FFM) is 75 kg − 18.9 kg = 56.1 kg.

Although, in general, this technique works very well and is often used as the gold standard, it has several limitations. The calculations are based on a two-compartment model (fat mass and fat-free mass). The composition of the fat-free mass can change considerably after weight training. In very muscular persons, the Siri equations will overestimate body fat and underestimate fat-free mass (Modlesky et al. 1996). A slightly modified equation may give more accurate results in this population:

% body fat = (521/body density) − 478

Measurements are usually made after the person has made a maximal exhalation and breath is held under water for 5 seconds to 10 seconds. This maximal exha-

© Laura Gilkey

Figure 11.3 With the underwater, or hydrostatic, weighing technique, a person's body density is determined using Archimedes' principle.

lation is performed to reduce the air remaining in the lungs, which would otherwise exert a buoyant effect. However, even with a maximal exhalation, a residual volume remains in the lungs and, therefore, residual lung volume must be measured and corrected for. Failure to correct for residual lung volume underestimates whole-body density and, thus, overestimates fat mass. Food intake and, especially, the intake of carbonated beverages, can also affect the measurement and should be avoided in the hours before a measurement.

Skinfolds

The most frequently used technique to estimate body fat is measuring the thickness of skinfolds. These measurements are based on the interrelationships between the fat located underneath the skin (subcutaneous fat), internal fat, and whole-body density. Skinfolds can be measured using a calliper, which will usually indicate the thickness in millimeters (see figure 11.4). The skinfold should be taken and the measurement read within 2 seconds to avoid skinfold compression. Considerable experience is necessary to produce accurate skinfold measurements. When comparing skinfold thicknesses, measurements should always be taken by the same person to guarantee consistency.

Figure 11.4 Skinfold measurement using callipers (subscapular site).

Several anatomical sites can be used for skinfold measurements. The four most common sites are the biceps, triceps, subscapular, and abdominal. These sites are shown in figure 11.5. Sometimes other sites on the upper thigh and chest are used. Often the sum of 4 skinfolds is chosen, but other methods have taken the sum of 7 or even 10 skinfolds.

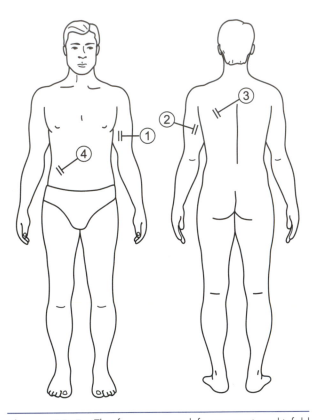

Figure 11.5 The four sites used for measuring skinfold thickness.

Adapted, by permission, from A.S. Jackson, and M.L. Pollock, 1978, "Generalized equations for predicting body density of men," *British Journal of Nutrition* 40(3): 497-504.

The sum of skinfolds can then be used to predict body density and, thence, body-fat percentage. This prediction is usually based on previous research in which the skinfold measurements were compared with the results of underwater weighing. Various experimenters have put forward equations that are used either with skinfold thickness alone or in conjunction with other measurements such as body circumference or limb lengths. Two of the most common sets of equations used are attributable to Durnin and Womersley (1974) (skinfolds alone) and to Jackson and Pollock (1978) (skinfolds and body measurements).

Once skinfold thickness has been measured using the sum of four skinfold measurements, body density can be calculated based on the equation and values

Table 11.2 Linear Regression Equations for the Calculation of Body Density

	17–19 y	20–29 y	30–39 y	40–49 y	50 y+
C	1.1620 (male)	1.1631 (male)	1.1422 (male)	1.1620 (male)	1.1715 (male)
	1.1549 (female)	1.1599 (female)	1.1423 (female)	1.1333 (female)	1.1339 (female)
M	0.0630 (male)	0.0632 (male)	0.0544 (male)	0.0700 (male)	0.0779 (male)
	0.0678 (female)	0.0717 (female)	0.0632 (female)	0.0612 (female)	0.0645 (female)

Body density = C–[M(log$_{10}$ sum of all four skinfolds)]
From Durnin & Wormersley 1974.

shown in table 11.2 (Durnin and Womersley 1974). Read the appropriate values of C and M from the table, and solve the equation to determine body density (g/cm³) according to gender, age, and sum of the four skinfolds (in millimeters).

Percentage body fat is calculated using the Siri equation. For ease of reference, tables have also been generated for percentage body fat values for both males (see table 11.3) and females (see table 11.4)

across the whole age range based on the sum of 4 skinfold measurements, with the results shown for each 2-mm increment of skinfold thickness.

Measurements at three skinfold sites in the body (different ones for males and females as illustrated in figures 11.6 and 11.7, respectively) can also be used to estimate percentage body fat. When using three skinfold measurements, the body density equations of Jackson and Pollock are used:

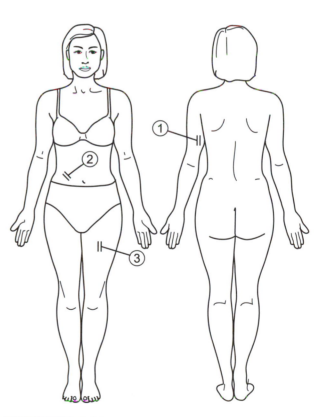

Figure 11.6 The three-site skinfold measuring system for male subjects.

Adapted, by permission, from A.S. Jackson, and M.L. Pollock, 1978, "Generalized equations for predicting body density of men," *British Journal of Nutrition* 40(3): 497-504.

Figure 11.7 The three-site skinfold measuring system for female subjects.

Adapted, by permission, from A.S. Jackson, and M.L. Pollock, 1978, "Generalized equations for predicting body density of men," *British Journal of Nutrition* 40(3): 497-504.

Table 11.3 Percentage Body Fat for Male Subjects According to Age and Skinfold Thickness

Skinfold thickness*	Age (years)				
	17–19	20–29	30–39	40–49	50+
10 mm	0.41	0.40	5.05	3.30	2.63
12 mm	2.46	2.1	6.86	5.61	5.20
14 mm	4.21	3.85	8.40	7.58	7.39
16 mm	5.74	5.38	9.74	9.31	9.31
18 mm	7.10	6.74	10.93	10.84	11.02
20 mm	8.32	7.96	12.00	12.22	12.55
22 mm	9.43	9.07	12.98	13.47	13.95
24 mm	10.45	10.09	13.87	14.62	15.23
26 mm	11.39	11.03	14.69	15.68	16.42
28 mm	12.26	11.91	15.46	16.67	17.53
30 mm	13.07	12.73	16.17	17.60	18.56
32 mm	13.84	13.49	16.84	18.47	19.53
34 mm	14.56	14.22	17.47	19.28	20.44
36 mm	15.25	14.90	18.07	20.06	21.31
38 mm	15.89	15.55	18.63	20.79	22.13
40 mm	16.51	16.17	19.17	21.49	22.92
42 mm	17.10	16.76	19.69	22.16	23.66
44 mm	17.66	17.32	20.18	22.80	24.38
46 mm	18.20	17.86	20.65	23.41	25.06
48 mm	18.71	18.37	21.10	24.00	25.72
50 mm	19.21	18.87	21.53	24.56	26.35
52 mm	19.69	19.35	21.95	25.10	26.96
54 mm	20.15	19.81	22.35	25.63	27.55
56 mm	20.59	20.26	20.73	26.13	28.11
58 mm	21.02	20.69	23.11	26.62	28.66
60 mm	21.44	21.11	23.47	27.09	29.20
62 mm	21.84	21.51	23.82	27.55	29.71
64 mm	22.23	21.90	24.16	28.00	30.21
66 mm	22.61	22.28	24.49	28.43	30.70
68 mm	22.98	22.65	24.81	28.85	31.17
70 mm	23.34	23.01	25.13	29.26	31.63
72 mm	23.69	23.36	25.43	29.66	32.07
74 mm	24.03	23.70	25.73	30.04	32.51
76 mm	24.36	24.03	26.01	30.42	32.93
78 mm	24.68	24.36	26.30	30.79	33.35
80 mm	25.00	24.67	26.57	31.15	33.75

*Sum of all four skinfolds.

Table 11.4 Percentage Body Fat for Female Subjects According to Age and Skinfold Thickness

Skinfold thickness*	Age (years)				
	17–19	20–29	30–39	40–49	50+
10 mm	5.34	4.88	8.72	11.71	12.88
12 mm	7.60	7.27	10.85	13.81	15.10
14 mm	9.53	9.30	12.68	15.59	16.99
16 mm	11.21	11.08	14.27	17.15	18.65
18 mm	12.71	12.66	15.68	18.54	20.11
20 mm	14.05	14.08	16.95	19.78	21.44
22 mm	15.28	15.38	18.10	20.92	22.64
24 mm	16.40	16.57	19.16	21.95	23.74
26 mm	17.44	17.67	20.14	22.91	24.76
28 mm	18.40	18.69	21.05	23.80	25.71
30 mm	19.30	19.64	21.90	24.64	26.59
32 mm	20.15	20.54	22.70	25.42	27.42
34 mm	20.95	21.39	23.45	26.16	28.21
36 mm	21.71	22.19	24.16	26.85	28.95
38 mm	22.42	22.95	24.84	27.51	29.65
40 mm	23.10	23.67	25.48	28.14	30.32
42 mm	23.76	24.36	26.09	28.74	30.96
44 mm	24.38	25.02	26.68	29.32	31.57
46 mm	24.97	25.65	27.24	29.87	32.15
48 mm	25.54	26.26	27.78	30.39	32.71
50 mm	26.09	26.84	28.30	30.90	33.25
52 mm	26.62	27.40	28.79	31.39	33.77
54 mm	27.13	27.94	29.27	31.86	34.27
56 mm	27.63	28.47	29.74	32.31	34.75
58 mm	28.10	28.97	30.19	32.75	35.22
60 mm	28.57	29.46	30.62	33.17	35.67
62 mm	29.01	29.94	31.04	33.58	36.11
64 mm	29.45	30.40	31.45	33.98	36.53
66 mm	29.87	30.84	31.84	34.37	36.95
68 mm	30.28	31.28	32.23	34.75	37.35
70 mm	30.67	31.70	32.60	35.11	37.74
72 mm	31.06	32.11	32.97	35.47	38.12
74 mm	31.44	32.51	33.32	35.82	38.49
76 mm	31.81	32.91	33.67	36.15	38.85
78 mm	32.17	33.29	34.00	36.48	39.20
80 mm	32.52	33.66	34.33	36.81	39.54

*Sum of all four skinfolds.

male body density = 1.0990750 − 0.0008209 (X2) + 0.0000026 (X2)² − 0.0002017 (X3) − 0.005675 (X4) + 0.018586 (X5)

where X2 = sum of the chest, abdomen, and thigh skinfolds in mm; X3 = age in years; X4 = waist circumference in cm; and X5 = forearm circumference in cm.

female body density = 1.1 470292 − 0.0009376 (X3) + 0.0000030 (X3)² − 0.0001156 (X4) − 0.0005839 (X5)

where X3 = sum of triceps, thigh, and suprailiac skinfolds, in mm; X4 = age in years; and X5 = gluteal circumference in cm.

Again, percentage body fat is then calculated using the Siri equation.

The correct tables must be used because the relationship between skinfold thickness and body fat may vary depending on gender, age, and ethnicity of the individual. Populations other than the population the equations were based on may result in large errors. Skinfold measurements, when properly taken, correlate very highly (r = 0.83 to 0.89) with hydrostatic weighing, with a standard error of only about 3% or 4%. This error should always be kept in mind when using tables or equations to convert skinfold thickness to a percentage body fat. Often sport scientists stay with the skinfold thickness measurement rather than convert it to a percentage body fat. This method is especially useful when repeated and regular measurements are made of the same athlete.

Bioelectrical Impedance Analysis

Bioelectrical impedance analysis (BIA) is based on the principle that different tissues and substances have a different impedance (resistance) to an electrical current. For example, impedance or conductivity is very different for fat tissue and water (see figure 11.8).

Electrodes are placed on different parts of the body, often the hand and foot, and if a current is applied to one of those electrodes, it can be measured at the other electrode. The less the measured resistance, the higher the body water content. Adipose tissue has a very high resistance, or impedance, whereas muscle—of which 75% is water—has a very low resistance. Based on these differential effects of applied electrical cur-

Figure 11.8 Bioelectrical impedance analysis (BIA). *(a)* If the resistance is measured to a known current in a tube with a salt solution and a known length (30 cm), the volume can be calculated. *(b)* If the same tube contains oil in addition to the salt solution, the resistance changes and a new calculation of volume is obtained. *(c)* The same principle can be applied to the human body, which can be viewed as 5 tubes (2 arms, 2 legs, and 1 trunk).

rent, BIA can be used to estimate percentage body fat, percentage lean-body mass, and percentage body water. Often BIA is used to measure body composition, but it can also be used to estimate fluid levels in different body segments.

A simple example of a device for measuring impedance is a tube containing a highly conductive salt solution and electrodes inserted at each end (see figure 11.8a). An electrical current is sent through one of the electrodes, and a resistance (Z) is measured between the two electrodes. If the length of the tube (L) and the specific resistivity (ρ) of the salt solution are known, the volume (V) can be calculated using the formula

$$V = \rho \times L^2/Z$$

If some of the salt solution is replaced with oil, the measured resistance increases and the new volume of the salt solution is calculated. By deduction the percentage of oil in the solution can be determined (see figure 11.8b). The principle is exactly the same when measuring body impedance and calculating body composition. For this purpose the measured body impedance and the subject's height are used.

Most BIA devices are tetrapolar, meaning they have 4 electrodes: 2 that apply the current and 2 that receive a signal. The device applies a current of 500 μA to 800 μA at a single frequency of 50 kHz or more, too weak to be felt by the subject.

The subject lies down on a nonconducting surface with arms not touching the trunk and legs at least 20 cm apart. Shoes and socks are removed, as well as metal objects (jewelry). The contact surfaces on the hand and ankle should be cleaned with alcohol. The resistance measured can then be used in various formulas in a similar manner to the tube examples. The body can be viewed as 5 tubes: 2 arms, 2 legs, and 1 trunk (see figure 11.8c).

The example of the tubes is an oversimplification. In reality, several factors can affect impedance and invalidate the assumptions. A larger tube increases the conductivity. Warming the tube also increases conductivity. Changes in the skin temperature, in particular, alter whole-body conductivity and have a profound effect on the measurement. A higher skin temperature results in an underestimate of the body fat content (Baumgartner et al. 1990). Often, when the measurements are performed, the subject may sweat more; a wet surface reduces impedance and underestimates body-fat content.

In humans, factors such as hydration status and distribution of water can also affect impedance. Even small changes in the hydration level can have a marked effect on the accuracy of the measurement and can influence the calculated body-fat content (Koulmann et

al. 2000; Saunders et al. 1998). If a person is dehydrated, the impedance decreases, whereas if someone drank a lot of fluid before the measurement, impedance could increase. Thus, losing body water through prior exercise or voluntary fluid restriction will overestimate body-fat content. Hyperhydration has the opposite effect and will underestimate body-fat content.

Body position is important, and the fluid shifts that occur can also affect impedance. The orientation of tissues can affect impedance. For example, a current is more easily transported along muscle fibers than against muscle fibers. The testing conditions under which BIA is run should be extremely well controlled. Usually subjects are advised as follows:

- Abstain from alcohol for 8 hours to 12 hours before the measurement.

- Avoid vigorous exercise for 8 hours to 12 hours before the measurement.

- Measurements are performed at least 2 hours after the last meal (or drink),

- Measurements are performed within 5 minutes of lying down.

BIA seems a convenient technique that needs considerable experience, expertise, and especially, control of the testing conditions. When BIA is performed in the best possible way, the results are very reliable but may not be as accurate as skinfold measurements (Broeder et al. 1997; Stolarczyk et al. 1997).

Dual Energy X-Ray Absorptiometry

Dual energy X-ray absorptiometry (DEXA or DXA) has become the clinical standard for measuring bone density. The principle is based on absorption of low-energy X-rays. The short duration of exposure gives only a minimal radiation dose.

During the measurement, the subject lies supine on a table and a source and detector probe pass across the body at relatively low speed (about 60 cm/min; a whole-body scan may take 15 minutes). The subject is exposed to these low-energy X-rays, and the loss of signal in various parts of the tissue are recorded. The measurement is performed at two different intensities, so that the instrument's software can distinguish not only between soft tissues and bone mineral content but also between lean-body mass and fat mass.

DEXA seems to be a fairly accurate technique that shows excellent agreement with other independent techniques to measure bone mineral content (Going et al. 1993: Heymsfield et al. 1990). Also, small changes in body composition can be detected with this method (Going et al. 1993).

277

However, DEXA may underestimate body-fat content somewhat compared with underwater weighing. In addition, with DEXA test conditions must be standardized (Kohrt 1995) because factors such as hydration status can influence the results (Elowsson et al. 1998). The software and hardware of the various commercially available DEXA scanners is different, which is also a source of error (Van Loan et al. 1995). Although DEXA has limitations, it appears to be one of the better ways to measure body composition, and it has the advantages over other methods in that it not only can distinguishes between lean-body mass and fat mass it also can assess bone density.

Computed Tomography

Computed tomography (CT) uses ionizing radiation via an X-ray beam to create images of body segments. The CT scan produces qualitative and quantitative information about the total area of the tissue investigated and the thickness and volume of tissues within an organ. With this method, fat surrounding a tissue as well as fat within a tissue can be measured.

Magnetic Resonance Imaging

With **magnetic resonance imaging** (MRI), pictures can be obtained from body tissues and compartments. The results are somewhat similar to those obtained by CT scan, but with MRI, electromagnetic radiation is used rather than ionizing radiation. Generally, MRI shows good agreement with other methods. A study found excellent agreement between MRI and underwater weighing estimates in both overweight and nonoverweight women, suggesting that MRI may be a satisfactory substitute for the more established methods of body-fat estimation in adult women. In fact, MRI showed the smallest day-to-day variation in the measurement within an individual (see figure 11.9). However, calculations of body fat from MRI scans are highly dependent on software, and this dependency can introduce an error.

Air Displacement Plethysmography

A relatively new and promising method to estimate whole-body volume is a small chamber in which air displacement is measured. The technique is called air displacement plethysmography and is marketed commercially as BOD POD (see figure 11.10). The advantage of this technique is that it is convenient for the subject because it takes place while the subject is sitting in a small chamber, measurements take only 3 minutes to 5 minutes, and the reproducibility is good.

The subject is first weighed accurately outside the BOD POD. He or she then sits in the 750 L volume

Figure 11.9 Comparison of typical in vivo magnetic resonance images obtained on 2 separate days from the same subject at the level of the midthigh. Regression between cross-sectional adipose tissue–free skeletal muscle (ATFSM) areas from 42 pairs of magnetic resonance images (6 subjects × 7 images each). SEE = SE of estimate; *N* = number of images. Solid line is regression line.

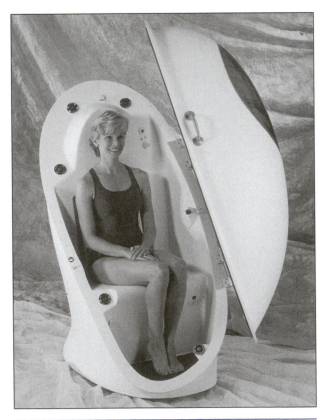

Figure 11.10 The BOD POD.

Reprinted, by permission, from Life Measurement, Inc.

BOD POD, which consists of a dual chamber made out of fiberglass (see figure 11.10). The person's volume is the original volume in the chamber minus the air that has been displaced with the subject inside. The subject breathes into an air circuit to assess pulmonary gas volume, which, when subtracted from measured body volume, yields true body volume. Body density can then be calculated from body mass and body volume. Although this technique has good reproducibility, it generally gives lower percentages of body fat compared with hydrostatic weighing and DEXA (Collins et al. 1999; Wagner et al. 2000; Weyers et al. 2002).

Multicomponent Models

Multicomponent models use a combination of methods such as hydrostatic weighing, BIA, and DEXA to reduce the errors associated with using a single method (Wagner et al. 2000). While the traditional 2-component model is based on separating fat mass and FFM to determine body composition, these models assume that the density of fat-free mass is 1.1 g/cm^3 and the components that constitute the FFM (water, protein, and minerals) are constant for all individuals. These assumptions may not always hold true, and accuracy can, therefore, be improved by measuring these different components. These multicomponent models can combine measures of whole-body density with measures of body water and bone-mineral density. This approach is generally believed to give the most accurate results.

Normal Ranges of Body Weight and Body Fat

Body fat consists of essential body fat and storage fat. Essential body fat is present in the nerve tissues, bone marrow, and organs (all membranes), and we cannot lose this fat without compromising physiological function. Storage fat, on the other hand, represents an energy reserve that accumulates when excess energy is ingested and decreases when more energy is expended than consumed. Essential body fat is approximately 3% of body mass for men and 12% of body mass for women. Women are believed to have more essential body fat than men because of childbearing and hormonal functions. In general, the total body fat percentage (essential plus storage fat) is between 12% and 15% for young men and between 25% and 28% for young women (Lohman and Going 1993).

Different sports have different requirements in terms of body composition. In some contact sports such as American football or rugby, a higher body weight is generally seen as an advantage. In sports such as gymnastics, marathon running, and other weight-bearing activities, a lower body weight and high power-to-weight ratio are extremely important. Therefore, in these sports both low body fat and low body weight are necessary. In sports such as bodybuilding, increasing lean-body mass and increasing body weight without increasing body fat are desirable.

No accepted percentage body fat standards exist for athletes. The ideal body composition is highly dependent on the particular sport or discipline and should be discussed on an individual basis with the coach, physiologist, and nutritionist or dietician. Body weight and body composition should be discussed in relation to functional capacity and exercise performance.

Genetics

A significant portion of the variation in body-fat levels of individuals is genetically determined. Perhaps 25% to 40% of adiposity is the result of our genes (Bouchard 1994). Evidence from both genetic epidemiology and molecular epidemiology studies suggests that genetic factors determine the susceptibility to gaining or losing body fat in response to dietary energy intake (Perusse and Bouchard 2000). To study the influence of genetics on the effects of overfeeding, identical twins were investigated. In one study, monozygotic twins were submitted to an energy surplus of 4.2 kJ/day (1,000 kcal/day) 6 days a week for 100 days (Bouchard et al. 1990). The excess energy intake over the entire period was 353 MJ (84,000 kcal). The average gain in body mass was 8.1 kg, but considerable interindividual variation occurred. Interestingly, the variation between pairs was more than 3 times greater than the variation within pairs, suggesting an important genetic component. The variation between pairs was even greater for changes in abdominal visceral fat, indicating that the site of storage is also genetically determined.

Similarly, when identical twins completed a negative energy balance protocol by exercising over a period of 93 days without increasing energy intake, more variation occurred between pairs than within pairs. The energy deficit was estimated to be 244 MJ (58,000 kcal), and the mean body-weight loss was 5 kg. The range of weight loss, however, was 1.0 kg to 8.0 kg (see figure 11.11).

These classical early studies demonstrate a genetic factor in the development of obesity. This link has been confirmed by molecular epidemiology studies, and now more than 250 genes are believed to have the potential to influence body fatness (Rankinen et al. 2002).

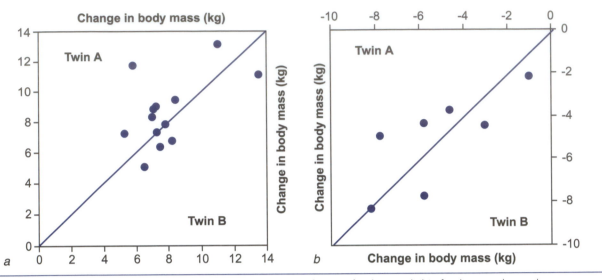

Figure 11.11 Changes in body mass in identical twins *(a)* after overfeeding and *(b)* after being subjected to a negative energy balance by exercise. Considerably more variation occurred between pairs than within pairs, strongly suggesting a genetic component in the regulation of body mass.

Adapted, by permission, from C. Bouchard et al., 1990, "The response to long-term over-feeding in identical twins," *New England Journal of Medicine* 322: 1477-1482.

Weight Loss

Many athletes, although not overweight, seek to lose body weight, particularly body fat. For some this weight loss is an advantage because it increases the power-to-weight ratio (jumping events). For others, weight loss means they can reduce the energy expenditure when competing (such as when running). Weight reduction is also common in weight-category sports in which athletes often compete well below their normal weight. Another reason why athletes want to get rid of some body fat is simply for physical appearance and to live up to the stereotype of the lean, toned, and strong athlete.

Weight loss is not always a good idea and can even be detrimental to performance. A reduction in body mass is usually accompanied by a reduction in muscle mass, and it may also reduce muscle glycogen stores. Excessive weight loss has also been associated with chronic fatigue and increased risk of injuries. Too much emphasis on losing weight can lead to the development of eating disorders, which are discussed in chapter 12. Many mistakes can be made in the weight management of the athlete, and the purpose of this chapter is to make the reader aware of some of these mistakes and to provide some guidelines on how to lose the weight in a responsible way.

Defining Goals

In conjunction with the coach and a nutritionist weight-loss goals should be established. These goals should be carefully thought out and well defined. Whether it is a good idea or not depends primarily on the current body-fat percentage. Although individual differences exist, a body-fat percentage less than 5% for men and 12% for women is not recommended. As discussed earlier, some fat is essential, and we can only lose some of the storage fat without affecting physiological function.

Goals also have to be defined with a time schedule in mind. How much weight must be lost and how soon? A realistic weight loss is about a 1 kg (2 lb) every 2 weeks, so to lose 3 kg at least 6 weeks are needed. This means reducing the energy intake by about 2,000 kJ (500 kcal) a day. A more rapid weight loss will make training difficult or impossible.

Energy and Substrate Balances

A negative energy balance is necessary to lose weight and it can be induced by reducing energy intake, by increasing energy expenditure, or by a combination of these two. However, these alterations in energy balance are just part of the picture. The macronutrient (carbohydrate, fat, and protein) intake and the expenditure of these substrates must also be considered. Excess intakes of carbohydrate and protein can be converted to fat, although this process requires energy and does not easily occur. The body increases the oxidation rate of carbohydrate and protein immediately when excess amounts are ingested. Fat, however, is different. Generally, fat is not converted into protein or carbohydrate.

Also, when excess amounts are ingested, the oxidation rates are not increased immediately, making fat more likely to be stored in adipose tissue (Abbott et al. 1988; Westerterp 1993).

The macronutrient composition of the diet, therefore, plays a very important role in the daily energy intake and expenditure (Westerterp et al. 1995), and to maintain body weight and body composition, individuals must not only be in energy balance but also be in carbohydrate, fat, and protein (and alcohol) balance. These substrate balances are influenced by a variety of genetic, environmental, cultural, and socioeconomic factors (Flatt 1995). For example, dietary intake is different in different socioeconomic classes, with the lower socioeconomic classes typically having a higher fat intake and lower carbohydrate intake than the higher socioeconomic classes. Also, clear cultural differences exist in diets as well as on acceptability of exercise. Some African countries, for example, have a very high carbohydrate intake (>70%), whereas the carbohydrate intake in the Western world is typically around 40% to 50%.

A simple example illustrates the importance of substrate balances. Someone who eats 50 g of sugar (e.g., by drinking half a liter of a soft drink) daily in addition to the normal diet is in positive energy balance by approximately 800 kJ/day (200 kcal/day). This level of intake means 292,000 kJ (73,000 kcal) a year, which over the course of 30 years amounts to 8,760 MJ (2,190,000 kcal). Assuming an energy density of adipose tissue of 19.0 kJ/g (7.7 kcal/g) this person should experience a weight gain of 284 kg (625 lb) in those 30 years. Clearly, this amount of weight gain is not reality, and this person would probably only gain a few kilograms.

The increased body weight results in an increased metabolic rate and an increased oxidation of energy substrates. Also, some of the energy ingested as carbohydrate is lost in the conversion to fat. Reducing dietary fat intake can be very effective for several reasons:

- Fat is very energy dense. It has more than twice the amount of energy as the same weight of carbohydrate or protein.

- High-fat foods generally taste good, which leads to a tendency to eat more. Studies show that increasing the fat content of the diet increases the spontaneous intake of food.

- Fat is efficiently stored and requires very little energy for digestion.

- Fat intake does not immediately increase fat oxidation.

Common Mistakes

When trying to lose weight, athletes make the following common mistakes:

- Trying to lose weight too rapidly. Like most people, athletes are impatient about weight loss. They want to see results within a couple of weeks, but unfortunately this expectation is not realistic. Although rapid weight loss is possible, this reduction is mostly dehydration, which reduces performance and the ability to train. Weight loss without performance loss has to occur slowly.

- Trying to lose weight during the on-season. Athletes often try to lose weight during the competitive season, and this effort may result in underperformance. Because hard training is difficult when the energy intake is reduced, weight loss best accomplished during the off-season.

- Not eating breakfast or lunch. Another weight-loss approach athletes have tried is skipping breakfast and sometimes also skipping lunch. Although this approach may work for some, it increases hunger feelings later in the day, and one very large evening meal, can easily compensate for the daytime reduction in food intake. Also, exercise capacity and, thus, the ability to train may be reduced without a breakfast, when liver glycogen stores may be low (see chapter 5).

- Too little carbohydrate intake. When losing body weight (being in negative energy balance), athletes risk also losing some muscle mass. However, this risk can partly be reduced by consuming relatively large amounts of carbohydrate. Carbohydrate has a protein-sparing effect.

Decreased Resting Energy Expenditure

Losing body weight becomes increasingly difficult because the body responds to the weight loss by becoming more efficient. Resting energy expenditure, or resting metabolic rate (RMR), decreases in response to weight loss (Dulloo and Jacquet 1998). This decrease in resting metabolism cannot simply be attributed to the decrease in body mass or fat-free mass. Rather, it is an autoregulatory feedback mechanism by which the body tries to preserve energy. This "food efficiency" may occur independently of a person's body mass or dieting history. It usually causes a plateau in weight loss and is a common source of frustration for dieters.

In an elegant study by Leibel et al. (1995), maintenance of a 10% reduced body weight was associated with a reduction in total energy expenditure of 25 kJ/kg FFM/day (6 kcal/kg FFM/day) in nonobese subjects (see figure 11.12). Resting energy expenditure and nonresting energy expenditure each decreased 13 kJ/kg FFM/day to 17 kJ/kg FFM/ day (3 kcal/ kg FFM/day to 4 kcal/kg FFM/day). Maintenance of a 10% higher body weight was associated with an increase in total energy expenditure of 38 kJ/kg FFM/day (9 kcal/kg FFM/day). Maintenance of a reduced or elevated body weight is associated with compensatory changes in energy expenditure, which oppose the maintenance of a body weight that is different from the usual weight. This study shows that the body has compensatory mechanisms that try to maintain the normal body weight.

Female athletes, especially runners, sometimes have very low energy intakes. Despite their training load (30 km to 90 km of running a week), they may have energy intakes similar to their sedentary counterparts (Drinkwater et al. 1984; Myerson et al. 1991). Amenorrheic runners (those whose menstrual cycles are currently absent) had a significantly lower RMR than their eumenorrheic runners (those with normal monthly menstrual cycles), and their energy intake was similar, despite higher activity levels (Lebenstedt et al. 1999; Myerson et al. 1991). These findings suggest that energy efficiency or food efficiency exists. However, other reasons may account for the negative energy balance or low energy intake and expenditure in these female athletes. Not all studies of these athletes have found a reduced RMR (Beidleman et al.

1995; Wilmore et al. 1992). Alternative explanations could include inaccuracies and underreporting of food intake by these athletes or reduced physical activity in the hours they are not training.

The concept of food efficiency fits in with the theory that the body has a weight "set point." Although the interindividual differences in body weight of humans are very large, the body weight of an individual is usually fairly constant and typically varies only 0.5% over periods of 6 weeks to 10 weeks (350 g for an individual with a body mass of 70 kg). If rats are given an energy-restricted diet for several weeks, they lose body mass rapidly. However, upon being permitted to eat freely again, they restore this body mass within weeks and their weight becomes identical to their counterparts who had free access to food for the entire period. A similar change happens when rats are overfed. Evidence also exists for such a "set point" for body weight in humans (Keesey and Hirvonen 1997).

Weight Cycling: The Yo-Yo Effect

Often, weight loss is achieved with considerable effort but maintaining the new lower body weight is even more difficult. After the weight is lost, it is regained in a relatively short period of time. This effect is usually referred to as the yo-yo effect. Studies in animals have documented this pattern of **weight cycling.** After a period of food restriction and weight reduction, animals tend to regain the

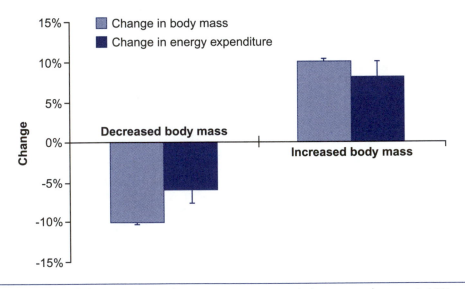

Figure 11.12 Changes in daily energy expenditure in response to weight loss or weight gain. A 10% reduction in body weight resulted in a 6% decrease in energy expenditure, and a 10% gain in body weight resulted in a 8% increase in energy expenditure. This shows that the body has compensatory mechanisms that try to maintain a normal body weight.

weight very quickly if they are allowed free access to food.

Several prospective studies have shown weight fluctuation (gain-loss or loss-gain) or weight variability to be associated with increased mortality, independent of the direction of weight change. However, when taking limited account of preexisting disease, studies show little evidence of negative side effects of weight cycling (Field et al. 1999; Wannamethee et al. 2002). From a public health perspective, the risks from overweight and obesity far exceed the potential risks of weight cycling.

Gender Differences in Weight Loss

Meta-analyses of studies on weight loss after aerobic-type exercise training showed that weight loss, although modest, was greater for males (Ballor and Keesey 1991). These findings confirm earlier research in males concerning exercise-training effects on body mass and body composition and extend them both to females and to a broader range of exercise types. These gender differences have been related to the differences in body-fat distribution. Women store more fat in the gluteal-femoral region, whereas men store more fat in the visceral (abdominal) depot. Fat located in the upper body and abdominal regions (central fat) is more metabolically active and, therefore, has higher rates of lipolysis in response to adrenergic stimulation. During exercise, FAs are preferentially mobilized from these regions (Wahrenberg et al. 1991). Also, postprandial fat storage may be higher in subcutaneous adipose tissue in women than in men. All of these differences may play a role in the variation in net regional fat storage between men and women (Blaak 2001) and women's greater resistance to weight loss.

Weight-Loss Methods

The various ways to lose body weight include pharmacological and surgical procedures (see figure 11.13), but here we focus on the weight-loss strategies that involve diet, exercise, or a combination of the two. Several different diets exist, some of which have been commercialized. Some diets have proved to be effective, whereas others are a list of erroneous assumptions and claims. For the athlete, distinguishing between the facts and the fallacies is often difficult. This section reviews some of the most common dietary regimens and weight-loss methods.

Energy Restriction and Reduced Fat Intake

Debate continues over whether weight loss can be achieved by reducing energy intake or by reducing fat intake only. Epidemiological evidence suggests that reducing the percentage of fat in the diet is more effective in reducing body weight than is reducing the absolute amount of fat (Sheppard et al. 1991). The most important factor, however, is the reduction in energy intake. Although both energy restriction and low-fat eating results in weight loss, energy restriction usually results in a larger reduction in energy intake than does ad libitum low-fat eating. Therefore, energy restriction may initially result in a larger weight loss, although studies show that both diets are effective over the long term (Jeffery et al. 1995; Schlundt et al. 1993).

The advantage of reduced fat intake is that relatively high carbohydrate content can be maintained, resulting in reasonable glycogen stores and better recovery. Many athletes adopt a diet that is low in fat with small reductions in the energy intake, so they can still replenish the carbohydrate stores. This type

Dietary methods

Fasting

Energy restriction

Low-fat diet

High-protein diet

High-carbohydrate diet

Low-carbohydrate ketogenic diet (Atkins diet, Sugarbusters)

Zone diet

Food-combining diet

Exercise

Regular exercise

Endurance exercise

Surgical procedures

Stomach stapling

Removal of a section of the small intestine

Liposuction

Pharmacological methods

Stimulants

Appetite suppressants

Drugs that reduce fat absorption

Figure 11.13 Methods to achieve weight loss.

of diet seems to be a sensible way of reducing weight, although suboptimal carbohydrate intake can still interfere with normal training. Thus, weight reduction should occur slowly and in the off-season.

Very-Low-Energy Diets

Very-low-energy diets (VLEDs) or very-low-calorie diets (VLCDs) diets are used as a therapy to achieve rapid weight loss in the obese. They are usually in the form of liquid meals that contain the recommended daily intakes of micronutrients but with only 1,600 kJ/day to 3,200 kJ/day (400 kcal/day to 800 kcal/day). These liquid meals contain a relatively large amount of protein to reduce muscle wasting and a relatively small amount of carbohydrate (less than 100 g/day). Such diets are very effective in reducing body weight rapidly. In the first week, the weight loss is predominantly glycogen and water. Fat and protein are lost as well during the initial phase, but these losses are a relatively small proportion of the total weight loss. After the initial rapid weight loss, the weight reduction is mainly from adipose tissue, with some losses of body protein. The increased fat oxidation results in ketosis (formation of ketone bodies, acetoacetate, and β-hydroxybutyrate). Ketone bodies have a very specific odor and can easily be detected on the breath (bad breath). Once ketosis is initiated, hunger feelings may be reduced somewhat.

Because carbohydrate intake is low, the blood glucose concentration is maintained by gluconeogenesis from various precursors (glycerol and alanine). Although increased physical activity is also encouraged when very-low-energy diets are prescribed to the obese, the diets are effective without the exercise component. Because of the associated chronic glycogen depletion, exercise capacity is severely impaired. For this reason, such diets are not advised for athletes, who would unlikely be able to complete their normal training sessions. Even in the off-season such diets are not advised, because the loss of body protein can be significant. Side effects of such diets include nausea, halitosis (bad breath), hunger (which may decrease after the initiation of ketosis), lightheadedness, and hypotension. Dehydration is also common with such diets, and electrolyte imbalances may occur.

Food-Combination Diets

Food-combination diets are based on a philosophy that certain foods should *not* be combined. Although a wide variety exists, most of these diets warn against the combination of protein and carbohydrate foods. Such combinations cause a "buildup of toxins" with "negative side effects such as weight gain." These diets are often very tempting because they promise an easy way to rapid weight loss, and these diets have worked for many individuals. When these diets are strictly followed, energy and fat intake are very likely to be reduced compared with the normal diet. The reduction in energy and fat is the reason for the success of the diet rather than the fact that certain foods were not combined. Because energy and carbohydrate intake are lower, glycogen stores are reduced, and performance as well as recovery may be impaired.

High-Protein Diets

Recommendations for increased protein consumption are among the most common approaches of popular or fad diets. Some have argued that high-protein diets suppress the appetite, which might be a mechanism for facilitated weight loss. Protein also has a larger thermic effect and a relatively low coefficient of digestibility compared with a mixed, equicaloric (isoenergetic) meal. In short-term studies, dietary protein modulates energy intake via the sensation of satiety and increases total-energy expenditure by increasing the thermic effect of feeding. Whereas these effects did not contribute to weight and fat loss in the studies in which energy intake was fixed, one ad libitum study suggests that a high-protein diet results in a greater decrease in energy intake and, therefore, greater weight and fat loss.

In terms of safety, little long-term information is available on the health effects of high-protein diets. The available data, however, indicates that consumption of protein greater than 2 times to 3 times the recommended intake contributes to urinary calcium loss and may, in the long term, predispose to bone mineral loss. Caution with these diets is recommended for individuals who may be predisposed to kidney disease and, particularly, individuals with diabetes mellitus.

The Zone Diet

The Zone diet was proposed by Barry Sears in his book, *The Zone: A Dietary Road Map* (Sears 1995). The diet opposes the traditional recommendations of a high-carbohydrate, low-fat diet for athletes. By reducing the carbohydrate intake, insulin responses are reduced and a favorable insulin to glucagon ratio is established. The benefits are increased lipolysis and improved regulation of eicosanoids, hormone-like derivatives of FAs in the body that act as cell-cell signaling molecules. The diet increases the "good" eicosanoids and decreases the "bad" eicosanoids. The "good" eicosanoids improve blood flow to the working muscle and enhance the delivery of oxygen and nutrients, eventually resulting in improved performance. To "enter the zone" the diet should consist of 40% carbohydrate, 30% fat, and 30% protein divided into a regimen of 3 meals and 2 snacks a day. The diet is also referred to as the 40:30:30 diet.

Although some arguments by Sears are scientifically sound, the book has problems, pitfalls, and errors in assumptions, and it also contains some contradictory information. Many of the promised benefits of the Zone diet are based on selective information about hormonal influences on eicosanoid metabolism. Opposing evidence is conveniently left out.

Eicosanoid metabolism is extremely complex and highly unpredictable, and previous diet manipulation studies have been unsuccessful in stimulating the synthesis of good eicosanoids relative to bad eicosanoids. Very small changes in insulin concentration are sufficient to reduce lipolysis significantly. Such effects persist for up to 6 hours after a meal. To avoid reductions in lipolysis after a meal, the carbohydrate intake must be extremely small, even less than proposed by the Zone diet. Meals with the 40:30:30 combination are very difficult to compose, unless you buy the 40:30:30 energy bars marketed by Sears.

Nevertheless, the Zone diet seems to work for some people, and anecdotal evidence indicates weight loss with the diet. The successes are expected because the Zone diet is essentially low in energy (4,000 kJ/day to 8,000 kJ/day [1,000 kcal/day to 2,000 kcal/day]). Even for athletes who train hard, the energy intake does not increase much and they are in a relatively large energy deficit.

The principle of vasodilating muscle arterioles by altering eicosanoid production is correct in theory. However, the little evidence available from human studies does not support any significant contribution of eicosanoids to active muscle vasodilation. In fact, the key eicosanoid reportedly produced in the Zone and responsible for improved muscle oxygenation is not found in skeletal muscle. Based on the best available scientific evidence, the Zone diet is more ergolytic than ergogenic to performance.

Low-Carbohydrate Diets

Some of the best-known low-carbohydrate ketogenic diets are the Atkins diet (Atkins 1992) and Sugarbusters (Andrews et al. 1998). These diets are based on the premise that reducing the carbohydrate intake results in increased fat oxidation. Ketone body production will increase, which may suppress appetite.

Ketones may also be present in urine, which could result in loss of "calories" via urine. Although all of the above may be true, the losses achieved in this diet are extremely small. The excretion of ketone bodies in urine is small and is at most 400 kJ/day to 600 kJ/day (100 kcal/day and 150 kcal/day). Such diets can be effective but not more effective than a well-balanced, energy-restricted diet. These low-carbohydrate diets are not recommended because of the relatively high fat content, which may raise blood lipids. For athletes, this diet is detrimental because of reduced glycogen stores and exercise capacity.

Exercise to Lose Weight

Exercise is another way to create a negative energy balance. In obese individuals, the effectiveness of exercise programs to achieve weight loss has been questioned because of problems with motivation, compliance with the program, and the fact that the ability to exercise is often impaired. In athletes, these factors are unlikely to be a problem. Most athletes can include exercise sessions with the specific aim of increasing energy expenditure, and they can exercise at a high enough intensity to significantly increase energy expenditure. However, athletes may have different problems. For example, coaches of athletes who compete in explosive events (e.g., sprints and jumps) are often reluctant to include aerobic exercise in their training programs. Athletes may have difficulty finding more time to exercise in addition to their normal training without compromising recovery.

Generally, however, adding exercise to a weight-loss program results in weight loss that is fat loss (Ballor and Keesey 1991; Kraemer et al. 1995; McMurray et al. 1985). The combination of exercise and diet is the most effective way to maintain a lower body weight after weight reduction. Some argue that the optimal exercise intensity is related to fat oxidation and should be the intensity with the highest fat-oxidation rates. As discussed in chapter 6, fat oxidation increases as exercise increases from low to moderate intensities, even though the percentage contribution of fat may actually decrease (see figure 6.8). The increased fat oxidation is a direct result of the increased energy expenditure when going from light-intensity to moderate-intensity exercise. At high exercise intensities (>75% $\dot{V}O_2max$), fat oxidation is inhibited, and both the relative rate and the absolute rate of fat oxidation decreases to negligible values (Achten et al. 2002). Maximal rates of fat oxidation are generally observed between 55% and 65% $\dot{V}O_2max$.

The type of exercise also affects maximal rates of fat oxidation and is significantly higher during uphill walking and running compared with cycling (Achten, Venables, Jeukendrup, et al. 2003; Arkinstall et al. 2001; Houmard et al. 1991; Nieman et al. 1998a, Nieman et al. 1998b; Snyder et al. 1993). No long-term studies have been conducted to compare different types of exercise and their effectiveness in achieving or maintaining weight loss. Also, whether exercises that optimize fat oxidation are indeed an effective way to reduce body fat remains to be determined.

Comparisons of resistance training with endurance training have demonstrated favorable effects on body composition (Broeder et al. 1997; Van Etten et al. 1994) or similar effects of resistance training compared with aerobic exercise in facilitating body-fat loss (Ballor and Keesey 1991). Resistance training seems more effective in preserving or increasing fat-free mass. In turn, the amount of metabolically active tissue also increases, and the increase is suggested to be one of the mechanisms by which exercise helps to maintain a lower body weight after weight loss through energy restriction. The exercise preserves (or even increases) muscle mass, resulting in a smaller reduction of the RMR.

Very few studies have compared the effectiveness of various types of exercise. From the current evidence, however, resistance training is at least as effective in reducing body fat as aerobic exercise. Most of the existing evidence is from studies in sedentary and obese individuals with almost no information about active individuals and trained athletes. One important factor is, of course, the duration of exercise, which largely determines the energy expended during exercise. Athletes who can spend more time exercising at relatively high exercise intensities likely have a greater opportunity to achieve a negative energy balance and, thus, lose body weight. Following are guidelines to help athletes achieve weight loss.

- Determine a realistic body-weight goal. The help of a sports dietician is likely to be needed to identify a realistic target weight.

- Do not try to lose more than about 0.5 kg/week (about 1 lb/week), and do not restrict energy intake by more than 500 kcal/day to 750 kcal/day.

- Eat more fruit and vegetables.

- Choose low-fat snacks.

- Study food labels and try to find substitutes for high-fat foods. Look not only at fat content but also at the energy content per serving.

- Limit fat add-ons such as sauces, sour cream, and high-fat salad dressings, or choose the low-fat versions of these products.

- Try to structure your eating into 5 or 6 smaller meals.

- Avoid eating very large meals.

- Make sure carbohydrate intake is high and consume carbohydrates immediately after training.

- A multivitamin and mineral supplement may be useful during periods of energy restriction. You should seek the advice of a nutritionist or dietician.

- Measure body weight daily and get measurements of body fat regularly (every 2 months). Keep a record of the changes

Making Weight and Rapid Weight-Loss Strategies

Sports in which making weight is important are those with weight categories, including judo, wrestling, rowing, and boxing. In horse racing, jockeys are weighed before and after competition to ensure that each horse will carry the precise assigned weight. In these sports, weight classes are clearly defined, and to compete in a particular weight class, body weight must be within the limits for that category at the weigh-in. Rowing, for instance, has a lightweight and a heavyweight division. In the lightweight division, male athletes are not permitted to exceed 72.5 kg (160 lb), with a crew average of 70 kg (155 lb). For females, the maximum individual weight is 59 kg (130 lb) with a crew average of 57 kg (125 lb). Weigh-ins can happen from 30 minutes to about 20 hours before competition, although sometimes the weigh-in is performed the day before the competition. Athletes commonly compete at a weight that is 2 kg to 6 kg (4 lb to 13 lb) below their normal weight, which implies that they must lose weight rapidly in the days or weeks before competition.

Most rapid weight loss is by dehydration, and athletes use various techniques to achieve it. The most common methods are energy or fluid restriction; dehydration by exercise, sauna, hotrooms, or steam rooms; diuretics, stimulants, and laxatives. Exercise is often performed in a hotroom, wearing plastic or rubber garments. This rapid weight loss mainly affects body water, glycogen content, and lean-body mass, with very little or no loss of body fat (Kelly et al. 1978; Oppliger et al. 1991). Wrestlers experience these weight-loss/weight-gain cycles about 7 to 15 times each year and approximately 100 times during a wrestling career (Tipton and Oppliger 1993).

The rapid weight loss may result in reductions in plasma volume, central blood volume, and blood flow to active tissues and increased core temperature and heart rate. The cardiovascular changes can be observed with a weight loss of approximately 2% of body weight (see chapter 8). These rapid weight-loss strategies have also been reported to alter hormone status, impede normal growth and development, affect psychological state, impair academic performance, and affect immune function. Severe dehydration can result in heat illness and even death.

In 1997, three previously healthy collegiate wrestlers in the United States died while each was engaged in a rapid weight-loss program to qualify for competition (Anonymous 1998). In the hours preceding the official weigh-in, all three wrestlers engaged in a similar rapid weight-loss regimen that promoted dehydration through perspiration and resulted in hyperthermia. The wrestlers restricted food and fluid intake and attempted to maximize sweat losses by wearing vapor-impermeable suits under cotton warm-up suits and exercising vigorously in hot environments. In response to these deaths, the National Collegiate Athletic Association (NCAA) rules were changed, and a wresting weight certification program was made mandatory to create a safer competitive environment (Davis et al. 2002). Other changes included establishing a weight class system that better reflected the wrestling population, weigh-ins close to competition (1 hour before), weigh-ins for each day of a multiple-day tournament, and eliminating tools that are used for rapid dehydration (Davis et al. 2002). The current NCAA rules are now in line with the recommendations by the American College of Sports Medicine (ACSM) (Oppliger et al. 1996).

Weight gain is a concern for athletes in sports where a higher body weight and increased muscle mass are advantages, such as hammer throwing, discuss throwing, shotput, weightlifting, American football, and rugby. The key to gaining weight is to have a higher energy intake than energy expenditure. To increase lean-body mass rather than just fat mass, one must increase carbohydrate intake and not fat intake. Whereas the body counteracts a decrease in body weight that occurs with energy restriction by decreasing resting energy expenditure (see previous section), the body increases resting energy expenditure when the energy intake is increased in excess of the expenditure. Just as expecting large weight losses in a short period of time is unrealistic, so is expecting large weight gains within days. Realistic weight gains are between 0.2 kg/week and 1.0 kg/week (0.4 lb/week to 2 lb/week), depending on the increase in energy intake. Protein synthesis is a slow process, and even with intake of excess amounts of protein, synthesis of muscle protein takes a long time and only takes place if combined with an adequate training program. For more information on protein synthesis and gaining muscle mass, see chapter 7.

Key Points

- Standard height-weight tables do not provide information about body composition and can be misleading when applied to individual athletes.

- Body mass index (BMI) is often used as a rough measure of body composition. However, although BMI can be useful in epidemiological and clinical studies, it does not distinguish between muscle mass and fat mass.

- The technique of densitometry is based on the "Archimedes principle" that the loss of weight in water is equal to the volume of the displaced water. Because body fat is less dense than water, it lets one float, whereas the fat-free mass, which is denser than water, makes one sink. After correcting for residual volume, percent fat can be calculated based on the underwater weight.

- The sum of skinfolds can be used to estimate body fat percentage. For accuracy, values from tables that have been established for specific populations (e.g., same gender, same age range, or same ethnicity) must be used.

(continued)

(continued)

■ Bioelectrical impedance analysis (BIA) is a convenient technique that needs considerable experience, expertise, and, especially, control of the environmental conditions to get reliable results. When BIA is performed in the best possible circumstances, the results may be reliable, but they may still be less accurate than skinfold measurements.

■ Dual energy X-ray absorptiometry (DEXA or DXA) is based on the principle that compartments with different densities will absorb different amounts of low-energy X-rays. The advantage of DEXA is that it can distinguish not only fat mass and fat-free mass but also bone density. DEXA has become the clinical standard to measure bone density.

■ Imaging technologies, such as computed tomography (CT) and magnetic resonance imaging (MRI) can visualize body fat of different parts of the body.

■ An average body-fat percentage for young adults is between 12% and 15% for males and between 25% and 28% for females. Approximately 3% of body mass of males and 12% of body mass of females is essential body fat.

■ A negative energy balance is required to lose weight. In addition, a negative fat balance will promote fat loss. However, the resting metabolic rate (RMR) decreases in response to weight loss. This effect is referred to as "food efficiency" and makes losing weight more difficult. A common problem is the so-called yo-yo effect, or weight cycling. After weight loss is achieved, the weight is often regained in a relatively short period of time.

■ Common diet strategies to lose weight include a very-low-energy diet (VLED), low carbohydrate diets, food-combination diets, and high-protein diets. For athletes seeking to lose weight, energy restriction and reduced fat intake are recommended. This strategy allows a reasonable carbohydrate intake, enabling the athletes to perform high-intensity training without major reductions in lean-body mass (LBM).

■ Exercise can help to create a negative energy balance, can help to maintain muscle mass, and may compensate for the reductions in RMR seen after weight loss.

■ In weight-category sports such as judo, wrestling, rowing, and boxing, the need to "make weight" encourages athletes to try to lose weight in a relatively short period of time. Athletes should be aware of the risks of rapid weight loss. Rapid weight loss (mainly dehydration) can affect both health and performance.

■ The recommended method to gain weight is maintaining a positive energy balance without increasing fat intake. Most of the excess energy intake should come from carbohydrate.

Key Terms

bioelectrical impedance analysis (BIA) 276

body mass index (BMI) 268

computed tomography 278

densitometry 269

dual energy X-ray absorptiometry 277

magnetic resonance imaging (MRI) 278

very-low-energy diets (VLED) 284

weight cycling 282

Recommended Readings

Bouchard, C. 1994. Genetics of obesity: Overview and research directions. In *The Genetics of Obesity*, ed. C. Bouchard, 223-233. CRC Press: Boca Raton, FL.

Bouchard, C., A. Tremblay, J.P. Despres, A. Nadeau, P.J. Lupien, G. Theriault, J. Dussault, S. Moorjani, S. Pinault, and G. Fournier. 1990. The response to long-term over-feeding in identical twins. *New England Journal of Medicine* 322:1477-1482.

Flatt, J.-P. 1995. Use and storage of carbohydrate and fat. *American Journal of Clinical Nutrition* 61:952S-959S.

Roche, A.F., S.B. Heymsfield, and T.G. Lohman. 1996. *Human Body Composition*. Human Kinetics: Champaign, IL.

Chapter 12

Eating Disorders in Athletes

© Dan Wendt

Objectives

After studying this chapter, you should be able to do the following:

- Describe the characteristics of anorexia nervosa and bulimia nervosa

- Describe the prevalence of eating disorders in athletes

- Describe the risk factors for eating disorders

- Describe the effects of eating disorders on sports performance

- Describe the effects of eating disorders on the health of the athlete

- Describe some effective strategies for the treatment and prevention of eating disorders

For people consuming 8 MJ/day to 12 MJ/day (1,900 kcal/day to 2,900 kcal/day) of dietary energy, a typical pattern of eating might be two or three main meals (e.g., breakfast, lunch, and dinner), with the occasional snack (e.g., biscuit or chocolate bar) between meals. For endurance athletes with higher energy intakes (e.g., typically 15 MJ/day to 20 MJ/day [3600 kcal/day to 4800 kcal/day]), a grazing pattern of eating is common, with a substantial proportion of daily energy intake consumed between meals. In most cases, athletes are in energy balance, meaning that over the course of several days or weeks, energy intake generally matches energy expenditure. However, some athletes (and nonathletes) experience eating disorders characterized by gross disturbances of eating behaviors. The major disorders are associated with abnormally low food intakes or bouts of binge eating followed by purging the stomach contents. If undiagnosed and untreated, eating disorders not only can have detrimental effects on sports performance but also can have damaging, long-lasting effects on the health of the individual and can even be fatal.

Evidence suggests that the prevalence of eating disorders is more common in certain athletic groups than in the general population, and the role of the sport nutritionist working with athletes who are susceptible to eating disorders is crucial to prevention. Often the best treatment is education concerning the health risks of eating disorders and counseling the athlete on wise food choices and good eating habits. This chapter reviews the characteristics of different eating disorders, the prevalence of eating disorders in different sports, risk factors for eating disorders, and the effects of eating disorders on sports performance and health. Some practical guidelines on diagnosis, treatment, and prevention of eating disorders are also given.

Types of Eating Disorders

The major classified eating disorders include anorexia nervosa, bulimia nervosa, and an eating disorder not otherwise specified (American Psychiatric Association 1987). For athletes who show significant symptoms of eating disorders but who do not meet the criteria of the *Diagnostic and Statistical Manual of Mental Disorders* (American Psychiatric Association 1987) for anorexia or bulimia, a subclinical eating disorder separately classified as anorexia athletica has been proposed (Sundgot-Borgen 1994a).

Anorexia nervosa is characterized by an abnormally small food intake and a refusal to maintain a normal body weight (according to what is expected for gender, age, and height), a distorted view of body image, an intense fear of being fat or overweight and gaining weight or "feeling fat" when the individual is clearly below normal weight, and the absence of at least three successive **menstrual cycles** in females **(amenorrhea)**. The physical symptoms of individuals experiencing anorexia nervosa or anorexia athletica can be summarized as follows (Thompson and Trattner-Sherman 1993; Sundgot-Borgen 1994b):

- Weight loss beyond that normally required for adequate sports performance
- Amenorrhea or some manifestation of menstrual dysfunction
- Dehydration
- High level of fatigue (beyond that normally expected after training or competition)
- Gastrointestinal problems (e.g., constipation, diarrhea, or distress after a meal)
- Hyperactivity
- **Hypothermia** (lower than normal body temperature)
- Low resting heart rate
- Muscle weakness
- Susceptible to overuse injuries
- Reduced bone mineral density and susceptibility to stress fractures
- Frequent infections, skin sores, and poor wound healing
- Low blood hemoglobin and **hematocrit** and low serum albumin, serum ferritin, glucose, HDL cholesterol, and estradiol levels.

The psychological characteristics of individuals suffering from anorexia nervosa or anorexia athletica can be summarized as follows (Thompson and Trattner-Sherman 1993):

- General anxiety
- Avoidance of eating and absence from meal situations
- Claims of "being fat" or "feeling fat" despite being thin and underweight
- Resistance to recommendations for weight gain
- Unusual weighing behaviors (e.g., excessive weighing, avoidance of weighing, negative reaction to being weighed, or refusal to be weighed)
- Excessive training beyond that required for a particular sport or exercising while injured

or when prohibited by coaching and medical staff

- Obsessed about their body image and compulsive behaviors regarding eating and physical activity
- Restlessness and inability or unwillingness to relax
- Social withdrawal
- Depression
- Tiredness and irritability
- **Insomnia** (difficulty with sleeping)

Most individuals experiencing anorexia do not seem to realize they have a problem and, therefore, are unlikely to seek treatment. Hence, for the susceptible athlete, the role of the coach, team doctor, physiologist, sport psychologist, and sport nutritionist is crucial in identifying the problem and persuading the athlete to get medical attention. In many cases, anorexic athletes only consider seeking help when their sports performances decline.

Bulimia nervosa is characterized by repeated episodes of binge eating (consumption of large amounts of usually energy-dense foods), soon followed by purging the stomach contents (vomiting) before many of the nutrients from the heavy meal can be absorbed. The food is often eaten in secrecy, and the individual will commonly disappear from view shortly after a meal to purge the stomach contents. Bulimic athletes do not usually volunteer information about their abnormal behavior until they feel the situation is getting out of control, or their habit detrimentally affects their sports performance. Bulimics may also use **laxatives** (drugs that promote defecation) and **diuretics** (drugs that promote urine formation) to achieve short-term weight loss. However, unlike anorexics, most bulimic athletes are not grossly underweight. Therefore, the athlete's support team must be aware of the physical symptoms and psychological characteristics associated with bulimia nervosa. The physical symptoms are as follows (Thompson and Trattner-Sherman 1993):

- Callus, sores, or abrasions on fingers or back of hand used to induce vomiting
- Dehydration
- Dental or gum problems
- Edema, complaints of bloating, or both
- Serum electrolyte abnormalities
- Gastrointestinal problems
- Low weight despite apparent intake of large amounts of food

- Frequent and often extreme weight fluctuations
- Muscle cramps, muscle weakness, or both
- Swollen parotid salivary glands
- Menstrual irregularities in females

The psychological characteristics associated with bulimia nervosa are as follows (Thompson and Trattner-Sherman 1993):

- Binge eating
- Secretive eating and agitation when bingeing is interrupted
- Disappearing after eating meals
- Evidence of vomiting unrelated to illness
- Dieting
- Excessive exercise beyond that required for the athlete's sport
- Depression
- Self-critical, especially concerning body image, body weight, and sport performance
- Substance abuse
- Use of laxatives, diuretics, or both that are unsanctioned by medical or coaching support staff

Prevalence of Eating Disorders in Athletes

Currently, data on the prevalence of eating disorders in athletes are limited and equivocal, mainly because few studies have applied strict classification criteria (such as those in the *Diagnostic and Statistical Manual of Mental Disorders,* American Psychiatric Association 1987) to both athletes and nonathlete control subjects. Rather, most studies have looked at a limited number of symptoms of eating disorders such as a preoccupation with body weight, body image, and food intake or the use of pathogenic means of weight control.

Some athlete populations exhibit a significantly greater preoccupation with body weight than nonathlete populations, particularly in sports emphasizing body shape, leanness, or body weight (Davis 1992). However, some studies have relied exclusively on the use of questionnaires, which is likely to result in underreporting of eating disorders and underreporting of the use of purging methods such as vomiting, laxatives, and diuretics (Sundgot-Borgen 1994a, 2000). Questionnaires also tend to result in overreporting of the incidence of binge eating compared with clinical evaluation by structured interviews (Sundgot-Borgen 1994a, 2000). Indeed, estimates of the prevalence of eating disorders among female athletes range from less than 1% to as high as 75% (Gadpalle et al. 1987; Burckes-Miller and Black 1988; Warren et al. 1990; Sundgot-Borgen 1994a, 1994b) and similarly among athletic males estimates vary from 0% to 57% (Dummer et al. 1987; Burckes-Miller and Black 1988; Rosen and Hough 1988; Rucinski 1989).

Studies generally indicate a substantially higher incidence of eating disorders among athletes compared with nonathletes and greater prevalence among females compared with males. Some studies report that eating disorders are at least 10 times more prevalent among females than among males (Andersen 1995). Classically defined anorexia nervosa does not seem to be much more prevalent (1.3%) in the female athletic population than in the general female population (Andersen 1990), whereas bulimia nervosa (8.2%) and subclinical eating disorders (8.0%) seem to be more prevalent among female athletes than among female nonathletes. The prevalence of eating disorders appears to be higher among female athletes who compete in endurance and weight-category sports and, as can be seen in figure 12.1, is especially high in aesthetic sports (e.g., gymnastics and dance) compared with games players, power sports, and technical sports, presumably because of the relative importance of leanness to success in these different sports or the

perceived advantage to be gained by competing in a lower weight category.

Risk Factors

Although the precise causes of eating disorders are unknown, several factors that increase the risk of eating disorders can be identified. These include gender, lifestyle, dieting, and certain personality traits.

Gender and Lifestyle

Clearly, the biggest risk factor is gender, with females having a 10 times greater risk of eating disorders compared with males (Andersen 1995). However, some recent evidence indicates that the incidence of male eating disorders is on the rise (Byrne and McLean 2002). For example, body dysmorphic disorder is a condition in which males are not happy with their bodies, They want more muscle and to look leaner with ripped midsections and are quite prepared to go to excessive lengths through exercise, supplement use, and drug abuse to achieve this end.

Athletes seem to be more susceptible to eating disorders than the general population. Both male and female athletes competing in sports that emphasize a lean body shape or low body weight have a significantly higher prevalence of eating disorders and eating-disorder symptoms than do other athletes and

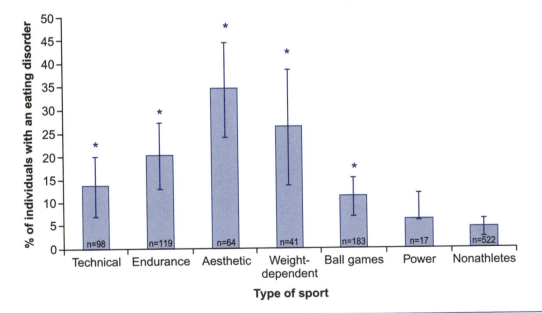

Figure 12.1 Prevalence of eating disorders among elite female athletes in different sports. Data are shown as mean and 95% confidence intervals. Asterisk (*) indicates significantly higher than nonathletes (P < 0.05).

Reprinted, by permission, from J. Sundgot-Borgen, 2000, "Eating disorders in athletes." In Nutrition in sport, 510-522, (Oxford, United Kingdom: Blackwell Science).

nonathletes. However, being an athlete does not place an individual at increased risk for an eating disorder. Rather, athletes who compete in sports where being thin is considered essential or having a low body weight is necessary to be successful are particularly vulnerable (Byrne and McLean 2002). This vulnerability may be a result of the additional physical, psychological, and social stresses associated with the athletic environment and lifestyle.

Studies suggest that a high training load may induce a negative energy balance in endurance athletes, which in turn may elicit physiological and social reinforcements leading to eating disorders. According to this hypothesis, elite athletes should be more prone to eating disorders because they do more training and are under more intense pressure to be lean than subelite athletes. Garner et al. (1987) reported a higher prevalence of eating disorders among top-level dancers compared with dancers in lower competitive levels. However, heavy training loads cannot be the prime cause of eating disorders, as female cyclists, marathon runners, and triathletes expend more energy in their training than do dancers and gymnasts. Nevertheless, there is no evidence to suggest that endurance athletes are more prone to the development of eating disorders than dancers or gymnasts. Another possibility is that young athletes who take up serious sport at a prepubertal age may not select the sport that is most suitable for their adult body types, and hence are subject to greater pressure to maintain different (i.e., leaner, smaller) body types than is natural for them. Indeed, Sundgot-Borgen (1994) found that athletes with eating disorders begin sport-specific training at an earlier age than athletes who do not have eating disorders.

Dieting

Dieting is an established risk factor for eating disorders (Polivy and Herman 1995). Sudden periods of enforced inactivity (e.g., because of injury) or longer periods of positive energy balance (e.g., during the off-season) may result in weight gain, which the athlete is then told to lose. The athlete may begin to diet excessively or may develop an irrational fear of additional weight gain. Guidance to athletes as to how best to lose weight is important at this point. In some cases, athletes may be asked to lose weight very rapidly to remain on the team. As a result, they may undergo periods of restricted eating and weight cycling. This type of behavior has been suggested as an important factor in triggering eating disorders in athletes (Brownell et al. 1987; Sundgot-Borgen 1994b).

Personality Traits

Certain personality traits may predispose individuals to eating disorders. Most affected individuals are reported to have low self-esteem and to be overly self-critical, particularly about body image (Sundgot-Borgen 2000). Bulimics consistently show high levels of impulsivity (DaCosta and Halmi 1992), and their addictiveness scores resemble those of drug addicts (DeSilva and Eysenck 1987). Athletes—at least the most successful ones—are, by nature, compulsive and focused. The same traits that encourage good sports performance in many athletes—perfectionism, dedication, and willingness to work hard and withstand discomfort—may lead to preoccupation with body image and body fat.

Exercise Dependence and Eating Disorders

Excessive exercising is widely reported to coexist with eating disorders, particularly among those practicing dietary restraint (Brewerton et al. 1995). Indeed, many of the reported characteristics of "exercise dependence" are evident in athletes with eating disorders (Touyz et al. 1987). A study described 28% of female eating-disorder patients as "compulsive exercisers" (Brewerton et al. 1995), and another study reported that the prevalence of excessive exercising among such patients was as high as 78% (Davis et al. 1994).

Overactivity in eating disorders appears either as deliberate exercise to increase energy expenditure and promote fat loss or as involuntary and persistent restlessness, often associated with sleep disturbance (Beumont 1995). Where the former is manifest, exercise is considered a secondary symptom of the disorder, and for athletes, distinguishing this motivation to exercise from the need to train for a particular sport may be impossible. Restless hyperactivity, on the other hand, may be a central feature of the eating disorder (Kron et al. 1978). This notion is supported by evidence of reduced food consumption in rats forced to exercise excessively and increased voluntary wheel running in food-deprived rats (Epling and Pierce 1988). Accordingly, a combination of excessive exercise and food restriction may be a self-perpetuating and mutually reinforcing cycle with potentially serious consequences. As yet, the precise role of exercise in the etiology of eating disorders remains unclear. Dieting is an established risk factor for eating disorders (Polivy and Herman 1995), but high levels of physical activity may play an important role in the perpetuation of an eating disorder. Davis et al. (1994)

found that 75% of eating-disorder patients were most active during the period of lowest food intake and greatest weight loss.

Effects of Eating Disorders on Sports Performance

The effect of an eating disorder on exercise performance is determined by how long the disorder has been manifest and the severity of the disorder. Whether an eating disorder affects performance in a specific sport is also determined by the nature of the sport (i.e., whether the predominant requirement of the sport is power, strength, endurance, or motor skills). In anorexia nervosa, a gradual loss of body weight may actually increase maximal oxygen uptake when expressed as ml/min/kg b.w. (Sundgot-Borgen 2000). As in the early stages of dieting, the body adapts and uses up stored fat and certain minerals (e.g., iron) and vitamins. A decreased performance may not be seen for some time, and the athlete may wrongly believe that the disordered eating behavior is harmless. However, endurance performance is likely to be impaired if liver and muscle glycogen levels are low or if the athlete becomes dehydrated or anemic (i.e., the blood hemoglobin concentration falls below normal).

Dehydration is common in both anorexia nervosa and bulimia nervosa (Sundgot-Borgen 2000), and acute dehydration has other consequences for sports performance, such as loss of motor skill and coordination (Fogelholm 1994b). A reduced plasma volume in the dehydrated state impairs the ability to thermoregulate during exercise, which can also contribute to impaired exercise performance, particularly in the heat (see chapter 8 for further details). Electrolyte disturbances are also likely to be detrimental to muscle function, and with time, a loss of lean-body (muscle) mass will reduce strength and power. Both short-term anaerobic performance and muscle strength are impaired after rapid weight loss, and performance is not restored with 1 hour to 3 hours of rehydration, but 5 hours to 24 hours of rehydration (Fogelholm, Koskinen, et al. 1993).

Effects of Eating Disorders on the Athlete's Health

The health problems that can arise from chronic eating disorders are the effects of semistarvation in anorexia nervosa and of the binge-purge cycle in bulimia nervosa, both of which result in micronutrient deficiencies that are detrimental to the health of the athlete. For female athletes in particular, inadequate intakes of calcium, iron, and B-vitamins are a serious concern. Energy and macronutrient deficiency in anorexic individuals may affect mood, endocrine status, growth, reproductive function, and bone health.

Psychological Mood State

Depression is a common symptom of eating disorders (Thompson and Trattner-Sherman 1993). Increased fatigue, anxiety, anger, and irritability are associated with low levels of energy and carbohydrate intake during periods of dieting to achieve rapid weight loss. Studies on the effects of eating disorders on mood state in athletes are currently lacking.

Growth and Maturation

Stunted growth in adolescent athletes may occur during prolonged periods of inadequate energy, protein, and micronutrient intake. The onset of puberty may be delayed in child athletes and poor bone development can lead to increased susceptibility to fractures and problems in later life, particularly in females.

Reproductive Function

Female reproductive function is affected by the negative energy balance that results from disordered eating coupled with intense training. Psychological stress and low body-fat content can be other contributing factors that lead to amenorrhea. The production of **gonadotrophic hormones** (follicle-stimulating hormone and luteinizing hormone) from the anterior pituitary gland is inhibited during prolonged energy deficits, and the ovarian production of the sex steroid hormones estrogen and progesterone drops to very low levels. Menstrual irregularity ensues, which may be followed by amenorrhea and absence of **ovulation.** In this state, the female is infertile, and her endocrine status is akin to that of a postmenopausal woman.

The long-term effects of athletic amenorrhea on fertility are still unclear, although some evidence suggests that the reproductive deficiencies associated with amenorrhea are reversible when the problem is treated (Mishell 1993). Although low body fat levels per se have not been implicated as the specific cause of menstrual dysfunction, evidence suggests that low energy intake is a risk factor. Studies show that restricting energy intake below a critical threshold amount causes metabolic and hormonal adaptations. These changes may be mediated, at least in part, by the hormone leptin.

Athletic amenorrhea represents the most extreme form of menstrual dysfunction. However, even less severe disturbances of the menstrual cycle, including a reduced frequency of periods (oligomenorrhea) and luteal-phase deficiency can result also result in depressed estrogen levels. Furthermore, in adolescent female athletes, the onset of puberty and **menarche** can be delayed (Manore 2002).

Osteoporosis

Because ovarian steroid hormones, particularly estradiol, facilitate calcium uptake into bone, amenorrhea may predispose female athletes to osteoporosis, a premature loss of bone quality and quantity. This condition can occur despite the fact that load-bearing physical activity induces greater bone mineral density. However, this effect is specific to the bones that receive the most impact stress during exercise, and even this degree of protection may not be enough to prevent net demineralization of bone. Athletes with eating disorders have decreased spinal vertebral bone mineral densities compared with normal values, but higher densities than nonathletes with eating disorders. Thus, exercise training may lessen the amount of bone loss, but exercise will not completely protect the athlete from osteoporosis. Abnormal and restrictive eating behaviors seem to be related to a greater likelihood of fractures (Bennell et al. 1999; Golden 2002).

The withdrawal of estrogens at any age is associated with bone loss that could lead to osteoporosis if prolonged and is more critical than low progesterone levels for the onset of bone demineralization (Cumming 1996). The absence of menstrual cycles and the associated low plasma estradiol levels may decrease bone mineral density to such an extent that fractures occur under minimal impact loading (Snow-Harter 1994; Cumming 1996). Bone development normally continues up to 25 years of age and is then followed by a gradual loss of bone with advancing age.

As shown in figure 12.2, bone loss is accelerated in females after menopause, when the ovaries stop producing estrogens. Thus, child and adolescent female athletes who experience eating disorders are at very high risk for osteoporosis later in life. All physically active women who lose their periods as a result of heavy training or eating disorders are strong candidates for premature bone loss, with typically 2% to 6% of bone lost each year, possibly resulting in the loss of 25% of total bone mass (Snow-Harter 1994).

Peak bone mass is reached during the first 3 decades of life, with 95% of maximum density reached by 18 years of age, and all women experiencing age-related bone loss after this time. Therefore, maximizing peak bone mass during the formative years is of utmost importance. Because the two years to three years that constitute the pubertal growth

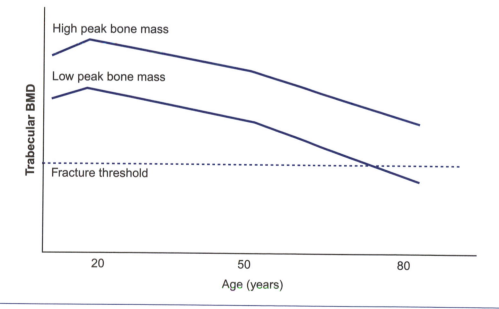

Figure 12.2 Age and peak bone mass in relation to trabecular bone mineral density (BMD) in females. Peak bone mass is reached in the early 20s, with all women experiencing age-related bone loss after this time. Individuals with a low peak bone mass reach the "critical threshold" for fractures at an earlier age.

Adapted, by permission, from C.M. Snow-Harter, 1994, "Bone health and prevention of osteoporosis in active and athletic women," *Clinical Sport Medicine* 13: 389-404.

spurt are accompanied by deposition of 60% of the final bone mass, any dietary inadequacy and disruption of the normal menstrual cycle at this time may more severely impair bone formation than at any other time (Snow-Harter 1994; Sabatini 2001; Golden 2002).

The three conditions that are prevalent in female athletes—amenorrhea, disordered eating, and osteoporosis—are collectively known as the **female athlete triad syndrome** (see figure 12.3). Any female athlete is at risk from this triad, but women who participate in sports in which low body fat is advantageous (e.g., endurance running and gymnastics) or a requirement (i.e., weight-category sports such as rowing and martial arts) are at highest risk for the syndrome.

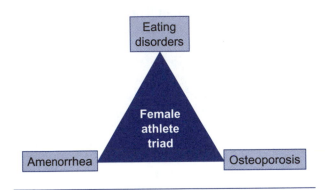

Figure 12.3 The female athlete triad syndrome.

Studies report that the total number of years of regular **menstrual cycles** predicts lumbar spine bone mineral density more accurately than any other training, dietary, or menstrual factor (Montagnani et al. 1992; Myburgh et al. 1993). Indeed over the past 15 years, numerous studies have reported that women with menstrual-cycle irregularities have bone mineral density values that are significantly lower than those of normally menstruating women athletes and non-athletes (Kazis and Iglesias 2003). Consequently, the present concern is that many female athletes whose rigorous training schedules and restricted dietary practices have led to extended periods of amenorrhea may have suffered irreversible bone loss.

The development of osteoporosis is also accelerated by inadequate dietary intake of calcium (see chapter 9), which must be another concern for athletes with eating disorders (Manore 2002). When amenorrhea is present, increasing the consumption of calcium to 120% of the RDA appears to help bones to maintain density and develop properly. Such nutrition guidance should be given to low-body-weight amenorrhoeic women.

Mortality

Death rates from eating disorders among athletes are not known, but among patients with anorexia nervosa in the general population mortality has been reported to range from less than 1% to as high as 18% (Thompson and Trattner-Sherman 1993). In patients with anorexia nervosa, death is usually caused by excessive fluid and electrolyte disturbance or is the result of suicide. Information on mortality in bulimia nervosa is not available, but clearly some deaths do occur, either as a complication of vomiting behavior or as suicide. The abuse of drugs, including diuretics, laxatives, **emetics** (which promote vomiting), and diet pills that commonly contain stimulants (e.g., amphetamines) is frequently reported among athletes with eating disorders (Sundgot-Borgen and Larsen 1993), and excessive or inappropriate use of some of these drugs may contribute to health problems and mortality in some cases. If dehydration or electrolyte disturbances are present as a result of an eating disorder, the athlete is at risk for cardiac arrest during exercise.

Treatment and Prevention of Eating Disorders

Perhaps the most effective means of preventing or treating eating disorders among athletes is education of the athletes. Most eating disorders persist because of a lack of understanding of the effect they can have on health. Individuals with eating disorders do not seem to remember what constitutes a balanced meal or a normal pattern of eating. Because of misconceptions and poor understanding of nutritional principles, athletes may have an irrational fear of admitting (even to themselves) that they have a problem. Early diagnosis is, therefore, vital because eating disorders are more difficult to treat the longer they progress. The coexistence of exercise dependence and depression is common among athletes with eating disorders. Some evidence suggests that a coincidence of an eating disorder and depression is most effectively treated by addressing the depressive illness first, via combination of cognitive-behavioral therapy and antidepressant medication (Roth and Fonagy 1998). Managing depression is the immediate concern because it is the most life-threatening. Treatment of the eating disorder would follow, generally in the form of cognitive-behavioral therapy for bulimia nervosa or interpersonal therapy for anorexia nervosa (Roth and Fonagy 1998).

For athletes with long-term conditions, the readiness to listen and accept advice should be assessed in conjunction with a mental health professional.

After the athlete's cooperation is gained, nutritional counseling can begin. The athlete's body weight and percent body fat should be measured to establish realistic goals, which also depend on the nature of the athlete's sport. An athlete who agrees to comply with all treatment regimens can continue to train and compete, but the athlete must be monitored closely, and effective treatment must always take precedence over sport.

Excessive exercising can aggravate medical complications of eating disorders (Pomeroy and Mitchell 1992) by, for example, worsening electrolyte disturbances through sweating. However, exercise is employed in the treatment of depression and eating disorders in nonathletes (Beumont et al. 1994; Byrne and Byrne 1993), so a continued level of moderate exercise is preferable to stopping the athlete from exercising altogether. Nevertheless, the benefits of continued exercising should be weighed against the potential risks in each case. Furthermore, the exercise should be supervised and signs of exercise dependence closely monitored. The treatment of an athlete with an eating disorder should follow a team approach, incorporating not only a physician and dietician but also a physiologist and psychologist. This approach gives the athlete encouragement to practice healthy eating habits from several sources, and the message that the consequences of the con-

dition are deterioration of both health and sports performance is reinforced by all.

According to Thompson and Trattner-Shermann (1993), athletes should maintain a minimum body weight that is no less than 90% of "ideal" health-related body weight. It is also recommended that the athlete should eat three balanced meals a day containing sufficient dietary energy to sustain the desired body weight set by the dietician. Athletes who have been amenorrheic for more than six months should be assessed for bone mineral density and considered for hormone replacement therapy.

Coaches should understand the influence they can have on their athletes' eating and weight-control behaviors. Although the exact causes of eating disorders remain unknown, the pressure of wanting to succeed and satisfy the coach's demands by highly motivated but uninformed young athletes seems a likely scenario that can first result in dieting followed by unhealthy eating behaviors. If such behavior is reinforced by success and praise from the coach, it could lead to a full-blown eating disorder. Coaches should, therefore, not comment on an athlete's body size, weight, or percent body fat. Such comments should be left to the dietician who, at the same time, can advise the athlete on healthy eating and set up a structured, supervised weight-loss program, where this is deemed necessary.

Key Points

- Eating disorders are characterized by gross disturbances of eating behavior. The major disorders are associated with abnormally low food intakes (anorexia nervosa) and bouts of binge-eating followed by vomiting (bulimia nervosa). If undiagnosed and untreated, eating disorders can have detrimental effects on sports performance and can also have damaging long-lasting effects on the health of the individual.

- A higher incidence of eating disorders seems to occur among athletes compared with nonathletes, and female athletes have a much greater prevalence compared with male athletes. Classically defined anorexia nervosa does not seem to be much more prevalent in the female athlete population compared with the general population, whereas bulimia nervosa and subclinical eating disorders seem to be more prevalent among female athletes than among female nonathletes.

- The prevalence of eating disorders appears to be higher among female athletes who compete in endurance and weight-category sports and is especially high in aesthetic sports such as gymnastics and dance compared with games players, power sports, and technical sports. Presumably, the higher prevalence is related to the importance of leanness to success in these different sports or to the perceived advantage of competing in a lower weight category.

- Risk factors for eating disorders include female gender, dieting, participation in an athletic lifestyle, and certain personality traits.

(continued)

299

(continued)

- Eating disorders are commonly associated with exercise dependence and depression.

- The precise causes of eating disorders are not known but probably progress from an initial desire or requirement to lose weight that develops into a pathological fear of gaining weight. Highly motivated but uninformed young female athletes are probably most at risk.

- Eating disorders are likely to be detrimental to sports performance, although this consequence depends on the severity and duration of the disorder and the nature of the sport. Athletes experiencing eating disorders may have low glycogen stores, be dehydrated, or exhibit electrolyte disturbances, so both high intensity and endurance exercise performance can be affected.

- Prolonged episodes of negative energy balance or of bingeing and purging are likely to result in micronutrient deficiencies that are detrimental to the health of the athlete. For female athletes in particular, inadequate intakes of calcium, iron, and B-vitamins are a serious concern. Energy and macronutrient deficiency are likely to affect mood, endocrine status, growth, reproductive function, and bone health in anorexic individuals.

- Athletic amenorrhea may predispose female athletes to premature osteoporosis because of the failure of the ovaries to produce estrogen. This condition can occur despite the fact that load-bearing physical activity induces greater bone mineral density.

- Amenorrhea, disordered eating, and osteoporosis are collectively known the "female athlete triad" syndrome. Any female athlete is at risk for this syndrome, but women who participate in sports in which a low body fat is advantageous or a requirement are at highest risk.

Key Terms

amenorrhea 292

anorexia nervosa 292

bulimia nervosa 293

diuretics 293

emetics 298

female athlete triad syndrome 298

gonadotrophic hormones 296

hematocrit 292

hypothermia 292

insomnia 293

laxatives 293

menarche 297

menstrual cycles 298

ovulation 296

Recommended Readings

Beumont, P.J.V., J.D. Russell, and S.W. Touyz. 1993. Treatment of anorexia nervosa. *Lancet* 26:1635-1640.

Brownell, K.D., and J. Rodin. 1992. Prevalence of eating disorders in athletes. In *Eating, Body Weight and Performance in Athletes: Disorders of Modern Society*, ed. K.D. Brownell, J. Rodin, and J.H. Wilmore, 128-143, Lea and Febiger: Philadelphia.

Byrne, S., and N. McLean. 2001. Eating disorders in athletes: A review of the literature. *Journal of Science and Medicine in Sport* 4:145-159

Clark, N. 1993. How to help the athlete with bulimia: Practical tips and case study. *International Journal of Sport Nutrition* 3:450-460.

Garner, D.M., L.W. Rosen, and D. Barry. 1998. Eating disorders among athletes. Research and recommendations. *Child and Adolescent Psychiatric Clinics of North America* 7:839-857.

Sundgot-Borgen J. 1993. Prevalence of eating disorders in female elite athletes. *International Journal of Sport Nutrition* 3:29-40.

Torstveit, G., C.G. Rolland, and J.Sundgot-Borgen. 1998. Pathogenic weight control methods and self-reported eating disorders among elite athletes. *Medicine and Science in Sports and Exercise* 5 (suppl):181.

Wilmore, J.H. 1991. Eating and weight disorders in female athletes. *International Journal of Sport Nutrition* 1:104-117.

Chapter 13

Nutrition and Immune Function in Athletes

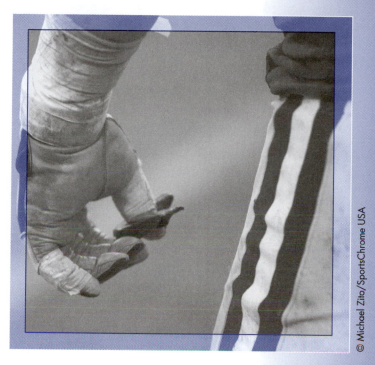

© Michael Zito/SportsChrome USA

Objectives

After studying this chapter, you should be able to do the following:

- Describe the main components and functional mechanisms of the immune system

- Describe the effects of exercise and training on immune function and susceptibility to infection

- Describe the mechanisms by which nutrition may influence immune function

- Describe the roles of several vitamins and minerals that are required to maintain immune function

- Discuss nutritional strategies that may be effective in reducing exercise-induced immunodepression

- Comment on studies that have investigated the effects of nutritional supplements on exercise-induced immunodepression

- Describe particular groups of athletes who may be at increased risk for immunodepression and susceptibility to infection

The **immune system** is involved in tissue repair after injury and in the protection of the body against potentially damaging (pathogenic) microorganisms such as bacteria, viruses, and fungi. In some circumstances, the immune system can become functionally depressed (known as **immunodepression**), which may result in an increased susceptibility to infection. Several forms of stress, including a heavy schedule of training and competition, can lead to immunodepression in athletes, placing them at a greater risk for opportunistic infections, particularly upper respiratory tract infections (URTIs). An abundance of epidemiological evidence and clinical data suggest that nutritional deficiencies impair immune function and increase the risk of infection, and even medically harmless infections may significantly impair athletic performance.

Many factors influence exercise-induced immunodepression (e.g., physical, environmental, and psychological stresses), but nutrition is a factor that plays a critical role. This chapter examines the role of nutrition in exercise-induced immunodepression and the effect of both excessive and insufficient nutrient intake on immune function. Because much of the present literature concerning nutrition and immune function is based on studies with sedentary subjects, the need for research that directly investigates the interrelationship between exercise immunology and nutrition is emphasized. Some important questions that must be answered include the following:

- Which aspects of nutrition are crucial to normal immune function? Are the reported dietary practices of athletes optimal for immune function?

- Do any specific nutritional practices impair immune function or exacerbate the temporary immunodepression that follows an acute bout of prolonged strenuous exercise?

- Does feeding of supplements (e.g., carbohydrate, amino acids, or vitamins) during and after prolonged exercise reduce the stress on the immune system?

- Can nutrient supplements reduce the risk of infection after heavy exertion?

Because the readers of this book are unlikely to have a detailed knowledge of the physiology of the immune system, the following section provides a brief summary of the main components of the immune system and their role in defending the body against pathogenic microorganisms.

Functions of the Immune System and Its Cellular Components

Simply put, the immune system recognizes, attacks, and destroys things that are foreign to the body. In actuality, the functions of this homeostatic system are far more complex, involving the precise coordination of many different cell types and molecular messengers. Yet, like any other homeostatic system, the immune system is composed of redundant mechanisms to ensure that essential processes are carried out.

The immune system has two broad functions, innate (natural, or nonspecific) and adaptive (acquired, or specific) immunity, which work synergistically. The attempt of an infectious agent to enter the body immediately activates the innate system. This so-called "first-line of defense" comprises three general mechanisms (see figure 13.1) with the common goal of restricting microorganism entry into the body:

- Physical/structural barriers, (skin, epithelial linings, and mucosal secretions)

- Chemical barriers (pH of bodily fluids and soluble factors)

- Phagocytic cells (e.g., **neutrophils** and **monocytes/macrophages**)

Failure of the innate system and the resulting infection activates the adaptive system, which aids recovery from infection. Adaptive immunity is helped greatly by T-**lymphocyte** and B-lymphocyte acquisition of receptors that recognize the foreign molecules (called antigens), engendering specificity and "memory" that enable the immune system to mount an augmented response when the host is reinfected by the same **pathogen.**

The components of the immune system comprise both cellular and soluble elements, which are listed in table 13.1. The white blood cells **(leukocytes)** have diverse functions, despite their common origin from the stem cells of the bone marrow. Leukocytes consist of the granulocytes (60% to 70%), monocytes (10% to 15%), and lymphocytes (20% to 25%). Various subsets of the latter can be identified through the use of monoclonal antibodies, which are used to identify specific proteins (clusters of differentiation or cluster designators [CD]) that are expressed on the cell surface of a particular cell type. For example, T-lymphocytes all express the protein CD3 on the cell surface. B-lymphocytes do not express CD3, but express CD19, CD20, and CD22. A particular subset of T-

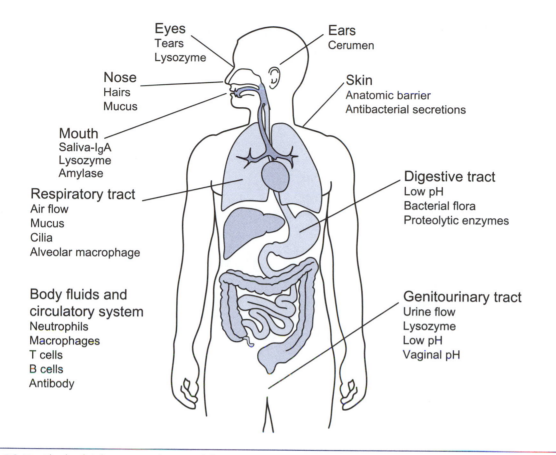

Figure 13.1 The body's barriers and innate defenses against invading microorganisms.

lymphocytes called helper T-cells specifically express the CD4 protein, whereas the cytotoxic T-cells express CD8. T-cells recognize short peptide sequences from antigens only if they are held on the cell's surface and complexed with a major histocompatibility complex (MHC) molecule. The characteristics of the various cells of the immune system are summarized in tables 13.2 and 13.3. The ability of the immune system to distinguish self from nonself depends largely on the MHC, a group of protein markers that are present on the surface of every cell and are slightly different in each individual person.

Table 13.1 Main Components of the Immune System

Innate components	Adaptive components
Cellular	**Cellular**
Natural killer cells (CD16+ and CD56+) Phagocytes (neutrophils, eosinophils, basophils, monocytes, and macrophages)	T-cells (CD3+, CD4+, and CD8+) B-cells (CD19+, CD20+, and CD22+)
Soluble	**Soluble**
Acute-phase proteins Complement Lysozymes Cytokines (interleukins (IL), interferons (IFN), colony-stimulating factors (CSF), tumor necrosis factors (TNF))	Immunoglobulins (IgA, IgD, IgE, IgG, and IgM)

CD = Clusters of differentiation or cluster designators.

Table 13.2 Characteristics of Leukocytes

Leukocyte	Main characteristics
Granulocytes Neutrophils	• 60%–70% of leukocytes • >90% of granulocytes • Phagocytose (i.e., ingest and destroy) bacteria and other foreign material (antigens) • Have a receptor for antibody: phagocytose antigen-antibody complexes • Display little or no capacity to recharge their killing mechanisms once activated
Eosinophils	• 2%–5% of granulocytes • Phagocytose parasites • Triggered by IgG to release toxic lysosomal products
Basophils	• 0%–2% of granulocytes • Produce chemotactic factors • Tissue equivalent = the mast cell, which releases an eosinophil chemotactic factor
Monocytes/macrophages	• 10%–15% of leukocytes • Egress into tissues (e.g., liver and spleen) and differentiate into the mature form: the macrophage • Phagocytose bacteria and viruses enabling antigen presentation • Secrete immunomodulatory cytokines • Retain their capacity to divide after leaving the bone marrow
Lymphocytes	• 20%–25% of leukocytes • Activate other lymphocyte subsets • Produce lymphokines • Recognize antigens • Produce antibody • Exhibit memory • Exhibit cytoxicity

Soluble factors of the immune system activate leukocytes, neutralize (kill) foreign agents, and regulate the immune system. The factors include the **cytokines,** proteins that act as chemical messenger substances (like hormones) to stimulate the growth, differentiation, and functional development of immune system cells via specific receptor sites on either secretory cells (autocrine function) or on immediately adjacent cells (paracrine function). Cytokine action is not confined to the immune system; they also influence the central nervous system and the neuroendocrine system.

Other soluble factors include **complement,** lysozyme, and the specific antibodies formed by the reaction of B-cell–derived **immunoglobulins** (Ig) with specific antigens. The actions of the innate soluble factors are summarized in table 13.4. The immunoglobulins are defined by the structure of the constant region of their heavy chains, which are associated with differences in biological activity and function.

General Mechanism of the Immune Response

The introduction of an infectious agent to the body initiates an inflammatory response that augments the response of the immune system. Acute **inflammation** increases local blood flow in the infected area, which, coupled with increased permeability of blood capillaries, facilitates the entry of leukocytes and plasma proteins into the infected tissue (see figure 13.2). The immune response itself varies according to the nature of the infectious agent (parasitic, bacterial, fungal, and viral), but a general response pattern is evident, as illustrated in figure 13.3. The key player is the macrophage, which ingests foreign material and presents antigens on its cell surface that, in turn, activates T-lymphocytes and B-lymphocytes specific for the antigen. Infectious agents also activate non-specific (innate) host defense mechanisms, including complement, phagocytic cells (e.g., neutrophils), and natural killer (NK) cells.

Table 13.3 Lymphocyte Functions and Characteristics

Lymphocyte subset	Main function and characteristic
T-cells (CD3+) TH (CD4+) TC/TS (CD8+)	• 60%–75% of lymphocytes • 60%–70% of T-cells • "Helper" T-cells • Recognize antigen to coordinate the acquired response • Secrete cytokines that stimulate T-cell and B-cell proliferation and differentiation • 30%–40% of T-cells • TS (suppressor T-cells) involved in the regulation B-cell and other T-cell proliferation by suppressing certain functions • TS may be important in "switching off" the immune response • TC (cytotoxic T-cells) kill a variety of targets, including some tumor cells
B-cells (CD19+, CD20+, and CD22+)	• 5%–15% of lymphocytes • Produce and secrete Ig specific to the activating antigen • Exhibit memory
Natural killer (NK) cells (CD16+ and CD56+)	• 10%–20% of lymphocytes • Large, granular lymphocytes • Express spontaneous cytolytic activity against a variety of tumor-infected and virus-infected cells • MHC-independent • Do not express the CD3 cell-surface antigen • Triggered by IgG • Control foreign materials until the antigen-specific immune system responds

The action of the macrophage on the invading microorganism initiates a chain of events. The macrophage first ingests the foreign organism and isolates it within a membranous vesicle (vacuole) inside the cell (phagocytosis). Digestive enzymes (e.g., lysozyme and elastase) and oxidizing agents (e.g., hydrogen peroxide) are secreted by the macrophage. The foreign proteins (antigens) normally found on the microorganism's surface are digested and processed by the macrophage and incorporated into its own cell surface. The antigen can now be presented to the other cellular immune components. Helper T-cells (CD4+) coordinate the response via cytokine release to activate other immune cells. Mature B-cell stimulation results in proliferation and differentiation into immunoglobulin-secreting (antibody-secreting)

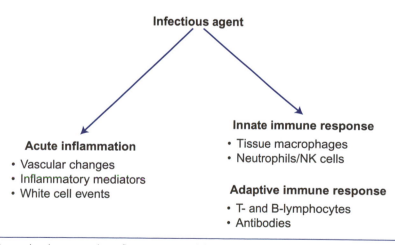

Figure 13.2 The relationship between the inflammatory and the immune response. NK = natural killer.

Table 13.4 Producers and Actions of the Innate Soluble Factors

Soluble factor	Producer(s) and immune actions
Cytokines IL-1	• Produced mainly from activated macrophages • IL-1α tends to remain cell associated • IL-1β acts as a soluble mediator • Stimulates IL-2 production from CD3+ and CD4+ cells • Increases IL-1 and IL-2 receptor expression • Increases B-cell proliferation • Increases TNF-α, IL-6, and CSF levels • Stimulates secretion of prostaglandins
IL-2	• Produced mainly by CD4+ cells • Stimulates T-cell and B-cell proliferation and expression of IL-2 receptors on their surfaces • Stimulates release of IFN • Stimulates NK cell proliferation and killing
IL-6	• Produced by activated helper T-cells, fibroblasts, and macrophages; also released from exercising muscle • Stimulates the differentiation of B-cells, inflammation, and the acute-phase response • Endogenous pyrogen (induces fever)
TNF-α	• Produced from monocytes, T-cells, B-cells, and NK cells • Enhances tumor cell killing and antiviral activity
Acute-phase proteins (APP)	• Made in the liver, secreted into the blood • Encourage cell migration to sites of injury and infection • Activate complement • Stimulate phagocytosis
Complement	• Found in the serum • Consists of 20 or more proteins • Stimulates phagocytosis, antigen presentation, and neutralization of infected cells • Amplifies the response

CSF = colony stimulating factor; IFN = interferon; IL = interleukin; NK = natural killer; TNF = tumor necrosis factor.

plasma cells. Reaction of the immunoglobulin with a specific antigen forms an antibody-antigen complex. Antibodies are essential to antigen recognition and memory of earlier exposure to specific antigens.

Clonal Selection and Immunological Memory

An antigen entering the body selectively activates only a tiny fraction of the quiescent lymphocytes, which then grow and divide to form a clone of identical effector cells (clonal selection). Each antigen (usually a foreign protein or lipopolysaccharide) carries several antigenic determinants, each activating a different clone, and an invading bacterium carries a number of antigens. So a particular species of bacterium invading the body activates a number of clones of lymphocytes.

The first encounter with any antigen causes the primary immune response to that antigen. After several days, clones of lymphocytes selected by the antigen multiply and differentiate to become effector B-cells and T-cells. After several more days specific antibodies from B-cells appear in the blood, as illustrated in figure 13.4. During the lag time, pathogenic organisms may enter the body and multiply in sufficient numbers to cause illness.

A second exposure to the same antigen (even years later) produces a much more rapid, stronger, and longer lasting secondary response. This response depends on memory cells, which are produced at the same time as effector cells during the primary response. Effector cells usually only last for a few days, but memory cells may last for decades. When a second exposure to an antigen occurs, memory cells rapidly multiply and differentiate to create

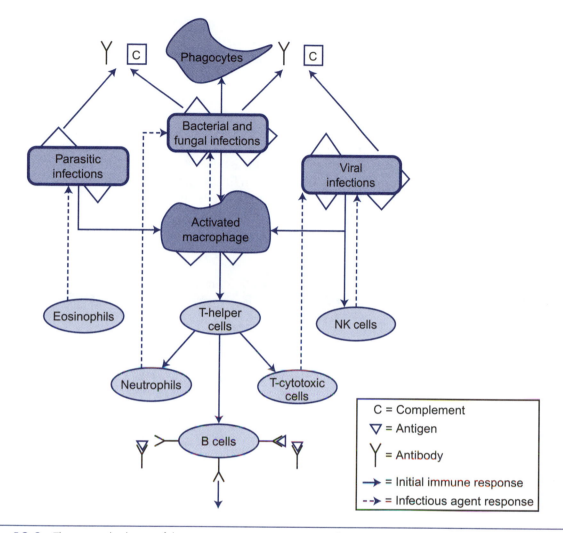

Figure 13.3 The general scheme of the immune response to various infectious agents.

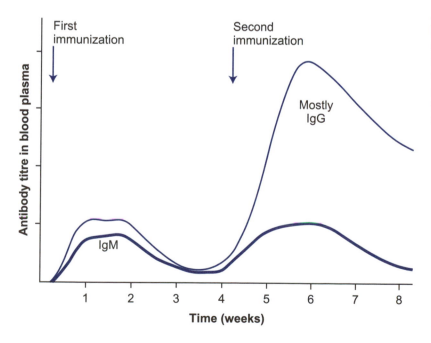

Figure 13.4 Specific antibody production (IgM and IgG subclasses) after first exposure to an antigen (at time = 0 weeks) and on subsequent exposure to the same antigen (at time = 4 weeks). Note the markedly larger and more rapid IgG response after the second exposure.

large numbers of effector cells and large quantities of antibodies dedicated to attacking the antigen. This enhanced antibody response usually prevents symptoms of infection from developing (i.e., immunity to the antigen has been acquired).

Cellular Immune Response

Many pathogens, including all viruses, are parasites that can only reproduce within host body cells. The cellular immune response fights pathogens that have already entered cells. Activated T-lymphocytes include memory cells and cytotoxic T-cells (killer

cells), that attack infected host cells or foreign cells. Helper T-cells and suppressor T-cells are also very important in mobilizing and regulating the whole immune response.

When helper T-cells bind to specific antigenic determinants displayed with MHC proteins on the cell surface of macrophages, the macrophage is stimulated to release a cytokine called **interleukin**-1 (IL-1), which causes the T-cells to grow and divide. The activated T-cells release another cytokine, IL-2, which further stimulates proliferation and growth of helper T-cells and cytotoxic T-cells (see figure 13.5). IL-2 and other cytokines from helper T-cells also

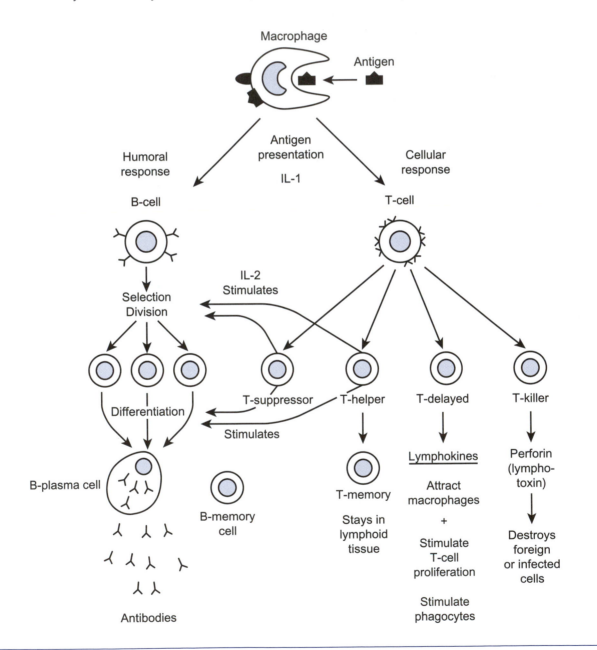

Figure 13.5 The cellular immune response (showing interaction with humoral response).

stimulate B-cells to respond to specific antigens by differentiating into antibody-forming plasma cells. Cytotoxic T-cells recognize and attach to cells that have on their surface appropriate antigenic determinants coupled with the MHC complex. Cytotoxic T-cells then release perforin, a protein that causes puncture of the cell membrane so that a lethal cocktail of digestive enzymes can be passed from the T-cell into the infected cell, causing cell necrosis (death) and lysis (break up) of the infected host cell. Natural killer (NK) cells exert cytotoxic activity in a similar way. The fragments of the lysed cell are then ingested and digested by **phagocytes.**

Humoral (Fluid) Immune Response

B-lymphocytes are also coated with receptors that are specific for particular antigenic determinants. Most antigens activate B-cells only when the B-cells are stimulated by cytokines from helper T-cells; they are T-cell–dependent antigens. Some antigens are T-cell independent. They usually have a repetitive structure and bind with several receptors on the B-cell surface at once (capping). As shown in figure 13.6, the antigen is taken into the cell and activates it. Exposure to an antigen causes appropriate clones of B-cells to proliferate and differentiate into memory

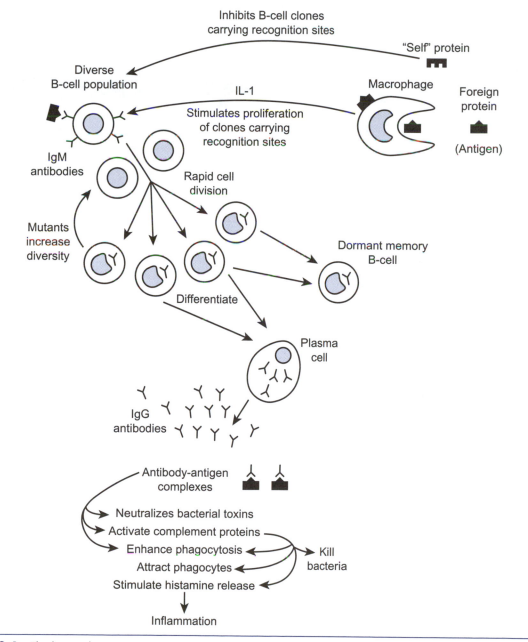

Figure 13.6   The humoral immune response.

cells and plasma cells. The latter are the effector cells of **humoral** immunity and are capable of secreting large amounts of antibody during their brief life of 4 days to 5 days.

The antibodies circulate in the blood and lymph, binding to antigen and contributing to the destruction of the organism bearing it. Antibodies belong to a class of proteins called immunoglobulins (Ig). Each antibody molecule has the ability to bind to a specific antigen and assist with the destruction of the antigen. Every antibody has separate regions for each of these two functions. The regions that bind the antigen differ from molecule to molecule, and are called variable regions. Only a few humoral effector mechanisms exist to destroy antigens, so only a few kinds of regions, the constant regions,

are involved. An antibody molecule consists of 2 pairs of polypeptide chains: 2 short, identical light (L) chains and 2 longer, identical heavy (H) chains. The chains are joined together to form a Y-shaped molecule (see figure 13.7). The variable regions of H chains and L chains are located at the ends of the arms of the Y, where they form the antigen-binding sites. Thus, each antibody molecule has 2 antigen-binding sites, 1 at each tip of the antibody's 2 arms. The rest of the antibody molecule, consisting of the constant regions of the H and L chains, determines the antibody's effector function. Along with the 5 types of constant region are 5 major classes of antibody called IgM, IgG, IgA, IgD, and IgE. Their different roles in the immune response are described in table 13.5. Within each class is a multitude of

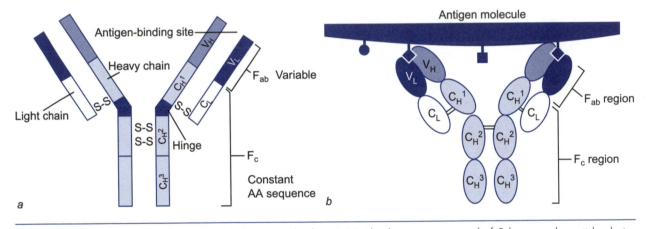

Figure 13.7 The structure of immunoglobulins or antibodies. *(a)* Antibodies are composed of 2 heavy polypeptide chains (H) and 2 light heavy polypeptide chains (L). *(b)* Different regions within the heavy and light chains. V indicates the variable regions and C indicates constant regions. Antigens combine with the variable regions, as shown in *(b)*. Each antibody molecule is divided into an Fab (antigen-binding) fragment and an Fc (constant) fragment.

Table 13.5 Physiological Properties of the Five Classes of Ig in Extracellular Fluid

Class	Mean adult serum level (g/L)	Serum half-life (days)	Physiological function
IgM	1.0	5	• Complement fixation • Early immune response • Stimulation of ingestion by macrophages
IgG	12	25	• Complement fixation • Placental transfer • Stimulation of ingestion by macrophages
IgA	1.8	6	• Localized protection in external secretions (e.g., saliva)
IgD	0.03	3	• Function unknown
IgE	0.0003	2	• Stimulation of mast cells • Parasite expulsion

subpopulations of antibodies, each specific to a particular antigen.

Antibodies cannot destroy antigen-bearing invaders directly. Instead, they tag foreign molecules and cells for destruction by various effector mechanisms. Each mechanism is triggered by the selective binding of antigens to antibodies to form antigen-antibody complexes. The antibodies may simply block the potential toxic actions of some antigens (neutralization), or they may cause clumping together of antigens or foreign cells (agglutination), which can then be ingested by phagocytes (see figure 13.8). Precipitation is a similar mechanism, in which soluble antigen molecules are cross-linked to form inactive and immobile precipitates that are captured by phagocytes. Antibody-antigen complexes on the surfaces of invading microorganisms usually cause complement activation. Complement proteins then attack the membrane of the invader, or, by coating the surface of foreign material, make it attractive to phagocytes (opsonization).

Effects of Exercise on the Immune System

Athletes engaged in heavy training programs, particularly endurance events, appear to be more

Figure 13.8 Types of antibody-antigen reactions.

susceptible to infection than the general population. For example, sore throats and flulike symptoms are more common in athletes. Some convincing evidence suggests that this increased susceptibility to infection arises because of a depression of immune system function (for detailed reviews, see Shephard [1997], Mackinnon [1999], and Gleeson and Bishop [1999]).

The main component of the immune system consists of the white blood cells, or leukocytes. The circulating numbers and functional capacities of leukocytes may be decreased by repeated bouts of intense, prolonged exercise. The cause may be increased levels of stress hormones during exercise and entry into the circulation of less mature leukocytes from the bone marrow. Drops in the blood concentration of glutamine have also been suggested as a possible cause of the immunodepression associated with heavy training, although the evidence for this is less compelling. Inflammation caused by muscle damage may be another factor.

During exercise, exposure to airborne bacteria and viruses increases because of the higher rate and depth of breathing. An increase in gut permeability may also allow entry of gut bacterial endotoxins into the circulation, particularly during prolonged exercise in the heat. Hence, the cause of the increased incidence of infection in athletes is most likely multifactorial. A variety of stressors (physical, psychological, environmental, and nutritional) suppress immune function, and these effects, together with increased exposure to potentially disease-causing pathogens, make the athlete more susceptible to infection (see figure 13.9).

The relationship between exercise and susceptibility to infection has been modeled in the form of a J-curve (Nieman 1994). This model suggests that, whereas engaging in moderate activity may enhance immune function above sedentary levels, excessive amounts of prolonged, high-intensity exercise induce detrimental effects on immune function. Although the literature provides strong evidence in support of the latter point, relatively little evidence is available to suggest any clinically significant difference in immune function between sedentary and moderately active persons. Thus, the portion of the J-curve representing this part of the relationship perhaps should be flattened out, as shown in figure 13.10. Matthews et al. (2002) reported that the regular performance of about 2 hours of moderate exercise a day is associated with a 29% reduction in risk of URTI compared with a sedentary lifestyle. This finding emphasizes that the benefit of regular, moderate exercise in improving resistance to infection is quite small.

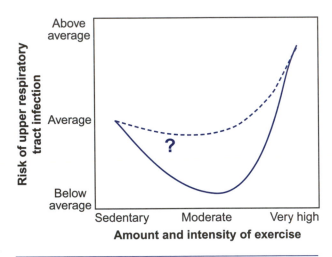

Figure 13.10 The J-curve model implies that risk of upper respiratory tract infection (URTI) is reduced by moderate activity but progressively elevated by heavier training loads. The dashed line between the two levels of exercise may be a more appropriate representation of the relationship between training load and URTI risk.

Acute Effects of Exercise on Immune Function

Prolonged strenuous exercise has a temporary depressive effect on immune function, and this effect has been associated with an increased incidence of infection. For example, both Peters and Bateman (1983) and Nieman et al. (1990) described a substantially higher (2-fold to 6-fold) frequency of self-reported symptoms of URTI in athletes who completed long-distance foot races compared with control runners who did not compete in the events.

An acute bout of physical activity is accompanied by responses that are similar in many respects to those induced by infection. A substantial increase

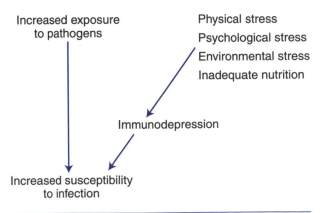

Figure 13.9 Factors contributing to infection incidence in athletes.

in the number of circulating leukocytes (mainly lymphocytes and neutrophils) occurs, the magnitude of which is related to both the intensity and duration of exercise. Increases also occur in the plasma concentrations of various substances that influence leukocyte functions, including **acute-phase proteins** such as C-reactive protein, activated complement fragments, and inflammatory and anti-inflammatory cytokines such as interferon-α, tumor necrosis factor, IL-1, IL-2, and IL-6. Hormonal changes also occur in response to exercise, including rises in the plasma concentration of several hormones (e.g., adrenaline, cortisol, growth hormone, and prolactin) that have immunomodulatory effects.

Acute exercise temporarily increases NK cell lytic activity but diminishes the proliferative response of lymphocytes to mitogens (see figure 13.11). Phagocytic neutrophils appear to be activated by an acute bout of exercise but show a diminished response to stimulation by bacterial lipopolysaccharide and reduced oxidative burst (killing capacity) after exercise, which can last for many hours (see figure 13.12).

During recovery from exercise, NK cell numbers and activity fall below pre-exercise levels (see figure 13.13), and if the exercise bout was high intensity or very prolonged, the number of circulating lymphocytes may be decreased below pre-exercise levels for several hours and the T-lymphocyte CD4+/CD8+

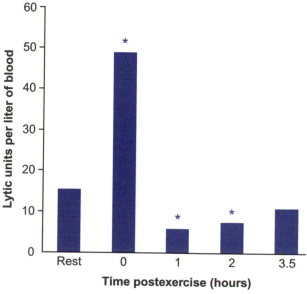

Figure 13.12 Changes in the in-vitro lipopolysaccharide (LPS)-stimulated neutrophil degranulation response (elastase release per cell) after 3 hours of cycling at 55% $\dot{V}O_2$max and after cycling to fatigue at 80% $\dot{V}O_2$max (mean exercise duration, 38 minutes) in 10 well-trained cyclists. Data are means and SEM. *$P < 0.05$ compared with pre-exercise. $P < 0.05$: 55% $\dot{V}O_2$max *versus* 80% $\dot{V}O_2$max.

International Journal of Sports Medicine: From P.J. Robson et al., "Effects of exercise intensity, duration, and recovery on in vitro neutrophil function in male athletes," 1999; 20: 128-135. Reprinted by permission.

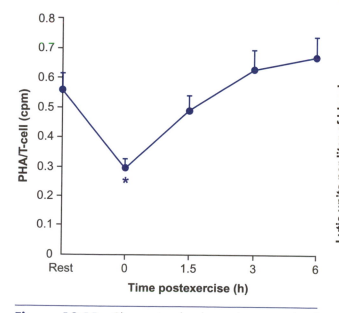

Figure 13.11 Change in phytohemaglutinin-stimulated (PHA-stimulated) lymphocyte proliferation after 2.5 hours of running.

International Journal of Sports Medicine: From D.A. Henson et al., "Carbohydrate supplementation and the lymphocyte proliferative response to long endurance running," 1998; 19: 574-580. Reprinted by permission.

Figure 13.13 Change in natural killer cell cytotoxic activity (NKCA, expressed as lytic units per liter of blood) after 2.5 hours of running.

Data from D.C. Nieman et al., 1993.

(helper/suppressor) ratio is decreased. After prolonged strenuous exercise, the production of immunoglobulins by B-lymphocytes is inhibited and the plasma concentration of glutamine falls by about 20% and may remain depressed for some time.

These changes during early recovery from exercise appear to weaken the potential immune response to pathogens and possibly provide an "open window" for infection at this most vulnerable time for an athlete (Pedersen and Bruunsgard 1995). Certainly, at this time, a temporary reduction in several aspects of innate immune function occurs, and athletes should be encouraged to adopt the following practices to minimize the risk of infection:

- Avoid contact with people with symptoms of infection.

- Minimize contact with children of school age, and avoid large crowds.

- Wash hands regularly, particularly after touching surfaces that are frequently handled by the public, such as doorknobs, handrails, and telephone receivers.

- Avoid hand-to-eye and hand-to-mouth contact to prevent transferring microbes to sensitive mucosal tissues.

- Maintain good oral hygiene.

- Avoid getting a dry mouth, both during competition and at rest, by drinking at regular intervals and maintaining hydration status.

- Never share drink bottles or cutlery.

- Use properly treated water for consumption and swimming.

- Avoid shared saunas, showers, and jacuzzis.

- Be aware that you may be particularly vulnerable after training or competition.

- Remember that good personal hygiene and thoughtfulness are the best defenses against respiratory infection.

Chronic Effects of Exercise Training on Immune Function

Exercise training also modifies immune function, with most changes suggesting an overall decrease in immune system function, particularly when training loads are high. Circulating numbers of leukocytes are generally lower in athletes at rest compared with sedentary people (see table 13.6). A low blood leukocyte count may arise from the hemodilution (expansion of the plasma volume) associated with training, or it may represent altered leukocyte kinetics, including a diminished release from the bone marrow. Indeed, the large increase in circulating neutrophil numbers that accompanies a bout of prolonged exercise could, over periods of months or years of heavy training, deplete the bone marrow reserve of these important cells. The blood population of these cells seems to be less mature than that found in sedentary individuals, and the phagocytic activity of blood neutrophils has been reported to be markedly lower in well-trained cyclists compared with age-matched and weight-matched sedentary control subjects.

Levels of secretory immunoglobulins, such as salivary IgA, are lower in well-trained subjects, as are T-lymphocyte CD4+/CD8+ ratios and in vitro mitogen-stimulated lymphocyte proliferation responses. Thus, with chronic periods of heavy training, both innate and adaptive immunity are depressed. Several causes of the diminution of immune function associated with heavy training are possible. One mechanism may simply be the cumulative effects of repeated bouts of intense exercise, with the consequent elevation of stress hormones, particularly glucocorticoids such as cortisol, causing temporary immunodepression. Frequently repeated exercise may not allow sufficient time for the immune system to recover fully. Furthermore, plasma glutamine levels can change substantially after exercise and may become chronically depressed

Table 13.6 Numbers of Circulating Leukocytes in Endurance-Trained Males and Sedentary Males

Blood cell count ($\times 10^9$/L)	Sedentary (n = 8)	Trained* (n = 8)
Leukocytes	6.62 (0.87)	4.36 (1.15)
Neutrophils	3.83 (0.86)	2.46 (0.87)
Lymphocytes	2.02 (0.27)	1.36 (0.20)

* $P < 0.01$ Trained versus sedentary subjects.

Subjects were matched for age and body mass.

Data from A.K. Blannin et al., 1996, "Effects of submaximal cycling and long-term endurance training on neutrophil phagocytic activity in middle aged men," *British Journal of Sports Medicine* 30: 125-129.

after repeated bouts of prolonged strenuous training. Complement activation also occurs during exercise, and a diminution of the serum complement concentration with repeated bouts of exercise, particularly when muscle damage is incurred, can also contribute to decreased nonspecific immunity in athletes. Well-trained individuals have a lower serum complement concentration compared with sedentary control subjects.

Nutritional Manipulations to Decrease Immunodepression in Athletes

Poor nutritional practices may contribute to impaired immunity in athletes. Some athletes adopt diets that are very high in carbohydrate content at the expense of protein and fat. By avoiding foods high in animal fat, athletes are also reducing their intake of fat-soluble vitamins and essential FAs. Many sports have strict weight categories, leading some competitors to follow energy-restricted diets that are often unbalanced, placing themselves at risk of several nutrient deficiencies.

Anecdotal and media reports promote the supposed performance benefits of certain vitamins and minerals, but most athletes do not realize that micronutrient supplementation is only beneficial when correcting a deficiency and that excessive intakes of individual micronutrients can be toxic or can limit the absorption of other essential trace elements. Deficiencies or excesses of various dietary components have substantial impact on immune function and may exacerbate the immunodepression associated with heavy training loads.

Mechanisms of Nutritional Influences on Immune Function in Athletes

Nutrient availability potentially affects almost all aspects of the immune system because many nutrients are involved in energy metabolism and protein synthesis. Most immune responses involve cell replication and the production of proteins with specific functions (e.g., cytokines, antibodies, and acute phase proteins). Immune system functions that may be compromised include the humoral and secretory antibody production, cell-mediated immunity, bactericidal capacity of phagocytes, complement formation, and T-lymphocyte proliferative response to mitogens.

A nutritional deficiency is said to have a direct effect when the nutritional factor has primary activity within the lymphoid system and an indirect effect when the primary activity affects all cellular material or an organ system that functions as an immune regulator. For example, carbohydrate availability directly affects a number of leukocyte functions but also indirectly affects the lymphoid system through its influence on circulating levels of the catecholamines, adrenocorticotrophic hormone (ACTH), and cortisol. Changes in plasma levels of these stress hormones are probably mostly responsible for the observed changes in immune function after an acute bout of exercise (see figure 13.14).

The impact of a nutrient deficiency on the immune system depends upon the duration of the deficiency as well as on the athlete's nutritional status as a whole. The severity of the deficiency is also factor, although even a mild deficiency of a single nutrient can alter the immune response. Because the availability of one

Figure 13.14 Nutrition and the stress-hormone response. Various stressors, including inadequate nutrition, prior exercise with inadequate recovery, psychological anxiety, and environmental extremes (e.g., heat and altitude) modify the hormonal response to exercise.

nutrient may enhance or impair the action of another, and nutrient deficiencies often occur together, nutrient-nutrient interactions on immune function are also an important consideration. Athletes who are training hard eat to satisfy their energy demands, consuming more macronutrients (carbohydrate, protein, and fat) and micronutrients (vitamins and minerals) than their sedentary counterparts and potentially ingesting excessive amounts of some nutrients. Excessive amounts of specific nutrients (e.g., omega-3 polyunsaturated FAs, iron, and zinc) can have detrimental effects on immune function.

The 1991 Consensus Conference on Foods, Nutrition, and Sports Performance gave the following dietary advice: "In the optimum diet for most sports, carbohydrate is likely to contribute about 60% to 70% of the total energy intake and protein about 12%, with the remainder coming from fat."

Athletes are generally advised to eat a well-balanced diet consisting of a variety of foods in sufficient quantity to cover their energy expenditures. However, diets high in protein or carbohydrate or fat, very-low-energy diets, fasting, or megadoses of vitamins and minerals are some of the many dietary alterations commonly used by athletes. Such dietary extremes may in fact compromise immune function. For example, diets that are excessively high in carbohydrate, favored by many athletes to keep glycogen stores high, are generally low in meat products and, thus, consequently low in protein (an important nutrient for immune function) and vitamin B_{12} (essential for DNA and RNA synthesis). Many athletes avoid dairy produce to minimize intake of saturated fat, but consequently, they are omitting from their diet major sources of vitamin D, B-group vitamins, and calcium, all of which play roles of varying importance in maintaining immune function.

Energy-restricted diets are not uncommon in sports where leanness or low body mass confers a performance advantage (e.g., gymnastics, figure skating, and endurance running) or is required to meet certain body-weight criteria (e.g., boxing, martial arts, weightlifting, and rowing). Indeed, such demands have led to the identification of a new subclinical eating disorder, anorexia athletica, which is associated with an increased susceptibility to infection (see chapter 12). Even short-term dieting can influence immune function in athletes. For example, a loss of 2 kg body mass over a 2-week period adversely affects macrophage phagocytic function.

Carbohydrate

The importance of adequate carbohydrate availability for maintenance of heavy training schedules and successful athletic performance is unquestionable (see chapter 3). During periods of heavy training, athletes should consume sufficient carbohydrate to cover about 60% of their energy costs. The recommended daily intake is 8 g/kg b.w. to 10 g/kg b.w. of carbohydrate for athletes who train for more than 2 h/day. These recommendations are principally aimed at restoring muscle and liver glycogen stores to ensure sufficient carbohydrate availability for skeletal muscle contraction for training on successive days.

Glucose is also an important fuel for cells of the immune system, including lymphocytes, neutrophils, and macrophages. Phagocytes utilize glucose at a rate 10 times greater than they utilize glutamine when both substrates are present in a culture medium at normal physiological concentrations. The importance of glucose for the proper functioning of lymphocytes and macrophages is further emphasized in a study that found that mitogen-stimulated proliferation of these cells in vitro depends on a glucose concentration over the physiological range. Cells of the immune system have very high metabolic rates, and this finding highlights the importance for adequate nutrition for the provision of fuels to maintain immunocompetence.

Recent studies have examined the impact of dietary carbohydrate on immune responses to exercise and have found that when subjects perform prolonged exercise after several days on very-low-carbohydrate diets (typically <10% of dietary energy intake from carbohydrate), the magnitude of the stress hormone and cytokine response is markedly higher than on a normal-carbohydrate or a high-carbohydrate diets as illustrated in figure 13.15 (Gleeson et al. 1998; Mitchell et al. 1998). Furthermore, the postexercise fall in plasma glutamine concentration is greater than on the normal-carbohydrate and high-carbohydrate diets. Athletes deficient in carbohydrate are believed to be placing themselves at risk for the immunosuppressive effects of cortisol and falls in glutamine availability, including the suppression of antibody production, lymphocyte proliferation, and NK cell cytotoxic activity.

Consumption of carbohydrate during prolonged exercise attenuates rises in plasma epinephrine, cortisol, and cytokines (Nehlsen-Cannarella et al. 1997); attenuates the trafficking of most leukocyte and lymphocyte subsets, including the rise in the neutrophil: lymphocyte ratio (see figure 13.16); prevents the exercise-induced fall in neutrophil function (see figure 13.17); and reduces the extent of the diminution of mitogen-stimulated T-lymphocyte proliferation (on a per cell basis) after prolonged exercise (Henson et al. 1998) (see figure 13.18).

The consumption of carbohydrate in beverages during exercise may also have the additional benefit of helping to maintain saliva flow rate during exercise. Saliva contains several proteins with antimicrobial properties, including IgA, lysozyme, and α-amylase. During periods of heavy training, athletes have lower levels of IgA in their saliva and this condition may contribute to their increased incidence of URTI (Mackinnon 1999). Saliva secretion is under neural control. The sympathetic nervous system stimulation that occurs during exercise causes vasoconstriction of the blood vessels to the salivary glands and results in a reduction in saliva secretion. Regular fluid intake during exercise prevents this effect, and a recent

a

b

(continued)

Figure 13.15 Changes in the concentrations of *(a)* plasma cortisol, *(b)* plasma interleukin-6 (IL-6), *(c)* plasma interleukin-1 receptor antagonist (IL-1 ra), and *(d)* the blood neutrophil:lymphocyte ratio after 1 hour of cycling at 60% $\dot{V}O_2$max immediately followed by a half hour time trial (work rate around 80% $\dot{V}O_2$max). For the 3 days before the exercise trial, subjects (n = 12) consumed either a high-carbohydrate (carbohydrate) diet (open circles) or a low-carbohydrate diet. Data are presented as mean and SEM. Significantly, different from low carbohydrate, *$P < 0.05$, **$P < 0.01$. Unpublished observations.

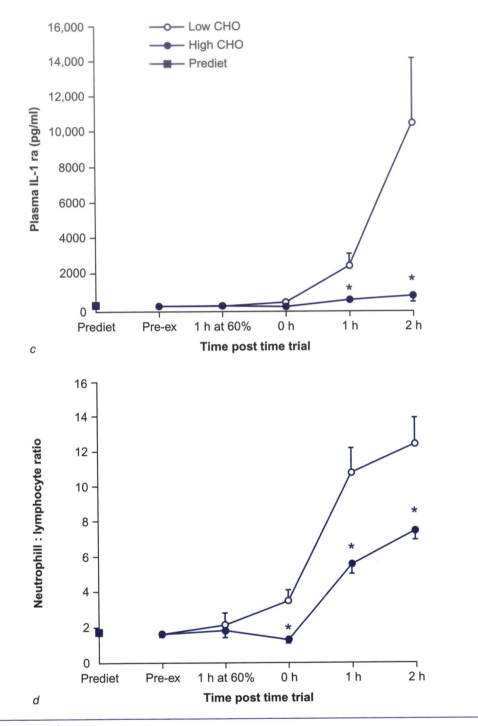

Figure 13.15 *(continued)*

study (Bishop et al. 2000) has confirmed that regular consumption of carbohydrate-containing drinks helps maintain saliva flow rate and, hence, saliva IgA secretion rate during prolonged exercise.

Although carbohydrate feeding during exercise appears to be effective in minimizing some of the immune perturbations associated with prolonged strenuous exercise, it does not prevent the fall in the plasma glutamine concentration and seems less effective for less-demanding exercise such as football (Bishop et al. 1999c) or rowing (Nieman et al. 1999) training. Carbohydrate feeding is not as effective in reducing immune-cell trafficking and functional depression when exercise is performed to the point

Figure 13.16 Changes in the neutrophil:lymphocyte ratio after 2 hours of cycling at 60% V̇O₂max when fed a 6% w/v carbohydrate solution (closed circles), the same volume of an artificially sweetened placebo solution (open circles), or a restricted fluid intake (open triangles). Significantly different from placebo trial, *P < 0.05, **P < 0.01.

Data from N.C. Bishop et al., 1999b.

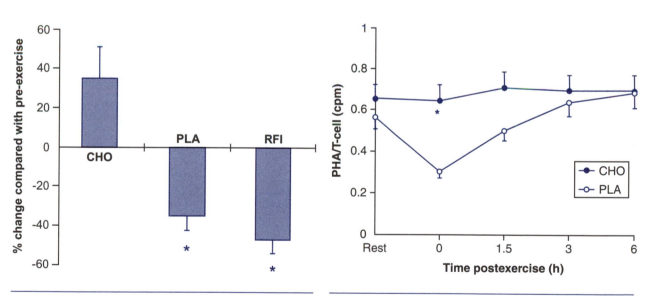

Figure 13.17 Percentage change (compared with pre-exercise) in the lipopolysaccharide-stimulated neutrophil degranulation response immediately after 2 hours of cycling at 60% V̇O₂max when fed a 6% w/v carbohydrate solution (CHO), the same volume of an artificially sweetened placebo solution (PLA), or a restricted fluid intake (RFI). Significant change from pre-exercise, *P < 0.05.

Data from N.C. Bishop et al., 1999b.

Figure 13.18 Change in phytohemaglutinin-stimulated (PHA-stimulated) lymphocyte proliferation after 2.5 hours running when fed a 6% w/v carbohydrate (CHO) solution (closed circles) or the same volume of an artificially sweetened placebo (PLA) solution (open circles). Significantly different from PLA, *P < 0.05.

Data from D. Henson et al., 1998.

of fatigue (Bishop et al. 2001). Pre-exercise feeding of carbohydrate is not very effective in limiting exercise-induced changes in leukocyte trafficking or depression of neutrophil function. Evidence that the beneficial effect of feeding carbohydrate on immune responses to exercise actually translates into a reduced incidence of URTI after prolonged exercise such as marathon races is currently lacking.

Fat

The International Consensus Conference on Foods, Nutrition, and Sports Performance advised athletes that 20% of energy intake should come from fat. The type of dietary fat is also important. In 1994, the UK Department of Health recommended that saturated fats contribute no more than 10% of our daily energy intake (the 2000 Dietary Guidelines for Americans made an identical recommendation), with the remainder of fat intake provided by monounsaturated FAs (15%), polyunsaturated FAs (PUFAs [6%]), linoleic acid (1%), linolenic acid (0.2%), and trans FAs (<2%). Two groups of PUFAs are essential to the body: the omega-6 (n-6) series, derived from linoleic acid, and the omega-3 (n-3) series, derived from linolenic acid. These FAs cannot be synthesized in the body and, therefore, must be derived from the diet. Diets rich in either of these PUFAs improve the conditions of patients suffering from diseases characterized by an overactive immune system, such as rheumatoid arthritis. These PUFAs, thus, have immunomodulatory functions.

Although FAs are utilized as fuels by lymphocytes, their oxidation does not appear to be crucial for lymphocyte function, because the inhibition of FA oxidation does not affect the ability of lymphocytes to proliferate in response to mitogens. FAs exert either direct effects (by altering cell membrane fluidity) or indirect effects (as precursors of cell-signaling molecules called eicosanoids) on immune function, generally resulting in reduced IL-2 production and suppressed mitogen-induced lymphocyte proliferation. However, supplementation with vitamin E or vitamin C appears to partly protect against some of these immunosuppressive effects.

Relatively little is known about the potential contribution of FAs to the regulation of exercise-induced modification of immune function. Although no study has been done in athletes, an excessive intake of PUFA could possibly further potentiate the exercise-induced suppression of IL-2 production and lymphocyte proliferation. High intakes of arachidonic acid relative to intakes of FA of the n-3 group may also exert an undesirable influence on inflammation and immune function during and after exercise. Alteration of essential FA distribution via dietary changes or nutritional supplementation is already being applied in the treatment of chronic inflammatory diseases. More research is needed on the effects of altering essential FA intake on immune function after exercise and during periods of heavy training. A study that investigated the effects of endurance training for 7 weeks on carbohydrate-rich (65% of dietary energy) or fat-rich (62% of dietary energy) diets concluded that diet during training may influence natural immunity because NK cell activity increased on the carbohydrate-rich diet compared with the fat-rich diet (Pedersen et al. 2000). The results of this study suggest that a fat-rich diet is detrimental to immune function compared with a carbohydrate-rich diet but do not clarify whether this effect is actually the result of a lack of dietary carbohydrate or an excess of a specific dietary fat component.

Protein and Amino Acids

The daily protein requirement is approximately doubled in athletes compared with the sedentary population. An intake of less than 1.6 g /kg b.w./day of protein is likely to be associated with a negative nitrogen balance in athletes who are training hard, particularly endurance athletes. Provided that athletes consume a well-balanced diet that meets their requirement for energy, the increased requirement for protein will be met. Those individuals at most risk for protein deficiency are athletes undertaking a program of food restriction to lose weight, vegetarian athletes, and athletes consuming unbalanced diets (e.g., with an excessive amount of carbohydrate at the expense of protein).

An inadequate intake of protein impairs host immunity, with particularly detrimental effects on the T-cell system, resulting in increased incidence of opportunistic infections. One of the most dramatic manifestations of this development is widespread atrophy of lymphoid tissue. In humans, protein-energy malnutrition (PEM) depresses the number of mature, fully differentiated T-lymphocytes and the in vitro response to T-lymphocyte mitogens, although the latter is reversible with nutritional repletion. Additionally, the T-lymphocyte CD4+/CD8+ ratio is markedly decreased in PEM. Essentially all forms of immunity are affected by PEM in humans, depending on the severity of the protein deficiency relative to energy intake. These effects include impaired phagocytic cell function, decreased cytokine production, and reduced complement formation. Although athletes are unlikely to reach a state of such extreme malnutrition unless dieting very severely, some impairment of host-defense mechanisms is observed even in moderate protein deficiency.

Too much dietary protein could also be potentially harmful to immune function. A diet rich in protein (24% protein, 72% fat, and 3% carbohydrate) consumed for 4 days caused a 25% lowering of muscle and plasma glutamine levels. This decline was attributed to an increased renal uptake of glutamine to reestablish normal acid-base balance because a high intake of protein combined with a low intake of carbohydrate induces a chronic metabolic acidosis. Furthermore, falls in the plasma glutamine concentration after prolonged strenuous exercise are greater when consuming a low-carbohydrate diet compared with a normal diet. However, feeding carbohydrate during exercise does not prevent the postexercise fall in plasma glutamine.

Glutamine is the most abundant free amino acid in human muscle and plasma and is utilized at very high rates by leukocytes to provide energy and optimal conditions for nucleotide biosynthesis. Indeed, glutamine is important, if not essential to lymphocytes and other rapidly dividing cells, including the gut **mucosa** and bone marrow stem cells. Glutamine is also required for optimal macrophage phagocytic activity. Prolonged exercise is associated with a fall in the plasma concentration of glutamine, and such a decrease has been hypothesized to impair immune function. The overtraining syndrome is associated with a chronic reduction in plasma glutamine levels, which may be partly responsible for the immunodepression apparent in this condition. Interestingly, evidence indicates that an additional intake of 20 g/day to 30 g/day of protein can restore depressed plasma glutamine levels in overtrained athletes.

Several scientists have suggested that exogenous provision of glutamine supplements may be beneficial by preventing the impairment of immune function after prolonged exercise. However, the evidence that oral glutamine supplements reduce the incidence of URTI after endurance events is very limited (Castell et al. 1996). Several studies that have investigated the effect of glutamine supplementation during and after exercise on various indices of immune function have failed to find any beneficial effect. A glutamine solution (0.1 g/kg b.w.) given at 0 minutes, 30 minutes, 60 minutes, and 90 minutes after a marathon race prevented the fall in the plasma glutamine concentration but did not prevent the fall in mitogen-induced lymphocyte proliferation and lymphocyte-activated NK cell activity (Rohde et al. 1998). Similarly, maintaining the plasma glutamine concentration by consuming glutamine in drinks taken both during and

after 2 hours of cycling at 60% $\dot{V}O_2$max did not affect leukocyte subset trafficking or prevent the exercise-induced fall in neutrophil function (Walsh et al. 2000). Unlike the feeding of carbohydrate during exercise, glutamine supplements do not seem to affect immune function perturbations, and a review article (Hiscock and Pedersen 2002) concluded that falls in plasma glutamine are not responsible for exercise-induced immunodepression.

Bassit and colleagues (2002) reported that supplementation of BCAAs (6 g/day for 15 days) before a triathlon or 30-kilometer run prevented the approximately 40% decline in mitogen-stimulated lymphocyte proliferation observed in the placebo control group after exercise. BCAAs are precursors for glutamine, and BCAA supplementation prevented the postexercise fall in plasma glutamine concentration and was also associated with increased IL-2 and interferon production. More research is needed to resolve these conflicting findings of BCAA and glutamine supplementation on immune responses to exercise.

Vitamins

Vitamins are essential organic molecules that cannot be synthesized in the body and, therefore, must be obtained from food (see chapter 9). Several vitamins are essential for normal immune function: fat-soluble vitamins A and E and water-soluble vitamins B_{12} and C. Other vitamins (e.g., B_6 and folic acid) also play important roles in immune function, but dietary deficiencies in humans are extremely rare.

No indications in the literature suggest that vitamin intake among athletes in general is insufficient. Athletes tend to ingest above-average quantities of these micronutrients, and, as with dietary protein requirements, any increase in need may be countered by increased dietary intake. On the other hand, perhaps the requirement for most vitamins is simply not increased in athletes. For example, vitamin loss via sweat during exercise is negligible.

Antioxidant Vitamins

Vitamins with antioxidant properties, including vitamins C, E, and β-carotene (provitamin A), may be required in increased quantities in athletes to inactivate the products of exercise-induced lipid peroxidation (Packer 1997). Oxygen free-radical formation that accompanies the dramatic increase in oxidative metabolism during exercise (see chapter 9) could potentially inhibit immune responses.

Reactive oxygen species (ROS) inhibit locomotory and bactericidal activity of neutrophils, reduce the proliferation of T-lymphocytes and B-lymphocytes, and inhibit NKCA. Sustained endurance training appears to be associated with an adaptive up-regulation of the antioxidant defense system. However, such adaptations may be insufficient to protect athletes who train extensively, and these individuals should consider increasing their intakes of nutritional antioxidants such as vitamins C, E, and β-carotene to reduce free radical damage.

Vitamin C (ascorbic acid) occurs in high concentration in leukocytes and is implicated in a variety of anti-infective functions, including promotion of T-lymphocyte proliferation, prevention of corticosteroid-induced suppression of neutrophil activity, production of interferon, and inhibition of virus replication. It is also a major water-soluble antioxidant that is effective as a scavenger of ROS in both intracellular and extracellular fluids. It can act as an antioxidant both directly (e.g., in the prevention of auto-oxidative dysfunction of neutrophil bactericidal activity) and indirectly via its regeneration of reduced vitamin E (α-tocopherol). Vitamin C occurs in high concentration in the adrenal glands and is necessary for the production of several hormones that are secreted in response to stress, such as epinephrine, norepinephrine, and cortisol.

Studies report that daily supplementation of large doses of vitamin C reduce the incidence of symptoms of URTI in athletes after participation in ultramara-

thon races (Peters et al. 1993, 1996). The results of one of these studies are illustrated in figure 13.19, which also shows that the supplementation of additional dietary antioxidants (vitamin E and β-carotene) does not confer any additional beneficial effect. The doses of vitamin C used in these studies (600 mg/day to 1,000 mg/day) are considerably higher than the daily dosage of 200 mg that is associated with accelerated clinical improvement in elderly patients hospitalized with acute respiratory infection after 4 weeks of daily supplementation (Hunt et al. 1994).

Animal studies show an increased oxidation of vitamin E during exercise that could result in reduced antioxidant protection. Dietary vitamin E stimulates mononuclear cell production of IL-Iβ via its influence on the arachidonic acid metabolic pathways, and cytokine production is further facilitated by a vitamin E–influenced inhibition of PGE_2 production. Severe vitamin E deficiency results in impaired cell-mediated immunity and decreased antibody synthesis.

Vitamin A is also essential for immunocompetence. Vitamin A deficiency in animals and humans results in atrophy of the thymus, decreased lymphocyte proliferation in response to mitogens, and increased bacterial binding to respiratory tract epithelial cells and impaired secretory IgA production. Consequently, vitamin A–deficient humans have a higher incidence of spontaneous infection. Vitamin A–defi-

Figure 13.19 The incidence of upper respiratory tract infection (URTI) in the week after the 1993 Comrades Ultramarathon (90 kilometers) in South Africa. Different groups of runners or control subjects received different combinations of antioxidant supplements or placebo for 3 weeks before the ultramarathon.

Adapted, by permission, from E.M. Peters et al., 1996, "Vitamin C as effective as combinations of anti-oxidant nutrients in reducing symptoms of upper respiratory tract infections in ultramarathon runners," *South African Journal of Sports Medicine* 11: 23-27.

cient experimental animals also demonstrate reduced NKCA, lower production of interferon and antibodies, impaired delayed cutaneous hypersensitivity, and less-effective macrophage activity.

β-carotene (provitamin A) acts as an immunostimulant, increasing the number of CD4+ helper T-cells in healthy human volunteers and stimulating NKCA when added in vitro to human lymphatic cultures. Furthermore, elderly men who had been taking β-carotene supplements (50 mg on alternate days) for 10 years to 12 years were reported to have significantly higher NKCA than elderly men on placebo. β-carotene also functions as an antioxidant; thus, the requirement may be increased in athletes involved in heavy training schedules that stimulate an increased production of ROS. However, supplementing ultramarathon runners with β-carotene had an insignificant effect on the incidence of URTI after the 90-kilometer Comrades Ultramarathon in South Africa (see figure 13.19).

Vitamin B$_{12}$ and Folic Acid

Vitamin B$_{12}$ and folic-acid deficiencies have profound effects on immune function. Both of these vitamins are essential for the synthesis of nucleic acids and, hence, are required for the normal production of red and white blood cells in the bone marrow. Vitamin B$_{12}$ can only be absorbed from the gut in the presence of the glycoprotein intrinsic factor. Lack of this factor or deficiency of vitamin B$_{12}$ causes pernicious anemia, with detrimental effects on immune function. For example, impaired lymphocyte proliferative responses to mitogens and a modest reduction in the phagocytic and bactericidal capacity of neutrophils have been reported in individuals with primary pernicious anemia. The only natural sources of vitamin B$_{12}$ are of animal origin. As such, vegetarian athletes and athletes avoiding dairy produce to minimize saturated fat intake are at a high risk for deficiency of this vitamin.

Vitamin Supplements and Megadoses

In general, supplementation with individual vitamins or consumption of large doses of simple antioxidant mixtures is not recommended. Athletes should obtain complex mixtures of antioxidant compounds from consumption of fruits and vegetables. A suitable alternative is commercially available capsules of dried fruit and vegetable juice.

Consuming megadoses of individual vitamins is likely to do more harm than good. Because most vitamins function mainly as coenzymes in the body, once the enzyme systems are saturated, the vitamins

in free form can have toxic effects. For example, 300 mg of vitamin E (as α-tocopherol acetate), given daily to 18 men for 3 weeks, produced a significant depression in the bactericidal activity of peripheral blood leukocytes and mitogen-induced lymphocyte proliferation. Prolonged intake of very large doses (>1,000 mg/day) of vitamin C is associated with kidney oxalate stone formation, impaired absorption of copper, and excessive absorption of iron and predisposition to gout in susceptible individuals. However, these side effects seem to be quite rare. Megadoses of vitamin A may impair the inflammatory response and complement formation as well as having other pathological effects, including causing fetal abnormalities when consumed by pregnant women.

Minerals

Minerals are classified as macrominerals or microminerals (trace elements), based upon the extent of their occurrence in the body (see chapter 9). Of importance here are the trace elements that constitute less than 0.01% of total-body mass, of which 14 have been identified as essential for maintenance of health. Of these 14, several are known to exert modulatory effects on immune function, including zinc, iron, selenium, and copper (see table 13.7). Yet, with the exception of zinc and iron, isolated deficiencies are rare. Indeed, iron deficiency is reported to be the most widespread nutrient deficiency in the world, and field studies consistently associate iron deficiency with increased morbidity from infectious disease. Exercise has a pronounced effect on both zinc and iron metabolism.

Zinc

The role of zinc in immune function has received increasing attention in recent years. Zinc is essential for the development of the immune system and more than 100 metalloenzymes are dependent on it, including those involved in the transcription of DNA and synthesis of proteins. For example, zinc is a cofactor for the enzyme terminal deoxynucleotidyl transferase, which is required by immature T-cells for their replication and functioning. The effects of zinc deficiency on immune function include lymphoid atrophy, decreased delayed-hypersensitivity cutaneous responses, decreased IL-2 production, impaired mitogen-stimulated lymphocyte proliferative responses, and decreased NKCA. Zinc availability affects superoxide free-radical production by stimulated phagocytes, although in the laboratory, this effect seems to depend on the actual molecular form of zinc.

Table 13.7 Roles of Minerals in Immune Function and the Effects of Dietary Deficiency or Excess

Mineral	Role in immune function	Effect of deficiency	Effect of excess
Iron	Oxygen transport and cofactor of metalloenzymes	Anemia and increased infections	Hemochromatosis, liver cirrhosis, heart disease, and increased infections
Zinc	Cofactor of metalloenzymes, protein synthesis, and antioxidant	Impaired growth, healing, increased infections, and anorexia	Impaired absorption of Fe and Cu, increased HDL cholesterol/LDL cholesterol ratio, anemia, nausea, vomiting, and immune system impairment
Selenium	Cofactor of glutathione peroxidase (antioxidant)	Cardiomyopathy, cancer, heart disease, impaired immune function, and erythrocyte fragility	Nausea, vomiting, fatigue, and hair loss
Copper	Promotes normal iron absorption and cofactor of superoxide dismutase (antioxidant)	Anemia and impaired immune function	Nausea and vomiting
Magnesium	Protein synthesis and cofactor of metalloenzymes	Muscle weakness, fatigue, apathy, muscle tremor, and cramp	Nausea, vomiting, and diarrhea

Vegetarian athletes are at risk for zinc deficiency because meat and seafood are the richest zinc sources (see table 13.8), and although nuts, legumes, and whole grains are good sources of zinc, the high levels of fiber in these foods can decrease zinc absorption. Zinc deficiency can also be a problem for athletes in sports where a low body mass confers a performance advantage. Very-low-energy or starvation-type diets may induce significant zinc losses. Because zinc is lost from the body mainly in sweat and urine (see table 13.9), and these losses are increased by exercise, a heavy schedule of exercise training could induce a zinc deficiency in athletes. Certainly, highly trained women have significantly higher urinary zinc excretion compared with untrained control subjects, and an acute bout of high-intensity exercise increases daily urinary zinc excretion by 34% compared with resting values in well-trained male games players.

Table 13.8 Dietary Sources and Daily RDA or AI of Important Minerals for Immune Function

Mineral	Source	RDA or AI*	Absorbed (%)
Iron	Liver, kidney, eggs, red meats, seafood, oysters, bread, flour, molasses, dried legumes, nuts, leafy green vegetables, broccoli, figs, raisins, and cocoa	8 mg (M) 18 mg (F)	10–30 (heme iron); 2–10 (nonheme iron)
Zinc	Oysters, shellfish, beef, liver, poultry, dairy products, whole grains, wheat germ, vegetables, asparagus, and spinach	11 mg (M) 8 mg (F)	20–50
Selenium	Meat, liver, kidney, poultry, fish, dairy produce, seafood, and whole grains and nuts from selenium-rich soil	55 µg (M, F)	Unknown
Copper	Liver, kidney, shellfish, meat, fish, poultry, eggs, bran cereals, nuts, legumes, broccoli, banana, avocado, and chocolate	0.9 mg (M, F)	20–50
Magnesium	Seafood, nuts, green leafy vegetables, fruits, whole-grain products, milk, and yogurt	420 mg (M) 320 mg (F)	25–60
Manganese	Whole grains, peas and beans, leafy vegetables, and bananas	2.3 mg* (M) 1.8 mg* (F)	Unknown

RDA = Recommended daily allowance; AI* = adequate intake. M = males; F = females.

Table 13.9   Body Content and Body Fluid Concentrations of Important Minerals for Immune Function

Mineral	Symbol	Total amount in body (mg)	Body fluid concentration (mg/L)		
			Plasma	Sweat	Urine
Iron	Fe	5,000	0.4–1.4	0.3–0.4	0.1–0.15
Zinc	Zn	2,000	0.7–1.3	0.7–1.3	0.2–0.5
Selenium	Se	13	0.05–0.10	<0.01	<0.01
Copper	Cu	100	0.7–1.7	0.2–0.6	0.03–0.04
Magnesium	Mg	25,000	16–30	4–15	60–100
Manganese	Mn	12	0.02	<0.01	<0.01

Male and female athletes have lower plasma zinc concentrations compared with untrained individuals.

Studies concerning the relationship between immune function, exercise, and zinc status in athletes are lacking. However, a study of male runners found that 6 days of zinc supplementation (25 mg of zinc and 1.5 mg of copper, twice a day) inhibited the exercise-associated increase in superoxide free-radical formation by activated neutrophils (as shown in figure 13.20) and exaggerated the exercise-induced suppression of T-lymphocyte proliferation in response to mitogens. Such effects might temporarily predispose athletes to opportunistic infection. Megadoses of zinc have further detrimental effects on immune function. The administration of zinc (150 mg twice a day) to 11 healthy males for 6 weeks was associated with reduced T-lymphocyte proliferative responses to mitogen stimulation and impaired neutrophil phagocytic activity. Hence, megadoses of zinc are not recommended. Athletes should be encouraged to consume zinc-rich foods (e.g., poultry, meat, fish, and dairy produce). Vegetarians have been advised to take a 10 mg to 20 mg supplement of zinc daily (the RDA is 10 mg and 12 mg for females and males, respectively), but in view of the above findings supplements, at the lower end of this range may be more suitable for vegetarian athletes.

The efficacy of zinc supplementation as a treatment for the common cold has been investigated in at least 11 studies published since 1984. The findings have been equivocal, and recent reviews of this topic conclude that further research is necessary before the use of zinc supplements to treat the common cold can be recommended (Macknin 1999; Marshall 2000). Although only limited evidence suggests that taking zinc supplements reduces the incidence of URTI (McElroy and Miller 2002), in the studies that have reported a beneficial effect of zinc in treating the common cold (i.e., reduction of symptom duration, severity, or both) zinc had to be taken within 24 hours of the onset of symptoms to be of any benefit. Potential problems with zinc supplements include nausea, bad taste reactions, lowering of HDL cholesterol, depression of some immune cell functions (e.g., neutrophil oxidative burst), and interference with the absorption of copper (Gleeson 2000).

Figure 13.20   The effect of zinc and copper supplementation versus placebo on the exercise-induced change in neutrophil respiratory burst activity.

Data from Singh et al. 1994.

Iron

Iron deficiency is prevalent throughout the world, and, by some estimates, as much as 25% of the world's population is iron deficient. Endurance athletes risk potential iron deficiency because of increased iron losses in sweat, urine, and feces. However, the incidence of iron depletion among athletes is no greater than that in the general population. Nevertheless, exercise may contribute to an iron-depleted state. The acute-phase host response to stress (including exercise) involves the depression of circulating free iron levels. Stress-induced elevation of IL-1 causes granulocyte release of the iron-binding protein lactoferrin within the circulation. Lactoferrin is then thought to bind (chelate) iron from transferrin, forming lactoferrin-iron complexes, leading to a depression of plasma iron concentration that is independent of plasma volume changes.

The immune system itself appears to be particularly sensitive to the availability of iron, although iron deficiency has neither completely harmful nor enhancing effects on immune function. On the one hand, free iron is necessary for bacterial growth. Removal of iron with the help of chelating agents such as lactoferrin reduces bacterial multiplication, particularly in the presence of specific antibody. A study reported that iron-deficient mice had a lower mortality after infection with *Salmonella* compared with iron-replete mice. Thus, iron deficiency may actually protect an individual from infection, whereas supplementation may predispose the individual to infectious disease, particularly because iron catalyzes the production of hydroxyl free radicals, and a high intake of iron can impair gastrointestinal zinc absorption. On the other hand, iron deficiency depresses various aspects of immune function, including macrophage IL-1 production, the lymphocyte proliferative response to mitogens, NKCA, neutrophil phagocytic activity, and delayed cutaneous hypersensitivity (an index of cell-mediated immune function).

A number of causes of iron deficiency in endurance athletes involved in heavy training have been suggested. Exercise may cause reductions in gastrointestinal iron absorption and iron is lost in sweat, which contains 0.3 mg/L (see table 13.9). This process can cause losses of up to 1.0 mg/day of iron in athletes who are training extensively. Because only about 10% of dietary iron is absorbed, such losses increase the dietary requirement by about 10 mg/day, which is approximately double the normal daily iron requirement (the RDA is 15 mg and 10 mg for females and males, respectively). In addition, some damage to red blood cells (hemolysis) may occur with foot strike, with subsequent loss of hemoglobin in the urine, although this loss is thought to be a negligible drain on iron stores. Some athletes are also susceptible to gastrointestinal bleeding during exercise, which may increase fecal iron losses.

The bioavailability of iron is lower in vegetarian diets because of the lack of heme iron, which is more easily absorbed. The general consensus is that all athletes should be aware of heme iron–rich foods such as lean red meat, poultry, and fish and include them in the daily diet. Iron requirements in endurance athletes may be double the RDA, although these requirements can be met through the diet without the need for artificial supplements. Vegetarian athletes should ensure that plant food choices are iron dense (e.g., green leafy vegetables). Breakfast cereals are usually fortified with iron and provide a good source. Megadoses of iron are not advised, and routine oral supplements of iron should not be taken without medical advice.

Selenium

Selenium deficiency can affect all components of the immune system. Selenium is a cofactor of glutathione peroxidase/reductase and, thus, influences the quenching of ROS. As such, requirement of selenium is possibly increased in athletes involved in regular intensive training programs. However, any selenium supplement should be taken with caution. Supplements with doses up to the RDA appear nontoxic. However, the safety of larger doses has not been confirmed, and intakes of 25 mg (approximately 40 times the RDA) have been associated with vomiting, abdominal pain, hair loss, and fatigue.

Copper

The effects of copper deficiency on immune function include impaired antibody formation, inflammatory response, neutrophil phagocytosis, NKCA, and lymphocyte stimulation responses. The results of changes in copper status as a result of exercise and training are controversial, perhaps reflecting the inadequacy of techniques used to measure copper status. With exercise there may be some redistribution of copper between body compartments, and athletes have been reported to lose copper in sweat collected after exercise. Even though copper deficiency is rare in humans, athletes who take zinc supplements may compromise the gastrointestinal absorption of copper because of the similar physicochemical properties of these two minerals.

Magnesium

Magnesium is an essential cofactor for many enzymes involved in biosynthetic processes and energy metabolism and is required for normal neuromuscular coordination. The total-body content of magnesium is about 25 g (see table 13.9). The RDA for magnesium is 350 mg/day for men and 280 mg/day for women; hence, magnesium is classified as a macromineral rather than a trace element. The main dietary sources of magnesium are listed in table 13.8. Most studies of dietary habits in athletes suggest that magnesium intake exceeds the RDA. However, the data used to determine RDAs for micronutrients often did not include athletes, or the activity levels of the subjects were not reported. Therefore, although the RDAs may apply to the sedentary population, they may not be an accurate means of evaluating the nutritional needs of athletes.

Several studies report low serum magnesium concentrations in athletes, and prolonged strenuous exercise is associated with increased losses of magnesium in urine and sweat. Although, as with zinc and iron, a single bout of exercise is unlikely to induce substantial magnesium losses, a state of mild magnesium deficiency may be induced during a period of heavy training, particularly in a warm environment where sweat losses are high.

Magnesium deficiency in both humans and animals is associated with neuromuscular abnormalities, including muscle weakness, cramps, and structural damage of muscle fibers and organelles. The structural damage may be caused by an impairment of calcium homeostasis secondary to an oxygen free radical–induced alteration in the integrity of the membrane of the sarcoplasmic reticulum. A lack of magnesium may also be associated with a depletion of selenium and reduced glutathione peroxidase activity, which increases the susceptibility to damage by free radicals. Hence, magnesium deficiency may potentiate exercise-induced muscle damage and stress responses, but direct evidence for this effect is lacking.

Manganese

Manganese is a cofactor of the enzyme superoxide dismutase, which aids in protection against free radicals. The RDA for manganese is 2.0 mg/day to 5.0 mg/day. Sources are whole-grain products, dried peas and beans, leafy vegetables, and bananas. The effects of exercise on manganese status are presently unknown, but training is associated with an increase in levels of antioxidant enzymes, suggesting an increased requirement for manganese during periods of increased training. As with other trace elements, losses of manganese in urine and sweat is likely higher in athletes than nonathletes.

Cobalt

Cobalt as a component of vitamin B_{12} promotes the development of red and white blood cells in the bone marrow. Deficiencies are associated with pernicious anemia, reduced blood leukocyte counts, impaired lymphocyte proliferation, and impaired bactericidal capacity of neutrophils. Major food sources of cobalt are meat, liver, and milk. Hence, athletes who avoid animal foods are at risk for cobalt/vitamin B_{12} deficiency.

Fluorine

Although not directly required for normal immune function, fluorine is needed for the normal formation of healthy bones and teeth, and it protects against dental caries (tooth decay by oral bacteria). Given the relatively high intake of sugary foods and sports drinks by athletes, good oral hygiene is important to maintaining healthy teeth. Frequent intakes of soft drinks and carbohydrates—particularly sugars—depress the oral pH with a resultant net demineralization of the teeth. Sugars are metabolized to organic acids by the bacteria in the plaque on teeth and gums. Therefore, all sports people should maintain good plaque control. The RDA for fluorine is 1.5 mg/day to 4.0 mg/day, and this trace element is found in milk, egg yolk, seafood, and drinking water. Several toothpastes and mouth rinses contain fluorine (as sodium fluoride), and in some countries, including the United States, fluoride is added to drinking water.

Dietary Immunostimulants

Several herbal preparations are reputed to have immunostimulatory effects, and consumption of products containing *Echinacea purpurea* is widespread among athletes. However, few controlled studies have examined the effects of dietary immunostimulants on exercise-induced changes in immune function. In a recent double-blinded, placebo-controlled study, the effect of a daily oral pretreatment for 28 days with pressed juice of *Echinacea purpurea* was investigated in 42 triathletes before and after a sprint triathlon. A subgroup of athletes was also treated with magnesium as a reference for supplementation with a micronutrient important for optimal muscular function. During the 28-day pretreatment period, none of the athletes in the *Echinacea* group fell ill, compared with 3 subjects in the magnesium group and 4 subjects in the placebo group who became ill. Pretreatment with *Echinacea purpurea* appeared to reduce the release of soluble IL-2 receptor before and after the race and increased the exercise-induced rise in IL-6.

Numerous experiments have shown that *Echinacea purpurea* extracts exert significant immunomodulatory effects. Among the many pharmacological properties reported, macrophage activation has been demonstrated most convincingly. Phagocytotic indices and macrophage-derived cytokine concentrations have been shown to be *Echinacea*-responsive in a variety of assays, and activation of polymorphonuclear leukocytes and NK cells has also been reasonably demonstrated (Barrett 2003). Changes in the numbers and activities of T-cell and B-cell leukocytes have been reported but are less certain. Despite this cellular evidence of immunostimulation, pathways leading to enhanced resistance to infectious disease have not been described adequately. Several dozen human experiments, including a number of blind, randomized trials, report health benefits. The most robust data come from trials testing *Echinacea purpurea* extracts in the treatment of acute URTI. Although suggesting a modest benefit, these trials are limited both in size and in methodological quality. In a recent randomized, double-blind, placebo-controlled trial, administering unrefined *Echinacea* at the onset of symptoms of URTI in 148 college students did not provide any detectable benefit or harm compared with placebo (Barrett et al. 2002). Hence, although a great deal of moderately good-quality scientific data regarding *Echinacea* has been gathered, its effectiveness in treating illness or in enhancing human health has not yet been proved beyond a reasonable doubt.

Probiotics are food supplements that contain "friendly" gut bacteria. A reasonable body of evidence indicates that regular consumption of probiotics can modify the population of the gut microflora and influence immune function (Gill and Cross 2002). Studies have shown that probiotic intake can improve rates of recovery from rotavirus diarrhea, increase resistance to enteric pathogens, and promote antitumor activity. Some evidence even suggests that probiotics may be effective in alleviating some allergic and respiratory disorders in young children (for a review see, Kopp-Hoolihan 2001). However, to date, no published studies have investigated the effectiveness of probiotic use in athletes.

Conclusions and Recommendations

Both heavy exercise and nutrition exert separate influences on immune function; these influences appear to be greater when exercise stress and poor nutrition act synergistically. Exercise training increases the body's requirement for most nutrients, and in many cases, these increased needs are countered by increased food consumption. However, some athletes adopt an unbalanced dietary regimen, and many surveys indicate that few athletes follow the best dietary pattern for optimal sport nutrition. Despite an abundance of studies investigating the effects of nutrition on immune function and the effects of nutrition on physical performance, relatively few have investigated the interrelationships between nutrition, performance, and immune function concurrently. Therefore, some of the conclusions drawn in this chapter remain speculative, relying on generalizations between sedentary and athletic populations. However, the poor nutritional status of some athletes very likely predisposes them to immunodepression. Although countering the effects of all of the factors that contribute to exercise-induced immunodepression is impossible, minimizing many of the effects is possible. Athletes can help themselves by eating well-balanced diets that include adequate carbohydrate, protein, and micronutrients.

Consumption of carbohydrate drinks during training and competition is recommended because this practice appears to attenuate some of the immunosuppressive effects of prolonged exercise. *Echinacea* supplements may provide some boost to immune function, but more studies are needed to confirm that taking this supplement can reduce the number of training days lost to infection.

The dangers of oversupplementation of vitamins and minerals should be emphasized because many micronutrients given in quantities beyond a certain threshold reduce immune responses. Other factors that may lower infection risk in athletes include reducing other life stresses, maintaining good oral and skin hygiene, obtaining adequate rest, and spacing prolonged training sessions and competitions as far apart as possible. The following practices are recommended:

- Allow sufficient time between training sessions for recovery. Include 1 or 2 days resting recovery in the weekly training program; more training is not always better.

- Avoid extremely long training sessions. Restrict continuous activity to less than 2 hours per session. For example, a 3-hour session might be better performed as two 1.5-hour sessions, one session in the morning and one session in the evening.

- Avoid training monotony by ensuring variation in the day-to-day training load. Follow a hard-training day with a light-training day.

- When increasing the training load, do so on the hard days. Do not eliminate the recovery days.

- When recovering from overtraining or illness, begin with very light training and build gradually.

- Monitor and record mood, feelings of fatigue, and muscle soreness during training; decrease the training load if the normal session feels harder than usual.
- Keep other life/social/psychological stresses to a minimum.
- Get regular and adequate sleep (at least 6 hours a night).
- Increase rest as needed after travel across time zones to allow circadian rhythms to adjust.
- Eat a well-balanced diet to obtain all the necessary vitamins and minerals, but if dieting to lose weight or if fresh fruit and vegetables are not readily available, multivitamin supplements should be considered.
- Ensure adequate total dietary energy, carbohydrate, and protein intake. Be aware that periods of carbohydrate depletion are associated with immunodepression.
- Drink carbohydrate "sports" drinks before, during, and after prolonged workouts to reduce some of the adverse effects of exercise on immune function.
- Consider discussing vaccination with your coach or doctor. Influenza vaccines take 5 weeks to 7 weeks to take effect. Intramuscular vaccines may have a few small side effects, so receiving vaccinations out of season is best. Do not get a vaccination before a competition or if symptoms of illness are present.

Key Points

- The immune system protects the body against potentially damaging microorganisms.
- Athletes engaged in heavy endurance training programs often have depressed immune function and suffer from an increased incidence of URTIs. Training and competitive surroundings may increase the athlete's exposure to pathogens and provide optimal conditions for pathogen transmission.
- Heavy, prolonged exertion is associated with numerous hormonal and biochemical changes, many of which potentially have detrimental effects on immune function. Improper nutrition can compound the negative influence of heavy exertion on immunocompetence.
- An athlete exercising in a carbohydrate-depleted state experiences larger increases in circulating stress hormones and a greater perturbation of several immune-function indices.
- Consuming carbohydrate (but not glutamine) during exercise attenuates rises in stress hormones such as cortisol and appears to limit the degree of exercise-induced immunodepression.
- The poor nutritional status of some athletes may predispose them to immunodepression. For example, dietary deficiencies of protein and specific micronutrients are associated with immune dysfunction.
- An adequate intake of iron, zinc, and B-vitamins is particularly important, but the dangers of oversupplementation should also be emphasized. Many micronutrients given in quantities beyond a certain threshold reduce immune responses and may have other toxic effects.
- Sustained endurance training appears to be associated with an adaptive up-regulation of the antioxidant defense system. However, such adaptations may be insufficient to protect athletes who train extensively, and these individuals should consider increasing their intakes of nutritional antioxidants.
- In general, supplementation of individual micronutrients or consumption of large doses of simple antioxidant mixtures is not recommended. Athletes should obtain complex mixtures of antioxidant compounds from consumption of fruits and vegetables. Consuming megadoses of individual vitamins is likely to do more harm than good.

(continued)

(continued)

■ Although countering the effects of all of the factors that contribute to exercise-induced immunodepression is impossible, minimizing many of the effects is possible. Athletes can help themselves by eating well-balanced diets that include adequate protein and carbohydrate to meet their energy requirements. Such diets ensure a more than adequate intake of trace elements without the need for special supplements.

■ By adopting sound nutritional practice, reducing life stresses, maintaining good hygiene, obtaining adequate rest, and spacing prolonged training sessions and competitions as far apart as possible, athletes can reduce their risk of infection.

Key Terms

acute-phase proteins 313

complement 304

cytokine 304

humoral 310

immune system 302

immunodepression 302

immunoglobulin (Ig) or antibody 304

inflammation 304

interleukin 308

leukocyte 302

lymphocyte 302

macrophage or monocyte 302

mucosa 321

neutrophil 302

pathogen 302

phagocyte 309

Recommended Readings

Calder P.C., C.J. Field, and H.S. Gill. 2002. *Nutrition and Immune Function*. CABI Publishing: Oxford.

Chandra, R.K. 1997. Nutrition and the immune system: An introduction. *American Journal of Clinical Nutrition* 66:460S-463S.

Gleeson, M., and N.C. Bishop. 2000. Elite athlete immunology: The importance of nutrition. *International Journal of Sports Medicine* 21(supplement 1):S44-S50.

Gleeson M., G.I. Lancaster, and N.C. Bishop. 2001. Nutritional strategies to minimise exercise-induced immunosuppression in athletes. *Canadian Journal of Applied Physiology* 26(supplement):635-647.

Konig, D., A. Berg, C. Weinstock, J. Keul, and H. Northoff.

1997. Essential fatty acids, immune function and exercise. *Exercise and Immunology Review* 3:1-31.

Nieman, D.C., and B.K. Pedersen (editors). 2000. *Nutrition and Exercise Immunology*. CRC Press: Boca Raton, FL.

Pedersen B.K., K. Ostrowski, T. Rohde, and H. Bruunsgaard. 1998. Nutrition, exercise and the immune system. *Proceedings of the Nutrition Society* 57:43-47.

Peters, E.M. 1997. Exercise, immunology and upper respiratory tract infections. *International Journal of Sports Medicine* 18(1 supplement):S69-S77.

Scrimshaw, N.S., and J.P. SanGiovanni. 1997. Synergism of nutrition, infection and immunity: An overview. *American Journal of Clinical Nutrition* 66:464S-477S.

Appendix A

Key Concepts in Biological Chemistry Relevant to Sport Nutrition

The study of sport nutrition requires an understanding of some simple biochemistry and physiology. The major components that make up the body and the diet—carbohydrates, lipids, proteins, and nucleic acids—are themselves composed of smaller building blocks. This appendix contains a short review of important chemical concepts, interactions, and processes involving biomolecules, together with a brief summary of membrane transport mechanisms, enzyme action, the structure and function of the various cellular organelles, and the characteristics of the four major tissue types found in the human body. This appendix can be used as a reference, but an understanding of what is covered is essential to most of the principles and mechanisms discussed elsewhere in this book. This appendix may be particularly useful for those readers who have little background in biology and chemistry. We begin with the smallest units that any substance can be broken down to: the atoms.

Matter, Energy, Atoms, and Molecules

The human body consists only of matter and energy in their various forms. Indeed, the same can be said of the entire universe. Matter occupies space and has a mass that represents the quantity of matter that is present. We often equate mass with weight, which is the force that gravity exerts upon the mass, but, technically, the two are different. The quantity or mass of an object does not change, regardless of its location, but its weight will vary according to the pull of gravity. For example, a rock weighing 6 kg (13.2 lb) on Earth weighs only about 1 kg (2.2 lb) on the surface of the Moon because the gravitational force of the Moon is only about one-sixth of that of the Earth. Of course, matter itself remains matter whether on the Earth or on the Moon.

Many thousands of different types of matter exist, and all can be reduced into smaller units. The smallest units into which a substance can be broken down

chemically are the elements, each of which has different and unique properties. Ninety-two elements are presently known to exist, but only about 12 are common in living organisms. The most abundant elements are oxygen, carbon, hydrogen, and nitrogen (in that order). These 4 elements compose 96% of the mass of a human.

Energy is the capacity of any system, including the living body, to do work (i.e., to produce a change of some sort in matter). Energy can exist in several forms, including light, heat, electrical, mechanical, and chemical energy. Energy can be transformed from one form to another. In the body, the potential chemical energy stored in foodstuffs is transformed to do various forms of work such as movement or the synthesis of large molecules from small molecules. Matter and energy are interrelated by Einstein's famous equation:

$$E = mc^2$$

where E is energy, m is mass, and c is the speed of light (about 299,744 km/s). Nothing is capable of moving faster than light. Einstein's equation can, in principle, go in either direction. Thus, energy can be transformed into matter, and matter can be transformed into energy.

Atoms are the smallest unit of an element that retains all the properties of the element. The atoms of all elements can be broken down physically into the same subatomic particles: protons, neutrons, and electrons. Hence, the atoms of the various elements differ only in the numbers of protons, neutrons, and electrons that they contain. Protons, which possess a positive charge, and neutrons, which are electrically neutral, are held together to form the nucleus of an atom. Electrons, which have negligible mass (only about 1/8,000 of that of a proton or a neutron) and possess a negative charge, spin around the atomic nucleus in discrete orbitals that may be spherical or dumbbell shaped. Some electrons move in orbitals close to the nucleus; others move in orbitals farther away. Electrons that are farther from the nucleus have more energy than those close to the nucleus, thus, the orbitals can be thought of as energy levels. Electrons normally stay at their particular energy level, but by gaining or losing energy, they jump from one energy level to another. Although electron orbitals can vary in shape, electrons at each energy level are usually depicted diagrammatically as moving in concentric and circular orbits, or shells, around the nucleus. A maximum of 2 electrons can be held in the innermost shell. The second and third shell can hold up to 8 electrons each. The fourth shell can hold up to 18 electrons.

The number of electrons equals the number of protons in the nucleus, resulting in an atom that is electrically neutral. The smallest atom is that of hydrogen, which is composed of just 1 proton and 1 electron (see figure A.1a). The carbon atom consists of 6 protons, 6 neutrons, and 6 electrons, whereas an oxygen atom is made up of 8 protons, 8 neutrons, and 8 electrons. Both oxygen and carbon have 2 electrons in their inner shells, but they differ in the number of electrons in the second shell. Oxygen has 6 electrons in the second shell, and carbon has 4 (see figure A.1, b and c).

The chemical properties of an element and the way it reacts with other elements depend on the number of electrons in its outer shell. If this shell is full, the element does not react with others and is said to be inert. Helium, with 2 electrons and neon with 18 electrons in their outer shells are examples of inert elements. Atoms whose outer shells are not full tend to move toward a more stable configuration by losing or gaining electrons or sharing electrons with other atoms. The atoms are bound together by attractive forces called chemical bonds. These bonds are a source of potential chemical energy. Breaking chemical bonds releases some energy that can be used to do work.

Nearly all the mass of an atom is in its protons and neutrons, so the combined number of these particles is the atomic mass of the element. An element's mass is indicated by a superscript in front of the element (e.g., ^{1}H, ^{12}C, ^{16}O). The number of protons in an atom is its atomic number, which is indicated as a subscript in front of the symbol for the atom (e.g. $^1_1$H, $^{12}_6$C, $^{16}_8$O).

All atoms of a given element contain the same number of protons and electrons (which determines the chemical properties of the element), but in some elements, the number of neutrons in the nucleus, and, hence, the atomic mass (but not the atomic number) varies. Atoms of an element that have a different number of neutrons are called isotopes. Some isotopes are unstable and emit radiation in the form of gamma rays, electrons, or a helium nucleus (2 protons and 2 neutrons). This radiation can be measured, and some unstable isotopes have proved useful as tracers. For example, normal carbon has an atomic mass of 12, but the radioactive isotope of carbon has a mass of 14. Glucose, a simple sugar, can be prepared using $^{14}_6$C, and its metabolism in the body can be followed by identifying the presence of $^{14}_6$C in intermediate compounds and in expired carbon dioxide. Nowadays, the presence and quantity of stable isotopes (those that do not decay by the emission of radiation) such as $^{13}_6$C can be detected, and these isotopes are increasingly used in place of the more dangerous radioactive isotopes in human metabolic studies.

Most elements in the body are not present as free atoms, but are combined with other atoms to form molecules. For example, a molecule of water contains 1 atom of oxygen bound to 2 atoms of hydrogen, symbolized as H_2O (see figure A.2). Even the oxygen in the air we breathe is made of molecular oxygen consisting of 2 atoms of oxygen bound together, symbolized as O_2. A molecule of a simple hexose sugar, glucose, contains 24 atoms: 6 of carbon, 12 of hydrogen, and 6 of oxygen. This formula can be expressed as $C_6H_{12}O_6$, which is known as the empirical chemical formula of glucose. The molecular mass is obtained by adding up the atomic masses present in the molecule. Thus, for glucose, we have $6 \times {}^{12}C + 12 \times {}^1H + 6 \times {}^{16}O = 72 + 12 + 96 = 180$. The molecular mass of a substance in grams is equal to 1 mole of that substance, and the number of molecules in a mole of any substance is the same and known as Avogadro's number, which is 6.022×10^{23}.

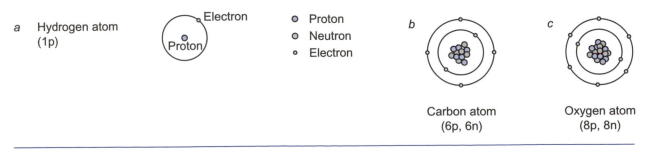

Figure A.1 Atoms of (a) hydrogen, (b) carbon, and (c) oxygen.

Molecule of water (H_2O)

Partial negative charge at oxygen end of molecule

Partial positive charge at hydrogen end of molecule

Can also be shown diagrammatically like this

or

Figure A.2 A molecule of water indicating the distribution of partial charges.

One mole of a substance dissolved in enough water to make 1 liter is known as a 1-molar (1.0 M) solution. Biochemists usually deal with smaller concentrations such as millimoles per liter (1 mM = 1 × 10^{-3} M) because many substances that are dissolved in the body fluids are found in this concentration range. For example, the concentration of glucose in blood is about 5 mM.

Chemical Bonds, Free Energy, and ATP

This section provides a brief review of chemical bonds, with emphasis on bonds between the six major elements found in the living body: hydrogen (H), carbon (C), nitrogen (N), oxygen (O), phosphorus (P), and sulfur (S).

- Covalent bonds hold together 2 or more atoms by the interaction of their outer electrons. Covalent bonds are the strongest chemical bonds. The energy of a typical covalent bond is approximately 330 kilojoules per mole (330 kJ/mol [79 kcal/mol]). However, this energy can vary from 210 kJ/mol to 460 kJ/mol (50 kcal/mol to 110 kcal/mol), depending on the elements involved. Once formed, covalent bonds rarely break spontaneously, because the thermal energy of a molecule at room temperature (20° C or 293° K [68° F]) is only about 2.5 kJ/mol (0.6 kcal/mol), much lower than the energy required to break a covalent bond. Covalent bonds are either single, double, or triple bonds (see table A.1).

- Carbon-carbon bonds are particularly strong and stable covalent bonds. The major organic

elements have standard bonding capabilities: C, N, and P can form up to 4 covalent bonds with other atoms, O and S can form 2 covalent bonds, and H can only form 1 covalent bond. In solution, O and S can lose a proton (or hydrogen ion, H^+), leaving the O or S with a negative charge (see figure A.3). Covalent bonds have partial charges when the atoms involved have different electronegativities. Water is one example of a molecule with partial charges. The symbols delta+ ($\delta+$) and delta– ($\delta-$) are used to indicate partial charges (see figure A.2). Oxygen, because of its high electronegativity, attracts the electrons away from the hydrogen atoms, resulting in a partial negative charge on the oxygen and a partial positive charge on each of the hydrogens. The possibility of hydrogen bonds is a consequence of these partial charges.

- Hydrogen bonds (H-bonds) are weak intramolecular or intermolecular attractions between a hydrogen atom and an electronegative atom possessing a lone pair of electrons (e.g., oxygen or nitrogen atoms). Hydrogen bonds are formed when a hydrogen atom is shared between 2 molecules (see figure A.4). Hydrogen bonds have polarity. A hydrogen atom covalently attached to a very electronegative atom (N, O, or P) shares its partial positive charge with a second electronegative atom (N, O, or P). Hydrogen bonds are 21 kJ/mol (5 kcal/mol) in strength. These bonds are frequently found in proteins and nucleic acids, and, by reinforcing each other, they keep the protein (or nucleic acid) structure secure. However, because the hydrogen atoms in the protein can also H-bond to the surrounding water, the relative strength of protein-protein H-bonds versus protein-H_2O bonds is smaller than 21 kJ/mol.

- Ionic bonds are formed when a complete transfer of electrons from one atom to another occurs. The valence (outer shell) electrons are either lost or gained, resulting in 2 ions, one positively charged and the other negatively charged. The ions, which are oppositely charged, are held together by electrostatic forces. For example, when a sodium atom (Na) donates the 1 electron in its outer valence shell to a chlorine atom (Cl), which needs 1 electron to fill its outer valence shell, NaCl (salt) results. The symbol for sodium chloride is Na^+Cl^-. Ionic bonds are 17 kJ/mol to 30 kJ/mol (4 kcal/mol to 7 kcal/mol) in strength.

- Nonpolar molecules cannot form H-bonds with water and are, therefore, very poorly soluble in water. These molecules are called hydrophobic (water hating) molecules, as opposed to hydrophilic (water loving) molecules, which can form H-bonds with water. Hydrophobic molecules tend to aggregate together in avoidance of water molecules, such as when a drop of oil is placed on water. The oil forms a thin layer over the surface of the water. If mixed together vigorously, the oil forms small globules but does not dissolve in the water. To understand the energetics driving this interaction, visualize the water molecules surrounding a single "dissolved" molecule attempting to form the greatest number of H-bonds with each other. The best energetic solution involves forcing all of the nonpolar molecules together, thus reducing the total surface area that breaks up the water's H-bond matrix.

During biochemical reactions that involve the breaking of chemical bonds, energy is released, some of which is available to do work. Some energy is also released as heat, which cannot be used to do work in the body, because body temperature is regulated within a very narrow range. The free energy released during the breaking of bonds, usually signified by the symbol G, can be used to do work because some of it is stored in the compound adenosine triphosphate (ATP). The free energy released when an inorganic phosphate group (Pi) is broken off ATP to form adenosine diphosphate (ADP) is used to drive several energy-requiring processes in the body, including the synthesis of macromolecules from smaller molecules (e.g., synthesis of proteins from free amino acids), membrane transport work (e.g., the movement of sodium ions out of a cell against the prevailing concentration gradient), and mechanical work (e.g., muscle contraction). Reactions involving the breaking of phosphate bonds and the liberation of Pi are catalyzed by enzymes called kinases. In the case of ATP breakdown, these kinases are commonly abbreviated as ATPases.

ATP is the only form of chemical energy that is convertible into other forms of energy used by living cells. Essentially, ATP is the energy currency of the cell. Fats and carbohydrates are the main storage forms of energy in the body, and when they are broken down by oxidation reactions to carbon dioxide and water, the energy released is used to resynthesize ATP from ADP and Pi.

All biochemical reactions are inefficient, which means that not all the energy released can be conserved or used to do work. Some energy is always lost as heat. This release of heat helps maintain body temperature at about 37°C (98.6° F). During exercise, when the rate of catabolic reactions is markedly increased in the active muscles to provide energy for contraction, the rate of heat production also increases substantially and muscle temperature rises by 1°C to 5°C (1.8° F to 9° F).

Table A.1 Single, Double, and Triple Covalent Bonds

Bond number	Example	Energy (kJ/mol and kcal/mol)
Single	(methane: $H-C-H$ with H above and below central C)	330 (79)
Double	(ethene: $H-C=C-H$ with H above and below each C)	630 (150)
Triple	$H-C\equiv C-H$	840 (200)

Lactic acid ⇌ Lactate anion + Hydrogen ion (proton)

Figure A.3 Dissociation of a proton (H^+ ion) from lactic acid, leaving an oxygen (O) with a negative charge.

Figure A.4 *(a)* Hydrogen bonding between water molecules. A hydrogen atom covalently attached to a very electronegative atom (N, O, or P) shares its partial positive charge with a second electronegative atom (N, O, or P). *(b)* More examples of hydrogen bonding.

Although ATP is considered the energy currency of the cell, it cannot be accumulated in large amounts, and the intramuscular ATP concentration is only about 5 mmol/kg of muscle tissue. During maximal exercise, ATP is sufficient to fuel about 2 seconds of muscle force generation. Experiments have shown that the muscle ATP store never becomes completely depleted, because it is efficiently resynthesized from ADP and Pi at the same rate at which it is degraded. During submaximal steady-state exercise, ATP resynthesis is achieved by mitochondrial oxidation of carbohydrates and lipids. This process is commonly referred to as aerobic metabolism because it requires oxygen. However, at the onset of exercise and in high-intensity exercise, ATP resynthesis is principally anaerobic (without the use of oxygen). Further details of the metabolic pathways involved can be found in chapter 2.

Chemical Reactions in the Body

A variety of different types of chemical reactions take place in the body. These reactions are defined in the following section together with a few illustrative examples.

- Oxidation is a reaction involving the loss of electrons from an atom. It is always accompa-

nied by a reduction (a reaction in which a molecule gains electrons). For example, pyruvate is reduced using hydrogen donated from the reduced form of the coenzyme nicotinamide adenine dinucleotide (NADH) to form lactate. In the reverse reaction, lactate is oxidized by NAD^+ (the oxidized form of the coenzyme) when pyruvate is reformed. This reaction is also known as dehydrogenation because it is a form of oxidation that involves the loss of hydrogen atoms:

Pyruvate CH_3-CO-COOH + NADH + H^+ $\leftrightarrow$
Lactate CH_3-CHOH-COOH + NAD^+

- Hydrolysis is a reaction in which an organic compound is split by interaction with water into simpler compounds. An example is the hydrolysis of phosphocreatine (PCr) to creatine (Cr) and phosphate, which is coupled to the resynthesis of ATP from ADP using the phosphate group liberated from phosphocreatine:

$$PCr + H_2O \rightarrow Cr + P$$

$$P + ADP + H^+ \rightarrow ATP + H_2O$$

- Phosphorylation is the addition of a phosphate (PO_3^{2-}) group to a molecule. Many enzymes are activated by the covalent bonding of a phosphate group. The phosphorylation of ADP forms ATP:

$$ADP + P_i \rightarrow ATP + H_2O$$

- Condensation is the union of 2 or more molecules with the elimination of a simpler group such as H_2O. An example is the joining of 2 amino acid molecules to form a dipeptide.
- Hydroxylation is the addition of a hydroxyl (OH) group to a molecule.
- Carboxylation is the addition of CO_2, catalyzed by an enzyme using biotin as its prosthetic group.
- Deamination is the loss of an amino (NH_2) group, liberating free ammonia (NH_3). This is important in the metabolism of amino acids such as alanine:

$$\text{Alanine} \rightarrow \text{Pyruvate} + NH_3$$

- Transamination is the transfer of an amino (NH_2) group from an amino acid to a keto-acid. An example is the transfer of an amino group from the amino acid glutamate to the keto-acid pyruvate, forming a new amino acid alanine and another keto-acid α-ketoglutarate:

$$\text{Glutamate} + \text{Pyruvate} \rightarrow \text{Alanine} + \text{α-ketoglutarate}$$

- Denaturation is the alteration of the physical properties and 3-dimensional structure of a protein by a chemical or physical treatment that does not disrupt the primary structure, but generally results in the inactivation of the protein (e.g., the inactivation of an enzyme by the addition of a strong acid or excessive heat).

Hydrogen Ion Concentrations and Buffers

Free hydrogen ions are produced in many chemical reactions in the body. Problems such as decreased activity or even complete inactivation of enzymes and inhibition of several biological processes, including muscle contraction, can arise when free hydrogen ions accumulate inside cells. Hence, the body has several mechanisms that help to limit changes in the free hydrogen ion concentration in the fluids inside and outside cells.

An acid is a compound able to donate a hydrogen ion (H^+); for example, hydrochloric acid (HCl), carbonic acid (H_2CO_3), and lactic acid (CH_3-CHOH-COOH). A base is a compound able to accept a hydrogen ion; for example, hydroxyl ions (OH^-), and bicarbonate ions (HCO_3^-). The pH is a measure of the concentration of hydrogen ions. These values are derived, for example, from the dissociation of an acid, such as HCl, when it is dissolved in water (HCl $\rightarrow H^+ + Cl^-$). The pH value is defined as the negative decimal logarithm of the free H^+ concentration or [H^+]; that is, $pH = -\log_{10}[H^+]$, where [H^+] is expressed in moles per liter (mol/L or M), so the concentration of free H^+ increases 10-fold for each decrease of 1 pH unit. The [H^+] in pure water is 10^{-7} mol/L. Therefore, the pH of pure water is

$$pH = -\log_{10}(10^{-7}) = -(-7) = 7$$

pH 7 is often referred to as neutral pH. Everything below pH 7 has a higher concentration of H^+ and is considered acidic. Everything above pH 7 has a lower concentration of H^+ and is considered basic (you can also think of this as a higher concentration of OH^-). Most body fluids are close to neutral pH. For example, blood plasma has a pH of 7.4, and resting muscle intracellular fluid (sarcoplasm) has a pH of 7.0. The pH of the body fluids is tightly regulated, and even in the most severe metabolic disturbances—such as high-intensity exercise—the pH of blood does not change by more than about 0.3. Even in the exercising muscle where the additional hydrogen ions are first appearing because of the increased lactic acid production, the pH does not fall below 6.5. As previously mentioned, this stability is important because if the pH falls too low, the activity of enzymes can be inhibited, which can have fatal consequences for the cell.

Buffers act as a reservoir for hydrogen ions and so limit, or buffer, changes in free H^+ concentration. Buffering is passive and virtually instantaneous. A buffer consists of a weak acid and its conjugate base. In solution, some, but not all, molecules of the weak acid dissociate into the conjugate base and hydrogen ions:

$$BH \leftrightarrow B^- + H^+$$

where BH is the weak acid and B^- is its conjugate base. The relationship between the concentrations of weak acid, base, and hydrogen ions can be expressed as an equation:

$$K_a.[BH] = [H^+].[B^-]$$

where K_a is the dissociation constant of the acid; that is, the concentration of H^+ at which the concentrations of the base and acid are equal. The equation can be rearranged to give the Henderson equation:

$$[H^+] = K_a.[BH]/[B^-]$$

or, alternatively, by taking the negative logarithm of each side of the equation, it becomes the Henderson-Hasselbach equation:

$$-\log_{10}[H^+] = -\log_{10}K_a + \log_{10}[B^-]/[BH]$$

which is the same as

$$pH = pK_a + \log_{10}[B^-]/[BH]$$

which tells us that optimal buffering (minimum change in pH when H^+ ions are added) occurs at pH $= pK_a$, and that this effect occurs when the concentrations of weak acid (BH) and base (B^-) are equal.

Carbonic acid/bicarbonate (H_2CO_3/HCO_3^-) is the most important extracellular buffer, with a pK_a of 6.1. Hemoglobin and other proteins and peptides containing the amino acid histidine (pK_a usually 6.0 to 8.0) and phosphates ($HPO_4^{2-}/H_2PO_4^-$), whose pK_a is 6.8, are important intracellular buffers. Because the pH of most body fluids is about 7.4, buffers with a pK_a of between 6 and 8 are the most effective.

In exercising muscle, large amounts of hydrogen ions are produced from the dissociation of lactic acid to H^+ and the lactate anion (see figure A.3). The resting intracellular pH of muscle is 7.0. A large fall in pH is undesirable because it would denature enzymes and is prevented by the presence of intracellular buffers, including carnosine (a dipeptide consisting of alanine and histidine), phosphocreatine, phosphates, and histidine-containing proteins. As the hydrogen ions diffuse out of the muscle into the blood, they are buffered by bicarbonate (in plasma) and hemoglobin (in the red blood cells). An increase in the blood lactic acid concentration of 10 mmol/L only changes the blood pH by about 0.1; this concentration of lactic acid dissolved in water alone causes the pH to drop from 7.0 to 2.0. Clearly, the body's buffer systems are very effective.

Enzymes

Enzymes act as controllable catalysts. These proteins speed up the rate of specific chemical reactions and allow them to be regulated in ways that permit the body to control the interactions between the different metabolic pathways. The direction in which the reactions proceed and the equilibrium point that is reached in a nonbiological system are governed by the laws of thermodynamics. The characteristics of enzymes that allow them to act as catalysts are briefly described.

Mechanisms of Enzyme Action and Enzyme Kinetics

The laws of thermodynamics tell us that chemical reactions proceed spontaneously only in the direction that results in the products of the reaction

having a lower energy status than the substrates (see figure A.5). Enzymes act as reusable catalysts, which involves the formation of an enzyme substrate complex as an intermediate step in the reaction. The formation of this substrate lowers the energy of activation. Because less energy is now needed, the reaction is more likely to proceed. Although the enzyme participates in the reaction, it is not consumed and is, therefore, required in only small amounts.

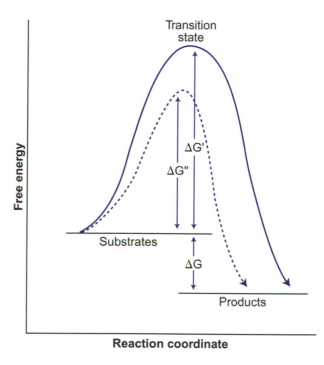

Figure A.5 Energy status of substrates and products.

The energetics of formation of the enzyme substrate complex are not well understood, but clearly some kind of weak bond forms between the substrate and the enzyme. This bond involves one or more active sites on the enzyme, and these sites have a particular shape and charge distribution that allows them to interact with the substrate. These characteristics allow enzymes to promote the rates of specific reaction in a number of different ways. Where two or more substrates are involved, attachment to binding sites on the enzyme allows the substrates to be brought into close proximity in the correct orientation, thus increasing the chances of a reaction taking place. Alternatively, binding to the enzyme can cause changes in the shape of the substrate molecule that increase its susceptibility to reaction.

Enzyme Kinetics

Enzyme kinetics is the measurement of the change in substrate or product concentration as a function of time. The first stage in an enzyme-catalyzed reaction is the binding of the substrate (S) to the active site of the enzyme (E) to form an enzyme-substrate complex (ES). The substrate then reacts to form the product (P), which is released. Release of the product restores the enzyme to its original free form:

$$E + S \leftrightarrow ES \rightarrow E + P$$

The assumption is that the first stage of the process is reversible but the second is not. In almost all reactions, the substrate concentration is far in excess of the enzyme concentration. This difference means that formation of the ES complex does not result in an appreciable change in the substrate concentration, but does reduce the concentration of the free enzyme.

The progress curve for the reaction is initially linear, decreasing in slope as the reaction proceeds and substrate is used up, as shown in figure A.6. The initial velocity during the linear part of the curve is called V_0. The relationship between V_0 and the substrate concentration ([S]) is described by the Michaelis-Menten equation:

$$V_0 = V_{max} [S] / K_m + [S]$$

where V_{max} is the maximum velocity of the reaction at infinite [S], and K_m is the Michaelis constant, equivalent to the substrate concentration in which the initial reaction velocity (V_0) is equal to one-half the maximal velocity (i.e., K_m = [S] where $V_0 = V_{max}/2$).

Figure A.6 Progress of an enzyme-catalyzed reaction.

This relationship is depicted graphically in figure A.7 and clearly shows that at low concentrations of substrate, the initial reaction rate increases linearly in response to increasing substrate concentration, but the rate approaches a limit above which it is constant and independent of substrate concentration. At this point, all of the enzyme molecules are effectively saturated with substrate. The V_{max} is, therefore, a function of the amount of enzyme present.

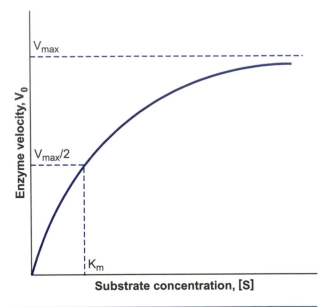

Figure A.7 Relationship between the initial reaction velocity and substrate concentration for an enzyme-catalyzed reaction.

When the substrate concentration is equal to K_m, the reaction rate is equal to half of the V_{max}. The K_m value is, therefore, equal to the substrate concentration that will result in the reaction proceeding at one-half of the maximum rate. A high K_m value is, therefore, an indication of low affinity of the enzyme for its substrate. A high substrate concentration is necessary to achieve a reaction rate equal to one-half the maximum rate. High reaction rates are only achieved when the substrate concentration is relatively high. If [S] is equal to 10 times the K_m, substituting these values into the Michaelis-Menten equation tells us that the reaction rate is 91% of V_{max}, and 99% of the maximum rate will only be achieved when the substrate concentration is 100 times the K_m.

Factors Influencing Enzyme Activity

The activity of enzymes can be assessed by the rate of substrate utilization or product formation under standardized conditions. The most common unit

338

of measurement is the International Unit (IU or U). This measure is the amount of enzyme that converts 1μmole of substrate to product in 1 minute under the conditions specified for that reaction. Although this measure is generally used among physiologists, the appropriate SI unit should be used. This unit is the katal (kat), which is the amount of enzyme that converts 1 mole of substrate to product in 1 second under optimum conditions. At least part of the reason for the persistence of the IU is the difficulty in defining optimum conditions for the activity of individual enzymes.

Effects of Temperature and pH

Enzyme activity is particularly sensitive to temperature and increases as the temperature increases. Any expression of enzyme activities must, therefore, specify the temperature at which measurements are made. Temperatures of 25° C and 37° C (77° F and 98.6° F) are normally used as standards. At high temperatures, however, enzyme activity falls sharply and irreversibly because of structural changes caused by denaturation of the protein, as shown in figure A.8. Although body core temperature is usually about 37° C (98.6° F), the temperature of muscle tissue may be as low as 30° C (86° F) in a resting person on a cold day and can rise to 42° C (108° F) during high-intensity exercise. Hence, warming up before an event has important implications for maximizing reaction rates and optimizing muscle performance. Except in extreme cases of heat illness, body core temperature seldom exceeds 41° C (106°F), but this temperature is close to the level at which some enzymes and other proteins are affected.

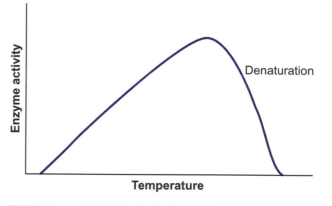

Figure A.8   Effect of temperature on enzyme activity.

Changes in the ionization state of an enzyme caused by a change in pH of the cell affects its affinity for its substrate because of changes in structure or charge distribution at the active site, as illustrated in figure A.9. The local pH may also affect the ionization state of the substrate. All enzymes have an optimum pH (where enzyme activity is at its highest, as shown in figure A.10), but optimum pH differs among different enzymes and may also be influenced by the presence of other activators and inhibitors. Variations in pH are generally small in most tissues, with skeletal muscle showing the largest changes in response to very-high-intensity exercise: pH may fall from the resting value of about 7.0 to 6.5 or even less. Many enzymes normally function in an environment that is close to their pH optimum. For example, pepsin, which has a pH optimum of about 2.0, seems well adapted for the acid conditions of the stomach, where

Figure A.9   Change in charge distribution of enzyme molecules caused by change in pH.

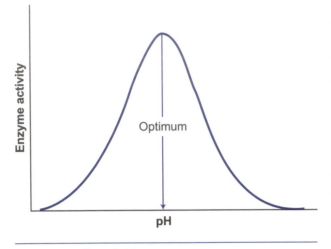

Figure A.10   Effect of pH on enzyme activity.

it hydrolyzes proteins into smaller fragments (peptides) and amino acids that can be absorbed in the small intestine. Some enzymes, however, have a pH optimum, at least in their isolated and purified form, that is far from their normal environment. Glycerol kinase has maximum activity at a pH of 9.8, a condition that is never reached in the cell.

Coenzymes, Prosthetic Groups, Cofactors, and Activators

Many enzymes require the presence of one or more coenzymes if the reaction is to proceed. For example, the conversion of lactate to pyruvate involves the removal of two hydrogen atoms from lactate and is catalyzed by lactate dehydrogenase, which requires that the coenzyme nicotinamide adenine dinucleotide (NAD$^+$) participate in the reaction. Coenzymes are chemically altered by participation in the reaction, in this case by conversion of NAD$^+$ to its reduced form, NADH. The coenzyme is, therefore, essentially a substrate for or product of the reaction, but a characteristic of coenzymes is that they are readily regenerated by other reactions within the cell. Some coenzymes, such as NAD$^+$, are loosely bound to the enzyme, but others, such as biotin, are tightly bound and are referred to as prosthetic groups.

Many enzymes have low activities in the absence of cofactors, and the presence of one or another metal ion, especially the divalent metals calcium, magnesium, manganese, and zinc, is essential for activation of many enzymes. Binding to these ions alters the charge distribution and shape of the active site of the enzyme. For example, the release of calcium into the cytoplasm in response to the nerve impulse is important in the activation of phosphorylase, which allows acceleration of the glycolytic pathway.

Competitive and Noncompetitive Inhibition

Substances with a chemical structure similar to that of the normal substrate may also bind to the active site on the enzyme and, thus, interfere with enzyme function by reducing the number of active sites available to the proper substrate. These substances compete with the substrate for access to the active site and are, therefore, known as competitive inhibitors. The effect of competitive inhibition is to increase K_m. Increasing the concentration of substrate to a sufficient level will, however, swamp the effects of the inhibitor, and V_{max} is not affected by competitive inhibition.

Noncompetitive inhibitors bind to the enzyme at other sites, leaving the active site of the enzyme available to the substrate, but they have the effect of altering the conformation of the protein and, thus, reducing the catalytic activity of the active site. The V_{max} is reduced, but the same substrate concentration still produces one-half of the new maximum activity (i.e., K_m remains unchanged).

Allosteric and Covalent Modulation

Allosteric modulation of enzyme activity is the reversible binding of small molecules to the enzyme at sites other than the active site, producing a conformational change in the structure of the enzyme molecule. This change in shape and charge distribution results in a change (either an increase or a decrease) in the affinity of the enzyme for its substrates or products and, hence, in its activity (see figure A.11a). The effect may either increase the activity of the enzyme, speeding up the rate of the reaction it catalyzes, or inhibit the activity of the enzyme, essentially preventing the reaction it catalyzes from taking place. Covalent modulation involves phosphorylation or dephosphorylation (i.e., the addition or removal of a phosphate group, respectively) of an enzyme, usually affecting the hydroxyl (-OH) group of a serine residue in the polypeptide chain (see figure A.11b). As with allosteric effects, covalent modulation may either activate or inhibit enzyme activity. A good example is the activity of glycogen phosphorylase, which catalyzes the breakdown of muscle glycogen. This enzyme needs to be activated at the onset of exercise to allow the muscle glycogen store to be used as an energy source, and this increase in enzyme activity is achieved by the covalent attachment of a phosphate group by a protein kinase that was itself activated by a rise in the intracellular calcium ion concentration (for further details, see chapter 2).

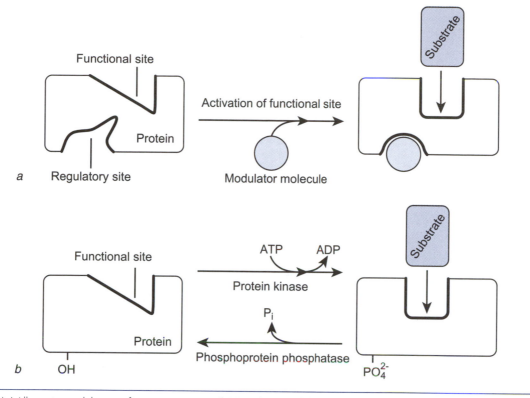

Figure A.11 *(a)* Allosteric modulation of enzyme activity. *(b)* Covalent modulation of enzyme activity.

Enzyme Isoforms

Some enzymes exist in more than one form. These isoforms catalyze the same reaction but are generally found in different tissues and may have different specificities or catalytic capabilities. Lactate dehydrogenase exists in 2 forms, each made up of 4 subunits. The subunits exist in 1 of 2 forms: the H form, predominantly in cardiac muscle, and the M form, predominantly in skeletal muscle. Five different combinations of these subunits are possible. In muscle, the H form is associated with tissues having a high capacity for oxidative metabolism and which, therefore, have a high capacity for lactate oxidation, whereas the M form is associated with tissues having a high anaerobic capacity relative to their oxidative capability. The M form favors the conversion of pyruvate to lactate, whereas the H form favors the conversion of lactate to pyruvate. Many other enzymes exist in a variety of isoforms, but their functional significance is not well understood.

Membrane Structure and Transport

Membranes set the limits of cell boundaries. To enter a cell from the extracellular fluid, a substance must pass through the cell membrane. For example, the simple sugars that are formed from the breakdown of complex carbohydrates in the gastrointestinal tract can only get into the bloodstream by passing through the cells that line the gut. The properties of cell membranes and the components within them determine which substances can and cannot enter or leave a cell.

Cell membranes are composed of a lipid bilayer containing mostly phospholipids and some cholesterol. Within these lipids are proteins, some of which are restricted to one side of the bilayer and some of which are embedded within the membrane from one side to the other (see figure A.12). These proteins have important structural roles as receptors, channels, or transporters.

Dissolved substances (solutes) move across these semipermeable membranes by simple diffusion, facilitated diffusion, or active transport. Osmosis is the movement of water across membranes.

Simple Diffusion

Solutes only move from high to low concentration by diffusion. Simple diffusion involves the movement of the solute across the lipid bilayer and, hence, is to a large degree influenced by the solubility of the

Figure A.12 Cell membranes. *(a)* A 2-dimensional cross section and *(b)* a 3-dimensional view.

substance in lipid. Most water-soluble substances (e.g., glucose) and charged particles (e.g., sodium ions) are poorly soluble in lipid. Large molecules such as proteins cannot pass across membranes. Very small molecules (e.g., O_2, CO_2, H_2O, and NH_3) diffuse easily across cell membranes. Rates of diffusion are affected by temperature and the concentration difference on either side of the membrane.

Facilitated Diffusion

In facilitated diffusion, solutes move only from high to low concentration by diffusion but use a specific protein carrier molecule to pass through the membrane. The protein may be a mobile carrier or a gated channel, as illustrated in figure A.13. As shown in the example of glucose membrane transport in figure A.14, the rate of transport across the membrane is far greater in facilitated diffusion compared with simple diffusion, but at high glucose concentrations, facili-

tated transport exhibits saturation kinetics. The maximum speed of facilitated transport (V_{max}), indicated by the dashed line, is limited by the number of protein transporters available in the membrane. When all the transporters are full, additional movement can only occur by simple diffusion. In muscle, glucose is transported into the fibers by a protein carrier called GLUT4. The number of GLUT4 transporters in the muscle fiber membrane is influenced by exercise and the hormone insulin.

Active Transport

In active transport, substances are moved against their concentration gradient by a specific protein carrier and energy supplied directly by ATP or indirectly by ion electrochemical gradients. The sodium/potassium pump, or Na^+-K^+-ATPase pump, is a good example of an active cellular transport mechanism and is illustrated in figure A.15. Energy released from

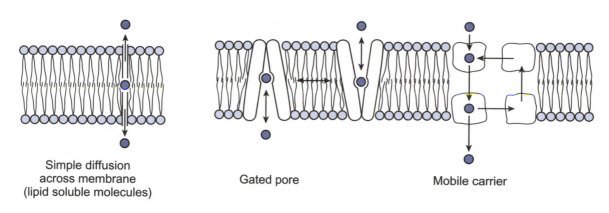

Simple diffusion
across membrane
(lipid soluble molecules)

Gated pore

Mobile carrier

Facilitated diffusion using a protein channel or transporter

Figure A.13   Diffusion and facilitated diffusion of substances across cell membranes. In both cases, net movement of the solute molecules occurs from a high concentration of solute to a low concentration of solute.

Figure A.14   Relative rates of glucose uptake into cells by simple diffusion and facilitated diffusion using a protein transporter in relation to the glucose concentration of the extracellular fluid.

the hydrolysis of ATP moves sodium and potassium ions across the cell membrane against the prevailing concentration gradients. For each molecule of ATP hydrolyzed to ADP, 3 sodium ions (Na$^+$) are transported out of the cell and 2 potassium ions (K$^+$) are transported into the cell. Because more positively charged ions are moved out of the cell than are transported in, an electrochemical gradient is established. Inside the cell becomes negative relative to outside, with a difference in electrical potential of about 70 millivolts. Inside the cell the Na$^+$ concentration is maintained at about 12 mM, whereas outside, it is about 145 mM. The K$^+$ concentration inside the cell is about 155 mM, whereas outside, it is only 4 mM. The presence of separate sodium and potassium ion channels in the membrane is also shown in figure

A.15. When these channels are open, the ions move by diffusion from high to low concentration. The selective opening of sodium channels (allowing a rapid influx of positively charged Na$^+$ ions) causes a temporary change in the resting membrane potential called depolarization. Depolarization is important in the generation and propagation of action potentials in excitable cells such as nerve and muscle.

Cotransport (or symport) mechanisms use the electrochemical gradient set up by the Na$^+$-K$^+$-ATPase pump to transport a substance against its concentration gradient. For example, the inward transport of dietary glucose from the gut lumen into intestinal epithelial cells is coupled to that of Na$^+$, as depicted in figure A.16. The Na$^+$-K$^+$-ATPase pump generates a large concentration difference for sodium across the membrane. The glucose-sodium symport protein uses that sodium gradient to transport glucose into the cell, followed by separate transport of glucose across the basal membrane into the blood by the action of a glucose transporter (GLUT2).

Osmosis

Water can readily diffuse across membranes, both through the lipid bilayer and through protein pores or channels in the membrane. Osmosis is the net movement of water as a consequence of a total-solute particle concentration difference across a membrane. Water moves across a semipermeable membrane from a region of low total-solute particle concentration (osmolarity) to a region of high total-solute particle concentration, until the total-solute particle concentration is equal on each side of the membrane (see figure A.17) or its movement is counteracted by the build-up of hydrostatic pressure.

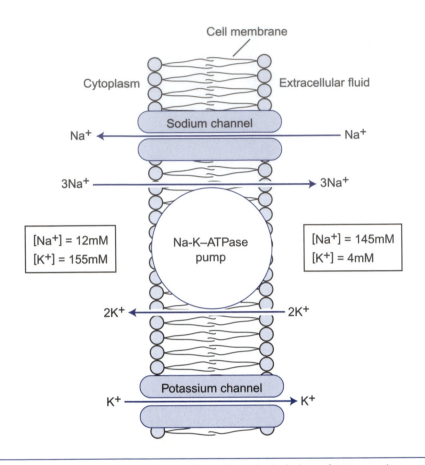

Figure A.15 The sodium-potassium ATPase pump. Energy released from the hydrolysis of ATP is used to move sodium and potassium ions across the cell membrane, against the prevailing concentration gradients.

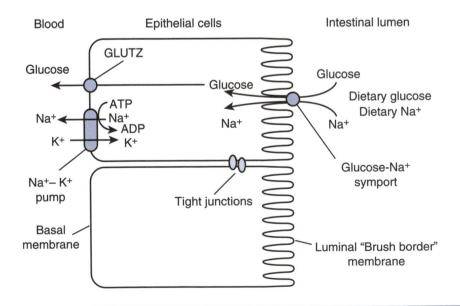

Figure A.16 Cotransport (symport) of glucose and sodium from the gut lumen into epithelial cells of the small intestine, followed by separate transport across the basal membrane into the blood by the action of a glucose transporter (GLUT2) and the sodium-potassium-ATPase pump.

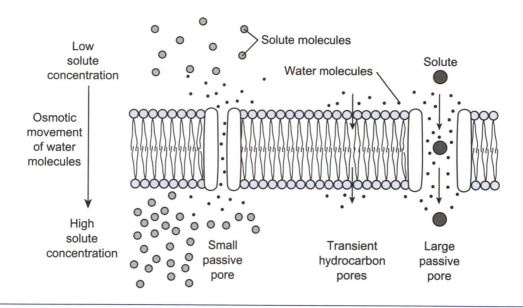

Figure A.17 Possible mechanisms for permeation of cell membranes by water. Water is a small molecule and, thus, permeates through the spaces between hydrophobic lipid molecules, specific water pores, or other pores (e.g., ion channels). Water molecules always move in the direction of a higher solute (dissolved particle) concentration.

Cells and Organelles

All tissues in the body are made of cells. Each cell contains several internal structures called organelles. These organelles include the nucleus, the mitochondrion, and other structures that are briefly described below. Not all cells contain all structures, because some cells are specialized for particular functions. For example, mature red blood cells are specialized for the transport of the respiratory pigment hemoglobin and oxygen and do not contain a nucleus or any mitochondria.

A typical cell is shown in figure A.18. The average diameter of a cell in the human body is about 10 μm (1/100th of a millimeter), although a wide variety of cell shapes and sizes exist. The cell is compartmentalized, and the organelles are distinct subcellular structures. In total, the adult human body contains about 10^{14} cells. Most cells (apart from those in adipose tissue) are 70% to 80% water.

- The nucleus is the largest organelle. It is usually round or oval shaped and surrounded by a nuclear envelope composed of 2 phospholipid membranes. This envelope contains pores through which messenger molecules pass to the cytoplasm. The nucleus stores genetic information in the form of deoxyribonucleic acid (DNA). That genetic information passes from the nucleus to the cytoplasm, where amino acids are assembled into proteins. The nucleolus is a densely staining region of the nucleus that expresses information required by ribosomal proteins.

- The rough granular endoplasmic reticulum is an extensive network of folded, sheetlike membranes that has ribosomes attached to its surface. Proteins are synthesized on the ribosomes. The smooth (agranular) endoplasmic reticulum is a highly branched tubular network that does not have attached ribosomes. It contains enzymes for fatty acid synthesis and stores and releases calcium, a process important in the regulation of contraction. The specialized smooth endoplasmic reticulum in muscle is called the sarcoplasmic reticulum.

- The Golgi apparatus is a series of cup-shaped flattened membranous sacs associated with numerous vesicles. It concentrates, modifies, and sorts newly synthesized proteins before their distribution, by way of vesicles, to other organelles, to the plasma membrane, or to secretions from the cell.

- The mitochondrion is an oval-shaped body surrounded by two membranes. The inner membrane folds into the matrix of the mitochondrion, forming cristae. This location is the major site of ATP production, oxygen utilization, and carbon dioxide production. It contains the enzymes of fatty acid oxidation, the tricarboxylic acid (Krebs) cycle, and the electron-transport chain.

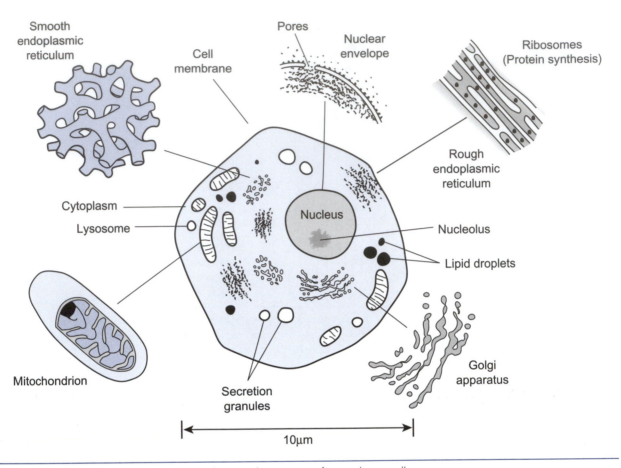

Figure A.18 A typical cell in cross section, showing the structure of several organelles.

- Lysosomes are small membranous vesicles containing digestive enzymes. After injury, these enzymes may be activated and cause necrosis (death) of the cell.

- The cytoplasm, or cytosol, is the fluid portion of the cell surrounding all the organelles. It stores energy in the form of glycogen granules and lipid droplets and contains the enzymes of anaerobic glycolysis.

Although the cell shape and size as depicted in figure A.18 is typical of many cells, other cells are distinctly specialized for the function they perform. For example, skeletal muscle cells are long, cylindrical striated fibers (see figure A.19). The cytoplasm of muscle fibers is the sarcoplasm, and the plasma membrane is the sarcolemma. Myofibrils are the contractile elements, composed of chains of sarcomeres containing thin (actin) and thick (myosin) filaments arranged in a regular array. Surrounding the myofibrils is the sarcoplasmic reticulum, an elaborate baglike membranous structure. Its interconnecting tubules lie in the narrow spaces between the myofibrils, surrounding and running parallel to them. It plays an important role in contraction by storing calcium ions, which when released into the sarcoplasm, initiate muscle contraction. Numerous mitochondria are located—mostly around the outer circumference of the muscle fiber—near the plasma membrane, close to the oxygen supply from the blood capillaries. Muscles contain a mixture of fiber types, classified according to their contractile speed and metabolic characteristics. Further details can be found in chapter 2.

Tissues, Organs, and Systems

The cells of the body form larger structures called tissues (e.g., muscle) and organs (e.g., heart, lungs, and liver). A tissue is a group of similar cells specialized to carry out particular functions. An organ is a distinct body part formed from the combination of all four major tissue groups and designed to carry out a more general function than the tissues within it.

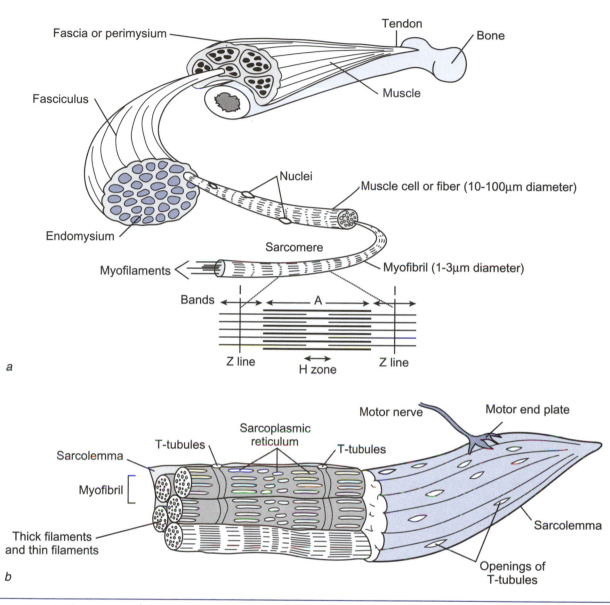

Figure A.19 (a) The structure of skeletal muscle and (b) the ultrastructure of a skeletal muscle fiber showing the location of the myofibrils (contractile proteins) and the sarcoplasmic reticulum.

Although all somatic cells of the body, except the germ cells (sperm in males, oocytes in females), contain the same genetic information, not all of this information in the DNA is expressed in the form of protein. Cellular specialization is possible because of the selective expression of genes by different cells. This specialization is what makes, for example, a skeletal muscle cell different from a nerve cell or a white blood cell. Cells can generally be classified as belonging to one of four groups of tissues: epithelial, connective, nerve, and muscle.

- Epithelial tissue generally forms sheets that protect against abrasion and the entry of potentially

harmful substances or microorganisms. Epithelial tissue comprises the skin surface, the internal linings of the gastrointestinal tract, blood and lymph vessels, the respiratory tract, kidney tubules, ureters, and bladder. Parts of many glands are also formed from epithelial tissue. Some epithelial tissues synthesize and release secretions, and others absorb nutrients.

- Connective tissue connects various body parts and forms supportive or protective structures within and around tissues and organs. Connective tissue forms cartilage and bone, holds bones together, and attaches skeletal muscles to bones and skin. Most connective tissue consists of cells surrounded by an organic, semifluid fibrous matrix. The latter is formed mostly from collagen, a fibrous protein that is synthesized and secreted by specialized epithelial cells called fibroblasts. Blood is a form of connective tissue. Normally the blood cells circulate within a fluid plasma, but after injury to a blood vessel, the plasma forms an insoluble clot by activating an insoluble fibrous protein called fibrinogen.

- Nerve tissue initiates and carries electrical signals that control the actions of many body tissues and organs. Nerve tissue is found in the brain, spinal cord, and nerves. Motor (efferent) nerves convey information from the central nervous system (brain and spinal cord) to the periphery. Information about changes in pressure, chemical composition, and temperature is conveyed from sensory organs in the periphery to the central nervous system by sensory (afferent) nerves.

- Muscle tissue is specialized to exert force by contracting (shortening in length). The three different types of muscle are skeletal muscle, smooth muscle, and cardiac muscle. Skeletal muscle produces body movement through its link to the bones of the skeleton and is under voluntary control. Skeletal muscle cells are long, striated, multinucleated fibers. Smooth muscle is found in internal organs such as the walls of arteries and veins, the esophagus, stomach, and intestines, the bladder, and the airways and is not under voluntary control. Smooth muscle cells are spindle-shaped and smaller than skeletal muscle cells. Cardiac muscle is found in the heart and in the large blood vessels very near the heart. It is involuntary like smooth muscle and striated like skeletal muscle. Cardiac muscle has branching fibers and specialized cell junctions called intercalated disks. These characteristics give it the ability to contract in a repetitive, synchronized manner that pumps blood to the lungs and other organs of the body.

An organ is a distinct body part formed from the combination of all four major tissue groups and designed to carry out a more general function than the tissues within it. For example, the stomach performs digestion. It contains epithelial tissue that forms a protective lining and produces digestive juices, acid, and mucus. Connective tissue supports the stomach wall and forms an outer protective layer. Smooth muscle within the stomach wall exerts forces that mix food with the digestive secretions and propel the food toward the small intestine. Nerve tissue conducts signals that coordinate the actions of the epithelial glands and muscle tissue within the stomach and with other parts of the digestive system.

Appendix B

Unit Conversion Tables

To measure energy, volume, weight, and length, a standardized system known as the System Internationale (S.I.) has been established. The S.I. units are based on the metric system. In many countries, however, the English system of measures is also used, and in the field of nutrition, both systems are utilized. The following tables define the S.I. units and provide equivalents that allow the reader to convert between the English system and the S.I. system.

Table B.1 Systeme Internationale (S.I.) Units

Physical quantity	Name of unit	Symbol	Definition of unit
Length	Meter	m	
Mass	Kilogram	kg	
Time	Second	s	
Temperature	Degrees Kelvin Degrees Celsius	°K °C	Temperature °K − 273.15
Amount of substance	Mole	mol	
Angle	Radian	rad	
Electric current	Ampere	A	
Potential difference	Volt	V	$kg \cdot m^2 \cdot s^{-3} \cdot A^{-1} = J \cdot A^{-1} \cdot s^{-1}$
Electric charge	Coulomb	C	$A \cdot s$
Resistance	Ohm	Ω	$kg \cdot m^2 \cdot s^{-3} \cdot A^{-2} = V \cdot A^{-1}$
Energy	Joule	J	$kg \cdot m^2 \cdot s^{-2}$
Force	Newton	N	$kg \cdot m \cdot s^{-2} = J \cdot m^{-1}$
Power	Watt	W	$kg \cdot m^2 \cdot s^{-3} = J \cdot s^{-1}$
Pressure	Pascal	Pa	$N \cdot m^{-2}$
Frequency	Hertz	Hz	$cycles \cdot s^{-1}$
Density	Kilogram per cubic meter		$kg \cdot m^{-3}$

Table B.2 S.I. Fractions and Multiples

	Prefix	Symbol	Examples
Fraction			
10^{-1}	Deci	d	Deciliter, dl
10^{-2}	Centi	c	Centimeter, cm
10^{-3}	Milli	m	Millisecond, ms
10^{-6}	Micro	μ	Micromole, μmol
10^{-9}	Nano	n	Nanometer, nm
10^{-12}	Pico	p	Picogram, pg
10^{-15}	Femto	f	Femtoliter, fl
Multiple			
10^{3}	Kilo	k	Kilogram, kg
10^{6}	Mega	M	Megajoule, MJ
10^{9}	Giga	G	Gigaohm, GΩ

Table B.3 Derived S.I Units and Non-S.I. Units Used in Biochemistry, Physiology, and Nutrition

Physical quantity	Name of unit	Symbol	Definition of unit
Length	Angstrom Inch Foot	Å in ft	10^{-10} m = 10^{-1} nm 0.0254 m 0.3048 m
Mass	Pound Ounce	lb oz	454 g 28.4g
Temperature	Degree Farenheit	°F	1.8 (°C) + 32
Energy	Erg Calorie Horsepower	erg cal h.p.	10^{-7} J 4.1868 J 745.7 W
Force	Dyne	dyn	10^{-5} N
Velocity		V	$m \cdot s^{-1}$ and $km \cdot h^{-1}$
Acceleration			$m \cdot s^{-2}$
Pressure	Bar Atmosphere Torricelli	bar atm torr	10^{5} $N \cdot m^{-2}$ 101.325 $kN \cdot m^{-2}$ 133.322 $N \cdot m^{-2}$
Volume	Liter Pint Fluid ounce	L pint fl oz	10^{-3} m^3 0.473×10^{-3} m^3 29.57×10^{-6} m^3
Density			$g \cdot cm^{-3}$ = $g \cdot ml^{-1}$
Enzyme activity	International unit	IU or U	$\mu mol \cdot min^{-1}$
Concentration	 Weight/volume%	[ ] %w/v	$mol \cdot l^{-1}$ or M $g \cdot dl^{-1}$ or $g \cdot 100$ ml^{-1}
Viscosity	Poise	P	10^{-1} $kg^{-1} \cdot s^{-1}$ = 10^{-1} $Pa \cdot s$
Radioactivity	Curie Roentgen	Ci R	37×10^{9} $counts \cdot s^{-1}$ 22.58×10^{-4} $counts \cdot kg^{-1}$

Table B.4 Useful Conversion Factors (Equivalents) for Units of Length, Mass (Weight), Temperature, Energy, and Volume

Physical quantity	Name of unit	Symbol	Approximate equivalent
Length	Inch	in	2.54 cm
	Foot	ft	0.3048 m
	Centimeter	cm	0.394 in
	Meter	m	3.28 ft
Mass	Ounce	oz	28.4 g
	Pound	lb	454 g
	Gram	g	0.035 oz
	Kilogram	kg	2.2 lb
Temperature	Degree Farenheit	°F	$1.8\ (°C) + 32$
	Degree Celsius	°C	$0.555\ (°F) - 32$
Energy	Calorie	cal	4.186 J
	Joule	J	0.239 cal
Volume	Fluid ounce	fl oz	29.57 ml
	Pint	pint	473 ml
	Milliliter	ml	0.034 fl oz
	Liter	L	33.8 fl oz or 2.112 pints
	1 teaspoon		5 ml or 0.17 fl oz
	1 tablespoon		15 ml or 0.51 fl oz
	1 glass or cup		240 ml or 8 fl oz

Appendix C

Recommended Daily Allowances for North America

Table C.1 Recommended Daily Allowances for Vitamins in North America

Age	Thiamin (mg/day)	Riboflavin (mg/day)	Niacin (mg/day)	Vitamin B₆ (mg/day)	Vitamin B₁₂ (µg/day)	Folate (µg/day)	Vitamin C (mg/day)	Vitamin A (µg/day)	Vitamin D (µg/day)
0–6 mo	0.2*	0.3*	2*	0.1*	0.4*	65*	40*	400*	5*
7–12 mo	0.3*	0.4*	4*	0.3*	0.5*	80*	50*	500*	5*
1–3 y	0.5	0.5	6	0.5	0.9	150	15	300	5*
4–8 y	0.6	0.6	8	0.6	1.2	200	25	400	5*
Males									
9–13 y	0.9	0.9	12	1.0	1.8	300	45	600	5*
14–18 y	1.2	1.3	16	1.3	2.4	400	75	900	5*
19–30 y	1.2	1.3	16	1.3	2.4	400	90	900	5*
31–50 y	1.2	1.3	16	1.3	2.4	400	90	900	5*
51–70 y	1.2	1.3	16	1.7	2.4	400	90	900	10*
70+ y	1.2	1.3	16	1.7	2.4	400	90	900	15*
Females									
9–13 y	0.9	0.9	12	1.0	1.8	300	45	600	5*
14–18 y	1.0	1.0	14	1.2	2.4	400	65	700	5*
19–30 y	1.1	1.1	14	1.3	2.4	400	75	700	5*
31–50 y	1.1	1.1	14	1.3	2.4	400	75	700	5*
51–70 y	1.1	1.1	14	1.5	2.4	400	75	700	10*
70+ y	1.1	1.1	14	1.5	2.4	400	75	700	15*
Pregnancy									
<18 y	1.4	1.4	18	1.9	2.6	600	80	750	5*
18–30 y	1.4	1.4	18	1.9	2.6	600	85	770	5*
31–50 y	1.4	1.4	18	1.9	2.6	600	85	770	5*
Lactation									
<18 y	1.4	1.6	17	2	2.8	500	115	1200	5*
18–30 y	1.4	1.6	17	2	2.8	500	120	1300	5*
31–50 y	1.4	1.6	17	2	2.8	500	120	1300	5*

* Adequate intakes

Table C.2 Recommended Daily Allowances for Minerals in North America

Age	Calcium (mg/day)	Phosphorus (mg/day)	Magnesium (mg/day)	Iron (mg/day)	Zinc (mg/day)	Copper (mg/day)	Selenium (mg/day)	Iodine (mg/day)
0–6 mo	210*	100*	30*	0.27*	2.0	0.2*	0.015*	0.11*
7–12 mo	270*	275*	75*	11.0	3.0	0.2*	0.02*	0.13*
1–3 y	500*	460	80*	7.0	3.0	0.34	0.02	0.09
4–8 y	800*	500	130*	10.0	5.0	0.34	0.03	0.09
Males								
9–13 y	1300*	1250	240*	8.0	8.0	0.70	0.04	0.12
14–18 y	1300*	1250	410*	11.0	11.0	0.89	0.055	0.15
19–30 y	1000*	700	400*	8.0	11.0	0.90	0.055	0.15
31–50 y	1000*	700	420*	8.0	11.0	0.90	0.055	0.15
51–70 y	1200*	700	420*	8.0	11.0	0.90	0.055	0.15
70+ y	1200*	700	420*	8.0	11.0	0.90	0.055	0.15
Females								
9–13 y	1300*	1250	240*	8.0	8.0	0.70	0.04	0.12
14–18 y	1300*	1250	360*	15.0	9.0	0.89	0.055	0.15
19–30 y	1000*	700	310*	18.0	8.0	0.90	0.055	0.15
31–50 y	1000*	700	320*	18.0	8.0	0.90	0.055	0.15
51–70 y	1200*	700	320*	8.0	8.0	0.90	0.055	0.15
70+ y	1200*	700	320*	8.0	8.0	0.90	0.055	0.15
Pregnancy								
<18 y	1300*	1250	400*	27	12	1.00	0.06	0.22
18–30 y	1000*	700	350*	27	11	1.00	0.06	0.22
31–50 y	1000*	700	360*	27.0	11.0	1.00	0.06	0.22
Lactation								
<18 y	1300*	1250	360*	10.0	13	1.30	0.07	0.29
18–30 y	1000*	700	310*	9.0	12	1.30	0.07	0.29
31–50 y	1000*	700	320*	9.0	12	1.30	0.07	0.29

*Adequate intakes

Table C.3 Recommended Daily Allowances for Protein in North America

Age	Reference nutrient intake (g/day)
0–6 mo	9.1*
7–12 mo	13.5
1–3 y	13.0
4–8 y	19.0
Males	
9–13 y	34.0
14–18 y	52.0
19–70 y	56.0
70+ y	56.0
Females	
9–13 y	34.0
14–18 y	46.0
19–70 y	46.0
70+ y	46.0
Pregnancy	
<18 y	71.0
18–30 y	71.0
31–50 y	71.0
Lactation	
<18 y	71.0
18–30 y	71.0
31–50 y	71.0

*Adequate intakes

Appendix D

Reference Nutrient Intakes for the United Kingdom

Table D.1   Reference Nutrient Intake for Vitamins in the United Kingdom

Age	Thiamin (mg/day)	Riboflavin (mg/day)	Niacin (mg/day)	Vitamin B₆ (mg/day)	Vitamin B₁₂ (µg/day)	Folate (µg/day)	Vitamin C (mg/day)	Vitamin A (µg/day)	Vitamin D (µg/day)
0–3 mo	0.2	0.4	3	0.2	0.3	50	25	350	8.5
4–6 mo	0.2	0.4	3	0.2	0.3	50	25	350	8.5
7–9 mo	0.2	0.4	4	0.3	0.4	50	25	350	7
10–12 mo	0.3	0.4	5	0.4	0.4	50	25	350	7
1–3 y	0.5	0.6	8	0.7	0.5	70	30	400	*
4–6 y	0.7	0.8	11	0.9	0.8	100	30	400	*
7–10 y	0.7	1.0	12	1.0	1.0	150	30	500	*
Males									
11–14 y	0.9	1.2	15	1.2	1.2	200	35	600	*
15–18 y	1.1	1.3	18	1.5	1.5	200	40	700	*
19–50 y	1.0	1.3	17	1.4	1.5	200	40	700	*
50+ y	0.9	1.3	16	1.4	1.5	200	40	700	*
Females									
11–14 y	0.7	1.1	12	1.0	1.2	200	35	600	*
15–18 y	0.8	1.1	14	1.2	1.5	200	40	600	*
19–50 y	0.8	1.1	13	1.2	1.5	200	40	600	*
50+ y	0.8	1.1	12	1.2	1.5	200	40	600	*
Pregnancy	+0.1	+0.3	*	*	*	*	*	*	*
Lactation									
0–4 mo	+0.2	+0.5	+2	*	+0.5	+60	+30	+350	10
4+ mo	+0.2	+0.5	+2	*	+0.5	+60	+30	+350	10

From Report on Health and Social Subjects: no 41. Dietary Reference Values for food energy and nutrients in the United Kingdom. Report of the Panel on Dietary Reference Values of the Committee on Medical Aspects of Food Policy. London: Her Majesty's Stationery Office, 1991. This is the UK's report Table 1.4.

*No recommendation.

Table D.2 Reference Nutrient Intake for Minerals in the United Kingdom

Age	Calcium (mg/day)	Phosphorus (mg/day)	Magnesium (mg/day)	Sodium (mg/day)	Potassium (mg/day)	Chloride (mg/day)	Iron (mg/day)	Zinc (mg/day)	Copper (mg/day)	Selenium (μg/day)	Iodine (μg/day)
0–3 mo	525	400	55	210	800	320	1.7	4.0	0.2	10	50
4–6 mo	525	400	60	280	850	400	4.3	4.0	0.3	13	60
7–9 mo	525	400	75	320	700	500	7.8	5.0	0.3	10	60
10–12 mo	525	400	80	350	700	500	7.8	5.0	0.3	10	60
1–3 y	350	270	85	500	800	800	6.9	5.0	0.4	15	70
4–6 y	450	350	120	700	1100	1100	6.1	6.5	0.6	20	100
7–10 y	550	450	200	1200	2000	1800	8.7	7.0	0.7	30	110
Males											
11–14 y	1000	775	280	1600	3100	2500	11.3	9.0	0.8	45	130
15–18 y	1000	775	300	1600	3500	2500	11.3	9.5	1.0	70	140
19–50 y	700	550	300	1600	3500	2500	8.7	9.5	1.2	75	140
50+ y	700	550	300	1600	3500	2500	8.7	9.5	1.2	75	140
Females											
11–14 y	800	625	280	1600	3100	2500	14.8	9.0	0.8	45	130
15–18 y	800	625	300	1600	3500	2500	14.8	7.0	1.0	60	140
19–50 y	700	550	270	1600	3500	2500	14.8	7.0	1.2	60	140
50+ y	700	550	270	1600	3500	2500	8.7	7.0	1.2	60	140
Pregnancy	*	*	*	*	*	*	*	*	*	*	*
Lactation											
0–4 mo	+550	+450	+50	*	*	*	*	+6.0	+0.3	+15	*
4+ mo	+550	+450	+50	*	*	*	*	+2.5	+0.3	+15	*

From Report on Health and Social Subjects: no 41. Dietary Reference Values for food energy and nutrients in the United Kingdom.

Report of the Panel on Dietary Reference Values of the Committee on Medical Aspects of Food Policy. London: Her Majesty's Stationary Office, 1991. This is the UK's report Table 1.5.

*No recommendations.

Table D.3 Reference Nutrient Intake for Protein in the United Kingdom

Age	Reference nutrient intake (g/day)
0–3 mo	12.5
4–6 mo	12.7
7–9 mo	13.7
10–12 mo	14.9
1–3 y	14.5
4–6 y	19.7
7–10 y	28.3
Males	
11–14 y	42.1
15–18 y	55.2
19–50 y	55.5
50+ y	53.3
Females	
11–14 y	41.2
15–18 y	55.2
19–50 y	55.5
50+ y	53.3
Pregnancy	+6
Lactation	
0–4 mo	+11
4+ mo	+8

From Report on Health and Social Subjects: no 41. Dietary Reference Values for food energy and nutrients in the United Kingdom.

Report of the Panel on Dietary Reference Values of the Committee on Medical Aspects of Food Policy. London: Her Majesty's Stationary Office, 1991.

This is the UK's report Table 1.4.

These figures assume complete digestibility.

Appendix E

Recommended Dietary Intakes for Australia

Table E.1 Recommended Dietary Intakes of Vitamins, Minerals, and Protein for Children Under 7 Years in Australia Expressed As Mean Daily Intake

	Infants 0–6 mo		Infants	Young children	
	Breast-fed	Bottle-fed	7–12 mo	1–3 y	4–7 y
Vitamin A (µg retinol equivalents)	425	425	300	300	350
Thiamin (mg)	0.15	0.25	0.35	0.5	0.7
Riboflavin (mg)	0.4	0.4	0.6	0.8	1.1
Niacin (mg niacin equivalents)	4	4	7	10	12
Vitamin B_6 (mg)	0.25	0.25	0.45	0.6–0.9	0.8–1.3
Total folate (µg)	50	50	75	100	100
Vitamin B_{12} (µg)	0.3	0.3	0.7	1.0	1.5
Vitamin C (mg)	25	25	30	30	30
Vitamin E (mg α tocopherol equivalents)	2.5	4.0	4.0	5.0	6.0
Zinc (mg)	3	3–6	4.5	4.5	6
Iron (mg)	0.5	3.0	9.0	6–8	6–8
Iodine (µg)	50	50	60	70	90
Magnesium (mg)	40	40	60	80	110
Calcium (mg)	300	500	550	700	800
Phosphorus (mg)	150	150	300	500	700
Selenium (µg)	10	10	15	25	30
Sodium (mmol)	6–12	6–12	14–25	14–50	20–75
(mg)	140–280	140–280	320–580	320–1,150	460–1,730
Potassium (mmol)	10–15	10–15	12–35	25–70	40–100
(mg)	390–580	390–580	470–1,370	980–2,730	1,560–3,900
Protein (g)	*	2.0 per kg b.w.	1.6 per kg b.w.	14–18	18–24

Asterisk (*) indicates no recommendation has been made for protein for breast-fed infants under the age of 6 months. Many observations show that infants breast-fed by healthy well-nourished mothers grow at a satisfactory rate for diet in the first 4 to 6 months. Therefore, protein requirements are assumed to be met if the volume of milk maintains growth at an acceptable rate.

Table E.2 Recommended Dietary Intakes of Vitamins, Minerals, and Protein for Children Over 7 Years in Australia Expressed As Mean Daily Intake

	Boys			Girls		
	8–11 y	12–15 y	16–18 y	8–11 y	12–15 y	16–18 y
Vitamin A (μg retinol equivalents)	500	725	750	500	725	750
Thiamin (mg)	0.9	1.2	1.2	0.8	1.0	0.9
Riboflavin (mg)	1.4	1.8	1.9	1.3	1.6	1.4
Niacin (mg niacin equivalents)	15	20	21	15	18	16
Vitamin B_6 (mg)	1.1–1.6	1.4–2.1	1.3–2.2	1.0–1.5	1.2–1.8	1.1–1.6
Total folate (μg)	150	200	200	150	200	200
Vitamin B_{12} (μg)	1.5	2.0	2.0	1.5	2.0	2.0
Vitamin C (mg)	30	30	40	30	30	30
Vitamin E (mg α-tocopherol equivalents)	8.0	10.5	11.0	8.0	9.0	8.0
Zinc (mg)	9	12	12	9	12	12
Iron (mg)	6–8	10–13	10–13	6–8	10–13	10–13
Iodine (μg)	120	150	150	120	120	120
Magnesium (mg)	180	260	320	160	240	270
Calcium (mg)	800	1,200	1,000	900	1,000	800
Phosphorus (mg)	800	1,200	1,100	800	1,200	1,100
Selenium (μg)	50	85	85	50	70	70
Sodium (mmol)	26–100	40–100	40–100	26–100	40–100	40–100
(mg)	600–2,300	920–2,300	920–2,300	600–2,300	920–2,300	920–2,300
Potassium (mmol)	50–140	50–140	50–140	50–140	50–140	50–140
(mg)	1,950–5,460	1,950–5,460	1,950–5,460	1,950–5,460	1,950–5,460	1,950–5,460
Protein (g)	27–38	42–60	64–70	27–39	44–55	57

Table E.3 Recommended Dietary Intakes of Vitamins, Minerals, and Protein for Adults in Australia Expressed As Mean Daily Intake

	Men			Women			
	19–64 y	64+ y	19–54 y	54+ y	Pregnant	Lactating
Vitamin A (µg retinol equivalents)	750	750	750	750	+0	+450
Thiamin (mg)	1.1	0.9	0.8	0.7	+0.2	+0.4
Riboflavin (mg)	1.7	1.3	1.2	1.0	+0.3	+0.5
Niacin (mg niacin equivalents)	19	16	13	11	+2	+5
Vitamin B$_6$ (mg)	1.3–1.9	1.0–1.5	0.9–1.4	0.8–1.1	+0.1	+0.7–0.8
Total folate (µg)	200	200	200	200	+200	+150
Vitamin B$_{12}$ (µg)	2.0	2.0	2.0	2.0	+1.0	+0.5
Vitamin C (mg)	40	40	30	30	+30	+45
Vitamin E (mg α-tocopherol equivalents)	10.0	10.0	7.0	7.0	+0	+2.5
Zinc (mg)	12	12	12	12	+4	+6
Iron (mg)	7	7	12–16	5–7	+10–20	+0
Iodine (µg)	150	150	120	120	+30	+50
Magnesium (mg)	320	320	270	270	+30	+70
Calcium (mg)	800	800	800	1,000	+300	+400
Phosphorus (mg)	1,000	1,000	1,000	1,000	+200	+200
Selenium (µg)	85	85	70	70	+10	+15
Sodium (mmol)	40–100	40–100	40–100	40–100	+0	+0
(mg)	920–2,300	920–2,300	920–2,300	920–2,300	+0	+0
Potassium (mmol)	50–140	50–140	50–140	50–140	+0	+0
(mg)	1,950–5,460	1,950–5,460	1,950–5,460	1,950–5,460	+0	+0
Protein (g)	55	55	45	55	+6	+16

National Health and Medical Research Council, Australia 1982-1989.

Glossary

α-amylase or amylase—A digestive enzyme found in saliva that begins the digestion of starches in the mouth (also called ptyalin). It catalyzes the hydrolysis of starch by cleaving the α-1-4-glycosidic linkages between the component glucose molecules. Amylase is also present in pancreatic juice.

1,3-DPG (1,3-diphosphoglycerate)—An intermediate compound in glycolysis.

2,3-DPG (2,3-diphosphoglycerate)—A highly anionic organic phosphate that is present in human red blood cells at about the same molar ratio as haemoglobin. It binds to deoxyhemoglobin but not the oxygenated form, therefore diminishing the oxygen affinity of haemoglobin. This is essential in enabling haemoglobin to unload oxygen in tissue capillaries.

3-methylhistidine—A metabolite of the amino acid histidine. Its urinary excretion is used as an index of contractile protein breakdown.

5-HT (5-Hydroxytryptamine)—A brain neurotransmitter. Also known as serotonin.

absorption—The transport of nutrients from the intestine into the blood or lymph system.

accelerometer—Small piece of equipment that can be attached to the body and register all accelerations the body makes. The number and the degree of the accelerations give an indication of someone's activity level.

acclimatization—Adaptation of the body to an environmental extreme (e.g., heat, cold, and altitude).

acetyl CoA—The major fuel for the oxidative processes in the body, being derived from the breakdown of glycogen, glucose, and fatty acids.

acid—A substance that tends to lose a proton (hydrogen ion).

acid-base balance—The relative balance of acid and base products in the body.

acidosis—A disturbance of the normal acid-base balance in which excess acids accumulate causing a fall in pH (e.g., when lactic acid accumulates in muscle and blood during high-intensity exercise).

ACSM—American College of Sports Medicine.

ACTH (adrenocorticotrophic hormone)—Hormone secreted from anterior pituitary gland, which stimulates release of cortisol from adrenal glands.

actin—One of the major contractile proteins in muscle found in the thin filaments.

active transport—The movement or transport across cell membranes by membrane carriers. An expenditure of energy (ATP) is required.

acute phase proteins—Several proteins released from liver (e.g., C-reactive protein) and leukocytes that aid body's response to injury or infection.

acyl carrier protein (ACP)—Protein that transports a fatty acyl-carnitine complex (a fatty acid linked to carnitine) across the inner mitochondrial membrane. Also known as the fatty acyl-carnitine translocase.

acyl group—The long hydrocarbon chain of a fatty acid.

adaptogen—A name used for substances that help the body to adapt to stress situations.

adenine (A)—A purine nucleotide found in DNA and several coenzymes.

Adequate Intake (AI)—Recommended dietary intake comparable to the RDA but based on less scientific evidence.

adipocyte—An adipose tissue cell whose main function is to store triacylglycerol (fat).

adipose tissue—White fatty tissue that stores triacylglycerol.

adipose tissue-free skeletal muscle (ATFSM)—Lean muscle tissue.

ADP (adenosine diphosphate)—Breakdown product of ATP.

adrenaline—A hormone secreted by the adrenal gland. It is a stimulant that prepares the body for "fight or flight" and an important activator of fat and carbohydrate breakdown during exercise. Also known as epinephrine.

aerobic—Occurring in the presence of free oxygen.

alanine—A nonessential amino acid.

alcohol—A colorless liquid with depressant and intoxicating effects. Ethyl alcohol or ethanol (C_2H_5OH) is the alcohol found in wines, spirits, and beers.

aldosterone—A steroid hormone secreted by the adrenal cortex. Primarily involved in fluid and electrolyte balance by controlling sodium and potassium excretion by the kidneys.

alimentary tract—See gastrointestinal tract.

alkalinizer—A group of substances with a buffering function (sodium bicarbonate, sodium citrate).

α-ketoisocaproate (α-KIC)—A metabolite of the amino acid leucine.

alpha-tocopherol—The most biologically active alcohol in vitamin E.

amenorrhea—The absence of at least 3 successive menstrual cycles in females.

amino acid (AA)—The chief structural molecule of protein, consisting of an amino group (NH_2) and a carboxylic acid group (CO_2H) plus another so-called R-group that determines the amino acid's properties. Twenty different amino acids can be used to make proteins.

ammonia (NH_3)—A metabolic by-product of the oxidation of amino acids. It may be transformed into urea for excretion from the body.

AMP (adenosine monophosphate)—Product of the breakdown of adenosine diphosphate.

amylase—See α-amylase.

amylopectin—A branched-chain starch (polymer of glucose).

amylose—A straight-chain starch that is more resistant to digestion compared with amylopectin.

anabolism—Constructive metabolism, the process whereby simple body compounds are formed into more complex ones.

anaerobic—Occurring in the absence of free oxygen.

androstenediol—A steroid metabolite.

androstenedione—An androgenic steroid produced in the body that is converted to testosterone. Marketed as a dietary supplement.

anemia—A condition defined by an abnormally low blood hemoglobin content resulting in a lowered oxygen carrying capacity.

anion—A negatively charged ion or electrolyte (e.g., chloride, Cl^-; phosphate, HPO_4^{2-}).

anorexia athletica—A form of anorexia nervosa observed in athletes who show significant symptoms of eating disorders but who do not meet the criteria of the *Diagnostic and Statistical Manual of Mental Disorders* (American Psychiatric Association 1987) for anorexia or bulimia nervosa.

anorexia nervosa—An eating disorder characterized by an abnormally small food intake and a refusal to maintain a normal body weight (according to what is expected for gender, age, and height), a distorted view of body image, an intense fear of being fat or overweight and gaining weight or "feeling fat" when clearly the individual is below normal weight, and the absence of at least three successive menstrual cycles in females (amenorrhea).

anthropometry—Use of body girths and diameters to evaluate body composition.

antibody—Soluble protein produced by B lymphocytes with antimicrobial effects. Also known as immunoglobulin.

antidiuretic hormone (ADH)—A hormone secreted by the posterior pituitary gland that influences water reabsorption by the kidneys.

antioxidant—Molecules that can prevent or limit the actions of free radicals usually by removing their unpaired electron and thus converting them into something far less reactive.

apoptosis—An internal program that allows damaged or obsolete cells to commit suicide.

appendix—A nonfunctional part of the small intestine that is short, thin, and outpouching from the cecum.

appetite—A desire for food for the purpose of enjoyment that is developed through previous experience. Believed to be controlled in humans by an appetite center in the hypothalamus.

arginine—An essential amino acid.

arteriosclerosis—Hardening of the arteries. Also see atherosclerosis.

arteriovenous (AV)—Refers to comparison of arterial and venous blood composition.

ascorbic acid—Vitamin C; major role is as a water-soluble antioxidant.

aspartame—An artificial sweetener made from amino acids.

aspartates—Salts of aspartic acid, an amino acid.

atherosclerosis—A specific form of arteriosclerosis characterized by the formation of fatty plaques on the luminal walls of arteries.

atom—The smallest unit of an element that retains all the properties of the element. The atoms of all elements can be broken down physically into the same subatomic particles: protons, neutrons, and electrons. Hence, the atoms of the various elements only differ in the numbers of protons, neutrons, and electrons that they contain.

ATP (adenosine triphosphate)—A high-energy compound that is the immediate source for muscular contraction and other energy-requiring processes in the cell.

ATPase (adenosine triphosphatase)—An enzyme that breaks down ATP to ADP and inorganic phosphate, releasing energy that can be used to fuel biological work.

atrophy—A wasting away, a diminution in the size of a cell, tissue, organ, or part.

Atwater factor—The average net energy values for carbohydrate, fat, and protein named after Wilbur Olin Atwater: 16 kJ/g (4 kcal/g) carbohydrate, 36 kJ/g (9 kcal/g) for fat, and 16 kJ/g (4 kcal/g) for protein.

autosome—Any chromosome occurring in a similar form in males and females and, therefore, able to pair fully during meiosis and mitosis. Distinguished from the sex chromosomes, which differ in the two sexes.

AV-differences—A difference between arterial and venous concentration of a substance, indicating net uptake or release of that substance.

average daily metabolic rate (ADMR)—The average energy expenditure over 24 hours.

base—A substance that tends to donate an electron pair or coordinate an electron.

BCAA (branched-chain amino acid)—Three essential amino acids that can be oxidized by muscle. Includes leucine, isoleucine, and valine.

β-carotene—A precursor for vitamin A found in plants. Also called provitamin A.

beta-hydroxy beta methylbutyrate (HMB)—Metabolite of the essential amino acid leucine. Marketed as a muscle growth promotor.

β-oxidation—Oxygen-requiring process in the mitochondria whereby 2-carbon units are sequentially removed from the hydrocarbon chain of a fatty acid in the form of acetyl-CoA, which can then enter the TCA cycle.

bile—Fluid produced by the liver and stored in the gall bladder that contains bile salts, bile pigments, cholesterol, and other molecules. The bile is secreted into the small intestine.

bile salts—Salts or derivatives of cholesterol in bile that are polar on one end and nonpolar on the other end of the molecule. Bile salts act to emulsify fat in the lumen of the small intestine.

bioavailability—In relation to nutrients in food, the amount that may be absorbed into the body.

bioelectrical impedance analysis (BIA)—A method to calculate percentage of body fat by measuring electrical resistance due to the water content of the body.

biopsy—A small sample of tissue taken for analysis.

b.m.—Body mass in kilograms (kg).

BMI (body mass index)—Body mass in kilograms divided by height in meters squared (kg/m^2). An index used as a measure of obesity.

BMR (basal metabolic rate)—Energy expenditure under basal, postabsorptive conditions representing the energy needed to maintain life under these basal conditions.

bomb calorimeter—An instrument to measure the energy content in which food is oxidized and the resulting heat production is measured.

breath-by-breath system—An automated system to analyse gas exchange to estimate energy expenditure and substrate utilization. These systems are able to measure CO_2 production and oxygen consumption from every breath.

brush border—Where the absorption of nutrients takes place in the intestine. The surface of the epithelial cells that line the intestinal wall is covered with microvilli that form the brush border.

buffer—A substance that, in solution, prevents rapid changes in hydrogen ion concentration (pH).

bulimia nervosa—An eating disorder characterized by repeated episodes of binge eating (consumption of large amounts of usually energy-dense foods) followed by purging of the stomach contents, allowing insufficient time for most of the nutrients from the heavy meal to be absorbed.

bulk flow—The transport of materials by the movement of the gas or liquid in which they are contained.

b.w.—Body weight.

caffeine—A stimulant drug found in many food products such as coffee, tea, and cola drinks. Stimulates the central nervous system and used as an ergogenic aid.

calorie (cal)—Traditional unit of energy. One calorie expresses the quantity of energy (heat) needed to raise the temperature of 1 g (1 ml) of water 1° C (from 14.5° C to 15.5° C).

calorimeter—An insulated chamber to estimate energy expenditure by measuring heat dissipation from the body. This method is called direct calorimetry.

cAMP (cyclic adenosine monophosphate)—An important intracellular messenger in the action of hormones.

C_aO_2 (content of oxygen in arterial blood)—The amount of oxygen per liter of arterial blood.

capillary—The smallest vessel in the cardiovascular system. Capillary walls are only one cell thick. All exchanges of molecules between the blood and tissue fluid occur across the capillary walls.

Carbohydrate (CHO)—A compound composed of carbon, hydrogen, and oxygen in a ration of 1:2:1 (i.e., CH_2O). Carbohydrates include sugars, starches, and dietary fibers.

carboloading—Eating large quantities of carbohydrate to optimize body glycogen stores. Common practice of endurance athletes.

carboxylation—A reaction involving the addition of CO_2, catalyzed by an enzyme using biotin as its prosthetic group.

carcinogen—A cancer-inducing substance.

carnitine—A compound used to assist the transport of fatty acyl-CoA molecules from the muscle sarcoplasm across the mitochondrial inner membrane into the mitochondria for subsequent oxidation.

catabolism—Destructive metabolism whereby complex chemical compounds in the body are degraded to simpler ones (e.g., glycogen to glucose; proteins to amino acids).

catalyst—A substance that accelerates a chemical reaction, usually by temporarily combining with the substrates and lowering the activation energy, and is recovered unchanged at the end of the reaction (e.g., an enzyme).

cation—A positively charged ion or electrolyte (e.g., sodium, Na^+; calcium Ca^{2+}).

CD (clusters of differentiation or cluster designators)—Proteins expressed on the cell surface of leukocytes (white blood cells) that can be used to identify different types of leukocyte or subsets of lymphocytes.

cecum—A blind pouch, open only at one end, at the beginning of the large intestine.

cell—The smallest discrete living unit of the body.

cellulose—A major component of plant cell walls and the most abundant nonstarch polysaccharide. Cannot be digested by human digestive enzymes.

cerebrospinal fluid (CSF)—The fluid found in the brain and spinal cord.

ceruloplasmin—A glycoprotein that binds copper and is thought to exert a protective effect against cellular damage caused by free radicals.

CHD (coronary heart disease)—Narrowing of the arteries supplying the heart muscle that can cause heart attacks.

cholecystokinin—A hormone secreted by the duo-denum that acts to stimulate the secretion of enzymes in pancreatic juice.

cholesterol—A lipid transported in the blood in high and low density lipoproteins (HDL and LDL, respectively). High HDL levels are somewhat protective against coronary heart disease.

choline—Can be found in phospholipids (phosphatidylcholine and sphingomyelin) and is a precursor for the neurotransmitter acetylcholine.

chromium—A trace element that plays a role in glucose metabolism.

chylomicrons—A class of lipoproteins that transport exogenous (dietary) cholesterol and triglycerides from the small intestine to tissues after meals.

chyme—The food in the gastrointestinal tract mixed with various secretions of the gastrointestinal tract, forming an homogenous souplike liquid.

cirrhosis—A degenerative disease of the liver. The most common cause is excessive consumption of alcohol.

cis-—A prefix indicating that geometrical isomer in which the two like groups are on the same side of a double bond with restricted rotation (e.g., in unsaturated fatty acids in which the hydrogen ions are on the same side of the double bond).

CK (creatine kinase)—An enzyme that catalyzes the transfer of phosphate from phosphocreatine to ADP to form ATP. Also known as creatine phosphokinase.

closed circuit spirometry—A method to measure resting energy expenditure in which the subject breathes through a mouthpiece into a closed system (spirometer) prefilled with 100% oxygen.

CO_2 (carbon dioxide)—Gas produced during oxidation of carbohydrates and fats.

CoA (coenzyme A)—A molecule that acts as a carrier for acyl or acetyl groups (A stands for acetylation).

CoA-SH—Free form of coenzyme A.

coefficient of digestibility—The percentage energy of food ingested that is actually digested, absorbed, and available for metabolic processes in the body.

coenzyme—Small molecules that are essential in stoichiometric amounts for the activity of some enzymes. Examples include nicotinamide adenine dinucleotide (NAD), flavin adenine dinucleotide (FAD), pyridoxal phosphate (PLP), thiamin pyrophosphate (TPP), and biotin.

colon—The large intestine. This part of the intestine is mainly responsible for forming, storing, and expelling feces.

complement—Soluble proteins found in body fluids and produced by the liver. Once activated, they exert several antimicrobial effects.

complex carbohydrates—Foods containing starch and other polysaccharides as found in bread, pasta, cereals, fruits, and vegetables in contrast to simple carbohydrates such as glucose, milk sugar, and table sugar.

concentration gradient—Difference in concentration of a substance on either side of a membrane.

condensation—A reaction involving the union of two or more molecules with the elimination of a simpler group such as H_2O.

conduction—In relation to body temperature, the transfer of heat from one substance to another by direct contact.

conformation—Shape of molecules determined by rotation about single bonds, especially in polypeptide chains about carbon-carbon links.

convection—Heat exchange that occurs between a solid medium (e.g., the human body) and one that moves (e.g., air or water).

COOH or CO_2H (carboxyl group)—Acidic group of amino acids and components of the TCA cycle.

CoQ (Coenzyme Q, Q10, or ubiquinone)—An electron carrier that mediates transfer of electrons from flavoprotein to cytochrome c in the electron-transport chain that is located in the inner mitochondrial membrane.

cortisol—A steroid hormone secreted from the adrenal glands.

covalent bond—A chemical bond in which two or more atoms are held together by the interaction of their outer electrons.

covalent regulation—Control of enzyme activity by covalent bonding of phosphate groups to sites other than the active site of the enzyme.

CPT (carnitine palmitoyl transferase)—Enzyme that links the fatty acid palmitate to carnitine so that it can be transported across the inner mitochondrial membrane for subsequent oxidation. Also known as carnitine acyl transferase (CAT).

creatine (Cr)—Compound synthesized from amino acids that is the precursor of phosphocreatine, an important anaerobic energy source for high-intensity exercise.

creatinine—A product of creatine breakdown that is found in the urine. Can be measured to assess overall kidney function. An abnormally elevated blood creatinine level is seen in those individuals with kidney insufficiency and kidney failure.

CSF (colony-stimulating factor)—A cytokine that stimulates increased production and release of leukocytes (white blood cells) from the bone marrow.

CT (computed tomography)—A method that uses ionizing radiation via an X-ray beam to create images of body segments. The CT scan produces qualitative and quantitative information about the total area of the tissue investigated, and the thickness and volume of tissues within an organ.

cutaneous—In the skin.

C_vO_2 (content of oxygen in venous blood)—The amount of oxygen per liter of venous blood (a bar over the v signifies mixed venous blood).

cytochrome—An iron-containing heme protein of the mitochondrial electron transport chain that can be alternately oxidized and reduced.

cytokine—Protein released from cells that acts as a chemical messenger by binding to receptors on other cells. Cytokines include interleukins (IL), tumor necrosis factors (TNF), colony-stimulating factors (CSF), and interferons (IFN).

cytosine (C)—A pyrimidine nucleotide found in DNA.

cytotoxic—Ability to kill other cells (e.g., those infected with a virus).

deamination—Reaction involving the loss of an amino (NH_2) group.

decarboxylation—Reaction involving the loss of a CO_2 group.

dehydration—Reaction involving the loss of a water molecule or loss of body water.

dehydroepiandrosterone (DHEA)—An androgen steroid sold as a nutrition supplement. It is often referred to as the "youth hormone."

dehydrogenation—A form of oxidation in which hydrogen atoms are removed from a molecule.

delta efficiency (DE)—The change in energy expended per minute relative to the change in actual work accomplished per minute.

denaturation—Alteration of the physical properties and 3-dimensional structure of a protein by a chemical or physical treatment that does not disrupt the primary structure but generally results in the inactivation of the protein (e.g., the inactivation of enzyme activity by the addition of a strong acid).

dental caries—Erosion or decay of tooth caused by the effects of bacteria in the mouth.

densitometry—Method used to estimate the density (mass per unit volume) of the tissues or the whole body.

DEXA (or DXA)—Dual energy X-ray absorptiometry is a high-tech technique that has become the clinical standard to measure bone density. The principle is based on absorption of low-energy X-rays.

DHA (dihydroxyacetone)—When linked to phosphate is a metabolite in glycolysis. In combination with pyruvate, it is marketed as an ergogenic aid.

DHEA (dehydroepiandrosterone)—A steroid hormone produced endogenously by the adrenal gland. May be marketed as a nutritional sports ergogenic as derived from herbal precursors.

DHEAS (dehydroepiandrosterone sulphate)—Sulphated form of DHEA, a steroid hormone produced endogenously by the adrenal gland.

diabetes mellitus—A disorder of carbohydrate metabolism caused by disturbances in production or utilization of insulin. Causes high blood glucose levels and loss of sugar in the urine.

diacylglycerol—Glycerol backbone with two fatty acids. Formed by the removal of one fatty acid from triacylglycerol. Also known as diglyceride.

diarrhea—Frequent passage of a watery fecal discharge because of a gastrointestinal disturbance or infection.

diastolic—The time, in between ventricular contractions (systole), at which ventricular filling occurs.

dietary reference intake (DRI)—The term used to encompass the latest nutrient recommendations by the Food and Nutrition Board of the National Academy of Sciences.

Dietary Supplement Health and Education Act (DSHEA)—Legislation passed by the United States Congress defining a dietary supplement and providing legislation to control advertising and marketing.

diet-induced thermogenesis (DIT)—The energy needed for the digestion, assimilation, and metabolism of food that is consumed (also referred to as thermic effect of food, or TEF).

diffusion—The movement of molecules from a region of high concentration to one of low concentration, brought about by their kinetic energy.

digestion—The process of breaking down food to its smallest components so it can be absorbed in the intestine.

dihydroxyacetone—An intermediate of glycolysis.

direct calorimetry—A method of determining energy expenditure by measuring heat dissipation from the body, usually using an insulated chamber or suit.

direct calorimetry suit—A suit to estimate energy expenditure by measuring heat dissipation from the body. This method is called direct calorimetry.

disaccharide—Sugars that yield two monosaccharides on hydrolysis. Sucrose is the most common and is composed of glucose and fructose.

diuretics—Drugs that act on the kidney to promote urine formation.

d.m. (dry matter, dry material, or dry mass)—Usually refers to tissue weight after removal of water.

DNA (deoxyribonucleic acid)—The compound that forms genes (i.e., the genetic material).

DOPA (dihydroxy phenylalanine)—A neurotransmitter in the brain.

Dopamine—A catecholamine neurotransmitter and hormone formed by decarboxylation of dehydroxyphenylalanine (dopa). A precursor of epinephrine (adrenaline) and norepinephrine (noradrenaline).

Douglas bag—A plastic bag (named after British scientist Claude Douglas) used to collect expired gases for a certain period of time and to measure the volume, the O_2 concentration, and the CO_2 concentration of this gas. From the measurements of inhaled and exhaled air, energy expenditure, and substrate utilization can be calculated.

DRV (daily reference value)—Recommended daily intakes for the macronutrients (carbohydrate, fat, and protein) as well as cholesterol, sodium, and potassium. On a food label, the DRV is based on a 2,000 kcal (8.3 MJ) diet.

duodenum—The first 20 cm to 30 cm of the small intestine.

DV (daily value)—A term used in food labeling that is based on a daily energy intake of 2,000 kcal (8.3 MJ) and for the food labeled. Gives the percentage of the RDI and the DRV recommended for healthy people in the United States.

d.w. (dry weight)—Usually refers to tissue weight after removal of water.

eating disorder—A psychological disorder centering on the avoidance or purging of food, such as anorexia nervosa and bulimia nervosa.

eccentric exercise—Types of exercise that involve lengthening of the muscle during activation, which can cause damage to some of the myofibers. Types of exercise that have a significant eccentric component include downhill running, bench stepping, and lowering of weights.

economy—Oxygen uptake needed to exercise at a certain work load or speed.

eicosanoids—Derivatives of fatty acids in the body that act as cell-cell signaling molecules. They include prostaglandins, thromboxanes, and leukotrienes.

electrolyte—A substance that, when dissolved in water, conducts an electric current. Electrolytes, which include acids, bases, and salts, usually dissociate into ions carrying either a positive charge (cation) or a negative charge (anion).

electron transport chain (ETC)—Proteins located on the inner mitochondrial membrane that transfer electrons from reduced coenzymes NADH and $FADH_2$ to oxygen and allow protons to be pumped into the space between the inner and outer mitochondrial membranes. The flow of H^+ ions (protons) back into the inner mitochondrial matrix through the ATP synthase complex is used to drive ATP synthesis.

element—The smallest units into which a substance can be broken down chemically are the elements, each of which has different and unique properties. Ninety-two different elements are presently known to exist, but only about 12 are common in living organisms. The most abundant are oxygen, carbon, hydrogen, and nitrogen (in that order). These four elements constitute 96% of the mass of a human.

emetics—Drugs that promote vomiting.

EMS—Eosinophilia-myalgia syndrome.

endocrine—Ductless glands that secrete hormones into the blood.

endogenous—From within the body.

energy—The ability to perform work. Energy exists in various forms, including mechanical, heat, and chemical energy.

energy balance—The balance between energy intake and energy expenditure.

energy expenditure (EE)—The energy expended per unit of time to produce power.

energy expenditure for activity (EEA)—The energy cost associated with physical activity (exercise).

enzyme—A protein with specific catalytic activity. They are designated by the suffix "-ase" frequently attached to the type of reaction catalyzed. Virtually all metabolic reactions in the body are dependent on and controlled by enzymes.

ephedrine—An α-adrenergic and β-adrenergic agonist that may also enhance release of norepinephrine. It has been used in the treatment of several disorders, including asthma, heart failure, rhinitis, and urinary incontinence and for its central nervous system stimulatory effects in the treatment of narcolepsy and depression. Ephedrine is on the IOC list of banned substances.

epimerization—A type of asymmetric transformation in organic molecules.

epinephrine—A hormone secreted by the adrenal gland. It is a stimulant and prepares the body for "fight or flight" and an important activator of fat and carbohydrate breakdown during exercise. Also known as adrenaline.

ergogenic—Performance enhancing.

ergogenic aids—Substances that improve exercise performance and are used in attempts to increase athletic or physical performance capacity.

ergolytic—Performance impairing.

erythrocyte—Red blood cell that contains hemoglobin and transports oxygen.

esophageal sphincter—A ring-like band of smooth muscle fibers that act as a valve between the esophagus and the stomach.

esophagus—Part of the intestinal tract located between mouth and stomach.

essential amino acids—Amino acids that must be obtained in the diet and cannot be synthesized in the body. Also known as indispensable amino acids.

essential fatty acids—Those unsaturated fatty acids that cannot be synthesized in the body and must be obtained in the diet (e.g., linoleic acid and linolenic acid).

estimated average requirement (EAR)—Nutrient intake value estimated to meet the requirements of an average individual in a certain age and gender group.

estimated mineral requirement (EMR)—Part of the RDA pertaining to the minimal daily requirement for sodium, chloride, and potassium.

estradiol—A hormone synthesized mainly in the ovary but also in the placenta, testis, and possibly adrenal cortex.

euhydration—Normal state of body hydration (water content).

eumenorrhea—Occurrence of normal menstrual cycles.

evaporation—The loss of water that occurs when water on a surface changes from a liquid to a gas.

excretion—The removal of metabolic wastes.

exogenous—From outside the body.

exogenous carbohydrate oxidation—Oxidation of carbohydrates that have been ingested or infused but are not from body stores.

extracellular fluid (ECF)—Body fluid that is located outside the cells, including the blood plasma, interstitial fluid, cerebrospinal fluid, synovial fluid, and ocular fluid.

F-6-P (fructose-6-phosphate)—A metabolic intermediate in glycolysis.

FA (fatty acid)—A type of fat having a carboxylic acid group (COOH) at one end of the molecule and a methyl (CH_3) group at the other end, separated by a hydrocarbon chain that can vary in length. A typical structure of a fatty acid is $CH_3(CH_2)_{14}COOH$ (palmitic acid or palmitate).

FABPc (cytosolic fatty acid–binding protein)—A protein found in liver and muscle that binds fatty acids in the cytosol of the cell. Involved in transport from plasma membrane to mitochondria.

FABPpm (plasma membrane fatty acid–binding protein)—A protein found in liver and muscle involved in transport of fatty acids across the plasma membrane.

FAD (flavin adenine dinucleotide, oxidized form)—A coenzyme important in energy metabolism.

FADH₂ (flavin adenine dinucleotide, reduced form)—Reduced form of the coenzyme FAD.

fasting—Starvation; abstinence from eating that may be partial or complete.

fat—Fat molecules contain the same structural elements as carbohydrates but with little oxygen relative to carbon and hydrogen and are poorly soluble in water. Fats are also known as lipids (derived from the Greek word *lipos*), and fat is a general name for oils, fats, waxes, and related compounds. Oils are liquid at room temperature, whereas fats are solid.

FAT/CD36—Fatty acid translocator involved in the transport of fatty acids across the plasma membrane

fatty acid–binding protein (FABP)—A protein found in liver and muscle that binds fatty acids in order to maintain a low intracellular free fatty acid concentration.

FDA—United States Food and Drug Administration.

FDP (fructose-1,6-diphosphate)—A metabolic intermediate in glycolysis.

FDPase (fructose-1,6-diphosphatase)—Enzyme that catalyzes the conversion of fructose-1,6-diphosphate to fructose-6-phosphate, a reaction involved in gluconeogenesis.

feces—The excrement discharged from the intestines, consisting of bacteria, cells from the intestines, secretions, and a small amount of food residue.

female athlete triad—A syndrome characterized by the three conditions prevalent in female athletes: amenorrhea, disordered eating, and osteoporosis.

ferritin—A protein that is used to store iron. Ferritin is mostly found in the liver, spleen and bone marrow. Soluble ferritin is released from cells into the blood plasma in direct proportion to cellular ferritin content. Hence the serum ferritin concentration can be used to indicate the status of the body's iron stores.

FFA (free fatty acid)—A fatty acid that is not esterified to glycerol or any other molecule. See FA (fatty acid).

FFM (fat-free mass)—Lean mass of a tissue or the whole body.

fiber—Indigestible carbohydrates.

fish oil—Oils high in unsaturated fats extracted from the bodies of fish or fish parts, especially the livers. The oils are used as dietary supplements.

flux—The rate of flow through a metabolic pathway.

FMN (flavin mononucleotide, oxidized form)—A coenzyme important in energy metabolism.

FMNH₂ (flavin mononucleotide, reduced form)—Reduced form of the coenzyme FMN.

folic acid or folate—A water-soluble vitamin required in the synthesis of nucleic acids. It appears to be essential in preventing certain types of anemia.

food diary—A written record of sequential food intake over a period of time. Details associated with the food intake are often recorded as well.

fractional breakdown rate (FBR)—The relative rate of protein breakdown, which is calculated from measurements using isotopic tracers.

fractional synthesis rate (FSR)—The relative rate of protein synthesis, which is calculated from measurements using isotopic tracers.

free radical—An atom or molecule that possess at least one unpaired electron in its outer orbit. Important free radicals include the superoxide (O_2^-), hydroxyl ($\cdot OH$), and nitric oxide ($\cdot NO$) radicals. They are highly reactive and may cause damage to lipid membranes, causing membrane instability and increased permeability. Free radicals can also cause oxidative damage to proteins, including enzymes and damage to DNA.

fTRP—Free tryptophan (used to distinguish from tryptophan that is bound to protein). Tryptophan is an essential amino acid and a precursor of the neurotransmitter serotonin in the brain.

G-1-P (glucose-1-phosphate)—Compound formed from the breakdown of glycogen.

G-6-P (glucose-6-phosphate)—Compound formed by the addition of a phosphate group to a glucose molecule by the action of hexokinase. Can also be formed from G-1-P by glucose phosphate isomerase. G-6-P is the starting substrate for glycolysis.

GABA (γ-amino butyric acid)—A neurotransmitter in the brain.

gall bladder—A digestive organ that stores bile (produced in the liver), which is used in the digestion and absorption of fats in the duodenum.

gastric emptying—The rate at which substances (food and fluids) leave the stomach into the small intestine. A high gastric emptying rate is desirable for sports drinks.

gastric juice—The secretions by the gastric mucosa. Gastric juice contains water, hydrochloric acid, and pepsinogen as major components.

gastrin—A hormone secreted by the stomach that stimulates gastric secretion of hydrochloric acid and pepsin.

gastrointestinal tract—Gastrointestinal system or alimentary tract. The main sites in the body used for digestion and absorption of nutrients. It consists of the mouth, esophagus, stomach, small intestine, large intestine, rectum, and anus.

GDP (guanosine diphosphate)—Compound formed from the breakdown of guanosine triphosphate (GTP).

gene—A specific sequence in DNA that codes for a particular protein. Genes are located on the chromosomes. Each gene is found in a definite position (locus).

genotype—The genetic composition or assortment of genes that together with environmental influences determines the appearance or phenotype of an individual.

geometrical isomerism—A form of stereoisomerism in which the difference arises because of hindered rotation about a double bond. An unsaturated fatty acid containing one carbon double bond has two isomers, depending on whether the hydrogen atoms are on the same (*cis*) or the opposite (*trans*) sides of the molecule.

ginseng—A root found in Asia and the United States, although the Asian variety is more easily obtainable. Ginseng has been a popular nutritional supplement and medication in Asia for centuries.

glandulars—Extracts from animal glands (such as the adrenals, thymus, pituitary, and testes) that are claimed to enhance the function of the equivalent gland in the human body. However, glandular extracts are degraded during the digestive process and so cannot exert a pharmacological effect.

glomerular filtration rates—Measure of the kidney's ability to filter and remove waste products.

gluconeogenesis—The synthesis of glucose from noncarbohydrate precursors such as glycerol, ketoacids, or amino acids.

GLUT—Glucose (or other monosaccharide) transporter found in cell membranes, including those of the muscle and liver.

GLUT-2—Isoform of the glucose transporter found in the liver and epithelial cell membranes of the gut.

GLUT-4—Isoform of the glucose transporter found in sarcolemma of muscle fibers.

GLUT-5—Isoform of the glucose transporter found in the epithelial cell membranes of the gut. This one is specific for fructose.

glutamate—Amino acid that acts as a neurotransmitter and a precursor of other neurotransmitters.

glutamine—One of the 20 amino acids commonly found in proteins.

glycemic index (GI)—Increase in blood glucose and insulin in response to a meal. The GI of a food is expressed against a reference food, usually glucose.

glycemic load (GL)—Increase in blood glucose and insulin response to a meal (like glycemic index) but does take into account the amount of that food that is normally consumed.

glycerokinase—Enzyme involved in phosphorylation of glycerol to glycerol-3-phosphate.

glycerol—3-carbon molecule that is the backbone structure of triglycerides.

glycogen—Polymer of glucose used as storage form of carbohydrate in the liver and muscles.

glycogenolysis—The breakdown of glycogen into glucose-1-phosphate by the action of phosphorylase.

glycolysis—The sequence of reactions that converts glucose (or glycogen) to pyruvate.

glycoprotein—A protein that is attached to one or more sugar molecules.

glycosidic bond—A chemical bond in which the oxygen atom is the common link between a carbon of one sugar molecule and the carbon of another. Glycogen, the glucose polymer, is a branched-chain polysaccharide consisting of glucose molecules linked by glycosidic bonds.

gonadotrophic hormones—Hormones released from the anterior pituitary gland that promote sex steroid hormone synthesis by the ovaries in females and the testes in males.

gross efficiency (GE)—The ratio of the total work accomplished to the energy expended. Humans are approximately 20% efficient.

gross energy value of food—The amount of energy in food when measured in a bomb calorimeter. This energy is more than the energy that would be available to the human body if the food was eaten.

GTP (guanosine triphosphate)—High-energy phosphate compound similar to ATP.

guanine (G)—A purine nucleotide base found in DNA.

gum—A form of water-soluble dietary fiber found in plants.

H⁺—Hydrogen ion or proton.

H₂O₂—Hydrogen peroxide.

half-life—Time in which half the quantity or concentration of a substance is eliminated or removed.

HCl—Hydrochloric acid; part of gastric digestive juices.

HCO₃⁻—Bicarbonate ion, the principal extracellular buffer.

HDL (high-density lipoprotein)—A protein-lipid complex in the blood plasma that facilitates the transport of triacylglycerols, cholesterol, and phospholipids.

HDL cholesterol (high-density lipoprotein cholesterol)—One way in which lipids are transported in the blood.

heart burn—Indigestion and a burning pain as a result of entering of acidic gastric juices into the esophagus.

heat stroke—Elevated body temperature of 41° C (105.8° F) or greater caused by exposure to excessive heat or high levels of heat production and diminished heat loss. May result in tissue damage and is potentially fatal.

heat syncope—Fainting caused by excessive heat exposure.

helix—A spiral having a uniform diameter and a periodic spacing between the coils. A common secondary structure of proteins and DNA.

hematocrit—Proportion of the blood volume that is occupied by the cellular elements (red cells, white cells, and platelets). Also known as the packed cell volume.

hematuria—Red blood cells or hemoglobin in the urine.

heme—Molecular ring structure that is incorporated in the hemoglobin molecule enabling this protein to carry oxygen.

hemicellulose—A form of dietary fiber found in plants. Differs from cellulose in that it can be hydrolyzed by acid outside of the body.

hemochromatosis—Presence of excessive iron in the body resulting in an enlarged liver and liver damage in susceptible individuals.

hemodilution—A thinning of the blood caused by an expansion of the plasma volume without an equivalent rise in red blood cells.

hemoglobin—The red, iron-containing respiratory pigment found in red blood cells. Hemoglobin is important in the transport of respiratory gases and in the regulation of blood pH.

hemolysis—Destruction of red blood cells within the circulation.

hemorrhage—Damage to blood vessel walls resulting in bleeding.

hemorrheology—Study of the viscous properties of blood.

hepatic glucose output—Liver glucose output. The glucose that is released from the liver as a result of glycogenolysis or gluconeogenesis.

hexokinase (HK)—Enzyme that catalyzes the phosphorylation of glucose to form glucose-6-phosphate.

HMB (beta-hydroxy-beta-methylbutyrate)—A metabolic by-product of the amino acid leucine

homeostasis—The tendency to maintain uniformity or stability of the internal environment of the cell or of the body.

hormone—An organic chemical produced in cells of one part of the body (usually an endocrine gland) that diffuses or is transported by the blood circulation to cells in other parts of the body, where it regulates and coordinates their activities.

hormone-sensitive lipase—Enzyme that splits triacylglycerols into fatty acids and glycerol. It is regulated by hormones (mainly by epinephrine and insulin).

humoral—Fluid borne.

hydration—A reaction involving the incorporation of a molecule of water into a compound or a term relating to the state of the body water content.

hydrogen bond—A weak intermolecular or intramolecular attraction resulting from the interaction of a hydrogen atom and an electronegative atom possessing a lone pair of electrons (e.g., oxygen or nitrogen). Hydrogen bonding is important in DNA and RNA and is responsible for much of the tertiary structure of proteins.

hydrolysis—A reaction in which an organic compound is split by interaction with water into simpler compounds.

hydroxylation—A reaction involving the addition of a hydroxyl (OH) group to a molecule.

hyperhydration—Increased body-water content above normal level.

hyperthermia—Elevated body temperature (> 37° C or 98.6° F).

hypertonic—Having a higher concentration of dissolved particles (osmolality) than that of another solution with which it is being compared (usually blood plasma, which has an osmolality of 290 mOsm/kg).

hyperventilation—A state in which an increased amount of air enters the pulmonary alveoli (increased alveolar ventilation), resulting in reduction of carbon dioxide tension and eventually leading to alkalosis.

hyponatremia—Below-normal serum sodium concentration (< 140 mmol/L).

hypothalamus—Region at base of brain responsible for integration of sensory input and effector responses in regulation of body temperature. Also contains centers for control of hunger, appetite, and thirst.

hypothermia—Lower than normal body temperature.

hypotonic—Having a lower concentration of dissolved particles (osmolality) than that of another solution with which it is being compared (usually blood plasma, which has an osmolality of 290 mOsm/kg).

hypovolemia—Reduced blood volume.

Hz—Unit of frequency in cycles per second.

IDL—Intermediate-density lipoproteins.

IFN (interferon)—A type of cytokine. Some interferons inhibit viral replication in infected cells.

Ig (immunoglobulin)—Same as antibody.

IGF—Insulin-like growth factor.

immune system—Cells and soluble molecules involved in tissue repair after injury and in the protection of the body against infection.

immunodepression—Lowered functional activity of the immune system.

IMP—Inosine monophosphate. A breakdown product of AMP.

IMTG (intramuscular triacylglycerol)—Storage form of fat found in muscle fibers.

in vitro—Within a glass, observable in a test tube, in an artificial environment.

in vivo—Within the living body.

incisors—Anterior teeth that are used for cutting food.

indirect calorimetry—A method to measure energy expenditure and substrate utilization on the basis of gas exchange measurements. The term *indirect* refers to the measurement of O_2 uptake and CO_2 production rather than the direct measurement of heat transfer.

inflammation—Body's response to injury, which includes redness (increased blood flow) and swelling (edema) caused by increased capillary permeability.

inosine—The fifth base of nucleic acids. Important because it fails to form specific pair bonds with the other bases. In transfer RNAs, this property is used in the anticodon to allow matching of a single tRNA to several codons.

insoluble fiber—Fiber that does not dissolve in water.

insomnia—Difficulty with sleeping.

insulin—A hormone secreted by the pancreas involved in carbohydrate metabolism, particularly, in the control of the blood glucose concentration.

interleukin—Type of cytokine produced by leukocytes and some other tissues. Acts as a chemical messenger, rather like a hormone, but usually with localized effects.

interstitial—Fluid-filled spaces that lie between cells.

IOC—International Olympic Committee.

ion—Any atom or molecule that has an electrical charge due to loss or gain of valency (outer shell) electrons. Ions may carry a positive charge (cation) or a negative charge (anion).

ionic bond—A bond in which valence electrons are either lost or gained, and atoms that are oppositely charged are held together by electrostatic forces.

ischemia—Reduced blood supply to a tissue or organ.

isoform—Chemically distinct forms of an enzyme with identical activities usually coded by different genes. Also called isoenzyme.

isomer—One of two or more substances that have an identical molecular composition and relative molecular mass but different structure because of a different arrangement of atoms within the molecule.

isotonicity—Having the same concentration of dissolved particles (osmolality) as that of another solution with which it is being compared (usually blood plasma, which has an osmolality of 290 mOsm/kg).

isotope—One of a set of chemically identical species of atom that have the same atomic number but different mass numbers (e.g., 12-isotopes,13-isotopes, and 14-isotopes of carbon whose atomic number is 12).

IU—International units.

jejunum—The middle and longest part of the small intestine where a lot of the absorption of nutrients takes place. The jejunum is approximately 1 m to 2 m long.

Joule (J)—Unit of energy according to the Systeme Internationale. One Joule is the amount of energy needed to move a mass of 1 g at a velocity of 1 m/s.

Ka—Rate constant of a reaction (e.g., for the dissociation of a weak acid into its conjugate base.

Kerckring, folds of—Folds in the intestinal mucosa of the gastrointestinal tract.

keto-acids—An acid containing a ketone group (-C=O) in addition to the acid group(s).

ketogenesis—The synthesis of ketones such as acetoacetate, 3-hydroxybutyrate, and acetone.

ketone bodies—Acidic organic compounds produced during the incomplete oxidation of fatty acids in the liver. Contain a carboxyl group (-COOH) and a ketone group (-C=O). Examples include acetoacetate and 3-hydroxybutyrate.

KIC—alpha-keto isocaproate; a metabolite of the amino acid leucine.

kinase—An enzyme that regulates a phosphorylation-dephosphorylation reaction (i.e., the addition or removal of a phosphate group). This process is one important way in which enzyme activity can be regulated.

kJ (kilojoule)—Unit of energy ($kJ = 10^3 J$).

KM—A kinetic parameter (called the Michaelis constant) used to characterize an enzyme, defined as the concentration of substrate that permits half maximal rate of reaction.

lactase—Enzyme responsible for the splitting of lactose into galactose and glucose.

lactate dehydrogenase (LDH)—Enzyme that catalyzes the reversible reduction of pyruvate to lactate.

lacteal—Lymphatic vessel that drains the villi in the gut wall.

lactic acid—Metabolic end product of anaerobic glycolysis.

lactose—Milk sugar, a disaccharide linking a molecule of glucose and a molecule of galactose.

lactovegetarian—A vegetarian who includes milk products in the diet.

laxatives—Drugs that act on the gut to promote defecation.

LCAT—Lecithin-cholesterol acyl-transferase.

LDL (low-density lipoproteins)—A protein-lipid complex in the blood plasma that facilitates the transport of triacylglycerols, cholesterol, and phospholipids.

LDL-C (low-density lipoprotein cholesterol)—A way in which cholesterol is transported in the blood. High blood levels are associated with increased incidence of coronary heart disease.

lean body mass (LBM)—All parts of the body, excluding fat.

lecithin—Common name for phosphatidyl choline, the most abundant phospholipid found in cell membranes.

lecithin (phosphatidyl choline)—A phospholipid that occurs naturally in a variety of food items (beans, eggs, and wheat germ).

legume—The high-protein fruit or pod of vegetables, including beans, peas, and lentils.

leptin—Regulatory hormone produced by fat cells. When released into the circulation, it influences the hypothalamus to control appetite.

leucine—An essential amino acid that is alleged to slow the breakdown of muscle protein during strenuous exercise and to improve gains in muscle mass with strength training.

leukocyte—White blood cell. Important in inflammation and immune defense.

leukocytosis—Increased number of leukocytes in the circulation.

lingual lipase—A fat-splitting enzyme secreted by cells at the base of the tongue.

linoleic acid—An essential fatty acid.

linolenic acid—An essential fatty acid.

lipase—An enzyme that catalyzes the hydrolysis of triacylglycerols into fatty acids and glycerol.

lipid—A compound composed of carbon, hydrogen, and oxygen and sometimes other elements. Lipids dissolve in organic solvents but not in water and include triacylglycerol, cholesterol, and phospholipids. Lipids are commonly called fats.

lipid peroxidation—Oxidation of fatty acids in lipid structures (e.g., membranes) caused by the actions of free radicals.

lipolysis—The breakdown of triacylglycerols into fatty acids and glycerol.

lipoprotein lipase (LPL)—Enzyme that catalyzes the breakdown of triacylglycerols in plasma lipoproteins.

LNAA—Large neutral amino acid.

long-chain fatty acid (LCFA)—Part of triacylglycerols. Hydrocarbon chains with 12 or more carbon atoms and the most abundant type of fatty acids. Palmitic acid and oleic acid are the most abundant long-chain fatty acids in humans.

long-chain triacylglycerols—Triacylglycerol consisting of glycerol and three long-chain fatty acids

LRNI—Lower reference nutrient intake.

lymphocyte—Type of white blood cell important in the acquired immune response. Includes both T cells and B cells. The latter produce antibodies.

lysis—The process of disintegration of a cell.

lysosome—A membranous vesicle found in the cell cytoplasm. Lysosomes contain digestive enzymes capable of autodigesting the cell.

lysozymes—Enzymes that break down proteins and attack bacteria.

mol (molar)—Unit of concentration (nmol: nanomolar = 10^{-9} mol; μmol: micromolar = 10^{-6} mol; mmol: millimolar = 10^{-3} mol).

macromineral—Dietary elements essential to life processes that each constitute at least 0.01% of total body mass. The seven macrominerals are potassium, sodium, chloride, calcium, magnesium, phosphorus, and sulfur.

macronutrients—Nutrients ingested in relatively large amounts (carbohydrate, fat, protein, and water).

macrophage or monocyte—Type of white blood cell that can ingest and destroy foreign material and initiate the acquired immune response.

maltodextrin—A glucose polymer (commonly containing 6 to 12 glucose molecules) that exerts lesser osmotic effects compared with glucose and is used in a variety of sports drinks as the main source of carbohydrate.

maltose—A disaccharide that yields two molecules of glucose upon hydrolysis.

masticating—Chewing of food.

McArdle's disease—A glycogen phosphorylase deficiency resulting in an inability to break down glycogen.

mechanical digestion—Breaking down food by chewing.

medium-chain fatty acid (MCFA)—A fatty acid with 8 or 10 carbon atoms.

medium-chain triacylglycerol (MCT)—Triacylglycerol (triglyceride) containing fatty acids with hydrocarbon chain lengths of 6 to 12 carbons.

megadose—An excessive amount of a substance in comparison to a normal dose (such as the RDA). Usually used to refer to vitamin supplements.

menarche—The onset of menstruation in adolescent girls.

menstruation—Monthly bleeding and discharge of the outer uterine wall in healthy females.

metabolic acidosis—A metabolic derangement of acid-base balance where the blood pH is abnormally low.

metabolite—A product of a metabolic reaction.

metalloenzyme—An enzyme that needs a mineral component (e.g., copper, iron, magnesium, and zinc) to function effectively.

METS (metabolic equivalents)—A measurement of energy expenditure expressed as multiples of the resting metabolic rate. One MET equals an oxygen uptake rate of approximately 3.5 ml O_2/kg b.w./ min.

micromineral or trace element—Those dietary elements essential to life processes that each comprise less than 0.01% of total-body mass and are needed in quantities of less than 100 mg a day. Among the 14 trace elements are iron, zinc, copper, chromium, and selenium.

micronutrients—Organic vitamins and inorganic minerals that must be consumed in relatively small amounts in the diet to maintain health.

microvilli—Very small (1 μm) fingerlike projections of a cell membrane. They occur on the luminal surface of the cells in the small intestine.

min (minute)—Unit of time; 60 seconds.

mineral—An inorganic element found in nature though the term is usually reserved for those elements that are solid. In nutrition, the term mineral is usually used to classify those dietary elements essential to life processes. Examples are calcium and iron.

mitochondrial matrix—The substance occupying the space enclosed by the inner membrane of a mitochondrion. It contains enzymes, filaments of DNA, ribosomes, granules, and inclusions of protein crystals, glycogen, and lipid.

mitochondrion—Oval or spherical organelle containing the enzymes of the tricarboxylic acid cycle and electron transport chain. Site of oxidative phosphorylation (resynthesis of ATP involving the use of oxygen).

mitogen—Chemical that can stimulate lymphocytes to proliferate (undergo rapid cell divisions).

mitosis—A type of cell division in which each of the two daughter cells receives exactly the same number of chromosomes present in the nucleus of the parent cell.

mole—The amount of a chemical compound whose mass in grams is equivalent to its molecular weight, the sum of the atomic weights of its constituent atoms.

molecule—An aggregation of at least two atoms of the same or different elements held together by special forces (covalent bonds) and having a precise chemical formula (e.g., O_2, $C_6H_{12}O_6$).

monoacylglycerol—Glycerol backbone with one fatty acid. Also known as monoglyceride.

monosaccharide—A simple sugar that cannot be hydrolyzed to smaller units (e.g., glucose, fructose, and galactose).

motility—The movement of food through the gastrointestinal tract by coordinated muscular contractions of the intestine.

motor unit—All the muscle fibers supplied by a single motor neuron.

MRI (magnetic resonance imaging)—An imaging technique that generates pictures of body tissues and compartments. The results are somewhat similar to those obtained by a CT scan, but with MRI electromagnetic radiation is used rather than ionizing radiation.

mucosa—Layer of cells lining the mouth, nasal passages, airways, and gut that present a barrier to pathogen entry into the body.

myofibril—Threadlike 1-μm to 3-μm thick structures containing the contractile proteins and continuous from end to end in the muscle fiber.

myoglobin—A protein that functions as an intracellular respiratory pigment that is capable of binding oxygen and only releasing it at very low partial pressures.

myosin—One of the major contractile proteins in muscle found in the thick filaments.

NAD+ (nicotinamide adenine dinucleotide, oxidized form)—A coenzyme important in energy metabolism.

NADH (nicotinamide adenine dinucleotide, reduced form)—Reduced form of the coenzyme NAD.

NADP+ (nicotinamide adenine dinucleotide phosphate, oxidized form)—A coenzyme important in energy metabolism.

NADPH (nicotinamide adenine dinucleotide phosphate, reduced form)—Reduced form of the coenzyme NAD.

nandrolone—A steroid with androgenic and anabolic properties.

NCAA—National Collegiate Athletic Association (United States).

NEFA—Nonesterified fatty acid. Same as free fatty acid (FFA) or fatty acid (FA).

net efficiency (NE)—The work accomplished divided by the energy expended minus resting energy expenditure.

neurotransmitters—Endogenous signaling molecules that transfer information from one nerve ending to the next.

neutrophil—Type of white blood cell that can ingest and destroy foreign material. Very important as a first line of defense against bacteria.

NH$_2$—Amino group.

NH$_4$+—Ammonium ion.

NIDDM—Non–insulin-dependent diabetes mellitus. Also know as type II diabetes.

nitrogen balance—A dietary state in which the input and output of nitrogen is balanced so that the body neither gains nor loses tissue protein.

NK (natural killer) cell—A type of lymphocyte important in eliminating viral infections and preventing cancer.

NKCA—Natural killer cytotoxic activity. The ability of NK cells to destroy virally infected cells and tumor cells.

NO—Nitric oxide.

NO·—Nitric oxide radical.

nonessential amino acids—Amino acids that can be synthesized in the body.

norepinephrine—Catecholamine neurohormone, the neurotransmitter of most of the sympathetic nervous system (of so-called adrenergic neurons). Also known as noradrenaline.

nutraceutical—A nutrient that may function as a pharmaceutical (drug) when taken in certain quantities.

nutrient—Substances found in food that provide energy or promote growth and repair of tissues.

nutrition—The total of the processes of ingestion, digestion, absorption, and metabolism of food and the subsequent assimilation of nutrient materials into the tissues.

nutrition density—Amount of essential nutrients expressed per unit of energy in the food.

O_2—Oxygen molecule.

O_2^- (superoxide radical)—A highly reactive free radical.

obesity—An excessive accumulation of body fat. Usually reserved for those individuals who are 20% or more above the average weight for their size.

OH—Hydroxyl group.

OH^- (hydroxyl radical)—A highly reactive free radical.

oligosaccharide—A saccharide of a small number of component sugars, either O or N, linked to the next sugar.

osmolality—A measure of the total dissolved particle concentration. Units are mOsm/kg.

osmolarity—A measure of the total concentration of a solution. The number of moles of solute per liter of solvent typically expressed in mOsm/L.

osmoreceptors—Sensory cells in the hypothalamus capable of detecting changes in osmolarity of the blood.

osmosis—The diffusion of water molecules from the lesser to the greater concentration of solute (dissolved substance) when two solutions are separated by a membrane that selectively prevents the passage of solute molecules but is permeable to water molecules.

osteoblasts—Cells responsible for mineralization of bone.

osteoclasts—Cells responsible for breakdown (demineralization) of bone.

osteoporosis—A weakening of the bone structure that occurs when the rate of demineralization exceeds the rate of bone formation.

ovolactovegetarian—A vegetarian who also consumes eggs and milk products.

ovulation—Monthly release of an ova (egg) from the ovaries in females.

oxidation—A reaction involving the loss of electrons from an atom. It is always accompanied by a reduction. For example, pyruvate is reduced by NADH to form lactate. In the reverse reaction, lactate is oxidized by NAD^+ when pyruvate is reformed.

oxidative phosphorylation—Resynthesis of ATP involving the use of oxygen.

Panax ginseng—Chinese or Korean ginseng.

Panax japonicum—Japanese ginseng from India, Southern China, and Japan.

Panax quinquefolium—American ginseng.

pancreas—An organ located below and behind the stomach. It secretes insulin and glucagon (involved in plasma glucose regulation) and pancreatic enzymes involved in the digestion of fats and protein in the small intestine.

pancreatic duct—The connecting tube between pancreas and duodenum through which pancreatic juice is transported into the duodenum.

pancreatic juice—The secretions of the pancreas that are transported by the pancreatic duct to the duodenum. Pancreatic juice contains bicarbonate and the digestive enzymes amylase, lipase, and trypsin.

parathyroid hormone (PTH)—Hormone secreted from the parathyroid glands and involved in regulation of the blood plasma calcium ion concentration.

pathogen—Microorganism that can cause symptoms of disease.

PCO_2—Partial pressure of carbon dioxide.

PCr—Phosphocreatine or creatine phosphate. An important energy source in very high intensity exercise.

PDH complex—pyruvate dehydrogenase complex, a complex multienzyme system that catalyzes the conversion of pyruvate to acetyl CoA + CO_2.

pectin—A form of soluble dietary fiber found in some fruits.

PEM (protein energy malnutrition)—Inadequate intake of dietary protein and energy.

pepsin—A protein digestive enzyme secreted in pancreatic juice.

pepsinogen—The inactive form (storage form) of pepsin. Pepsinogen is stored in the cells of the stomach wall.

peptide—Small compound formed by the bonding of two or more amino acids. Larger chains of linked amino acids are called polypeptides or proteins.

peptide bond—The bond formed by the condensation of the amino group and the carboxyl group of a pair of amino acids. Peptides are constructed from a linear array of amino acids joined together by a series of peptide bonds.

peristalsis—Waves of contraction in smooth muscle of the digestive tract. It involves circular and longitudinal muscle fibers at successive locations along the tract and serves to propel the contents of the tract in one direction.

pH—A measure of acidity/alkalinity. pH = $-\log_{10}[H^+]$.

phagocyte—Leukocyte capable of ingesting and digesting microorganisms.

phenotype—The appearance or physiological characteristic of an individual that results from the interaction of the genotype and the environment.

phosphagen—The term given to both high-energy phosphate compounds, adenosine triphosphate and phosphocreatine.

phosphodiesterase—An enzyme that cleaves phosphodiesters to give a phosphomonoester and a free hydroxyl group.

phosphoenol pyruvate (PEP)—A metabolic intermediate in glycolysis.

Phosphofructokinase (PFK)—The rate-limiting enzyme in glycolysis.

phospholipids—Fats containing a phosphate group that on hydrolysis yield fatty acids, glycerol, and a nitrogenous compound. Lecithin is an example. Phospholipids are important components of membranes.

phosphorylase—Enzyme that breaks down the glucose polymer glycogen into molecules of glucose-1-phosphate.

phosphorylation—A reaction that involves the addition of a phosphate (PO_3^{2-}) group to a molecule. Many enzymes are activated by the covalent bonding of a phosphate group. The oxidative phosphorylation of ADP forms ATP.

photosynthesis—Process by which green plants and algae absorb light energy and use it to synthesize organic compounds, including glucose.

P_i—Inorganic phosphate (HPO_4^{2-}).

PKU (phenyl ketonuria)—Congenital lack of an enzyme that metabolizes phenylalanine, an essential amino acid. This condition may lead to mental retardation if not detected early in life.

plaque—The material that accumulates on the inner layer of arteries and contributes to atherosclerosis. It contains cholesterol, lipids, platelets, and other debris. Plaque on the inner layers of the arterial wall is a cause of coronary heart disease.

plasma—The liquid portion of the blood in which the blood cells are suspended. Typically accounts for 55% to 60% of the total blood volume. Differs from serum in that it contains fibrinogen, the clot-forming protein.

PO_2—Partial pressure of oxygen.

polypeptide—A peptide that, upon hydrolysis, yields more than two amino acids.

polyphenols—A large class of naturally occurring compounds that include the flavonoids, flavonols, flavonones, and anthocyanidins. These compounds contain a number of phenolic hydroxyl (-OH) groups attached to ring structures, which confers them with powerful antioxidant activity.

polysaccharide—Polymers of (arbitrarily) more than about 10 monosaccharide residues linked glycosidically in branched or unbranched chains. Examples include starch and glycogen.

postabsorptive state—The period after a meal has been absorbed from the gastrointestinal tract.

power—Work performed per unit of time.

precursor—A substance from which another, usually more active or mature substance is formed.

prohormones—A protein hormone before processing to remove parts of its sequence and thus make it active.

prosthetic group—A coenzyme that is tightly bound to an enzyme.

protease—An enzyme that catalyzes the digestion or cleavage of proteins.

protein—Biological macromolecules composed of a chain of covalently linked amino acids. Proteins may have structural or functional roles.

protein breakdown—See protein degradation.

protein degradation—The process in which the individual amino acids from a protein are disconnected.

protein synthesis—The process in which individual amino acids, whether of exogenous or endogenous origin, are connected to each other in peptide linkage in a specific order dictated by the sequence of nucleotides in DNA.

ptyalin—A digestive enzyme found in saliva that begins the digestion of starches in the mouth (also called α-amylase).

PUFA (polyunsaturated fatty acid)—Fatty acid that contains more than one carbon-carbon double bond.

pyloric sphincter—See pylorus.

pylorus—A circular muscle that controls the entry of stomach contents into the duodenum.

pyrogen—A substance that causes body temperature to be elevated, as in fever, and be regulated at a higher set point.

pyruvate—3-carbon molecule that is the end product of glycolysis.

pyruvate dehydrogenase (PDH)—The enzyme catalysing the conversion of pyruvate to acetyl-CoA.

Q—Blood flow rate or cardiac output.

R (group)—Side chain of an amino acid.

R_a (rate of appearance)—Usually referring to the rate at which a substance enters the blood circulation.

radiation—Transfer of energy waves that are emitted by one object and absorbed by another (e.g., solar energy from sunlight).

radiolabeled isotopes—An isotope is a specific form of a chemical element. It differs from atoms of other forms (isotopes) of the same element in the number of neutrons in its nucleus. Radiolabeled isotopes will transmit radiation and are used as tracers.

rate-limiting enzyme—An enzyme in a metabolic pathway that regulates the slowest step in the pathway, and, hence, limits the rate of flux through the pathway.

rating of perceived exertion (RPE)—A subjective rating, on a numerical scale, used to express the perceived difficulty of a given exercise task.

RBC—Red blood cell (erythrocyte).

R_d (rate of disappearance)—Usually refers to the rate at which a substance leaves the blood circulation.

RDA (recommended daily allowance)—Recommended intake of a particular nutrient that meets the needs of nearly all (97%) healthy individuals of similar age and gender. The RDAs are established by the Food and Nutrition Boards of the National Academy of Sciences.

RDI (reference daily intake)—Nutrient intake standards set by the FDA based on the 1968 RDA for various vitamins and minerals. RDIs have been set for infants, toddlers, people over 4 years of age, and pregnant and lactating women.

reactive hypoglycemia—See rebound hypoglycemia.

rebound hypoglycemia—Reactive hypoglycemia. A decrease in blood glucose concentration to hypoglycemic levels (<3.5 mmol/L) in response to carbohydrate feeding before exercise.

rectum—Last portion of the colon, connected to the anus.

reduction—A reaction in which a molecule gains electrons.

re-esterification—Process during which fatty acids are not released into the circulation, but are used to form new triacylglycerols within the adipose tissue.

relative humidity—The percentage of moisture in the air compared with the amount of moisture needed to cause saturation, which is taken as 100%.

reperfusion—Restoration of the blood supply to a tissue or organ.

RER (respiratory exchange ratio)—The ratio of carbon dioxide produced divided by oxygen consumption, representing a measure of substrate utilization at the whole-body level.

respiration chamber—A chamber in which the exchange of CO_2 and O_2 is measured to estimate energy expenditure and substrate utilization.

ribosome—Very small organelle composed of protein and RNA that is either free in the cytoplasm or attached to the membranes of the endoplasmic reticulum of a cell. The site of protein synthesis.

RMR (resting metabolic rate)—Energy expenditure under resting conditions.

RNA (ribonucleic acid)—A nucleic acid essential for protein synthesis (mRNA: messenger RNA; tRNA: transfer RNA; rRNA: ribosomal RNA).

RNI (recommended nutrient intake)—Defined as the level of intake required to meet the known nutritional needs of more than 97.5% of healthy persons. In the UK the RNI is very similar to the original RDA.

ROS (reactive oxygen species)—Collective name for free radicals and other highly reactive molecules derived from molecular oxygen. ROS include superoxide radical (O_2^-), hydroxyl radical (OH^-), hydrogen peroxide (H_2O_2), and perchlorous acid (HOCl).

RQ (respiratory quotient)—The ratio of the rate of carbon dioxide production divided by the rate of oxygen consumption, which can be used to establish the approximate pattern of substrate utilization by an organ or tissue (e.g., muscle).

s (second)—A unit of time.

saccharine—An artificial sweetener made from coal tar.

saponins—One of the characteristic compounds in ginseng. Also referred to as ginsenosides or panaxosides.

sarcolemma—The cell membrane of a muscle fiber.

sarcomere—The smallest contractile unit or segment of a muscle fiber; defined as the region between two Z lines.

sarcoplasm—The cytoplasm or intracellular fluid within a muscle fiber.

sarcoplasmic reticulum—An elaborate bag-like membranous structure found within a muscle cell. Its interconnecting membranous tubules lie in the narrow spaces between the myofibrils, surrounding and running parallel to them.

SD (standard deviation)—A measure of variability about the mean; 68% of the population is within 1 standard deviation above and below the mean, and about 95% of the population is within 2 standard deviations of the mean.

SE **(standard error)**—A measure of variability about the mean.

SEE—Standard error of estimate.

serotonin—A brain neurotransmitter. Also known as 5-hydroxytryptamine (5-HT).

serum—Fluid left after blood has clotted.

SGLT—sodium-dependent glucose transporter.

short-chain fatty acid (SCFA)—A fatty acid containing 6 or fewer carbon atoms.

smooth muscle—A specialized type of nonstriated muscle tissue composed of single nucleated fibers. It contracts in an involuntary rhythmic fashion in the walls of visceral organs. Also found in the walls of blood vessels.

sodium glucose transporter (SGLT)—Carrier protein that cotransports sodium and glucose across a cell membrane.

sodium pump—Common name for the sodium-potassium-ATPase that helps to establish the resting membrane potential of a cell.

soluble fiber—Fiber that dissolves well in water.

solute—A substance dissolved in a solvent liquid such as water.

solvent—A liquid medium in which particles can dissolve.

specific heat—The amount of energy or heat needed to raise the temperature of a unit of mass, such as 1g of body tissue, by 1° Celsius. Units are $J/g/°C$.

sphingomyelin—Type of lipid found in the membranes of Schwann cells that provide an insulating sheath around nerve axons.

spirometry—A method to measure breathing.

stable isotope—An isotope is a specific form of a chemical element. It differs from atoms of other forms (isotopes) of the same element in the number of neutrons in its nucleus. "Stable" refers to the fact that the isotope is not radioactive, in contrast to some other types of isotopes.

starch—A carbohydrate made of multiple units of glucose attached together by bonds that can be broken down by human digestion processes. Starch is also known as a complex carbohydrate.

stereoisomerism—The existence of different substances whose molecules possess an identical connectivity but different arrangements of their atoms in space.

steroid—A complex molecule derived from the lipid cholesterol containing four interlocking carbon rings.

STPD—Standard conditions of temperature (0° C) and pressure (760 mmHg) and dry.

substrate—The reactant molecule in a reaction catalyzed by an enzyme.

Substrate-level phosphorylation—Synthesis of high-energy phosphate bonds through reaction of inorganic phosphate with an activated (usually) organic substrate.

succinate dehydrogenase (SDH)—An enzyme of the tricarboxylic acid cycle.

sucrose—A disaccharide consisting of a combination of glucose and fructose; table sugar.

suit calorimeter—See direct calorimetry suit.

supercompensation of muscle glycogen—Higher than normal muscle glycogen concentrations that can be achieved with a combination of exercise and diet.

superoxide dismutase (SOD)—An enzyme in body cells that helps neutralize free radicals.

Systeme Internationale (SI)—International Unit System, a worldwide agreed uniform system of units.

systolic—Indicating the maximum arterial pressure during contraction of the left ventricle of the heart.

TBARS (thiobarituric acid-reactive substances)—Stable compounds produced as a consequence of free radical actions on lipid structures, which are commonly used as a measure of oxidative stress.

TCA (tricarboxylic acid)—A compound such as citric acid containing three carboxyl (-COOH) groups.

TCA cycle (tricarboxylic acid cycle)—A series of reactions that are important in energy metabolism and take place in the mitochondrion. Also known as the Krebs cycle (after Hans Krebs, who first described the reactions involved, or the citric acid cycle), as citrate is one of the key intermediates in the process.

testosterone—The male sex hormone responsible for male secondary sex characteristics at puberty. It has anabolic and androgenic effects and is responsible for aggressive behavior.

thermic effect of exercise (TEE)—The energy required for exercise. Increased muscle contraction increases heat production.

thermic effect of food (TEF)—See diet-induced thermogeneisis.

thermogenesis—The production of heat. Metabolic processes in the body generate heat constantly.

thermoreceptors—Sensory cells capable of detecting changes in temperature.

thioester bond—A bond in which the oxygen has been replaced by sulfur. For example, the linking of CoA in acetyl-CoA is through a thioester bond.

thymine (T)—A pyrimidine nucleotide found in DNA.

tissue—An organized association of similar cells that perform a common function (e.g., muscle tissue).

TNF (tumor necrosis factor)—A cytokine that promotes inflammation.

tracee—The compound that is traced.

tracer—An element or compound containing atoms that can be distinguished from their normal counterparts by physical means (e.g., radioactivity assay or mass spectrometry) and can thus be used to follow (trace) the metabolism of the normal substances.

trafficking (of leukocytes)—Movements of leukocytes into or out of the circulation.

trans—A prefix indicating that geometrical isomer in which like groups are on opposite sides of a double bond with restricted rotation.

transamination—Reaction involving the transfer of an amino (NH_2) group from an amino acid to a keto-acid.

transcription—The process by which RNA polymerase produces single-stranded RNA complimentary to one strand of the DNA.

transit time—The time that food stays in the gastrointestinal tract.

translation—The process by which ribosomes and tRNA decipher the genetic code in mRNA in order to synthesise a specific polypeptide or protein.

triacylglycerol—The storage form of fat composed of three fatty acid molecules linked to a 3-carbon glycerol molecule. Also known as triglyceride.

triglyceride—The storage form of fat composed of three fatty acid molecules linked to a 3-carbon glycerol molecule. Also known as triacylglycerol.

triplet code—The sequences of 3 nucleotides that compose the codons, the units of genetic information in DNA or RNA that specify the order of amino acids in a peptide or protein.

tRNA (transfer ribonucleic acid)—Transports amino acids to ribosomes where protein synthesis takes place.

TRP (tryptophan)—An essential amino acid.

type I diabetes mellitus (insulin-dependent diabetes mellitus)—A chronic condition in which the pancreas makes little or no insulin because the beta cells have been destroyed. The body is then not able to use the glucose (blood sugar) for energy.

type I fibers—Small-diameter muscle cells that contain relatively slow-acting myosin ATPases and, hence, contract slowly. Their red color is caused by the presence of myoglobin. These fibers possess a high capacity for oxidative metabolism, are extremely fatigue resistant, and are specialized for the performance of repeated contractions over prolonged periods.

type II diabetes mellitus—Non–insulin-dependent diabetes mellitus.

type II fibers—Muscle cells that are much paler than type I fibers because they contain little myoglobin. They possess rapidly-acting myosin ATPases, and so their contraction (and relaxation) time is relatively fast. A high activity of glycogen phosphorylase and glycolytic enzymes endows type II fibers with a high capacity for rapid (but relatively short-lived) ATP production.

UDP (uridine diphosphate)—A coenzyme involved in glycogen synthesis.

UFA (unsaturated fatty acid)—Fatty acid (FA) containing at least one double bond within its hydrocarbon chain.

UK—United Kingdom.

UL—Tolerable upper intake level. The highest level of daily nutrient intake likely to not pose a health problem.

uracil (U)—A pyrimidine nucleotide found in RNA.

urea—End product of protein metabolism. Chemical formula $CO(NH_2)_2$.

uric acid—A breakdown product of nucleic acids, present in small quantity in the urine of man and most mammals.

urine—Fluid produced in the kidney and excreted from the body. Contains urea, ammonia, and other metabolic wastes.

URTI—Upper respiratory tract infections like colds and flu.

USDA—United States Department of Agriculture.

USNDB—United States Nutrient Data Bank.

UTP—Uridine triphosphate.

vanadium—A trace element with a role in glucose metabolism.

VCO_2—Rate of carbon dioxide production.

vegan—Vegetarian who eats no animal products.

vegetarian—One whose food is of vegetable or plant origin.

villi—Fingerlike folds (1 mm) of the mucosa of the small intestine.

vitamin—An organic substance necessary in small amounts for the normal metabolic functioning of the body. Must be present in the diet because the body cannot synthesize it (or cannot synthesize an adequate amount of it).

vitamin B_1—Thiamin.

vitamin B_2—Riboflavin.

vitamin B_6—Pyridoxine.

vitamin B_{12}—Cyanocobalamin.

vitamin C—Ascorbic acid.

vitamin D—Cholecalciferol, the product of irradiation of 7-dehydrocholesterol found in the skin.

vitamin E—Alpha tocopherol.

vitamin K—Menoquinone.

VLCD—Very-low-calorie diet. Same as VLED.

VLDL (very-low-density lipoproteins)—A protein-lipid complex in the blood plasma that transports triacylglycerols, cholesterol, and phospholipids; has a very low density.

VLED—Very-low-energy diet.

V_{max}—Maximal velocity of an enzymatic reaction when substrate concentration is not limiting.

$\dot{V}O_2$—Rate of oxygen uptake.

$\dot{V}O_2max$—Maximal oxygen uptake. The highest rate of oxygen consumption by the body that can be determined in an incremental exercise test to exhaustion.

W (watt)—Unit of power or work rate (J/s).

water—The universal solvent of life (H_2O). The body is composed of 60% water.

WBC—White blood cell (leukocyte); important cells of the immune system that defend the body against invading micro-organisms.

wet-bulb globe thermometer index (WBGT Index)—A heat-stress index based upon four factors measured by the wet-bulb globe thermometer.

weight cycling—A cycle in which weight loss is achieved with considerable effort but maintaining the new lower body weight is even more difficult. After the weight is lost, it is regained in a relatively short period of time. Also referred to as the yo-yo effect.

work efficiency (WE)—The work accomplished divided by the energy expended minus the energy cost in the unloaded condition.

w.w.—Wet weight.

yohimbine—An alkaloid substance derived from yohimbine bark, which functions as an α_2 adrenoreceptor blocker (monamine oxidase inhibitor).

yo-yo effect—See weight cycling.

References

Abbott, W.G., B.V. Howard, L. Christin, et al. 1988. Short-term energy balance: relationship with protein, carbohydrate, and fat balances. *Am J Physiol* 255(3): E332-337.

Achten, J., and A.E. Jeukendrup. 2002. Maximal fat oxidation during exercise in trained men. *Int J Sports Med* 24(8): 603-608.

Achten, J., M. Gleeson, and A.E. Jeukendrup. 2002. Determination of the exercise intensity that elicits maximal fat oxidation. *Med Sci Sports Exerc* 34(1): 2-97.

Achten, J., S.L. Halson, L. Moseley, M.P. Rayson, A.C. Casey, and A.E. Jeukendrup. 2004. Higher dietary carbohydrate content during intensified running training results in better maintenance of performance and mood state. *J Appl Physiol* 96: 1331-1340.

Achten, J., M.C. Venables, and A.E. Jeukendrup. 2003. Fat oxidation rates are higher during running compared to cycling over a wide range of intensities. *Metabolism* 52(6): 747-752.

Acker, S.A.B.E., M.N.J.L. Tromp, G.R.M.M. Haenen, J.F. Wim, V. Vijgh, and A. Bast. 1995. Flavonoids as scavengers of nitric oxide radical. *Bio Chem Res Rev* 3: 755-757.

Allen, J.D., J. McLung, A.G. Nelson, and M. Welsch. 1998. Ginseng supplementation does not enhance healthy young adults' peak aerobic exercise performance. *J Am Coll Nutr* 17(5): 462-466.

American College of Sports Medicine. 1996. Exercise and fluid replacement. *Med Sci Sports Exerc* 16: i-vii.

American Dietetic Association. 1997. Position of the American Dietetic Association: Health implications of dietary fiber. *J Am Diet Assoc* 97: 1157-1160.

American Psychiatric Association. 1987. *Diagnostic and Statistical Manual of Mental Disorders*, 3rd ed. American Psychiatric Association: Washington, DC.

Andersen, A.E. 1990. Diagnosis and treatment of males with eating disorders. In *Males with eating disorders*, ed. A.E. Andersen, 133-162. Brunner/Mazel: New York.

———. 1995. Eating disorders in males. In *Eating disorders and obesity: a comprehensive handbook*, ed. K.D. Brownell and C.G. Fairburn, 177-192. Guildford Press: London.

Anderson, M.J., J.D. Cotter, A.P. Garnham, D.J. Casley, and M.A. Febbraio. 2001. Effect of glycerol-induced hyperhydration on thermoregulation and metabolism during exercise in the heat. *Int J Sport Nutr Exerc Metab* 11(3): 315-333.

Anderson, R.A., and A.S. Kozlovsky. 1985. Chromium intake, absorption and excretion of subjects consuming self-selected diets. *Am J Clin Nutr* 41(6): 1177-1183.

Andrews, S., L.A. Balart, M.C. Bethea, et al. 1998. *Sugarbusters*. Vermillion: London.

Angus, D.J., M. Hargreaves, J. Dancey, and M.A. Febbraio. 2000. Effect of carbohydrate or carbohydrate plus medium-chain triglyceride ingestion on cycling time trial performance. *J Appl Physiol* 88(1): 113-119.

Anonymous. 1998. Hyperthermia and dehydration-related deaths associated with intentional rapid weight loss in three collegiate wrestlers—North Carolina, Wisconsin, and Michigan, November-December 1997. *Morb Mortal Wkly Rep* 47(6): 105-108.

Applegate, E. 1999. Effective nutritional ergogenic aids. *Int J Sport Nutr* 9(2): 229-239.

Applegate, E.A., and L.E. Grivetti. 1997. Search for the competitive edge: a history of dietary fads and supplements. *J Nutr* 127(5 Suppl): S869S-S873.

Ardawi, M.S.M., and E.A. Newsholme. 1994. *Glutamine metabolism in lymphoid tissues*, ed. D. Haussinger and H. Sies, 235-246. Springer-Verlag: Berlin.

Arkinstall, M.J., C.R. Bruce, V. Nikolopoulos, et al. 2001. Effect of carbohydrate ingestion on metabolism during running and cycling. *J Appl Physiol* 91(5): 2125-2134.

Armstrong, L.E. 2002. Caffeine, body fluid-electrolyte balance, and exercise performance. *Int J Sport Nutr Exerc Metab* 12(2): 189-206.

Armstrong, L.E., D.L. Costill, and W.J. Fink. 1985. Influence of diuretic-induced dehydration on competitive running performance. *Med Sci Sports Exerc* 17: 456-461.

Atkins, R.C. 1992. *Doctor Atkins' new diet revolution*. Avon Books: New York.

Aulin, K.P. 2000. Minerals: calcium. In *Nutrition in Sport*, ed. R.J. Maughan, 318-325. Blackwell Science: Oxford.

Bach, A.C., and V.K. Babayan. 1982. Medium-chain triglycerides: an update. *Am J Clin Nutr* 36: 950-962.

Bagby, G.J., H.J. Green, S. Katsuta, and P.D. Gollnick. 1978. Glycogen depletion in exercising rats infused with glucose, lactate or pyruvate. *J Appl Physiol* 45(3): 425-429.

Ballantyne, C.S., S.M. Phillips, J.R. MacDonald, M.A. Tarnopolsky, and J.D. MacDougall. 2000. The acute effects of androstenedione supplementation in healthy young males. *Can J Appl Physiol* 25(1): 68-78.

Ballor, D.L., and R.E. Keesey. 1991. A meta-analysis of the factors affecting exercise-induced changes in body mass, fat mass and fat-free mass in males and females. *Int J Obes* 15(11): 717-726.

Balsom, P.D., B. Ekblom, K. Soderlund, B. Sjodin, and E. Hultman. 1993. Creatine supplementation and dynamic high-intensity intermittent exercise. *Scand J Med Sci Sports* 3: 143-149.

Balsom, P.D., S.D.R. Harridge, K. Soderlund, B. Sjodin, and B. Ekblom. 1993. Creatine supplementation per se does not enhance endurance exercise performance. *Acta Physiol Scand* 149: 521-523.

Balsom, P.D., K. Wood, P. Olsson, and B. Ekblom. 1999. Carbohydrate intake and multiple sprint sports: with special reference to football (soccer). *Int J Sports Med* 20(1): 48-52.

Barnett, C., D.L. Costill, M.D. Vukovich, K.J. Cole, B.H. Goodpaster, S.W. Trappe, and W.J. Fink. 1994. Effect of L-carnitine supplementation on muscle and blood carnitine content and lactate accumulation during high-intensity sprint cycling. *Int J Sports Nutr* 4(3): 280-288.

Barrett, B. 2003. Medicinal properties of echinacea: critical review. *Phytomedicine* 10: 66-86.

Barrett, B.P., R.L. Brown, K. Locken, R. Maberry, J.A. Bobula, and D. D'Alessio. 2002. Treatment of the common cold with unrefined echinacea. A randomized, double-blind, placebo-controlled trial. *Ann Intern Med* 137: 939-946.

Barry, A., T. Cantwell, F. Doherty, J.C. Folan, M. Ingoldsby, J.P. Kevany, J.D. O'Broin, H. O'Connor, B. O'Shea, B.A. Ryan, and J. Vaughan. 1981. A nutritional study of Irish athletes. *Br J Sports Med* 5: 99.

Bassit, R.A., L.A. Sawada, R.F.P. Bacurau, F. Navarro, E. Martins, R.V.T. Santos, E.C. Caperuto, P. Rogeri, and L.F.B.P. Costa-Rosa. 2002. Branched-chain amino acid supplementation and the immune response of long-distance athletes. *Nutrition* 18: 376-379.

Baumgartner, R.N., W.C. Chumlea, and A.F. Roche. 1990. Bioelectric impedance for body composition. *Exerc Sport Sci Rev* 18: 193-224.

Beckers, E.J., A.E. Jeukendrup, F. Brouns, A.J.M. Wagenmakers, and W.H.M. Saris. 1992. Gastric emptying of carbohydrate medium-chain triglyceride suspensions at rest. *Int J Sports Med* 13(8): 581-584.

Beidleman, B.A., J.L. Puhl, and M.J. De Souza. 1995. Energy balance in female distance runners. *Am J Clin Nutr* 61(2): 303-311.

Below, P., R. Mora-Rodriguez, J. Gonzalez-Alonso, and E.F. Coyle. 1995. Fluid and carbohydrate ingestion independently improve performance during 1 h of intense cycling. *Med Sci Sports Exerc* 27: 200-210.

Bennell, K., G. Matheson, and W. Heevwisse. 1999. Risk factors for stress fractures. *Sports Med* 28: 91-122.

Bennet, W.M., A.A. Connacher, C.M. Scrimgeour, and M.J. Rennie. 1990. The effect of amino acid infusion on leg protein turnover assessed by L- [15N]phenylalanine and L-[1-13C]leucine exchange [published erratum appears in Eur J Clin Invest 20(4): 479]. *Eur J Clin Invest* 20(1): 41-50.

Bennet, W.M., and M.J. Rennie. 1991. Protein anabolic actions of insulin in the human body. *Diabetic Med* 8: 199-207.

Bergstrom, J., and E. Hultman. 1966. Muscle glycogen synthesis after exercise: an enhancing factor localized in muscle cells in man. *Nature* 210: 309-310.

————. 1967. Synthesis of muscle glycogen in man after glucose and fructose infusion. *Acta Med Scand* 182(1): 93-107.

Beumont, P.J.V. 1995. The clinical presentation of anorexia and bulimia nervosa. In *Eating disorders and obesity: a comprehensive handbook*, ed. K.D. Brownell and C.G. Fairburn, 151-158. Guildford Press: London.

Beumont, P.J.V., B. Arthur, J.D. Russell, and S.W. Touyz. 1994. Excessive physical activity in dieting disorder patients: proposals for a supervised exercise program. *Int J Eating Disorders* 15: 21-36.

Bierkamper, G.G., and A.M. Goldberg. 1980. Release of acetylcholine from the vascular perfused rat phrenic nerve-hemidiaphragm. *Brain Res* 202(1): 234-237.

Biolo, G., S.P. Maggi, B.D. Williams, K.D. Tipton, and R.R. Wolfe. 1995. Increased rates of muscle protein turnover and amino acid transport after resistance exercise in humans. *Am J Physiol* 268(3 pt 1): E514-E520.

Biolo, G., B.D. Williams, R.Y. Fleming, and R.R. Wolfe. 1999. Insulin action on muscle protein kinetics and amino acid transport during recovery after resistance exercise. *Diabetes* 48(5): 949-957.

Birch, R., D. Noble, and P.L. Greenhaff. 1994. The influence of dietary creatine supplementation on work output and metabolism during repeated bouts of maximal isokenetic cycling in man. *Eur J Appl Physiol* 69(3): 268-276.

Bishop, N.C., A.K. Blannin, and M.Gleeson. 2000. Effect of carbohydrate and fluid intake during prolonged exercise on saliva flow and IgA secretion. *Med Sci Sports Exerc* 32: 2046-2051.

Bishop, N.C., A.K. Blannin, L. Rand, R. Johnson, and M. Gleeson. 1999. Effects of carbohydrate and fluid intake on the blood leucocyte response to prolonged exercise. *J Sports Sci* 17: 26-27.

Bishop, N.C., A.K. Blannin, P.J. Robson, N.P. Walsh, and M. Gleeson. 1999. The effects of carbohydrate supplementation on neutrophil degranulation responses to a soccer-specific exercise protocol. *J Sports Sci* 17: 787-779.

Bishop, N.C., A.K. Blannin, N.P. Walsh, and M. Gleeson. 2001. Effect of dietary carbohydrate status on bacterial lipopolysaccharide-stimulated neutrophil degranulation response following cycling to fatigue. *Int J Sports Med* 22: 226-231.

Bishop, N.C., A.K. Blannin, N.P. Walsh, P.J. Robson, and M.Gleeson. 1999. Nutritional aspects of immunosuppression in athletes. *Sports Med* 28: 151-176.

Blaak, E. 2001.Gender differences in fat metabolism. *Curr Opin Clin Nutr Metab Care* 4(6): 499-502.

Blom, P.C.S., A.T. Høstmark, O. Vaage, K.R. Kardel, and S. Maehlum. 1987. Effect of different post-exercise sugar diets on the rate of muscle glycogen resynthesis. *Med Sci Sports Exerc* 19: 491-496.

Blomstrand, E., S. Andersson, P. Hassmen, B. Ekblom, and E.A. Newsholme. 1995. Effect of branched-chain amino acid and carbohydrate supplementation on the exercise-induced change in plasma and muscle concentration of amino acids in human subjects. *Acta Physiol Scand* 153(2): 87-96.

Blomstrand, E., P. Hassmen, S. Ek, B. Ekblom, and E.A. Newsholme. 1997. Influence of ingesting a solution of branched-chain amino acids on perceived exertion during exercise. *Acta Physiol Scand* 159(1): 41-49.

Blomstrand, E., P. Hassmen, B. Ekblom, and E.A. Newsholme. 1991. Administration of branched-chain amino acids during sustained exercise—effects on performance and on plasma concentration of some amino acids. *Eur J Appl Physiol* 63(2): 83-88.

Blot, W. 1997. Vitamin/mineral supplementation and cancer risk: international chemoprevention trials. *Proc Soc Exp Biol Med* 261: 291-296.

Blundell, J.E., C.L. Lawton, J.R. Cotton, and J.I. MacDiarmid. 1996. Control of human appetite: implications for the intake of dietary fat. *Annu Rev Nutr* 16: 285-319.

Boden, G., X. Chen, J. Ruiz, G.D. van Rossum, and S. Turco. 1996. Effects of vanadyl sulfate on carbohydrate and lipid metabolism in patients with non-insulin-dependent diabetes mellitus. *Metabolism* 45(9): 1130-1135.

Bond, V., R. Adams, B. Balkissoon, J. McRae, E. Knight, S. Robbins, and M. Banks. 1987. Effects of caffeine on cardiorespiratory function and glucose metabolism during rest and graded exercise. *J Sports Med* 27: 47-52.

Bonen, A., J.J. Luiken, Y. Arumugam, J.F. Glatz, and N.N. Tandon. 2000. Acute regulation of fatty acid uptake involves the cellular redistribution of fatty acid translocase. *J Biol Chem* 275(19): 14501-14508.

Bosch, A.N., S.C. Dennis, and T.D. Noakes. 1994. Influence of carbohydrate ingestion on fuel substrate turnover and oxidation during prolonged exercise. *J Appl Physiol* 76(6): 2364-2372.

Bouchard, C. 1994. Genetics of obesity: overview and research directions. In *The genetics of obesity*, ed. C. Bouchard, 223-233. CRC Press: Boca Raton, FL.

Bouchard, C., A. Tremblay, J.P. Despres, A. Nadeau, P.J. Lupien, G. Theriault, J. Dullault, S. Moorjani, S. Pinault, and G. Fournier. 1990. The response to long-term overfeeding in identical twins. *N Engl J Med* 322(21): 1477-1482.

Bowtell, J.L., K. Gelly, M.L. Jackman, A. Patel, M. Simeoni, and M.J. Rennie. 1999. Effect of oral glutamine on whole body carbohydrate storage during recovery from exhaustive exercise. *J Appl Physiol* 86: 1770-1777.

Bray, G.A., and B.M. Popkin. 1998. Dietary fat intake does affect obesity! [see comments]. *Am J Clin Nutr* 68(6): 1157-1173.

Bredle, D.L., J.M. Stager, W.F. Brechue, and M.O. Farber. 1988. Phosphate supplementation, cardiovascular function, and exercise performance in humans. *J Appl Physiol* 65(4): 1821-1826.

Bremer, J. 1983. Carnitine-metabolism and functions. *Phys Rev* 63(4): 1420-1479.

Brewerton, T.D., E.J. Stellefson, N. Hibbs, E.L. Hodges, and C.E. Cochrane. 1995. Comparison of eating disorder patients with and without compulsive exercising. *Int J Eating Disorders* 17: 413-416.

Brilla, L.R., and T.E. Landerholm. 1990. Effect of fish oil supplementation on serum lipids and aerobic fitness. *J Sports Med Phys Fitness* 30: 173-180.

Broeder, C.E., K.A. Burrhus, L.S. Svanevik, et al. 1997. Assessing body composition before and after resistance or endurance training. *Med Sci Sports Exerc* 29(5): 705-712.

Brooks, G.A. 1986. The lactate shuttle during exercise and recovery. *Med Sci Sports Exerc* 18(3): 360-368.

Brouns, F. 1991. Etiology of gastrointestinal disturbances during endurance events. *Scand J Med Sci Sports* 1: 66-77.

Brouns, F., and E. Beckers. 1993. Is the gut an athletic organ? Digestion, absorption and exercise. *Sports Med* 15(4): 242-257.

Brouns, F., W.H.M. Saris, and N.J. Rehrer. 1987. Abdominal complaints and gastrointestinal function during long-lasting exercise. *Int J Sports Med* 8: 175-189.

Brouns, F., W.H.M. Saris, J. Stroecken, E. Beckers, R. Thijssen, N.J. Rehrer, and F. ten Hoor. 1989a. Eating, drinking, and cycling. A controlled Tour de France simulation study, part I. *Int J Sports Med* 10(suppl 1): S32-S40.

———. 1989b. Eating, drinking, and cycling. A controlled Tour de France simulation study, part II: Effect of diet manipulation. *Int J Sports Med* 10(suppl 1): S41-S48.

Brouns, F., J. Senden, E.J. Beckers, and W.H.M. Saris. 1995. Osmolarity does not affect the gastric emptying rate of oral rehydration solutions. *JPEN* 19: 403-406.

Brownell, K.D., S.N. Steen, and J.H.Wilmore 1987. Weight regulation practices in athletes: analysis of metabolic and health effects. *Med Sci Sports Exerc* 6: 546-560.

Brownlie, T., V. Utermohlen, P.S. Hinton, C. Giordano, and J.D. Haas. 2002. Marginal iron deficiency without anemia impairs aerobic adaptation among previously untrained women. *Am J Clin Nutr* 75: 734-742.

Brune, M., B. Magnusson, H. Persson, and L. Hallberg. 1986. Iron losses in sweat. *Am J Clin Nutr* 43: 438-443.

Brutsaert, T. D., S. Hernandez-Cordero, J. Rivera, T. Viola, G. Hughes, and J.D. Haas. 2003. Iron supplementation improves progressive fatigue resistance during dynamic knee extensor exercise in iron-depleted, nonanemic women. *Am J Clin Nutr* 77: 441-448.

Bucci, L.R., J.F. Hickson, Jr., I. Wolinsky, and J.M. Pivarnik. 1992. Ornithine supplementation and insulin release in bodybuilders. *Int J Sport Nutr* 2(3): 287-291.

Burckes-Miller, M.E., and D.R. Black. 1988. Male and female college athletes: prevalence of anorexia nervosa and bulimia nervosa. *Athletic Training* 2: 137-140.

Burke, L.M. 2001. Nutritional practices of male and female endurance cyclists. *Sports Med* 31(7): 521-532.

Burke, L.M., D.J. Angus, G.R. Cox, K.M. Gawthorn, J.A. Hawley, M.A. Febbraio, and M. Hargreaves. 1999. Fat adaptation with carbohydrate recovery promotes metabolic adaptation during prolonged cycling. *Med Sci Sports Exerc* 31(5): 297.

Burke, L.M., A. Claassen, J.A. Hawley, and T.D. Noakes. 1998. Carbohydrate intake during prolonged cycling minimizes effect of glycemic index of preexercise meal. *J Appl Physiol* 85: 2220-2226.

Burke, L.M., and V. Deakin (eds). 2000. *Clinical Sports Nutrition.* McGraw-Hill: Sydney.

Burke, L.M., G.R. Collier, and M. Hargreaves. 1993. Muscle glycogen storage after prolonged exercise: effect of glycemic index of carbohydrate feedings. *J Appl Physiol* 75(2): 1019-1023.

Burke, L.M., D.B. Pyne, and R.D. Telford. 1996. Effect of oral creatine supplementation on single-effort sprint performance in elite swimmers. *Int J Sport Nutr* 6(3): 222-233.

Burke, L.M., and R.S.D. Read. 1993. Dietary supplements in sport. *Sports Med* 15(1): 43-65.

Burns, J.M., D.L. Costill, W.J. Fink, J.B. Mitchell, and J.A. Hol. 1988. Effects of choline on endurance performance. *Med Sci Sports Exerc* 20(2): S25.

Butterfield, G.E., and D.H. Calloway. 1984. Physical activity improves protein utilization in young men. *Br J Nutr* 51(2): 171-184.

Byrne, A., and D.G. Byrne. (1993). The effect of exercise on depression, anxiety, and other mood states: a review. *J Psychosomatic Res* 37: 565-574.

Byrne, S., and N. McLean. 2002. Elite athletes: effects of pressure to be thin. *J Sci Med Sport* 5: 80-94.

Cade, R., M. Conte, C. Zauner, D. Mars, J. Peterson, D. Lunne, N. Hommen, and D. Packer. 1984. Effects of phosphate loading on 2,3-diphosphoglycerate and maximal oxygen uptake. *Med Sci Sports Exerc* 16(3): 263-268.

Calle, E.E., M.J. Thun, J.M. Petrelli, et al. 1999. Body-mass index and mortality in a prospective cohort of U.S. adults. *N Engl J Med* 341(15): 1097-1105.

Cannon, J.G., S.F. Orencole, R.A. Fielding, M. Meydani, S.N. Meydani, M.A. Fiatarone, et al. 1990. Acute phase response in exercise: interaction of age and vitamin E on neutrophils and muscle enzyme release. *Am J Physiol* 259: R1214-R1219.

Carvalho, J.J., R.G. Baruzzi, P.F. Howard, N. Poulter, M.P. Alpers, L.J. Franco, L.F. Marcopito, V.J. Spooner, A.R. Dyer, P. Elliott, et al. 1989. Blood pressure in four remote populations in the intersalt study. *Hypertension* 14(3): 238-246.

Casey, A., D. Constantin-Teodosiu, S. Howell, E. Hultman, and P.L. Greenhaff. 1996. Creatine ingestion favorably affects performance and muscle metabolism during maximal exercise in humans. *Am J Physiol* 271(1 pt 1): E31-E37.

Casey, A., R. Mann, K. Banister, J. Fox, P.G. Morris, I.A. Macdonald, and P.L. Greenhaff. 2000. Effect of carbohydrate ingestion on glycogen synthesis in human liver and skeletal muscle, measured by (13) C MRS. *Am J Physiol* 278(1): E65-E75.

Casey, A., and P.L. Greenhaff. 2000. Does dietary creatine supplementation play a role in skeletal muscle metabolism and performance? *Am J Clin Nutr* 72(2 suppl): 607S-617S.

Castell, L.M., J.R. Poortmans, and E.A. Newsholme. 1996. Does glutamine have a role in reducing infections in athletes? *Eur J Appl Physiol* 73: 488-490.

Castell, L.M., and E.A. Newholme. 1997. The effects of oral glutamine supplementation on athletes after prolonged, exhaustive exercise. Nutrition 13(7-8): 738-742.

Ceesay, S.M., A.M. Prentice, K.C. Day, P.R. Murgatroyd, G.R. Goldberg, W. Scott, and G.B. Spurr. 1989. The use of heart rate monitoring in the estimation of energy expenditure: a validation study using indirect whole-body calorimetry. *Br J Nutr* 61: 175-186.

Chandler, J., and J. Hawkins. 1984. The effect of bee pollen on physiological performance. *Int J Biosci Res* 6: 107.

Chaouloff, F., G.A. Kennett, B. Serrurrier, D. Merino, and G. Curzon. 1986. Amino acid analysis demonstrates that increased plasma free tryptophan causes the increase of brain tryptophan during exercise in the rat. *J Neurochem* 46(5): 1647-1650.

Chasiotis, D. 1983. The regulation of glycogen phosphorylase and glycogen breakdown in human skeletal muscle. *Acta Physiol Scand Suppl* 518: 1-68.

Christensen, E.H. 1932. Der Stoffwechsel und die Respiratorischen Funktionen bei schwerer körperlicher Arbeit. *Skand Arch Physiol* 81: 160-171.

Christensen, E.H., and O. Hansen. 1939. Arbeitsfahigkeit und Ernahrung. *Scand Arch Physiol* 81: 160-171.

Clancy, S.P., P.M. Clarkson, M.E. DeCheke, K. Nosaka, P.S. Freedson, J.J. Cunningham, and B. Valentine. 1994. Effects of chromium picolinate supplementation on body composition, strength, and urinary chromium loss in football players. *Int J Sport Nutr* 4(2): 142-153.

Cohen, N., M. Halberstam, P. Shlimovich, C.J. Chang, H. Shamoon, and L. Rossetti. 1995. Oral vanadyl sulfate improves hepatic and peripheral insulin sensitivity in patients with non-insulin-dependent diabetes-mellitus. *J Clin Invest* 95: 2501-2509.

Collins, M.A., M.L. Millard-Stafford, P.B. Sparling, et al. 1999. Evaluation of the BOD POD for assessing body fat in collegiate football players. *Med Sci Sports Exerc* 31(9): 1350-1356.

Collomp, K., S. Ahmaidi, M. Audran, et al. 1991. Effects of caffeine ingestion on performance and anaerobic metabolism during the wingate test. *Int J Sports Med* 12(5): 439-443.

Conlay, L.A., R.J. Wurtman, K. Blusztajn, I.L. Coviella, T.J. Maher, and G.E. Evoniuk. 1986. Decreased plasma choline concentrations in marathon runners [letter]. *N Engl J Med* 315(14): 892.

Conlee, R.K., R.L. Hammer, W.W. Winder, M.L. Bracken, A.G. Nelson, and D.W. Barnett. 1990. Glycogen repletion and exercise endurance in rats adapted to a high fat diet. *Metabolism* 39(3): 289-294.

Constantin-Teodosiu, D., J.I. Carlin, G. Cederblad, R.C. Harris, and E. Hultman. 1991. Acetyl group accumulation and pyruvate dehydrogenase activity in human muscle during incremental exercise. *Acta Physiol Scand* 143(4): 367-372.

Costill, D.L., A. Bennett, G. Branam, and D. Eddy. 1973. Glucose ingestion at rest and during prolonged exercise. *J Appl Physiol* 34(6): 764-769.

Costill, D.L., R. Bowers, G. Branam, and K. Sparks. 1971. Muscle glycogen utilization during prolonged exercise on successive days. *J Appl Physiol* 31: 834-838.

Costill, D.L., E. Coyle, G. Dalsky, W. Evans, W. Fink, and D. Hoopes. 1977. Effects of elevated plasma FFA and insulin on muscle glycogen usage during exercise. *J Appl Physiol* 43(4): 695-699.

Costill, D.L., G.P. Dalsky, and W.J. Fink. 1978. Effects of caffeine ingestion on metabolism and exercise performance. *Med Sci Sports Exerc* 10(3): 155-158.

Costill, D.L., and W.J. Fink 1974. Plasma volume changes following exercise and thermal dehydration. *J Appl Physiol* 37: 521-525.

Costill, D.L., and J.M. Miller. 1980. Nutrition for endurance sport: carbohydrate and fluid balance. *Int J Sports Med* 1: 2-14.

Costill, D.L., and B. Saltin. 1974. Factors limiting gastric emptying during rest and exercise. *J Appl Physiol* 37(5): 679-683.

Costill, D.L., W.M. Sherman, W.J. Fink, C. Maresh, M. Witten, and J.M. Miller. 1981. The role of dietary carbohydrates in muscle glycogen resynthesis after strenuous running. *Am J Clin Nutr* 34: 1831-1836.

Coyle, E.F., and A.R. Coggan. 1984. Effectiveness of carbohydrate feeding in delaying fatigue during prolonged exercise. *Sports Med* 1: 446-458.

Coyle, E.F., A.R. Coggan, M.K. Hemmert, and J.L. Ivy. 1986. Muscle glycogen utilization during prolonged strenuous exercise when fed carbohydrate. *J Appl Physiol* 61(1): 165-172.

Coyle, E.F., A.R. Coggan, M.K. Hemmert, R.C. Lowe, and T.J. Walters. 1985. Substrate usage during prolonged exercise following a preexercise meal. *J Appl Physiol* 59(2): 429-433.

Coyle, E.F., J.M. Hagberg, B.F. Hurley, W.H. Martin, A.A. Ehsani, and J.O. Holloszy. 1983. Carbohydrate feeding during prolonged strenuous exercise. *J Appl Physiol* 55(1): 230-235.

Coyle, E.F., A.E. Jeukendrup, M.C. Oseto, B.J. Hodgkinson, and T.W. Zderic. 2001. Low-fat diet alters intramuscular substrates and reduces lipolysis and fat oxidation during exercise. *Am J Physiol Endocrinol Metab* 280(3): E391-E398.

Coyle, E.F, A.E. Jeukendrup, A.J.M. Wagenmakers, and W.H.M. Saris. 1997. Fatty acid oxidation is directly regulated by carbohydrate metabolism during exercise. *Am J Physiol* 273: E268-E275.

Craig, E.N., and E.G. Cummings. 1966. Dehydration and muscular work. *J Appl Physiol* 21: 670-674.

Crook, T.H., J. Tinklenberg, J. Yesavage, W. Petrie, M.G. Nunzi, and D.C. Massari. 1991. Effects of phosphatidylserine in age-associated memory impairment. *Neurology* 41(5): 644-649.

Cumming, D. 1996. Exercise-associated amenorrhoea, low bone density and oestradiol replacement therapy. *Arch Intern Med* 156: 2193-2195.

Curatolo, P.W., and D. Robertson. 1983. The health consequences of caffeine. *Ann Intern Med* 98(5 pt 1): 641-653.

DaCosta, M., and K.A. Halmi 1992. Classification of anorexia nervosa: question of subtypes. *Int J Eating Disorders* 11: 305-314.

Dahlstrom, M., E. Jansson, E. Nordevang, and L. Kaijser. 1990. Discrepancy between estimated energy intake and requirement in female dancers. *Clin Physiol* 10(1): 11-25.

Davies, K.J.A., A.T. Quintanilha, G.A. Brooks, and L. Packer 1982. Free radicals and tissue damage produced by exercise. *Biochem Physiol Res Communications* 107: 1198-1205.

Davis, C. 1992. Body image, dieting behaviours and personality factors: a study of high performance female athletes. *Int J Sport Psychol* 23: 179-192.

Davis, C., S.H. Kennedy, E. Ralevski, and M. Dionne. 1994. The role of physical activity in the development and maintenance of eating disorders. *Psycholog Med* 24: 957-967.

Davis, S.E., G.B. Dwyer, K. Reed, et al. 2002. Preliminary investigation: the impact of the NCAA Wrestling Weight Certification Program on weight cutting. *J Strength Cond Res* 16(2): 305-307.

Deakin, V. 2000. "Iron depletion in athletes." In *Clinical Sports Nutrition*, eds. L. Burke and V. Deakin (McGraw-Hill Companies), 273-311.

De Luca, L., and S. Ross 1996. Beta-carotene increases lung cancer incidence in cigarette smokers. *Nutr Rev* 54: 178-180.

DeSilva, P., and S.B.G. Eysenck. 1987. Personality and addictiveness in anorexic and bulimic patients. *Personality and Individual Differences* 8: 749-751.

DeFronzo, R.A., D. Thorin, J.P. Felber, D.C. Simonson, D. Thiebaud, E. Jequier, and A. Golay. 1984. Effect of beta and alpha adrenergic blockade on glucose-induced thermogenesis in man. *J Clin Invest* 73(3): 633-639.

Depaola, D.P., M.P. Faine, and C.A. Pamer. 1999. Nutrition in relation to dental medicine. In *Modern nutrition in health and disease*, ed. M.E. Shils, J.A. Olson, M. Shike, and A.C. Ross, 1099-1124. Williams & Wilkins: Baltimore.

Dietary Supplement Health and Education Act of 1994. 1994. Public law 103-417, 103rd congress. Available at http://www.fda.gov/opacom/laws/dshea.html.

Dill, D.B., H.T. Edwards, and J.H. Talbott. 1932. Factors limiting the capacity for work. *J Physiol* 1932: 49-62.

Dodd, S.L., E. Brooks, S.K. Powers, and R. Tulley. 1991. The effects of caffeine on graded exercise performance in caffeine naive versus habituated subjects. *Eur J Appl Physiol* 62: 424-429.

Dohm, G.L., R.T. Beeker, R.G. Israel, and E.B. Tapscott. 1986. Metabolic responses after fasting. *J Appl Physiol* 61(4): 1363-1368.

Dohm, G.L., E.B. Tapscott, H.A. Barakat, and G.J. Kasperek. 1983. Influence of fasting on glycogen depletion in rats during exercise. *J Appl Physiol* 55(3): 830-833.

Drinkwater, B.L., K. Nilson, C.H. Chesnut III, et al. 1984. Bone mineral content of amenorrheic and eumenorrheic athletes. *N Engl J Med* 311(5): 277-281.

Duchman, S.M., A.J. Ryan, H.P. Schedl, R.W. Summers, T.L. Bleiler, and C.V. Gisolfi. 1997. Upper limit for intestinal absorption of a dilute glucose solution in men at rest. *Med Sci Sports Exerc* 29(4): 482-488.

Duffy, D.J., and R.K. Conlee. 1986. Effects of phosphate loading on leg power and high intensity treadmill exercise. *Med Sci Sports Exerc* 18(6): 674-677.

Dulloo, A.G., and J. Jacquet 1998. Adaptive reduction in basal metabolic rate in response to food deprivation in humans: a role for feedback signals from fat stores. *Am J Clin Nutr* 68(3): 599-606.

Dummer, G.M., L.W. Rosen, and W.W. Heusner. 1987. Pathogenic weight-control behaviors of young competitive swimmers. *Physician Sports Med* 5: 75-86.

Dupre, J., J.D. Curtis, R.W. Waddell, and J.C. Beck. 1968. Alimentary factors in the endocrine response to administration of arginine in man. *Lancet* 2(7558): 28-29.

Durnin, J.V., and J. Womersley 1974. Body fat assessed from total body density and its estimation from skin fold thickness: measurements on 481 men and women aged from 16 to 72 years. *Br J Nutr* 32(1): 77-97.

Duthie, G.G. 1999. Determination of activity of antioxidants in human subjects. *Pro Nutr Soc* 58: 1015-1024.

Dyck, D.J., S.A. Peters, P.S. Wendling, A. Chesley, E. Hultman, and L.L. Spriet. 1996. Regulation of muscle glycogen phosphorylase activity during intense aerobic cycling with elevated FFA. *Am J Physiol* 265: E116-E125.

Dyck, D.J., C.T. Putman, G.J.F. Heigenhauser, E. Hultman, and L.L. Spriet. 1993. Regulation of fat-carbohydrate interaction in skeletal muscle during intense aerobic cycling. *Am J Physiol* 265: E852-859.

Edwards, H.T., R. Margaria, and D.B. Dill. 1934. Metabolic rate, blood sugar and the utilization of carbohydrate. *Am J Physiol* 108: 203-209.

Eichner, E.R. 2000. Minerals: Iron. In *Nutrition in sport*, ed. R.J. Maughan, 326-338. Blackwell Science: Oxford.

Elowsson, P., A.H. Forslund, H. Mallmin, et al. 1998. An evaluation of dual-energy X-ray absorptiometry and underwater weighing to estimate body composition by means of carcass analysis in piglets. *J Nutr* 128(9): 1543-1549.

Engels, H.J., and J. C. Wirth. 1997. No ergogenic effects of ginseng (*Panax ginseng* C.A. Meyer) during graded maximal aerobic exercise. *J Am Diet Assoc* 97(10): 1110-1115.

Epling, W.F., and W.D. Pierce. 1988. Activity based anorexia: a biobehavioural perspective. *Int J Eating Disorders* 7: 475-485.

Erickson, M.A., R.J. Schwarzkopf, and R.D. McKenzie. 1987. Effects of caffeine, fructose, and glucose ingestion on muscle glycogen utilization during exercise. *Med Sci Sports Exerc* 19(6): 579-583.

Essig, D., D.L. Costill, and P.J. Van Handel. 1980. Effects of caffeine ingestion on utilization of muscle glycogen and lipid during leg ergometer cycling. *Int J Sports Med* 1: 86-90.

Evain-Brion, D., M. Donnadieu, M. Roger, and J.C. Job. 1982. Simultaneous study of somatotrophic and corticotrophic pituitary secretions during ornithine infusion test. *Clin Endocrinol* 17(2): 119-122.

Evans, G.W. 1989. The effect of chromium picolinate on insulin controlled parameters in humans. *Int J Biosoc Med Res* 11: 163-180.

Fahey, T.D., J.D. Larsen, G.A. Brooks, W. Colvin, S. Henderson, and D. Lary. 1991. The effects of ingesting polylactate or glucose polymer drinks during prolonged exercise. *Int J Sport Nutr* 1(3): 249-256.

Falk, B., R. Burstein, I. Ashkenazi, et al. 1989. The effect of caffeine ingestion on physical performance after prolonged exercise. *Eur J Appl Physiol* 59: 168-173.

Fallowfield, J.L., Williams C., Booth J., Choo B.H., and S. Growns. 1996. Effect of water ingestion on endurance capacity during prolonged running. *J Sports Sci* 14: 497-502.

Fery, F., and E.O. Balasse. 1983. Ketone body turnover during and after exercise in overnight-fasted and starved humans. *Am J Physiol* 245: E18-E25.

Field, A.E., T. Byers, D.J. Hunter, et al. 1999. Weight cycling, weight gain, and risk of hypertension in women. *Am J Epidemiol* 150(6): 573-579.

Fielding, R.A., Manfredi T.J., Ding W., Fiatarone M.A., Evans W.J., and Cannon J.G. 1993. Acute phase response in exercise III. Neutrophil and IL-1 β accumulation in skeletal muscle. *Am J Physiol* 265: R166-R172.

Flatt, J-P. 1995. Use and storage of carbohydrate and fat. *Am J Clin Nutr* 61: 952S-959S.

Floyd, J.C., Jr., S.S. Fajans, J.W. Conn, R.F. Knopf, and J. Rull. 1966. Stimulation of insulin secretion by amino acids. *J Clin Invest* 45(9): 1487-1502.

Fogelholm, M. 1994a. Effects of body weight reduction on sports performance. *Sports Med* 4: 249-267.

Fogelholm, M. 1994b. Vitamins, minerals and supplementation in soccer. *J Sports Sci* 12: S23-S27.

Fogelholm, M., R. Koskinen, and J. Laasko. 1993. Gradual and rapid weight loss: effects on nutrition and performance in male athletes. *Med Sci Sports Exerc* 25: 371-377.

Fogelholm, G.M., H.K. Naveri, K.T. Kiilavuori, and M.H. Harkonen. 1993. Low dose amino acid supplementation: no effects on serum growth hormone and insulin in male weightlifters. *Int J Sports Nutr* 3: 290-297.

Food and Nutrition Board. 1989. *Recommended Daily Allowances*. 52-77. National Research Council: Washington, DC.

Foster, C., D.L. Costill, and W.J. Fink. 1979. Effects of preexercise feedings on endurance performance. *Med Sci Sports* 11(1): 1-5.

Foster-Powell, K., S.H. Holt, and J.C. Brand-Miller. 2002. International table of glycemic index and glycemic load values. Am J Clin Nutr 76(1): 5-56.

Frexes-Steed, M., D.B. Lacy, J. Collins, and N.N. Abumrad. 1992. Role of leucine and other amino acids in regulating protein metabolism in vivo. *Am J Physiol* 262(6 pt 1): E925-E935.

Gadpalle, W.J., C.F. Sandborn, and W.W. Wagner. 1987. Athletic amenorrhea, major affective disorders and eating disorders. *Am J Psychiatry* 144: 939-943.

Galbo, H. 1983. *Hormonal and metabolic adaptation to exercise*. Verlag: New York.

———. 1992. Exercise physiology: humoral function. *Sport Sci Rev* 1: 65-93.

Galloway, S.D.R., and R.J. Maughan. 2000. The effects of fluid and substrate provision on thermoregulatory and metabolic responses to prolonged exercise in a hot environment. *J Sports Sci* 18: 339-351.

Galloway, S.D., M.S. Tremblay, J.R. Sexsmith, and C.J. Roberts. 1996. The effects of acute phosphate supplementation in subjects of different aerobic fitness levels. *Eur J Appl Physiol* 72(3): 224-230.

Gardiner, J.E., and M.C. Gwee. 1974. The distribution in the rabbit of choline administered by injection or infusion. *J Physiol* [Lond] 239(3): 459-476.

Garner, M.D., P.E. Garfinkel, W. Rockert, and M.P. Olmsted. 1987. A prospective study of eating disturbances in the ballet. *Psychother Psychosomat* 48: 170-175.

Gibson, S.A. 1996. Are high-fat, high-sugar foods and diets conducive to obesity? *Int J Food Sci Nutr* 47(5): 405-415.

Gill, H.S., and M.L. Cross. 2002. Probiotics and immune function. In *Nutrition and immune function*, ed. P.C. Calder, C.J. Field, and H.S. Gill, 251-272. CABI Publishing: Oxford.

Girandola, R.N., R.A. Wiswell, and R. Bulbulian. 1980. Effects of pangamic acid (B-15) ingestion on metabolic response to exercise. *Biochem Med* 24(2): 218-222.

Gleeson, M. 1998. Temperature regulation during exercise. *Int J Sports Med* 19(suppl 2): S96-S99.

———. 2000. Minerals and exercise immunology. In *Nutrition and Exercise Immunology*, ed. D.C. Nieman and B.K. Pedersen, 137-154, CRC Press: Boca Raton.

Gleeson, M., and N.C. Bishop. 1999. Immunology. In *Basic and applied sciences for sports medicine*, ed. R.J. Maughan, 199-236. Butterworth Heinemann: Oxford.

———. 2000a. Elite athlete immunology: importance of nutrition. *Int J Sports Med* 21(suppl 1): S44-S50.

———. 2000b. Modification of immune responses to exercise by carbohydrate, glutamine and antioxidant supplements. *Immunol Cell Biol* 78: 554-561.

Gleeson, M., A.K. Blannin, N.P. Walsh, N.C. Bishop, and A.M. Clark. 1998. Effect of low and high carbohydrate diets on the plasma glutamine and circulating leukocyte responses to exercise. *Int J Sport Nutr* 8: 49-59.

Gleeson, M., R.J. Maughan, and P.L. Greenhaff. 1986. Comparison of the effects of pre-exercise feeding of glucose, glycerol and placebo on endurance and fuel homeostasis in man. *Eur J Appl Physiol* 55(6): 645-653.

Gleeson, M., J.D. Robertson, and R.J. Maughan. 1987. Influence of exercise on ascorbic acid status in man. *Clin Sci* 73: 501-505.

Goedecke, J.H., R. Elmer-English, S.C. Dennis, I. Schloss, T.D. Noakes, and E.V. Lambert. 1999. Effects of medium chain triacylglycerol ingested with carbohydrate on metabolism and exercise performance. *Int J Sports Nutr* 9(1): 35-47.

Going, S.B., M.P. Massett, M.C. Hall, et al. 1993. Detection of small changes in body composition by dual-energy X-ray absorptiometry. *Am J Clin Nutr* 57(6): 845-850.

Golay, A., and E. Bobbioni. 1997. The role of dietary fat in obesity. *Int J Obes Relat Metab Disord* 21(suppl 3): S2-S11.

Goldberg, A.L., and T.W. Chang. 1978. Regulation and significance of amino acid metabolism in skeletal muscle. *Fed Proc* 37: 2301-2307.

Golden, N.H. 2002. A review of the female athlete triad (amenorrhea, osteoporosis and disordered eating). *Int J Adolesc Med Health* 14: 9-17.

Gontzea, I., R. Sutzeescu, and S. Dumitrache. 1975. The influence of adaptation to physical effort on nitrogen balance in man. *Nutr Rep Internat* 11(3): 231-236.

Gonzalez-Alonso, J., J.A.L. Calbet, and B. Nielsen.1998. Muscle blood flow is reduced with dehydration during prolonged exercise in humans. *J Physiol* 513: 895-905.

Goodpaster, B.H., D.E. Kelley, F.L. Thaete, J. He, and R. Ross. 2000. Skeletal muscle attenuation determined by computed tomography is associated with skeletal muscle lipid content. *J Appl Physiol* 89(1): 104-110.

Gordon, D.J. 1995a. Cholesterol and mortality: What can meta-analysis tell us? In *Cardiovascular disease 2*, ed. L.L. Gallo, 333-340. Plenum Press: New York.

———. 1995b. Cholesterol lowering and mortality. In *Lowering cholesterol in high risk individuals and populations*, ed. B.M. Rifkind, 33-48. Marcel Dekker: New York.

Gould, A.L., J.E. Rossouw, N.C. Santanello, J.F. Heyse, and C.D. Furberg. 1998. Cholesterol reduction yields clinical benefit: impact of statin trials. *Circulation* 97(10): 946-952.

Graham, T.E., P.K. Pedersen, and B. Saltin. 1987. Muscle and blood ammonia and lactate responses to prolonged exercise with hyperoxia. *J Appl Physiol* 63(4): 1457-1462.

Graham, T.E., J.W. Rush, and M.H. van Soeren. 1994. Caffeine and exercise: metabolism and performance. *Can J Appl Physiol* 19(2): 111-138.

Graham, T.E., and L.L. Spriet. 1991. Performance and metabolic responses to a high caffeine dose during prolonged exercise. *J Appl Physiol* 71(6): 2292-2298.

———. 1995. Metabolic, catecholamine, and exercise performance responses to various doses of caffeine. *J Appl Physiol* 78(3): 867-874.

Graudal, N.A., A.M. Galloe, and P. Garred. 1998. Effects of sodium restriction on blood pressure, renin, aldosterone, catecholamines, cholesterols, and triglyceride: a meta-analysis. *JAMA* 279(17): 1383-1391.

Gray, M.E., and L.W. Titlow. 1982. The effect of pangamic acid on maximal treadmill performance. *Med Sci Sports Exerc* 14(6): 424-427.

Green, A.L., D.A. Sewell, L. Simpson, E. Hultman, and P.L. Greenhaff. 1995. Carbohydrate ingestion stimulates creatine uptake in human skeletal muscle. *J Physiol* 489: 27P.

Green, A.L., E.J. Simpson, J.J. Littlewood, I.A. MacDonald, and P.L. Greenhaff. 1996. Carbohydrate ingestion augments creatine retention during creatine feeding in humans. *Acta Physiol Scand* 158: 195-202.

Green, H.J. 1995. Metabolic determinants of activity induced muscular fatigue. In *Exercise metabolism*, ed. M. Hargreaves, 211-256. Human Kinetics: Champaign, IL.

Green, N.R., and A.A. Ferrando. 1994. Plasma boron and the effects of boron supplementation in males. *Environ Health Perspect* 102(suppl 7): 73-77.

Greenhaff, P.L. 1998. The nutritional biochemistry of creatine. *Nutr Biochem* 11: 1610-1618.

Greenhaff, P.L., K. Bodin, K. Soderlund, and E. Hultman. 1994. Effect of oral creatine supplementation on skeletal muscle phosphocreatine resynthesis. *Am J Physiol* 266: E725-E730.

Greenhaff, P.L., A. Casey, A.H. Short, R. Harris, K. Soderlund, and E. Hultman. 1993. Influence of oral creatine supplementation of muscle torque during repeated bouts of maximal voluntary exercise in man. *Clin Sci* 84: 565-571.

Greenhaff, P.L., and J.A. Timmons. 1998. Pyruvate dehydrogenase complex activation status and acetyl group availability as a site of interchange between anaerobic and oxidative metabolism during intense exercise. *Adv Exp Med Biol* 441: 287-298.

Greenleaf, J.E. 1979. Hyperthermia in exercise. In *International Review of Physiology: Environmental Physiology III*, vol. 20, ed. D. Robertshaw and M. D., 1-50. University Park Press: Baltimore.

Greer, F., C. McLean, and T.E. Graham. 1998. Caffeine, performance, and metabolism during repeated Wingate exercise tests. *J Appl Physiol* 85(4): 1502-1508.

Guezennec, C.Y., J.F. Nadaud, P. Satabin, F. Léger, and P. Lafargue. 1989. Influence of polyunsaturated fatty acid diet on the hemorrheological response to physical exercise in hypoxia. *Int J Sports Med* 10(4): 286-291.

Halberstam, M., N. Cohen, P. Shlimovich, L. Rossetti, and H. Shamoon. 1996. Oral vanadyl sulfate improves insulin sensitivity in NIDDM but not in obese nondiabetic subjects. *Diabetes* 45: 659-666.

Hallmark, M.A., T.H. Reynolds, C.A. DeSouza, C.O. Dotson, R.A. Anderson, and M.A. Rogers. 1996. Effects of chromium and resistive training on muscle strength and body composition. *Med Sci Sports Exerc* 28(1): 139-144.

Hambraeus, L., A. Sjodin, P. Webb, A. Forslund, K. Hambraeus, and T. Hambraeus. 1994. A suit calorimeter for energy balance studies on humans during heavy exercise. *Eur J Appl Physiol* 68(1): 68-73.

Harper, A.E. 1999. Nutritional essentiality: evolution of the concept. *Nutr Today* 36: 216-222.

Hargreaves, M. 1995. *Exercise metabolism*. Human Kinetics: Champaign, IL.

Hargreaves, K.M., and W.M. Pardridge. 1988. Neutral amino acid transport at the human blood-brain barrier. *J Biol Chem* 263(36): 19392-19397.

Harris, R.C., K. Soderlund, and E. Hultman. 1992. Elevation of creatine in resting and exercised muscle of normal subjects by creatine supplementation. *Clin Sci* 83: 367-374.

Hasten, D.L., E.P. Rome, B.D. Franks, and M. Hegsted. 1992. Effects of chromium picolinate on beginning weight training students. *Int J Sport Nutr* 2(4): 343-350.

Haubrich, D.R., P.F. Wang, D.E. Clody, and P.W. Wedeking. 1975. Increase in rat brain acetylcholine induced by choline or deanol. *Life Sci* 17(6): 975-980.

Havel, R.J., B. Pernow, and N.L. Jones. 1967. Uptake and release of free fatty acids and other metabolites in the legs of exercising men. *J Appl Physiol* 23(1): 90-99.

Hawley, J.A., A.N. Bosch, S.M. Weltan, S.C. Dennis, and T.D. Noakes. 1994. Glucose kinetics during prolonged exercise in euglycemic and hyperglycemic subjects. *Pflügers Arch* 426: 378-386.

Hawley, J.A., E.J. Schabort., T.D. Noakes, and S.C. Dennis. 1997. Carbohydrate loading and exercise performance. *Sports Med* 24(1): 1-10.

Heinonen, O.J. 1996. Carnitine and physical exercise. *Sports Med* 22(2): 109-132.

Helge, J.W., B. Wulff, and B. Kiens. 1998. Impact of a fat-rich diet on endurance in man role of the dietary period. *Med Sci Sports Exerc* 30: 456-461.

Helge, J.W., E.A. Richter, adn B. Kiens. 1996. Interaction of training and diet on metabolism and endurance during exercise in man. *J Physiol* 492(1): 293-306.

Henson, D.A., D.C. Nieman, J.C.D. Parker, M.K. Rainwater, D.E. Butterworth, B.J. Warren, A. Utter, J.M. Davis, O.R. Fagoaga, and S.L. Nehlsen-Cannarella. 1998. Carbohydrate supplementation and the lymphocyte proliferative response to long endurance running. *Int J Sports Med* 19: 574-580.

Herbert, V. 1979. Pangamic acid ("vitamin B15"). *Am J Clin Nutr* 32(7): 1534-1540.

Hertog, M.C.L., E.M. Feskens, P.C.H. Hollman, and M.B. Katan. 1993. Dietary antioxidant flavonoids and risk of coronary heart disease: the Zutphen elderly study. *Lancet* 342: 1007-1011.

Heymsfield, S.B., R. Smith, M. Aulet, et al. 1990. Appendicular skeletal muscle mass: measurement by dual-photon absorptiometry. *Am J Clin Nutr* 52(2): 214-218.

Hinton, P.S., C. Giordano, T. Brownlie, and J.D. Haas. 2000. Iron supplementation improves endurance after training in iron-depleted, nonanemic women. *J Appl Physiol* 88: 1103-1111.

Hiscock, N., and B.K. Pedersen. 2002. Exercise-induced immunosuppression—plasma glutamine is not the link. *J Appl Physiol* 93: 813-822.

Hogervorst, E., W.J. Riedel, E. Kovacs, F. Brouns, and J. Jolles. 1999. Caffeine improves cognitive performance after strenuous physical exercise. *Int J Sports Med* 20(6): 354-361.

Holloszy, J.O., and W. Booth. 1976. Biochemical adaptations to endurance exercise in muscle. *Ann Rev Physiol* 38: 273-291.

Holloszy, J.O., and E.F. Coyle. 1984. Adaptations of skeletal muscle to endurance exercise and their metabolic consequences. *J Appl Physiol* 56(4): 831-838.

Hopkins, W.G., J.A. Hawley, and L.M. Burke. 1999. Design and analysis of research on sport performance enhancement. *Med Sci Sports Exerc* 31(3): 472-485.

Horowitz, J.F., R. Mora-Rodriguez, L.O. Byerley, and E.F. Coyle. 1997. Lipolytic suppression following carbohydrate ingestion limits fat oxidation during exercise. *Am J Physiol* 273: E768-E775.

———. 2000. Preexercise medium-chain triglyceride ingestion does not alter muscle glycogen use during exercise. *J Appl Physiol* 88(1): 219-225.

Horswill, C.A. 1995. Effects of bicarbonate, citrate, and phosphate loading on performance. *Int J Sports Nutr* 5: S111-S119.

Houmard, J.A., P.C. Egan, R.A. Johns, et al. 1991. Gastric emptying during 1 h of cycling and running at 75% $\dot{V}O_2$max. *Med Sci Sports Exerc* 23(3): 320-325.

Hu, F.B., M.J. Stampfer, J.E. Manson, E. Rimm, G.A. Colditz, B.A. Rosner, C.H. Hennekens, and W.C. Willett. 1997. Dietary fat intake and the risk of coronary heart disease in women [see comments]. *N Engl J Med* 337(21): 1491-1499.

Hultman, E. 1967. Physiological role of muscle glycogen in man, with special reference to exercise. *Circ Res* 10: I99-I114.

Hultman, E., P.L. Greenhaff, J.M. Ren, and K. Soderlund. 1991. Energy metabolism and fatigue during intense muscle contraction. *Biochem Soc Trans* 19(2): 347-353.

Hultman, E., and L.H. Nilsson. 1971. Liver glycogen in man: effects of different diets and muscular exercise. In *Muscle metabolism during exercise, II*, ed. B. Pernow and B. Saltin, 143-151. Plenum: New York.

Hultman, E., K. Soderlund, J.A. Timmons, G. Cederblad, and P.L. Greenhaff. 1996. Muscle creatine loading in men. *J Appl Physiol* 81(1): 232-237.

Hunt, C., N.K. Chakaravorty, G. Annan, N. Habibzadeh, and C.J. Schorah. 1994. The clinical effects of vitamin C supplementation in elderly hospitalized with acute respiratory infections. *Int J Vit Nutr Res* 64: 202-207.

Hunt, J.N., and I. Donald. 1954. The influence of volume on gastric emptying. *J Physiol* 126: 459-474.

Inder, W.J., M.P. Swanney, R.A. Donald, T.C.R. Prickett, and J. Hellemans. 1998. The effect of glycerol and desmopressin on exercise performance and hydration in triathletes. *Med Sci Sports Exerc* 30: 1263-1269.

Issekutz, B., H.I. Miller, P. Paul, and K. Rodahl. 1964. Source of fat in exercising dogs. *Am J Physiol* 207(3): 583-589.

Isselbacher, K.J. 1968. Mechanisms of absorption of long and medium chain triglycerides. In *Medium chain triglycerides*, ed. J.R. Senior, 21-37. University of Pennsylvania Press: Philadelphia.

Ivy, J.L. 1998. Glycogen resynthesis after exercise: effect of carbohydrate intake. *Int J Sports Med* 19: S142-S145.

Ivy, J.L., D.L. Costill, W.J. Fink, and R.W. Lower. 1979. Influence of caffeine and carbohydrate feedings on endurance performance. *Med Sci Sports* 11: 6-11.

Ivy, J.L., A.L. Katz, C.L. Cutler, W.M. Sherman, and E.F. Coyle. 1988. Muscle glycogen synthesis after exercise: effect of time of carbohydrate ingestion. *J Appl Physiol* 64: 1480-1485.

Ivy, J.L., and C.-H. Kuo. 1998. Regulation of GLUT4 protein and glycogen synthase during musle glycogen synthesis after exercise. *Acta Physiol Scand* 162: 295-304.

Ivy, J.L., M.C. Lee, J.T. Brozinick, and M.J. Reed. 1988. Muscle glycogen storage after different amounts of carbohydrate ingestion. *J Appl Physiol* 65: 2018-2023.

Jackman, M., P. Wendling, D. Friars, and T.E. Graham. 1996. Metabolic catecholamine, and endurance responses to caffeine during intense exercise. *J Appl Physiol* 81(4): 1658-1663.

Jackson, A.S., and M.L. Pollock. 1978. Generalized equations for predicting body density of men. *Br J Nutr* 40(3): 497-504.

Jackson, M.J. 2000. Exercise and oxygen radical production by muscle. In *Handbook of oxidants and antioxidants in exercise*, ed. C.K. Sen, L. Packer, and O.P. Hanninnen Osmo, 297-321. Elsevier: Amsterdam.

Jakubowicz, D., N. Beer, and R. Rengifo. 1995. Effect of dehydro-epiandrosterone on cyclic-guanosine monophosphate in men of advancing age. *Ann N Y Acad Sci* 774: 312-315.

Jansson, E., and L. Kaijser. 1982. Effect of diet on the utilization of blood-borne and intramuscular substrates during exercise in man. *Acta Physiol Scand* 115: 19-30.

Jeffery, R.W., W.L. Hellerstedt, S.A. French, et al. 1995. A randomized trial of counseling for fat restriction versus calorie restriction in the treatment of obesity. *Int J Obes Relat Metab Disord* 19(2): 132-137.

Jentjens, R.L., C. Cale, C. Gutch, and A.E. Jeukendrup. 2003. Effects of pre-exercise ingestion of differing amounts of carbohydrate on subsequent metabolism and cycling performance. *Eur J Appl Physiol* 88(4-5): 444-452.

Jentjens, R.L., and A.E. Jeukendrup. 2002. Effect of acute and short-term administration of vanadyl sulphate on insulin sensitivity in healthy active humans. *Int J Sports Nutr Exerc Metab* 12: 434-443.

———. 2003a. Effects of pre-exercise ingestion of trehalose, galactose and glucose on subsequent metabolism and cycling performance. *Eur J Appl Physiol* 88(4-5): 459-465.

———. 2003b. Determinants of post-exercise glycogen synthesis during short-term recovery. *Sports Med* 33(2): 117-144.

Jentjens, R.L.P.G., L. Moseley, R.H. Waring, L.K. Harding, and A.E. Jeukendrup. 2003. Oxidation of combined ingestion of glucose and fructose during exercise. *J Appl Physiol* [online] at DOI, 10.1152/japplphysiol.00974.2003. Also pub. 2004, in *J Appl Physiol* 96: 1277-1284.

Jentjens, R.L., L.J. van Loon, C.H. Mann, A.J. Wagenmakers, and A.E. Jeukendrup. 2001. Addition of protein and amino acids to carbohydrates does not enhance postexercise muscle glycogen synthesis. *J Appl Physiol* 91(2): 839-846.

Jeukendrup, A.E., and R.L. Jentjens. 2000. Oxidation of carbohydrate feedings during prolonged exercise: current thoughts, guidelines and directions for future research. *Sports Med* 29(6): 407-424.

Jeukendrup, A.E., F. Brouns, A.J.M. Wagenmakers, and W.H.M. Saris. 1997. Carbohydrate feedings improve 1 h time trial cycling performance. *Int J Sports Med* 18(2): 125-129.

Jeukendrup, A.E., N.P. Craig, and J.A. Hawley. 2000. The bioenergetics of world class cycling. *J Sci Med Sport* 3(4): 414-433.

Jeukendrup, A.E., W.H.M. Saris, A.J.M. Wagenmakers. 1998. Fat metabolism during exercise Part I. Fatty acid mobilization and muscle metabolism. *Int J Sports Med* 19(4): 231-277.

Jeukendrup, A.E., W.H.M. Saris, F. Brouns, and A.D.M. Kester. 1996. A new validated endurance performance test. *Med Sci Sport Exerc* 28(2): 266-270.

Jeukendrup, A.E., W.H.M. Saris, P. Schrauwen, F. Brouns, and A.J.M. Wagenmakers. 1995. Metabolic availability of medium chain triglycerides co-ingested with carbohydrates during prolonged exercise. *J Appl Physiol* 79(3): 756-762.

Jeukendrup, A.E., J.J.H.C. Thielen, A.J.M. Wagenmakers, F. Brouns, and W.H.M. Saris. 1998. Effect of MCT and carbohydrate ingestion on substrate utilization and cycling performance. *Am J Clin Nutr* 67: 397-404.

Jeukendrup, A.E., K. Vet-Joop, A. Sturk, J.H. Stegen, J. Senden, W.H. Saris, and A.J. Wagenmakers. 2000. Relationship between gastro-intestinal complaints and endotoxaemia, cytokine release and the acute-phase reaction during and after a long-distance triathlon in highly trained men. *Clin Sci* [Colch] 98(1): 47-55.

Jeukendrup, A.E., A.J. Wagenmakers, J.H. Stegen, A.P. Gijsen, F. Brouns, and W.H. Saris. 1999. Carbohydrate ingestion can completely suppress endogenous glucose production during exercise. *Am J Physiol* 276(4 pt 1): E672-E683.

Jeukendrup, A.E., A.J.M. Wagenmakers, L.M.L.A. Van Etten, R.L.P. Jentjens, G.J. Oomen, J.H.C.H. Stegen, P.F. Schoffelen, and W.H.M. Saris. 2000. Negative fat balance in weight stable physically active humans on a low-fat diet. *J Physiol* 523: 223P.

Johannes, C.B., R.K. Stellato, H.A. Feldman, C. Longcope, and J.B. McKinlay. 1999. Relation of dehydroepiandrosterone and dehydroepiandrosterone sulfate with cardiovascular disease risk factors in women: longitudinal results from the Massachusetts Women's Health Study. *J Clin Epidemiol* 52(2): 95-103.

Johansson, L., K. Solvoll, G.E. Bjorneboe, and C.A. Drevon. 1998. Under- and overreporting of energy intake related to weight status and lifestyle in a nationwide sample. *Am J Clin Nutr* 68(2): 266-274.

Jones, D.A., and O.M. Rutherford. 1987. Human muscle strength training: the effects of three different regimens and the nature of the resultant changes. *J Physiol* [Lond] 391: 1-11.

Jowko, E., P. Ostaszewski, M. Jank, J. Sacharuk, A. Zieniewicz, J. Wilczak, and S. Nissen. 2001. Creatine and beta-hydroxy-beta-methylbutyrate (HMB) additively increase lean body mass and muscle strength during a weight-training program. *Nutrition* 17(7-8): 558-566.

Kagan, A., B.R. Harris, W. Winkelstein, Jr., K.G. Johnson, H. Kato, S.L. Syme, G.G. Rhoads, M.L. Gay, M.Z. Nichaman, H.B. Hamilton, and J. Tillotson. 1974. Epidemiologic studies of coronary heart disease and stroke in Japanese men living in Japan, Hawaii and California: demographic, physical, dietary and biochemical characteristics. *J Chronic Dis* 27(7-8): 345-364.

Kamada, T., S. Tokuda, S.-I. Aozaki, and S. Otsuji. 1993. Higher levels of erythrocyte membrane fluidity in sprinters and long-distance runners. *J Appl Physiol* 74(1): 354-358.

Kaminski, M., and R. Boal. 1992. An effect of ascorbic acid on delayed-onset muscle soreness. *Pain* 50: 317-321.

Kandelman, D. 1997. Sugar, alternative sweeteners and meal frequency in relation to caries prevention: new perspectives. *Br J Nutr* 77(suppl 1): S121-S128.

Karlsson, J., and B. Saltin. 1970. Lactate, ATP, and CP in working muscles during exhaustive exercise in man. *J Appl Physiol* 29(5): 596-602.

Kasperek, G.J., and R.D. Snider. 1989. Total and myofibrillar pro-tein degradation in isolated soleus muscles after exercise. *Am J Physiol* 257(1 pt 1): E1-E5.

Katch, F.I., and W.D. McArdle. 1998. Nutrition, Weight Control, and Exercise, 3rd Edition. Lea and Febiger: Philadelphia.

Kazis, K., and E. Iglesias 2003. The female athlete triad. *Adolesc Med* 14. 87-95.

Keeffe, E.B., D.K. Lowe, J.R. Goss, and R. Wayne. 1984. Gastro-intestinal symptoms of marathon runners. *West J Med* 141: 481-484.

Keesey, R.E., M.D. Hirvonen. 1997. Body weight set-points: determination and adjustment. *J Nutr* 127(9): 1875S-1883S.

Keizer, H., H. Kuipers, and G. van Kranenburg. 1987. Influence of liquid and solid meals on muscle glycogen resynthis, plasma fuel hormone response, and maximal physical working capacity. *Int J Sports Med* 8: 99-104.

Kelly, J.M., B.A.Gorney, and K.K. Kalm. 1978. The effects of a collegiate wrestling season on body composition, cardiovascular fitness and muscular strength and endurance. *Med Sci Sports* 10(2): 119-124.

Khatta, M., B.S. Alexander, C.M. Krichten, M.L. Fisher, R. Freudenberger, S.W. Robinson, and S. S. Gottlieb. 2000. The effect of coenzyme Q10 in patients with congestive heart failure. *Ann Intern Med* 132(8): 636-640.

King, D.S., R.L. Sharp, M.D. Vukovich, G.A. Brown, T.A. Reifenrath, N.L. Uhl, and K.A. Parsons. 1999. Effect of oral androstenedione on serum testosterone and adaptations to resistance training in young men: a randomized controlled trial [see comments]. *JAMA* 281(21): 2020-2028.

Klein, S., E.F. Coyle, and R.R. Wolfe. 1994. Fat metabolism during low-intensity exercise in endurance trained and untrained men. *Am J Physiol* 267: E934-E940.

Klein, S., J.-M. Weber, E.F. Coyle, and R.R. Wolfe. 1996. Effect of endurance training on glycerol kinetics during strenuous exercise in humans. *Metabolism* 45(3): 357-361.

Knapik, J.J., B.H. Jones, M.M. Toner, W.L. Daniels, and W.J. Evans. 1983. Influence of caffeine on serum substrate changes during running in trained and untrained individuals. *Bioch Exerc* 13: 514-519.

Knapik, J., C. Meredith, B. Jones, R. Fielding, V. Young, and W. Evans. 1991. Leucine metabolism during fasting and exercise. *J Appl Physiol* 70(1): 43-47.

Knapik, J.J., C.N. Meredith, B.H. Jones, L. Suek, V.R. Young, and W.J. Evans. 1988. Influence of fasting on carbohydrate and fat metabolism during rest and exercise in men. *J Appl Physiol* 64(5): 1923-1929.

Knopf, R.F., J.W. Conn, J.C. Floyd, Jr., S.S. Fajans, J.A. Rull, E.M. Guntsche, and C.A. Thiffault. 1966. The normal endocrine response to ingestion of protein and infusions of amino acids: sequential secretion of insulin and growth hormone. *Trans Assoc Am Physicians* 79: 312-321.

Kochan, R.G., D.R. Lamb, S.A. Lutz, C.V. Perrill, E.M. Reimann, and K.K. Schlender. 1979. Glycogen synthase activation in human skeletal muscle: effects of diet and exercise. *Am J Physiol* 5(6): E660-E666.

Koenigsberg, P.S., K.K. Martin, H.R. Hlava, and M.L. Riedesel. 1995. Sustained hyperhydration with glycerol ingestion. *Life Sci* 57(7): 645-653.

Kohrt, W.M. 1995. Body composition by DXA: tried and true? *Med Sci Sports Exerc* 27(10): 1349-1353.

Kopp-Hoolihan, L. 2001. Prophylactic and therapeutic uses of probiotics: a review. *J Am Diet Assoc* 101: 229-238.

Koubi, H.E., D. Desplanches, C. Gabrielle, J.M. Cottet-Emard, B. Sempore, and R.J. Favier. 1991. Exercise endurance and fuel utilization: a reevaluation of the effects of fasting. *J Appl Physiol* 70(3): 1337-1343.

Koulmann, N., C. Jimenez, D. Regal, et al. 2000. Use of bioelectrical impedance analysis to estimate body fluid compartments after acute variations of the body hydration level. *Med Sci Sports Exerc* 32(4): 857-864.

Kovacs, E.M.R., J.H.C.H. Stegen, and F. Brouns. 1998. Effect of caffeinated drinks on substrate metabolism, caffeine excretion, and performance. *J Appl Physiol* 85: 709-715.

Kraemer, W.J., J.F. Patton, S.E. Gordon, et al. 1995. Compatibility of high-intensity strength and endurance training on hormonal and skeletal muscle adaptations. *J Appl Physiol* 78(3): 976-989.

Kreider, R.B., M. Ferreira, M. Wilson, P. Grindstaff, S. Plisk, J. Reinardy, E. Cantler, and A.L. Almada. 1998. Effects of creatine supplementation on body composition, strength, and sprint performance. *Med Sci Sports Exerc* 30(1): 73-82.

Kreider, R.B., G.W. Miller, D. Schenck, C.W. Cortes, V. Miriel, C.T. Somma, P. Rowland, C. Turner, and D. Hill. 1992. Effects of phosphate loading on metabolic and myocardial responses to maximal and endurance exercise. *Int J Sport Nutr* 2(1): 20-47.

Kreider, R.B., G.W. Miller, M.H. Williams, C.T. Somma, and T.A. Nasser. 1990. Effects of phosphate loading on oxygen uptake, ventilatory anaerobic threshold, and run performance. *Med Sci Sports Exerc* 22(2): 250-256.

Krogh, A., and J. Lindhard. 1920. The relative value of fat and carbohydrate as sources of muscular energy. *Biochem J* 14: 290-363.

Kromhout, D., and C. de Lezenne Coulander. 1984. Diet, prevalence and 10-year mortality from coronary heart disease in 871 middle-aged men: the Zutphen study. *Am J Epidemiol* 119(5): 733-741.

Kromhout, D., A. Menotti, B. Bloemberg, C. Aravanis, H. Blackburn, R. Buzina, A.S. Dontas, F. Fidanza, S. Giampaoli, A. Jansen, et al. 1995. Dietary saturated and *trans* fatty acids and cholesterol and 25-year mortality from coronary heart disease: the Seven Countries study. *Prev Med* 24(3): 308-315.

Kron, L., J.L. Katz, G. Gorzynski, and H. Weiner. 1978. Hyperactivity in anorexia nervosa: a fundamental clinical feature. *Comp Psych* 19: 433-440.

Kuipers, H., D.L. Costill, D.A. Porter, W.J. Fink, and W.M. Morse. 1986. Glucose feeding and exercise in trained rats: mechanisms for glycogen sparing. *J Appl Physiol* 61(3): 859-863.

Kuipers, H., W.H.M. Saris, F. Brouns, H.A. Keizer, and C. ten Bosch. 1989. Glycogen synthesis during exercise and rest with carbohydrate feeding in males and females. *Int J Sports Med* 10(suppl.1): S63-S67.

Kumanyika, S.K., and J.A. Cutler. 1997. Dietary sodium reduction: Is there cause for concern? *J Am Coll Nutr* 16(3): 192-203.

Lambert, C.P., D. Ball, J.B. Leiper, and R.J. Maughan. 1999. The use of a deuterium tracer technique to follow the fate of fluids ingested by human subjects: effects of drink volume and tracer concentration and content. *Exp Physiol* 84(2): 391-399.

Lambert, M.I., J.A. Hefer, R.P. Millar, and P.W. Macfarlane. 1993. Failure of commercial oral amino acid supplements to increase serum growth hormone concentrations in male body-builders. *Int J Sport Nutr* 3(3): 298-305.

Lamont, L.S., A.J. McCullough, and S.C. Kalhan. 1999. Comparison of leucine kinetics in endurance-trained and sedentary humans. *J Appl Physiol* 86(1): 320-325.

Lang, F., G.L. Busch, M. Ritter, H. Volkl, S. Waldegger, E. Gulbins, and D. Haussinger. 1998. Functional significance of cell volume regulatory mechanisms. *Physiol Rev* 78(1): 247-306.

Latzka, W.A., M.N. Sawka, S.J. Montain, G.S. Skrinar, R.A. Fielding, R.P. Matott, and K.B. Pandolf. 1997. Hyperhydration: thermoregulatory effects during compensable exercise-heat stress. *J Appl Physiol* 83(3): 860-866.

———. 1998. Hyperhydration: tolerance and cardiovascular effects during uncompensable exercise-heat stress. *J Appl Physiol* 84: 1858-1864.

Lebenstedt, M., P. Platte, K.M. Pirke. 1999. Reduced resting metabolic rate in athletes with menstrual disorders. *Med Sci Sports Exerc* 31(9): 1250-1256.

Leenders, N.M., D.R. Lamb, and T.E. Nelson. 1999. Creatine supplementation and swimming performance. *Int J Sport Nutr* 9(3): 251-262.

Leibel, R.L., M. Rosenbaum, J. Hirsch. 1995. Changes in energy expenditure resulting from altered body weight. *N Engl J Med* 332(10): 621-628.

Leiper, J.B., N.P. Broad, and R.J. Maughan. 2001. Effect of intermittent high-intensity exercise on gastric emptying in man. *Med Sci Sports Exerc* 33(8): 1270-1278.

Leiper, J.B., A.S. Prentice, C. Wrightson, and R.J. Maughan. 2001. Gastric emptying of a carbohydrate-electrolyte drink during a soccer match. *Med Sci Sports Exerc* 33(11): 1932-1938.

Levine, S.A., B. Gordon, and C.L. Derick. 1924. Some changes in chemical constituents of blood following a marathon race. *JAMA* 82: 1778-1779.

Lichtenstein, A.H., L.M. Ausman, S.M. Jalbert, and E.J. Schaefer. 1999. Effects of different forms of dietary hydrogenated fats on serum lipoprotein cholesterol levels [see comments] [published erratum appears in N Engl J Med 341(11): 856]. *N Engl J Med* 340(25): 1933-1940.

Linderman, J.K., and K.L. Gosselink. 1994. The effects of sodium bicarbonate ingestion on exercise performance. *Sports Med* 18(2): 75-80.

Lohman, T.G., and S.B. Going. 1993. Multicomponent models in body composition research: opportunities and pitfalls. *Basic Life Sci* 60: 53-58.

Louard, R.J., E.J. Barrett, and R.A. Gelfand. 1990. Effect of infused branched-chain amino acids on muscle and whole-body amino acid metabolism in man. *Clin Sci* [Colch] 79(5): 457-466.

Loy, S.F., R.K. Conlee, W.W. Winder, A.G. Nelson, D.A. Arnall, and A.G. Fisher. 1986. Effect of 24-hour fast on cycling endurance time at two different intensities. *J Appl Physiol* 61(2): 654-659.

Lukaski, H.C., W.W. Bolonchuk, W.A. Siders, and D.B. Milne. 1996. Chromium supplementation and resistance training: effects on body composition, strength, and trace element status of men. *Am J Clin Nutr* 63(6): 954-965.

Luke, A., K.C. Maki, N. Barkey, R. Cooper, and D. McGee. 1997. Simultaneous monitoring of heart rate and motion to assess energy expenditure. *Med Sci Sports Exerc* 29(1): 144-148.

Lyons, T.P., M.L. Riedesel, L.E. Meuli, and T.W. Chick. 1990. Effects of glycerol-induced hyperhydration prior to exercise in the heat on sweating and core temperature. *Med Sci Sports Exerc* 22(4): 477-483.

Mackinnon, L.T. 1999. *Advances in exercise and immunology*. Human Kinetics: Champaign, IL.

Macknin, M.L. 1999. Zinc lozenges for the common cold. *Cleveland Clin J Med* 66: 27-32.

Madsen, K., D.A. MacLean, B. Kiens, and D. Christensen. 1996. Effects of glucose, glucose plus branched-chain amino acids, or placebo on bike performance over 100 km. *J Appl Physiol* 81(6): 2644-2650.

Malm, C., M. Svensson, B. Ekblom, and B. Sjodin. 1997. Effects of ubiquinone-10 supplementation and high intensity training on physical performance in humans. *Acta Physiol Scand* 161(3): 379-384.

Mannix, E.T., J.M. Stager, A. Harris, and M.O. Farber. 1990. Oxygen delivery and cardiac output during exercise following oral phosphate-glucose. *Med Sci Sports Exerc* 22(3): 341-347.

Manore, M.M. 2002. Dietary recommendations and athletic menstrual dysfunction. *Sports Med* 32: 887-901.

Marmy-Conus, N., S. Fabris, J. Proietto, and M. Hargreaves. 1996. Preexercise glucose ingestion and glucose kinetics during exercise. *J Appl Physiol* 81(2): 853-857.

Marshall, I. 2000. Zinc for the common cold. *Cochrane Database Syst Rev* CD001364.

Martin, B., S. Robinson, and D. Robertshaw. 1978. Influence of diet on leg uptake of glucose during heavy exercise. *Am J Clin Nutr* 31: 62-67.

Martin III, W.H., G.P. Dalsky, B.F. Hurley, D.E. Matthews, D.M. Bier, J.M. Hagberg, M.A. Rogers, D.S. King, and J.O. Holloszy. 1993. Effect of endurance training on plasma free fatty acid turnover and oxidation during exercise. *Am J Physiol* 265: E708-E714.

Matson, L.G., and Z. Vu Tran. 1993. Effects of sodium bicarbonate ingestion on anaerobic performance: a meta-analytic review. *Int J Sport Nutrition* 3: 2-28.

Matthews, C.E., I.S. Ockene, P.S. Freedson, M.C. Rosal, P.A. Merriam, and J.R. Hebert. 2002. Moderate to vigorous physical activity and the risk of upper-respiratory tract infection. *Med Sci Sports Exerc* 34: 1242-1248.

Matthews, D.E. 1999. Proteins and amino acids. In *Modern Nutrition in Health and Disease*, ed. M.E. Shils, J.A. Olson, M. Shike, and A.C. Ross, 11-48. Williams & Wilkins: Baltimore.

Maughan, R.J. 1985. Thermoregulation and fluid balance in marathon competition at low ambient temperature. *Int J Sports Med* 6: 15-19.

———. 1991. Fluid and electrolyte loss and replacement in exercise. *J Sports Sci* 9: 117-142.

Maughan, R.J., L. Bethell, and J.B. Leiper. 1996. Effects of ingested fluids on homeostasis and exercise performance in man. *Exper Physiol* 81: 847-859.

Maughan, R.J., A.E. Donnelly, M. Gleeson, P.H. Whiting, K.A. Walker, and P.J. Clough. 1989. Delayed-onset muscle damage and lipid peroxidation in man after a downhill run. *Muscle Nerve* 12: 332-336.

Maughan, R.J., C.E. Fenn, M. Gleeson, and J.B. Leiper. 1987. Metabolic and circulatory responses to the ingestion of glucose polymer and glucose/electrolyte solutions during exercise in man. *Eur J Appl Physiol* 56: 356-362.

Maughan, R.J., and M. Gleeson. 1988. Influence of a 36 h fast followed by refeeding with glucose, glycerol or placebo on metabolism and performance during prolonged exercise in man. *Eur J Appl Physiol* 57(5): 570-576.

Maughan, R.J., M. Gleeson, and P.L. Greenhaff. 1997. *Biochemistry of exercise and training*. Oxford University Press: Oxford.

Maughan, R.J., P.L. Greenhaff, J.B. Leiper, D. Ball, C.P. Lambert, and M. Gleeson. 1997. Diet composition and the performance of high-intensity exercise. *J Sports Sci* 15(3): 265-275.

Maughan, R.J., J.B. Leiper, and S.M. Shirreffs. 1996. Restoration of fluid balance after exercise-induced dehydration: effects of food and fluid intake. *Eur J Appl Physiol* 73: 317-325.

Maughan, R.J., and D.J. Sadler. 1983. The effects of oral administration of salts of aspartic acid on the metabolic response to prolonged exhausting exercise in man. *Int J Sports Med* 4(2): 119-123.

Maughan, R.J., C. Williams, D.M. Campbell, and D. Hepburn. 1978. Fat and carbohydrate metabolism during low intensity exercise: effects of the availability of muscle glycogen. *Eur J Appl Physiol* 39: 7-16.

Maughan, R.J., and R. Murray (eds.). 2000. *Sports drinks: Basic science and practical aspects*. CRC Press: Boca Raton.

McCarty, M.F. 1996. Chromium (III) picolinate (letter). *FASEB J* 10(2): 365-369.

McCrory, M.A., P.A. Mole, L.A. Nommsen-Rvers, and K.G. Dewey. 1997. Between-day and within-day variation in the relation between heart rate and oxygen consumption: effect on the estimation of energy expenditure by heart-rate monitoring. *Am J Clin Nutr* 66: 18-25.

McElroy, B.H., and S.P. Miller. 2002. Effectiveness of zinc gluconate glycine lozenges (Cold-Eeze) against the common cold in school-aged subjects: a retrospective chart review. *Am J Ther* 9: 472-475.

McGinnis, J.M., and W.H. Foege. 1993. Actual causes of death in the United States. *JAMA* 270(18): 2207-2212.

McMurray, R.G., V. Ben-Ezra, W.A. Forsythe, et al. 1985. Responses of endurance-trained subjects to caloric deficits induced by diet or exercise. *Med Sci Sports Exerc* 17(5): 574-579.

McNaughton, L.R. 1990. Sodium citrate and anaerobic performance: implications of dosage. *Eur J Appl Physiol* 61(5-6): 392-397.

McNaughton, L., and R. Cedaro. 1992. Sodium citrate ingestion and its effects on maximal anaerobic exercise of different durations. *Eur J Appl Physiol* 64(1): 36-41.

McNaughton, L., B. Dalton, and G. Palmer. 1999. Sodium bicarbonate can be used as an ergogenic aid in high-intensity, competitive cycle ergometry of 1 h duration. *Eur J Appl Physiol* 80(1): 64-69.

McNaughton, L., B. Dalton, and J. Tarr. 1999. Inosine supplementation has no effect on aerobic or anaerobic cycling performance. *Int J Sport Nutr* 9: 333-344.

Mensink, R.P., and M.B. Katan. 1990. Effect of dietary trans fatty acids on high-density and low-density lipoprotein cholesterol levels in healthy subjects. *N Engl J Med* 323(7): 439-445.

Merimee, T.J., D.A. Lillicrap, and D. Rabinowitz. 1965. Effect of arginine on serum-levels of human growth-hormone. *Lancet* 2(7414): 668-670.

Meydani, M., W.J. Evans, A. Handleman, R.A. Biddle, R.A. Fielding, and S.N. Meydani, et al. 1993. Protective effect of vitamin E on exercise-induced oxidative damage in young and older adults. *Am J Physiol* 264: R992-R998.

Miller, W.C., R. Bryce, and R.K. Conlee. 1984. Adaptation to a high-fat diet that increases exercise endurance in male rats. *J Appl Physiol* 56(1): 78-83.

Mishell, D.R. 1993. Non-contraceptive benefits of oral contraceptives. *J Reprod Med* 38: 1021-1029.

Mitchell, J.B., F.X. Pizza, A. Paquet, J.B. Davis, M.B. Forrest, and W.A. Braun.1998. Influence of carbohydrate status on immune responses before and after endurance exercise. *J Appl Physiol* 84: 1917-1925.

Mitsiopoulos, N., R.N. Baumgartner, S.B. Heymsfield, et al. 1998. Cadaver validation of skeletal muscle measurement by magnetic resonance imaging and computerized tomography. *J Appl Physiol* 85(1): 115-122.

Modlesky, C.M., K.J. Cureton, R.D. Lewis, et al. 1996. Density of the fat-free mass and estimates of body composition in male weight trainers. *J Appl Physiol* 80(6): 2085-2096.

Montagnani, G.F., B. Arena, and N. Maffulli. 1992. Oestradiol and progesterone during exercise in healthy untrained women. *Med Sci Sports Exerc* 24: 764-768.

Montain, S.J., M.K. Hopper, A.R. Coggan, and E.F. Coyle. 1991. Exercise metabolism at different time intervals after a meal. *J Appl Physiol* 70(2): 882-888.

Monteleone, P., L. Beinat, C. Tanzillo, M. Maj, and D. Kemali. 1990. Effects of phosphatidylserine on the neuroendocrine response to physical stress in humans. *Neuroendocrinology* 52(3): 243-248.

Monteleone, P., M. Maj, L. Beinat, M. Natale, and D. Kemali. 1992. Blunting by chronic phosphatidylserine administration of the stress-induced activation of the hypothalamo-pituitary-adrenal axis in healthy men. *Eur J Clin Pharmacol* 42(4): 385-388.

Morrison, M.A., L.L. Spriet, and D.J. Dyck. 2000. Pyruvate ingestion for 7 days does not improve aerobic performance in well-trained individuals. *J Appl Physiol* 89: 549-556.

Mortola, J.F., and S.S. Yen. 1990. The effects of oral dehydroepiandrosterone on endocrine-metabolic parameters in postmenopausal women. *J Clin Endocrinol Metab* 71(3): 696-704.

Morton, J.F., and J.F. Guthrie. 1998. Changes in children's total fat intakes and their group sources of fat, 1989-91 versus 1994-95: implications for diet quality. *Fam Econ Nutr Rev* 11: 44-57.

Moseley, L., and A.E. Jeukendrup. 2001. The reliability of cycling efficiency. *Med Sci Sports Exerc* 33(4): 621-627.

Moseley, L., G.I. Lancaster, R.L.P.G. Jentjens, J. Achten, and A.E. Jeukendrup. 2001. The effect of timing of pre-exercise carbohydrate feedings on metabolism and cycling performance. *Med Sci Sports Exerc* 34(5): S203.

Mujika, I., J.C. Chatard, L. Lacoste, F. Barale, and A. Geyssant. 1996. Creatine supplementation does not improve sprint performance in competitive swimmers. *Med Sci Sports Exerc* 28(11): 1435-1441.

Murray, R., D.E. Eddy, G.L. Paul, J.G. Seifert, and G.A. Halaby. 1991. Physiological responses to glycerol ingestion during exercise. *J Appl Physiol* 71(1): 144-149.

Myburgh, K.H., L.K. Bachrach, and B. Lewis, 1993. Low bone mineral density at axial and appendicular sites in amenorrhoeic athletes. *Med Sci Sports Exerc* 25: 1197-1202.

Myerson, M., B. Gutin, M.P. Warren, et al. 1991. Resting metabolic rate and energy balance in amenorrheic and eumenorrheic runners. *Med Sci Sports Exerc* 23(1): 15-22.

Nachtigall, D., P. Nielsen, R. Fischer, R. Engelgardt, and E.E. Gabbe. 1996. Iron deficiency in distance runners: a reinvestigation using 59Fe-labelling and non-invasive liver iron quantification. *Int J Sports Med* 17: 473-479.

Nadel, E.R., E. Cafarelli, M.F. Roberts, and C.B. Wenger. 1979. Circulatory regulation during exercise in different ambient temperatures. *J Appl Physiol* 46: 430-437.

Nadel, E.R., S.M. Fortney, and C.B. Wenger. 1980. Effect of hydration state on circulatory and thermal regulations. *J Appl Physiol* 49: 715-721.

Nair, K.S., D.E. Matthews, S.L. Welle, and T. Braiman. 1992. Effect of leucine on amino acid and glucose metabolism in humans. *Metabolism* 41(6): 643-648.

Nehlsen-Cannarella, S.L., O.R. Fagoaga, D.C. Nieman, D.A. Henson, D.E. Butterworth, R.L. Schmitt, E.M. Bailey, B.J. Warren, A. Utter, and J.M. Davis. 1997. Carbohydrate and the cytokine response to 2.5 h of running. *J Appl Physiol* 82: 1662-1667.

Nestler, J.E., C.O. Barlascini, J.N. Clore, and W.G. Blackard. 1988. Dehydroepiandrosterone reduces serum low density lipoprotein levels and body fat but does not alter insulin sensitivity in normal men. *J Clin Endocrinol Metab* 66(1): 57-61.

Neufer, P.D., D.L. Costill, M.G. Flynn, J.P. Kirwan, J.B. Mitchell, and J. Houmard. 1987. Improvements in exercise performance: effects of carbohydrate feedings and diet. *J Appl Physiol* 62(3): 983-988.

Neufer, P.D., Young, A.J., and Sawka M.N. 1989. Gastric emptying during exercise: effects of heat stress and hypohydration. *Eur J Appl Physiol* 58: 433-439.

Newsholme, E.A., I.N. Acworth, and E. Blomstrand. 1987. Amino acids, brain neurotransmitters and a functional link between muscle and brain that is important in sustained exercise. In *Advances in myochemistry*, ed. G. Benzi, 127-147. John Libby Eurotext: London.

Newsholme, E.A., E. Blomstrand, and B. Ekblom. 1992. Physical and mental fatigue: metabolic mechanisms and importance of plasma amino acids. *Brit Med Bull* 48(3): 477-495.

Nielsen, F.H. 1996. Other trace elements. In *Present knowledge of nutrition*, ed. E.E. Ziegler and L.J. Filer, 355-358. ILSI Press: Washington, DC.

Nielsen, F.H., C.D. Hunt, L.M. Mullen, and J.R. Hunt. 1987. Effect of dietary boron on mineral, estrogen, and testosterone metabolism in postmenopausal women. *FASEB J* 1(5): 394-397.

Nieman, D.C. 1994. Exercise, infection, and immunity. *Int J Sports Med* 15(suppl 3): S131-S141.

Nieman, D.C., L.M. Johansen, J.W. Lee, and K. Arabatzis. 1990. Infectious episodes in runners before and after the Los Angeles Marathon. *J Sports Med Phys Fitness* 30: 316-328.

Nieman, D.C., A.R. Miller, D.A. Henson, B.J. Warren, G. Gusewitch, R.L. Johnson, J.M. Davis, D.E. Butterworth, and S.L. Nehlsen-Cannarella. 1993. Effects of high- versus moderate-intensity exercise on natural killer activity. *Med Sci Sports Exerc* 25: 1126-1134.

Nieman, D.C., S.L. Nehlsen-Cannarella, O.R. Fagoaga, et al. 1998a. Effects of mode and carbohydrate on the granulocyte and monocyte response to intensive, prolonged exercise. *J Appl Physiol* 84(4): 1252-1259.

———. 1998b. Influence of mode and carbohydrate on the cytokine response to heavy exertion. *Med Sci Sports Exerc* 30(5): 671-678.

Nieman, D.C., S.L. Nehlsen-Cannarella, O.R. Fagoaga, D.A. Henson, M. Shannon, J.M. Davis, M.D. Austin, C.L. Hisey, J.C. Holbeck, J.M. Hjertman, M.R. Bolton, and B.K. Schilling. 1999. Immune response to two hours of rowing in elite female rowers. *Int J Sports Med* 20: 476-481.

Nieman, D.C., and B.K. Pedersen (eds.). 2000. *Nutrition and exercise immunology*. CRC Press: Boca Raton, FL.

Nilsson, L.H., and E. Hultman. 1973. Liver glycogen in man: The effects of total starvation or a carbohydrate-poor diet followed by carbohydrate feeding. *Scand J Clin Lab Invest* 32: 325-330.

Nissen, S.L., and R.L. Sharp. 2003. Effect of dietary supplements on lean mass and strength gains with resistance exercise: a meta-analysis. *J Appl Physiol* 94(2): 651-659.

Nissen, S., R.L. Sharp, L. Panton, M. Vukovich, S. Trappe, and J.C. Fuller, Jr. 2000. Beta-hydroxy-beta-methylbutyrate (HMB) supplementation in humans is safe and may decrease cardiovascular risk factors. *J Nutr* 130(8): 1937-1945.

Nissen, S., R. Sharp, M. Ray, J.A. Rathmacher, D. Rice, J.C. Fuller, Jr., A.S. Connelly, and N. Abumrad. 1996. Effect of leucine metabolite beta-hydroxy-beta-methylbutyrate on muscle metabolism during resistance-exercise training. *J Appl Physiol* 81(5): 2095-2104.

Noakes, T.D. 1986. *Lore of running*. Oxford University Press: Cape Town.

Noakes, T.D., N. Goodwin, B.L. Rayner, T. Branken, and R.K.N. Taylor. 1985. Water intoxication: a possible complication during endurance exercise. *Med Sci Sports Exerc* 17: 370-375.

Nose, H., G.W. Mack, X. Shi, and E.R. Nadel. 1988. Role of osmolality and plasma volume during rehydration in humans. *J Appl Physiol* 65: 325-331.

Notivol, R., I. Carrio, L. Cano, M. Estorch, and F. Vilardell. 1984. Gastric emptying of solid and liquid meals in healthy young subjects. *Scand J Gastroenterol* 19(8): 1107-1113.

Odland, L.M., G.J.F. Heigenhauser, G.D. Lopaschuk, and L.L. Spriet. 1996. Human skeletal muscle malonyl-COA at rest and during prolonged submaximal exercise. *Am J Physiol* 270: E541-E44.

Odland, L.M., R.A. Howlett, G.J. Heigenhauser, E. Hultman, and L.L. Spriet. 1998. Skeletal muscle malonyl-COA content at the onset of exercise at varying power outputs in humans. *Am J Physiol* 274(6 pt 1): E1080-E1085.

Oostenbrug, G.S., R.P. Mensink, T. De Vries, M.R. Hardeman, F. Brouns, and G. Hornstra. 1997. Exercise performance, red blood cell characteristics and lipid peroxidation: effect of fish oil and vitamin E. *J Appl Physiol* 83(3): 746-752.

Oppliger, R.A., H.S. Case, C.A. Horswill, G.L. Landry, and A.C. Shelter. 1996. American College of Sports Medicine position stand. Weight loss in wrestlers. *Med Sci Sports Exerc* 28(6): ix-xii.

Oppliger, R.A., D.H. Nielsen, and C.G. Vance. 1991. Wrestlers' minimal weight: anthropometry, bioimpedance, and hydrostatic weighing compared. *Med Sci Sports Exerc* 23(2): 247-253.

Oscai, L.B., D.A. Essig, and W.K. Palmer. 1990. Lipase regulation of muscle triglyceride hydrolysis. *J Appl Physiol* 69(5): 1571-1577.

Packer, L. 1997. Oxidants, antioxidant nutrients and the athlete. *J Sports Sci* 15: 353-363.

Paddon-Jones, D., A. Keech, and D. Jenkins. 2001. Short-term beta-hydroxy-beta-methylbutyrate supplementation does not reduce symptoms of eccentric muscle damage. *Int J Sport Nutr Exerc Metab* 11(4): 442-450.

Pagala, M.K., T. Namba, and D. Grob. 1984. Failure of neuromuscular transmission and contractility during muscle fatigue. *Muscle Nerve* 7(6): 454-464.

Pan, D.A., S. Lillioja, A.D. Kriketos, M.R. Milner, L.A. Baur, C. Bogardus, A.B. Jenkins, and L.H. Storlien. 1997. Skeletal muscle triglyceride levels are inversely related to insulin action. *Diabetes* 46: 983-988.

Panton, L.B., J.A. Rathmacher, S. Baier, and S. Nissen. 2000. Nutritional supplementation of the leucine metabolite beta-hydroxy-beta-methylbutyrate (Hmb) during resistance training. *Nutrition* 16(9): 734-739.

Papet, I., P. Ostaszewski, F. Glomot, C. Obled, M. Faure, G. Bayle, S. Nissen, M. Arnal, and J. Grizard. 1997. The effect of a high dose of 3-hydroxy-3-methylbutyrate on protein metabolism in growing lambs. *Br J Nutr* 77(6): 885-896.

Parry-Billings, M., R. Budgett, Y. Koutedakis, E. Blomstrand, S. Brooks, C. Williams, P.C. Calder, S. Pilling, R. Baigrie, and E.A. Newsholme. 1992. Plasma amino acid concentrations in the overtraining syndrome: possible effects on the immune system. *Med Sci Sports Exerc* 24(12): 1353-1358.

Pasman, W.J., M.A. van Baak, A.E. Jeukendrup, and A. deHaan. 1995. The effect of varied dosages of caffeine on endurance performance time. *Int J Sports Med* 16(4): 225-230.

Pedersen, B.K., and H. Bruunsgaard. 1995. How physical exercise influences the establishment of infections. *Sports Med* 19: 393-400.

Pedersen, B.K., J. Helge, E. Richter, T. Rhode, K. Ostrowski, and B. Kiens. 2000. Training and natural immunity: effects of diets rich in fat or carbohydrate. *Eur J Appl Physiol* 82: 98-102.

Pendergast, D.R., P.J. Horvath, J.J. Leddy, and J.T. Venkatraman. 1996. The role of dietary fat on performance, metabolism and health. *Am J Sports Med* 24(6): S53-S58.

Perusse, L., and C. Bouchard. 2000. Gene-diet interactions in obesity. *Am J Clin Nutr* 72(5 suppl): 1285S-1290S.

Peters, E.M., and E.D. Bateman. 1983. Ultramarathon running and URTI: an epidemiological survey. *S Afr Med J* 64: 582-584.

Peters, E.M., and J.M. Goetzsche. 1997. Dietary practices of South African ultradistance athletes. *Int J Sport Nutr* 7: 80-103.

Peters, E.M., J.M. Goetzsche, B. Grobbelaar, and T.D. Noakes. 1993. Vitamin C supplementation reduces the incidence of post-race symptoms of upper respiratory tract in ultramarathon runners. *Am J Clin Nutr* 57: 170-174.

Peters, E.M., J.M. Goetzsche, L.E. Joseph, and T.D. Noakes. 1996. Vitamin C as effective as combinations of anti-oxidant nutrients in reducing symptoms of upper respiratory tract infections in ultramarathon runners. *S Afr J Sports Med* 11: 23-27.

Peyrebrune, M.C., M.E. Nevill, F.J. Donaldson, and D.J. Cosford. 1998. The effects of oral creatine supplementation on performance in single and repeated sprint swimming. *J Sports Sci* 16(3): 271-279.

Phillips, S.M., K.D. Tipton, A. Aarsland, S.E. Wolf, and R.R. Wolfe. 1997. Mixed muscle protein synthesis and breakdown after resistance exercise in humans. *Am J Physiol* 273(1 pt 1): E99-E107.

Phillips, S.M., K.D. Tipton, A.A. Ferrando, and R.R. Wolfe. 1999. Resistance training reduces the acute exercise-induced increase in muscle protein turnover. *Am J Physiol* 276(1 pt 1): E118-E124.

Phinney, S.D., B.R. Bistrian, W.J. Evans, E. Gervino, and G.L. Blackburn. 1983. The human metabolic response to chronic ketosis without caloric restriction: preservation of submaximal exercise capability with reduced carbohydrate oxidation. *Metabolism* 32(9): 769-776.

Phinney, S.D., B.R. Bistrian, R.R. Wolfe, and G.L. Blackburn. 1983. The human metabolic response to chronic ketosis without caloric restriction: physical and biochemical adaptation. *Metabolism* 32(8): 757-768.

Phinney, S.D., E.S. Horton, E.A.H. Sims, J.S. Hanson, E. Danforth, and B.M. LaGrange. 1980. Capacity for moderate exercise in obese subjects after adaptation to a hypocaloric, ketogenic diet. *J Clin Invest* 66: 1152-1161.

Pinchan, G., R.K. Gauttam, O.S. Tomar, and A.C. Babaj. 1988. Effects of primary hypohydration on physical work capacity. *Int J Biometeorol* 32: 176-180.

Pirnay, F., J.M. Crielaard, N. Pallikarakis, M. Lacroix, F. Mosora, G. Krzentowski, A.S. Luyckx, and P.J. Lefebvre. 1982. Fate of exogenous glucose during exercise of different intensities in humans. *J Appl Physiol* 53: 1620-1624.

Pirnay, F., A.J. Scheen, J.F. Gautier, M. Lacroix, and P.J. Lefèbvre. 1995. Exogenous glucose oxidation during exercise in relation to the power output. *Int J Sports Med* 16(7): 456-460.

Polivy, J., and C.P. Herman. 1995. Dieting and its relation to eating disorders. In *Eating disorders and obesity: A comprehensive handbook*, ed. K.D. Brownell and C.G. Fairburn, 83-86. Guildford Press: London.

Pomeroy, C., and S.F. Mitchell. 1992. Medical issues in the eating disorders. In *Eating, body weight and performance in athletes: disorders of modern society*, ed. K.D. Brownell, J. Rodin, and J.H. Wilmore, 202-221. Lea & Febiger: Philadelphia.

Posner, B.M., L.A. Cupples, M.M. Franz, and D.R. Gagnon. 1993. Diet and heart disease risk factors in adult American men and women: the Framingham offspring-spouse nutrition studies. *Int J Epidemiol* 22(6): 1014-1025.

Potteiger, J.A., G.L. Nickel, M.J. Webster, M.D. Haub, and R.J. Palmer. 1996. Sodium citrate ingestion enhances 30 km cycling performance. *Int J Sports Med* 17(1): 7-11.

Powers, S.K., R.J. Byrd, R. Tulley, and T. Callender. 1983. Effects of caffeine ingestion on metabolism and performance during graded exercise. *Eur J Appl Physiol* 50: 301-307.

Randle, P.J., P.B. Garland, C.N. Hales, and E.A. Newsholme. 1963. The glucose fatty acid cycle: its role in insulin sensitivity and the metabolic disturbances of diabetes mellitus. *Lancet* 1: 786-789.

Rankinen, T., L. Perusse, S. J. Weisnagel, et al. 2002. The human obesity gene map: the 2001 update. *Obes Res* 10(3): 196-243.

Rasmussen, B.B., K.D. Tipton, S.L. Miller, S.E. Wolf, and R.R. Wolfe. 2000. An oral essential amino acid-carbohydrate supplement enhances muscle protein anabolism after resistance exercise. *J Appl Physiol* 88(2): 386-392.

Rasmussen, B.B., E. Volpi, D.C. Gore, and R.R. Wolfe. 2000. Androstenedione does not stimulate muscle protein anabolism in young healthy men. *J Clin Endocrinol Metab* 85(1): 55-59.

Rehrer, N.J., E.J. Beckers, F. Brouns, F. ten Hoor, and W.H. Saris. 1990. Effects of dehydration on gastric emptying and gastrointestinal distress while running. *Med Sci Sports Exerc* 22(6): 790-795.

Rehrer, N.J., M. van Kemenade, W. Meester, F. Brouns, and W.H.M. Saris. 1992. Gastrointestinal complaints in relation to dietary intake in triathletes. *Int J Sport Nutr* 2: 48-59.

Rehrer, N.J., A.J.M. Wagenmakers, E.J. Beckers, D. Halliday, J.B. Leiper, F. Brouns, R.J. Maugham, K. Westerterp, and W.H.M. Saris. 1992. Gastric emptying, absorption and carbohydrate oxidation during prolonged exercise. *J Appl Physiol* 72(2): 468-475.

Ren, J.M., C.F. Semenkovich, E.A. Gulve, J. Gao, and J.O. Holloszy. 1994. Exercise induces rapid increases in GLUT4 expression, glucose transport capacity, and insulin-stimulated glycogen storage in muscle. *J Biol Chem* 269(20): 14396-14401.

Rennie, M.J., P.A. MacLellan, H.S. Hundal, B. Weryl, K. Smith, P.M. Taylor, C. Egan, and P.W. Watt. 1989. Skeletal muscle glutamine concentration and muscle protein turnover. *Clin Exp* 38: 47-51.

Rennie, M.J., and K.D. Tipton. 2000. Protein and amino acid metabolism during and after exercise and the effects of nutrition. *Annu Rev Nutr* 20: 457-483.

Riley, M.L., R.G. Israel, D. Holbert, E.B. Tapscott, and G.L. Dohm. 1988. Effect of carbohydrate ingestion on exercise endurance and metabolism after 1-day fast. *Int J Sports Med* 9: 320-324.

Robson, P. J., A.K. Blannin, N.P. Walsh, L.M. Castell, and M. Gleeson. 1999. Effects of exercise intensity, duration and recovery on in vitro neutrophil function in male athletes. *Int J Sports Med* 20: 128-135.

Rohde, T., S. Asp, D. Maclean, and B.K. Pedersen. 1998. Competitive sustained exercise in humans, and lymphokine activated killer cell activity—an intervention study. *Eur J Appl Physiol* 78: 448-453.

Rolls, B.J., and E.A. Bell. 1999. Intake of fat and carbohydrate: role of energy density. *Eur J Clin Nutr* 53(suppl 1): S166-S173.

Rolls, B.J., E.A. Bell, V.H. Castellanos, M. Chow, C.L. Pelkman, and M.L. Thorwart. 1999. Energy density but not fat content of foods affected energy intake in lean and obese women. *Am J Clin Nutr* 69(5): 863-871.

Romer, L.M., J.P. Barrington, and A.E. Jeukendrup. 2001. Effects of oral creatine supplementation on high intensity, intermittent exercise performance in competitive squash players. *Int J Sports Med* 22(8): 546-552.

Romijn, J.A., E.F. Coyle, L.S. Sidossis, A. Gastaldelli, J.F. Horowitz, E. Endert, and R.R. Wolfe. 1993. Regulation of endogenous fat and carbohydrate metabolism in relation to exercise intensity. *Am J Physiol* 265: E380-E391.

Romijn, J.A., E.F. Coyle, X.-J. Zhang, L.S. Sidossis, and R.R. Wolfe. 1995. Fat oxidation is impaired somewhat during high intensity exercise by limited plasma FFA. *J Appl Physiol* 79(6): 1939-1945.

Rontoyannis, G.P., T. Skoulis, and K.N. Pavlou. 1989. Energy balance in ultramarathon running. *Am J Clin Nutr* 49(5 suppl): 976-979.

Rosen, L.W., and D. O. Hough. 1988. Pathogenic weight control behaviors of female college gymnasts. *Physician Sports Med* 9: 141-144.

Ross, S. 2000. Functional foods: The food and drug administration perspective. *Am J Clin Nutr* 71(6 suppl): 1735S-1738S.

Rossiter, H.B., E.R. Cannell, and P.M. Jakeman. 1996. The effect of oral creatine supplementation on the 1000-m performance of competitive rowers. *J Sports Sci* 14(2): 175-179.

Roth, A., and G. Fonagy. 1998. *What works for whom?* Guildford Press: New York.

Rucinski, A. 1989. Relationship of body image and dietary intake of competitive ice skaters. *J Am Dietetic Assoc* 89: 98-100.

Sabatini, S. 2001. The female athlete triad. *Am J Med Sci* 322: 193-195.

Saltin, B. 1973. Metabolic fundamentals in exercise. *Med Sci Sports Exerc* 5: 137-146.

Saltin, B., A.P. Gagge, and J.A.J. Stolwijk. 1968. Muscle temperature during submaximal exercise in man. *J Appl Physiol* 25: 679-688.

Sandage, B.W., R.N. Sabounjian, R. White, and R.J. Wurtman. 1992. Choline citrate may enhance athletic performance. *Physiologist* 35: 236A.

Saris, W.H.M., B.H. Goodpaster, A.E. Jeukendrup, F. Brouns, D. Halliday, and A.J.M. Wagenmakers. 1993. Exogenous carbohydrate oxidation from different carbohydrate sources during exercise. *J Appl Physiol* 755: 2168-2172.

Saris, W.H.M., M.A. van Erp-Baart, F. Brouns, K.R. Westerterp, and F. ten Hoor. 1989. Study on food intake and energy expenditure during extreme sustained exercise: the Tour de France. *Int J Sports Med* 10(1 suppl): S26-S31.

Sarna, S., and J. Kaprio. 1994. Life expectancy of former elite athletes. *Sports Med* 17(3): 49-51.

Sasaki, H., J. Maeda, S. Usui, and T. Ishiko. 1987. Effect of sucrose and caffeine ingestion on performance of prolonged strenuous running. *Int J Sports Med* 8: 261-265.

Saunders, M.J., J.E. Blevins, and C.E. Broeder. 1998. Effects of hydration changes on bioelectrical impedance in endurance trained individuals. *Med Sci Sports Exerc* 30(6): 885-892.

Sawka, M.N., and K.B. Pandolf. 1990. Effects of body water loss on physiological function and exercise performance. In *Perspectives in exercise science and sports medicine*, vol. 3, eds. C.V. Gisolfi, and D.R. Lamb, 1-38. Benchmark Press: Carmel, IN.

Sawka, M.N., and C.B. Wenger. 1988. Physiological responses to acute-exercise heat stress. In *Human performance physiology and environmental medicine at terrestrial extremes*, ed. K. Pandolf, M.N. Sawka, and R.R. Gonzalez, 97-151. Cooper Publishing: Indianapolis, IN.

Sawka, M.N., A.J. Young, B.S. Cadarette, L. Levine, and K.B. Pandolf. 1985. Influence of heat stress and acclimation on maximal aerobic power. *Eur J Appl Physiol*. 53: 294-298.

Sawka, M.N., A.J. Young, R.P. Francesconi, S.R. Muza, and K.B. Pandolf. 1985. Thermoregulatory and blood responses during exercise at graded hypohydration levels. *J Appl Physiol* 59: 1394-1401.

Sawka, M.N., A.J. Young, W.A. Latzka, P.D. Neufer, M.D. Quigley, and K.B. Pandolf. 1992. Human tolerance to heat strain during exercise: influence of hydration. *J Appl Physiol* 73: 368-375.

Schlundt, D.G., J.O. Hill, J. Pope-Cordle, et al. 1993. Randomized evaluation of a low fat ad libitum carbohydrate diet for weight reduction. *Int J Obes Relat Metab Disord* 17(11): 623-629.

Schoeller, D.A., E. Ravussin, Y. Schutz, K.J. Acheson, P. Baertschi, and E. Jequier. 1986. Energy expenditure by doubly labeled water: validation in humans and proposed calculation. *Am J Physiol* 250(5 pt 2): R823-R830.

Schoffelen, P.F., K.R. Westerterp, W.H.M. Saris, and F. ten Hoor. 1997. A dual respiration chamber system with automated calibration. *J Appl Physiol* 83: 2064-2072.

Sears, B. 1995. *The Zone: A dietary road map*. Harper Collins: New York.

Segura, R., and J.L. Ventura. 1988. Effect of L-tryptophan supplementation on exercise performance. *Int J Sports Med* 9: 301-305.

Seidell, J.C. 1997. Time trends in obesity: an epidemiological perspective. *Horm Metab Res* 29(4): 155-158.

———. 1998. Dietary fat and obesity: an epidemiologic perspective. *Am J Clin Nutr* 67(3 suppl): 546S-550S.

Shephard, R. J. 1997. *Physical activity, training and the immune response*. Cooper: Carmel, IN.

Sheppard, L., A.R. Kristal, L.H. Kushi. 1991. Weight loss in women participating in a randomized trial of low-fat diets. *Am J Clin Nutr* 54(5): 821-828.

Sherman, W.M., and D.L. Costill. 1984. The marathon: dietary manipulation to optimize performance. *Am J Sports Med* 12(1): 44-51.

Sherman, W.M., D.L. Costill, W.J. Fink, and J.M. Miller. 1981. The effect of exercise and diet manipulation on muscle glycogen and its subsequent utilization during performance. *Int J Sports Med* 2: 114-118.

Sherman, W.M., J.A. Doyle, D.R. Lamb, and R.H. Strauss. 1993. Dietary carbohydrate, muscle glycogen, and exercise performance during 7 d of training. *Am J Clin Nutr* 57: 27-31.

Shi, X., R.W. Summers, H.P. Schedl, S.W. Flanagan, R. Chang, and C.V. Gisolfi. 1995. Effects of carbohydrate type and concentration and solution osmolality on water absorption. *Med Sci Sports Exerc* 27(12): 1607-1615.

Shils, M.E., J.A. Olson, M. Shike, and A.C. Ross. 1999. *Modern nutrition in health and disease*. 9th ed. Williams & Wilkins: Baltimore.

Shirreffs, S.M., and R.J. Maughan. 1997. Restoration of fluid balance after exercise-induced dehydration: effects of alcohol consumption. *J Appl Physiol* 83: 1152-1157.

———. 1998. Volume repletion following exercise-induced volume depletion in man: replacement of water and sodium losses. *Am J Physiol* 274: F868-F875.

———. 2000. Rehydration and recovery of fluid balance after exercise. *Exer Sports Sci Rev* 28: 27-32.

Shirreffs, S.M., A.J. Taylor, J.B. Leiper, and R.J. Maughan. 1996. Post-exercise rehydration in man: effects of volume consumed and drink sodium content. *Med Sci Sports Exerc* 28: 1260-1271.

Sidossis, L.S., A. Gastaldelli, S. Klein, and R.R. Wolfe. 1997. Regulation of plasma fatty acid oxidation during low- and high-intensity exercise. *Am J Physiol* 272: E1065-1070.

Silva, A.C., M.S. Santos-Neto, A.M. Soares, M.C. Fonteles, R.L. Guerrant, and A.A. Lima. 1998. Efficacy of a glutamine-based oral rehydration solution on the electrolyte and water absorption in a rabbit model of secretory diarrhea induced by cholera toxin [see comments]. *J Pediatr Gastroenterol Nutr* 26(5): 513-519.

Simi, B., B. Sempore, M.-H. Mayet, and R.J. Favier. 1991. Additive effects of training and high-fat diet on energy metabolism during exercise. *J Appl Physiol* 71(1): 197-203.

Singh, A., M.L. Failla, and P.A. Deuster. 1994. Exercise-induced changes in immune function: effects of zinc supplementation. *J Appl Physiol* 76: 2298-2301.

Singh, R.B., M.A. Niaz, S. Ghosh, R. Beegom, P. Agarwal, S. Nangia, M. Moshiri, and E.D. Janus. 1998. Low fat intake and coronary artery disease in a population with higher prevalence of coronary artery disease: the Indian paradox. *J Am Coll Nutr* 17(4): 342-350.

Siri, W.E. 1956. The gross composition of the body. *Adv Biol Med Physiol* 4: 239-280.

Sirrs, S.M., and R.A. Bebb. 1999. DHEA: panacea or snake oil? *Can Fam Physician* 45: 1723-1728.

Sjodin, A.M., A.B. Andersson, J.M. Hogberg, and K.R. Westerterp. 1994. Energy balance in cross-country skiers: a study using doubly labeled water. *Med Sci Sports Exerc* 26(6): 720-724.

Slater, G., D. Jenkins, P. Logan, H. Lee, M. Vukovich, J.A. Rathmacher, and A.G. Hahn. 2001. Beta-hydroxy-beta-methylbutyrate (HMB) supplementation does not affect changes in strength or body composition during resistance training in trained men. *Int J Sport Nutr Exerc Metab* 11(3): 384-396.

Snow-Harter, C.M. 1994. Bone health and prevention of osteoporosis in active and athletic women. *Clin Sport Med* 13: 389-404.

Snyder, A.C., K.P. O'Hagan, P.S. Clifford, et al. 1993. Exercise responses to in-line skating: comparisons to running and cycling. *Int J Sports Med* 14(1): 38-42.

Sole, C.C., and T.D. Noakes. 1989. Faster gastric emptying for glucose-polymer and fructose solutions than for glucose in humans. *Eur J Appl Physiol* 58: 605-612.

Spector, S.A., M.R. Jackman, L.A. Sabounjian, C. Sakkas, D.M. Landers, and W.T. Willis. 1995. Effect of choline supplementation on fatigue in trained cyclists. *Med Sci Sports Exerc* 27(5): 668-673.

Spriet, L.L. 1991. Phosphofructokinase activity and acidosis during short-term tetanic contractions. *Can J Physiol Pharmacol* 69: 298-304.

———. 1995a. Anaerobic metabolism during high-intensity exercise. In *Exercise metabolism*, ed. M. Hargreaves, 1-39. Human Kinetics: Champaign, IL.

———. 1995b. Caffeine and performance. *Int J Sports Nutr* 5: S84-S99.

Spriet, L.L., D.A. McLean, D.J. Dyck, E. Hultman, G. Cederblad, and T.E. Graham. 1992. Caffeine ingestion and muscle metabolism during prolonged exercise in humans. *Am J Physiol* 262: E891-E898.

Spurr, G.B., A.M. Prentice, P.R. Murgatroyd, G.R. Goldberg, J.C. Reina, and N.T. Christman. 1988. Energy expenditure from minute-by-minute heart-rate recording: comparison with indirect calorimetry. *Am J Clin Nutr* 48: 552-559.

Stanko, R.T., R.J. Robertson, R.J. Spina, J.J. Reilly, Jr., K.D. Greenawalt, and F.L. Goss. 1990. Enhancement of arm exercise endurance capacity with dihydroxyacetone and pyruvate. *J Appl Physiol* 68(1): 119-124.

Stanko, R.T., R.J. Robertson, R.W. Galbreath, J.J. Reilly, K.D. Greenawalt, and F.L. Goss. 1990. Enhanced leg exercise endurance with a high-carbohydrate diet and dihydroxyacetone and pyruvate. *J Appl Physiol* 69(5): 1651-1656.

Starling, R.D., T.A. Trappe, K.R. Short, M. Sheffield-Moore, A.C. Jozsi, W.J. Fink, and D.L. Costill. 1996. Effect of inosine supplementation on aerobic and anaerobic cycling performance. *Med Sci Sports Exerc* 28(9): 1193-1198.

Starritt, E.C., R.A. Howlett, G.J. Heigenhauser, and L.L. Spriet. 2000. Sensitivity of CPT I to malonyl-CoA in trained and untrained human skeletal muscle. *Am J Physiol Endocrinol Metab* 278(3): E462-E468.

Stearns, D.M., J.J. Belbruno, and K.E. Wetterhahn. 1995. A prediction of chromium (III) accumulation in humans from chromium dietary supplements. *FASEB J* 9(15): 1650-1657.

Stensrud, T., F. Ingjer, H. Holm, and S.B. Strømme. 1992. L-tryptophan supplementation does not improve running performance. *Int J Sports Med* 13(6): 481-485.

Stewart, I., L. McNaughton, P. Davies, and S. Tristram. 1990. Phosphate loading and the effects on $\dot{V}O_2$max in trained cyclists. *Res Q Exerc Sport* 61(1): 80-84.

Stoecker, B.J. 1996. Chromium. In *Present knowledge in nutrition*, ed. E.E. Ziegler and L.J. Filer, 344-353. ILSI Press: Washington, DC.

Stolarczyk, L.M., V.H. Heyward, M.D. Van Loan, et al. 1997. The fatness-specific bioelectrical impedance analysis equations of Segal et al.: are they generalizable and practical? *Am J Clin Nutr* 66(1): 8-17.

Sundgot-Borgen, J. 1994a. Eating disorders in female athletes. *Sports Med* 3: 176-188.

———. 1994b. Risk and trigger factors for the development of eating disorders in female elite athletes. *Med Sci Sports Exerc* 4: 414-419.

———. 2000. Eating disorders in athletes. In *Nutrition in sport*, ed. R.J. Maughan, 510-522. Blackwell Science: Oxford.

Sundgot-Borgen, J., and S. Larsen. 1993. Pathogenic weight-control methods and self-reported eating disorders in female elite athletes and controls. *Scand J Med Sci Sports* 3: 150-155.

Sutton, J.R., and O. Bar-Or. 1980. Thermal illness in fun running. *Am Heart J* 100: 778-781.

Svensson, M., C. Malm, M. Tonkonogi, B. Ekblom, B. Sjodin, and K. Sahlin. 1999. Effect of Q10 supplementation on tissue Q10 levels and adenine nucleotide catabolism during high-intensity exercise. *Int J Sport Nutr* 9(2) : 166-180.

Swensen, T., G. Crater, D.R. Bassett, Jr., and E.T. Howley. 1994. Adding polylactate to a glucose polymer solution does not improve endurance. *Int J Sports Med* 15(7): 430-434.

Tarnopolsky, M.A., S.A. Atkinson, J.D. McDoughall, D.G. Sale, and J.R. Sutton. 1989. Physiological responses to caffeine during endurance running in habitual caffeine users. *Med Sci Sports Exerc* 21(4): 418-424.

Terjung, R.L., P. Clarkson, E.R. Eichner, P.L. Greenhaff, P.J. Hespel, R.G. Israel, W.J. Kraemer, R.A. Meyer, L.L. Spriet, M.A. Tarnopolsky, A.J. Wagenmakers, and M.H. Williams. 2000. American College of Sports Medicine roundtable. The physiological and health effects of oral creatine supplementation. *Med Sci Sports Exerc* 32(3): 706-717.

Thompson, R.A., and R. Trattner-Sherman. 1993. *Helping athletes with eating disorders*. Human Kinetics: Champaign, IL.

Timmons, J.A., S.M. Poucher, D. Constantin-Teodosiu, V. Worrall, I.A. Macdonald, and P.L. Greenhaff. 1996. Increased acetyl group availability enhances contractile function of canine skeletal muscle during ischemia. *J Clin Invest* 97: 879-883.

Tippett, K.S., and L.E. Cleveland (eds.). 1999. How current diets stack up—comparison with dietary guidelines. *Agricultulture Information Bulletin Number 750*, 51-70. United States Department of Agriculture, Economic Research Service: Washington, DC.

Tipton, C.M., and R.A. Oppliger. 1993. Nutritional and fitness considerations for competitive wrestlers. *World Rev Nutr Diet* 71: 84-96.

Tipton, K.D., A.A. Ferrando, S.M. Phillips, D. Doyle, Jr., and R.R. Wolfe. 1999. Postexercise net protein synthesis in human muscle from orally administered amino acids. *Am J Physiol* 276(4 pt 1): E628-634.

Toner, M.M., D.T. Kirkendall, D.J. Delio, J.M. Chase, P.A. Cleary, and E.L. Fox. 1982. Metabolic and cardiovascular responses to exercise with caffeine. *Ergonomics* 25: 1175-1183.

Touyz, S.W., P.J.V. Beumont, and S. Hook. 1987. Exercise anorexia: a new dimension in anorexia nervosa? *Handbook of Eating Disorders* 1: 143-157.

Tremblay, M.S., S.D. Galloway, and J.R. Sexsmith. 1994. Ergogenic effects of phosphate loading: physiological fact or methodological fiction? *Can J Appl Physiol* 19(1): 1-11.

Tsintzas, K., and C. Williams. 1998. Human muscle glycogen metabolism during exercise: effect of carbohydrate supplementation. *Sports Med* 25(1): 7-23.

Tsintzas, O.K., C. Williams, L. Boobis, and P. Greenhaff. 1995. Carbohydrate ingestion and glycogen utilisation in different muscle fibre types in man. *J Physiol* 489(1): 243-250.

Turcotte, L.P., E.A. Richter, and B. Kiens. 1995. Lipid metabolism during exercise. In *Exercise metabolism*, ed. M. Hargreaves, 99-130. Human Kinetics: Champaign, IL.

U.S. Department of Agriculture. 1991. United States Nutrition Labeling and Education Act of 1990. *Nutr Rev* 49: 273-276.

———. 2000. *Dietary Guidelines for Americans, 2000*. Available from http://www.usda.gov/cnpp/Pubs/DG2000/Index.htm.

———. 2003. *USDA national nutrient database for standard reference* (release 16). Available from http://www.nal.usda.gov/fnic/foodcomp/Data/index.html.

Van Der Meulen, J., A. McArdle, M. Jackson, and J.A. Faulkner 1997. Contraction-induced injury to the extensor digitorum longus muscles of rats: the role of vitamin E. *Eur J Appl Physiol* 83: 817-823.

van Erp-Baart, A.M.J., W.H.M. Saris, R.A. Binkhorst, J.A. Vos, and J.W.H. Elvers. 1989a. Nationwide survey on nutritional habits in elite athletes. Part I: Energy, carbohydrate, protein, and fat intake. *Int J Sports Med* 10(suppl 1): S3-S10.

———. 1989b. Nationwide survey on nutritional habits in elite athletes. Part II: Mineral and vitamin intake. *Int J Sports Med* 10(1): S11-S16.

Van Etten, L.M., F.T. Verstappen, K.R. Westerterp 1994. Effect of body build on weight-training-induced adaptations in body composition and muscular strength. *Med Sci Sports Exerc* 26(4): 515-521.

Van Hall, G., J.S.H. Raaymakers, W.H.M. Saris, and A.J.M. Wagenmakers. 1995. Ingestion of branched-chain amino acids and tryptophan during sustained exercise in man: failure to affect performance. *J Physiol* 486(3): 789-794.

Van Loan, M.D., N.L. Keim, K. Berg, et al. 1995. Evaluation of body composition by dual energy X-ray absorptiometry and two different software packages. *Med Sci Sports Exerc* 27(4): 587-591.

van Loon, L.J., W.H. Saris, M. Kruijshoop, and A.J. Wagenmakers. 2000. Maximizing postexercise muscle glycogen synthesis: carbohydrate supplementation and the application of amino acid or protein hydrolysate mixtures. *Am J Clin Nutr* 72(1): 106-111.

Van Soeren, M.H., and T.E. Graham. 1998. Effect of caffeine on metabolism, exercise endurance, and catecholamine responses after withdrawal. *J Appl Physiol* 85(4): 1493-1501.

Van Soeren, M.H., P. Sathasivam, L.L. Spriet, and T.E. Graham. 1993. Caffeine metabolism and epinephrine responses during exercise in users and nonusers. *J Appl Physiol* 75(2): 805-812.

Van Zeyl, C.G., E.V. Lambert, J.A. Hawley, T.D. Noakes, and S.C. Dennis. 1996. Effects of medium-chain triglyceride ingestion on carbohydrate metabolism and cycling performance. *J Appl Physiol* 80: 2217-2225.

Vandenberghe, K., M. Goris, P. Van Hecke, M. Van Leemputte, L. Vangerven, and P. Hespel. 1997. Long-term creatine intake is beneficial to muscle performance during resistance training. *J Appl Physiol* 83(6): 2055-2063.

Varnier, M., P. Sarto, D. Martines, L. Lora, F. Carmignoto, G.P. Leese, and R. Naccarato. 1994. Effect of infusing branched-chain

amino acid during incremental exercise with reduced muscle glycogen content. *Eur J Appl Physiol* 69(1): 26-31.

Vergauwen, L., F. Brouns, and P. Hespel. 1998. Carbohydrate supplementation improves stroke performance in tennis. *Med Sci Sports Exerc* 30(8): 1289-1295.

Verma, S., M.C. Cam, and J.H. McNeill. 1998. Nutritional factors that can favorably influence the glucose/insulin system: vanadium. *J Am Coll Nutr* 17: 11-18.

Vist, G.E., and R.J. Maughan. 1994. Gastric emptying of ingested solutions in man: effect of beverage glucose concentration. *Med Sci Sports Exerc* 26(10): 1269-1273.

———. 1995. The effect of osmolality and carbohydrate content on the rate of gastric emptying of liquids in man. *J Physiol* 486(pt 2): 523-531.

Volek, J.S., W.J. Kraemer, J.A. Bush, M. Boetes, T. Incledon, K.L. Clark, and J.M. Lynch. 1997. Creatine supplementation enhances muscular performance during high-intensity resistance exercise. *J Am Diet Assoc* 97(7): 765-770.

Volpe, S.L., L.J. Taper, and S. Meacham. 1993. The relationship between boron and magnesium status and bone mineral density in the human: a review. *Magnes Res* 6(3): 291-296.

von Allworden, H.N., S. Horn, J. Kahl, and W. Feldheim. 1993. The influence of lecithin on plasma choline concentrations in triathletes and adolescent runners during exercise. *Eur J Appl Physiol* 67(1): 87-91.

Vukovich, M.D., D.L. Costill, M.S. Hickey, S.W. Trappe, K.J. Cole, and W.J. Fink. 1993. Effect of fat emulsion infusion and fat feeding on muscle glycogen utilization during cycle exercise. *J Appl Physiol* 75(4): 1513-1518.

Vukovich, M.D., D.L. Costill, and W.J. Fink. 1994. Carnitine supplementation: effect on muscle carnitine and glycogen content during exercise. *J Appl Physiol* 26(9): 1122-1129.

Wagenmakers, A. J. 1999a. Amino acid supplements to improve athletic performance. *Curr Opin Clin Nutr Metab Care* 2(6): 539-544.

Wagenmakers, A.J.M. 1999b. Nutritional supplements: effects on exercise performance and metabolism. In Perspectives in Exercise Science and Sports Medicine. Vol. 12, eds. D.R. Lamb, and R. Murray, 2007-259. Cooper Publishing Group: Carmel, IN.

Wagenmakers, A.J.M., E.J. Beckers, F. Brouns, H. Kuipers, P.B. Soeters, G.J. van der Vusse, and W.H.M. Saris. 1991. Carbohydrate supplementation, glycogen depletion, and amino acid metabolism during exercise. *Am J Physiol* 260(6): E883-E890.

Wagenmakers, A.J.M., J.H. Brookes, J.H. Coakley, T. Reilly, and R.H.T. Edwards. 1989. Exercise-induced activation of branched-chain 2-oxo acid dehydrogenase in human muscle. *Eur J Appl Physiol* 59: 159-167.

Wagner, D.R., V.H. Heyward, and A.L. Gibson. 2000. Validation of air displacement plethysmography for assessing body composition. *Med Sci Sports Exerc* 32(7): 1339-1344.

Wahrenberg, H., J. Bolinder, P. Arner. 1991. Adrenergic regulation of lipolysis in human fat cells during exercise. *Eur J Clin Invest* 21: 534-541.

Wallace, M.B., J. Lim, A. Cutler, and L. Bucci. 1999. Effects of dehydroepiandrosterone vs androstenedione supplementation in men. *Med Sci Sports Exerc* 31(12): 1788-1792.

Waller, M.F., and E.M. Haymes. 1996. The effects of heat and exercise on sweat iron loss. *Med Sci Sports Exerc* 28: 197-203.

Walsh, N.P., A.K. Blannin, N.C. Bishop, P.J. Robson, and M. Gleeson. 2000. Oral glutamine supplementation does not attenuate the fall in human neutrophil lipopolysaccharide-stimulated degranulation following prolonged exercise. *Int J Sport Nutr* 10: 39-50.

Walsh, N.P., A.K. Blannin, P.J. Robson, and M. Gleeson. 1998. Glutamine, exercise and immune function: links and possible mechanisms. *Sports Med* 26: 177-191.

Wannamethee, S.G., A.G. Shaper, and M. Walker 2002. Weight change, weight fluctuation, and mortality. *Arch Intern Med* 162(22): 2575-2580.

Wapnir, R.A., M.C. Sia, and S.E. Fisher. 1996. Enhancement of intestinal water absorption and sodium transport by glycerol in rats. *J Appl Physiol* 81(6): 2523-2527.

Warren, B.J., A.L. Stanton, and D.L.Blessing. 1990. Disordered eating patterns in competitive female athletes. *Int J Eating Disorders* 5: 565-569.

Warren, J.A., R.R. Jenkins, L. Packer, E.H. Witt, and R.B.Armstrong. 1992. Elevated muscle vitamin E does not attenuate eccentric exercise-induced muscle injury. *J Appl Physiol* 72: 2168-2175.

Weaver, C., and S. Rajaram. 1992. Exercise and iron status. *J Nutrition* 122: 782-787.

Webb, P., W.H.M. Saris, P.F.M. Schoffelen, G.J. van Ingen Schenau, and F. ten Hoor. 1988. The work of walking: a calorimetric study. *Med Sci Sports Exerc* 20: 331-337.

Wee, S.L., C. Williams, S. Gray, and J. Horabin. 1999. Influence of high and low glycemic index meals on endurance running capacity. *Med Sci Sports Exerc* 31(3): 393-399.

Welle, S., R. Jozefowicz, and M. Statt. 1990. Failure of dehydroepi-androsterone to influence energy and protein metabolism in humans. *J Clin Endocrinol Metab* 71(5): 1259-1264.

Wemple, R.D., D.R. Lamb, and K.H. McKeever. 1997. Caffeine vs caffeine-free sports drinks: effects on urine production at rest and during prolonged exercise. *Int J Sports Med* 18(1): 40-46.

Westerterp, K.R. 1993. Food quotient, respiratory quotient, and energy balance. *Am J Clin Nutr* 57(5 suppl): 759S-764S.

Westerterp, K.R., J.H.H.L.M. Donkers, E.E.H.M. Fredrix, et al. 1995. Energy intake, physical activity and body weight: a simulation model. *Br J Nutr* 73: 337-347.

Westerterp, K.R., W.H. Saris, M. van Es, and F. ten Hoor. 1986. Use of the doubly labeled water technique in humans during heavy sustained exercise. *J Appl Physiol* 61(6): 2162-2167.

Weyers, A.M., S.A. Mazzetti, D.M. Love, et al. 2002. Comparison of methods for assessing body composition changes during weight loss. *Med Sci Sports Exerc* 34(3): 497-502.

Wiles, J.D., S.R. Bird, J. Hopkins, and M. Riley. 1992. Effect of caffeinated coffee on running speed, respiratory factors, blood lactate and perceived exertion during 1500-m treadmill running. *Br J Sports Med* 26(2): 116-191.

Willett, W.C. 2000. Diet and cancer. *Oncologist* 5: 393-404.

Williams, J.H., J.F. Signorile, W.F. Barnes, and T.W. Henrich. 1988. Caffeine, maximal power output and fatigue. *Br J Sports Med* 22(4): 132-134.

Williams, M.H. 1993. Nutritional supplements for strength trained athletes. *Sports Sci Exch* 6(6): 1-4.

Williams, M.H., R.B. Kreider, and J.D. Branch. 1999. *Creatine the power supplement*. Human Kinetics: Champaign, IL.

Williams, M.H., R.B. Kreider, D.W. Hunter, et al. 1990. Effect of inosine supplementation on 3-mile treadmill run performance and VO2 peak. *Med Sci Sports Exerc* 22(4): 517-522.

Wilmore, J.H., K.C. Wambsgans, M. Brenner, et al. 1992. Is there energy conservation in amenorrheic compared with eumenorrheic distance runners? *J Appl Physiol* 72(1): 15-22.

Winder, W.W. 1986. Effect of intravenous caffeine on liver glycogenolysis during prolonged exercise. *Med Sci Sports Exerc* 18(2): 192-196.

Wolfe, R.R. 1992. *Radioactive and stable isotope tracers in biomedicine*. Wiley-Liss: New York.

Wolfe, R.R., R.D. Goodenough, M.H. Wolfe, G.T. Royle, and E.R. Nadel. 1982. Isotopic analysis of leucine and urea metabolism in exercising humans. *J Appl Physiol* 52(2): 458-466.

Wolfe, R.R., S. Klein, F. Carraro, and J.-M. Weber. 1990. Role of triglyceride-fatty acid cycle in controlling fat metabolism in humans during and after exercise. *Am J Physiol* 258: E382-E389.

Wurtman, R.J., and M.C. Lewis. 1991. Exercise, plasma composition and neurotransmission. *Med Sport Sci* 32: 94-109.

Wyss, M., and R. Kaddurah-Daouk. 2000. Creatine and creatinine metabolism. *Physiol Rev* 80(3): 1107-1213.

Yaspelkis, B.B., J.G. Patterson, P.A. Anderla, Z. Ding, and J.L. Ivy. 1993. Carbohydrate supplementation spares muscle glycogen during variable-intensity exercise. *J Appl Physiol* 75(4): 1477-1485.

Zawadzki, K.M., B.B. Yaspelkis III, and J.L. Ivy. 1992. Carbohydrate-protein complex increases the rate of muscle glycogen storage after exercise. *J Appl Physiol* 72(5): 1854-1859.

Zeisel, S.H., K.A. Da Costa, P.D. Franklin, E.A. Alexander, J.T. Lamont, N.F. Sheard, and A. Beiser. 1991. Choline, an essential nutrient for humans [see comments]. *FASEB J* 5(7): 2093-2098.

Zeisel, S.H. 1998. *Choline and phosphatidylcholine*. ILSI Press: Washington, DC.

Zerba, E., T.E. Komorowski, and J.A. Faulkner. 1990. Free radical injury to skeletal muscles of young, adult, and old mice. *Am J Physiol* 258: C429-C435.

Zinker, B.A., K. Britz, and G.A. Brooks. 1990. Effects of a 36-hour fast on human endurance and substrate utilization. *J Appl Physiol* 69(5): 1849-1855.

Index

Note: The italicized *f* and *t* following page numbers refer to figures and tables, respectively. The italicized *ff* and *tt* following page numbers refer to multiple figures and tables, respectively.

About the Authors

Asker Jeukendrup, PhD, is a recognized authority on exercise biochemistry and physiology and sport nutrition. He was an invited speaker and author delegate to the International Olympic Committee Sports Nutrition Consensus Conference in 2003. He has served as scientific adviser to the Rabobank professional cycling team, one of the top cycling teams in the world, and as nutrition consultant to U.K. Athletics and numerous Olympic athletes. More than 100 of his papers and book chapters have been published over the past 10 years. He is also the editor of the *European Journal of Sport Science* and a fellow of the American College of Sports Medicine.

Jeukendrup received his PhD in health sciences in 1997 in Maastricht, Netherlands, and is currently a senior lecturer in the school of sport and exercise sciences at the University of Birmingham in the United Kingdom. He was already an avid cyclist when he first entered the fields of exercise physiology and sport nutrition. In his work, he not only performs cutting-edge research but also translates his findings into terms that are useful for athletes. In his free time, Jeukendrup enjoys cycling, traveling, and competing in triathlons. He and his wife, Antoinette, live in Birmingham, England.

Michael Gleeson, PhD, is a professor of sport and exercise sciences at Loughborough University in Leicestershire, England. He has taught sport nutrition and worked with coaches and elite athletes for many years.

An active researcher in sport nutrition and exercise metabolism, Dr. Gleeson has published more than 150 papers in exercise physiology and sport nutrition over the past 20 years. He was an invited speaker and author delegate to the International Olympic Committee Sports Nutrition Consensus Conference in 2003. He is the editor of *Exercise Immunology Review*.

Dr. Gleeson is a fellow of the European College of Sports Sciences. He is a member of the American College of Sports Medicine (ACSM), Physiological Society, British Association of Sport and Exercise Sciences, and International Society for Exercise and Immunology. At the University of Central Lancashire Dr. Gleeson completed his PhD on the effects of diet and exercise on energy metabolism.